Inflammatory and Neoplastic Diseases of Craniofacial Bones

Yue He
Editor

Inflammatory and Neoplastic Diseases of Craniofacial Bones

SSTP

Springer

Editor
Yue He
Department of Oral Maxillofacial-Head & Neck Oncology
Shanghai Ninth People's Hospital, Shanghai Jiao Tong University School of Medicine
Shanghai, China

ISBN 978-981-97-4154-0 ISBN 978-981-97-4155-7 (eBook)
https://doi.org/10.1007/978-981-97-4155-7

Jointly published with Shanghai Scientific and Technical Publishers
The print edition is not for sale in China (Mainland). Customers from China (Mainland) please order the print book from: Shanghai Scientific and Technical Publishers.

This Springer imprint is published by the registered company Springer Nature Singapore Pte Ltd.
The registered company address is: 152 Beach Road, #21-01/04 Gateway East, Singapore 189721, Singapore

Foreword

From the anatomical point of view, the cranial and maxillofacial development is integrated—starting from the neural crest and pharynx (branchia) arch. Therefore, the formation of cranial and maxillofacial bones is also inseparable. Except that the mandible is independent, other cranial and maxillofacial bones are firmly connected with each other. Cranial and maxillofacial bones can be either a single piece or bilaterally symmetric two pieces, with the former such as frontal bone and vomer, and the latter such as maxilla and mandible. If it is classified by anatomy, it can be divided into two categories: cranial and maxillofacial bones. There are 14 cranial bones (block number included in parentheses below), namely occipital bone (1), sphenoid bone (1), temporal bones (2), parietal bones (2), frontal bone (1), ethmoid bone (1), inferior turbinate (2), lacrimal bones (2), and nasal bones (2). There are 7 maxillofacial bones, namely maxilla (2), mandible (2), palate bones (2), zygomatic bones (2), and hyoid bone (1).

Clinically, if it is classified according to the surface anatomical marks, the skull mainly refers to the skull after the vertical line at the posterior margin of the frontal bone, such as the parietal bone and occipital bone, while the bones located in the posterior part of the posterior vertical line of the frontal bone are mostly regarded as maxillofacial bone and no longer subdivided into cranial or maxillofacial bones.

The book *Inflammatory and Neoplastic Diseases of Craniofacial Bones* edited by Professor He Yue is also written in accordance with this clinical anatomical concept.

Inflammatory and neoplastic diseases of cranial and maxillofacial bones (including tumor-like diseases) are common illness of maxillofacial surgery. There are still many problems in the options of diagnosis, differential diagnosis, and treatment methods that need to be further figured out.

One of the characteristics of this book is that it is guided by clinical cases, and then further analyzed with respect to the clinical cases, including diagnosis, differential diagnosis, treatment, and prognosis. This arrangement method is quite characteristic in clinical medical reference books, which is helpful to train the ability of clinicians in disease analysis and dialectical thinking.

The second feature of this book is that it is compiled based on the Classification of Head and Neck Tumors by WHO in 2017 and completes the clinical classification based on pathology. Clinical discussion in this way may benefit clinicians to review the pathological diagnosis. In addition to the pathological content, the book has also collected a large number of clinical imaging data, texts, and pictures for illustration.

With the progress of medicine and an increase in clinical application of drugs, the third feature of this book is that it adds some cutting-edge content, such as bisphosphonate-related osteonecrosis.

This book has its own distinctive features among many similar books, for which I am happy to recommend it to the general readers.

Shanghai, China
Aug. 2021

Wei Liu Qiu

Foreword

With the development and progress of China, the progress of modern medicine with each passing day. As an important part of modern medicine, stomatology has also experienced great changes and already broken through the category of traditional "Dentistry." Maxillofacial bone disease is often needed to be faced by dental doctors, especially oral and maxillofacial surgeons in daily diagnosis and treatment. In addition to the commonness with bone diseases in other parts of the body, it also has its own anatomical characteristics and complexity, especially odontogenic cysts and tumors, which are particularly close to the dentition, in particular for the germination, development, and eruption of teeth.

The department I work with is one of the largest oral and maxillofacial head and neck tumor diagnosis and treatment centers in China. It has accumulated rich clinical data and has a large number of common and difficult cases, as well as a considerable number of rare cases. Professor He Yue and his team have long been committed to the clinical and basic research of osteoradionecrosis of the jaws, medication-related osteonecrosis of jaw, various odontogenic and non-odontogenic lesions, and actively participated in the establishment and promotion of standardized diagnosis and treatment guidelines for related diseases, in order to better serve the majority of patients and reduce their pain. This book is a systematic summary and concise presentation of Professor He Yue on the precious case data collected for nearly 20 years. A total of 100 clinical cases and more than 860 images have been selected, combining clinical practice with basic theory closely. There is a summary of the key points of the latest relevant research progress at home and abroad behind each disease, with a total of 58 articles. It is the finishing touch of the book for the readers to think about and cause discussion. The long-term data accumulation, experience summary, and unremitting efforts of the chief editor together with the experts from relevant colleges and departments have contributed to the publication of this book. The editor team brings relevant discipline specialists, young and middle-aged physicians together from Oral and Maxillofacial Surgery, Oral Pathology Department, Radiology of Shanghai Ninth People's Hospital, Shanghai JiaoTong University School of Medicine, Hospital of Stomatology, Guanghua College of Stomatology, Sun Yat-sen University, Hospital of Stomatology Wuhan University, etc. They are energetic and knowledgeable all work in the first line of medical practice, teaching, and researching fields and study hard on their profession. Their participation has not only ensured the quality of the book, but also played a role in training new doctors, inheritance, and development. Writing the book is also open-ended. I believe that they will carry out more in-depth research in the future. They will have more discoveries, accumulate more experience, and have more gains and thoughts into the book, thereby making this book more informative and rich.

As an oral and maxillofacial surgeon, I am glad to recommend this book to the majority of physicians in related specialties such as oral and maxillofacial surgery, oncology, E.N.T department, head and neck surgery, radiology, microreconstructive surgery, and oral pathology department, as well as graduate students. I believe this book will give you a lot of inspiration and help, and let you benefit a lot. I hope this book plays a certain role in promoting the further development of stomatology in China.

Shanghai, China Zhi Yuan Zhang
Jul. 2021

Book Summary

There are 100 clinical cases of common diseases, rare diseases, and difficult diseases of cranial and maxillofacial bones selected in this book, taking into account both systemic and clinical practicability. It is divided into 13 parts. Through the complete introduction of the medical history, specialized examination, auxiliary examination, diagnosis, treatment and other contents of each patient, combined with a large number of clinical photographs, the detailed steps were interpreted during the operation. Therefore, the course of diagnosis and treatment and characteristics of each patient are truthfully present, highlighting the concept of clinical diagnosis and treatment. At the same time, these selected diseases are further investigated by specialists and scholars of oral and maxillofacial surgery, oral pathology, imaging, radiotherapy, oncology, and other related departments. It either summarizes the editor's research experience and clinical experience or brings together the latest research progress at home and abroad, which makes the physicians of oral and maxillofacial surgery, E.N.T. department, head and neck surgery, radiology, oral pathology, and microreconstructive surgery realize the key points of the diagnosis and treatment of cranial and maxillofacial bone lesions, so as to promote the development of the standardized treatment of related diseases, and ultimately to serve the patients.

Preface

May 2021
Shanghai, China

Cranial and maxillofacial bones include jaw bone, zygomatic bone, palate bone, nasal bone and vomer, etc. The lesions involving or occurring in the bones of these regions are often varying and heterogeneous due to embryological and anatomical properties. Some of these lesions are only limited to the cranial and maxillofacial bones, mainly related to the dentition, including odontogenic cysts and tumors. Other lesions are not limited to the cranial and maxillofacial bones, but they may cause unique differential diagnostic problems in this region, such as reactive bone diseases, fiber-bone lesions, giant cell lesions, and bone tumors. With the further research, people are increasing in understanding of the disease of cranial and maxillofacial bones and have also experienced different stages of change for some of these diseases. In 2017, the World Health Organization (WHO) released the 4th edition of disease classification. Relative to the 3rd edition classification, the head and neck tumors are changed in the new classification of neoplastic and nonneoplastic cystic lesions. For example, "keratocystic odontogenic tumor" and "calcifying cystic odontogenic tumor" return to their former names of "odontogenic keratocyst" and "calcifying odontogenic cyst." This also reflects the complexity of the diseases of cranial and maxillofacial bones from another side.

The oral and maxillofacial—head and neck oncology team I work with has always been committed to the basic and clinical studies of the osteoradionecrosis of the jaws, medication-related osteonecrosis of jaw, all kinds of odontogenic and non-odontogenic diseases, is long-term working in the forefront of clinical practice and exploration and committed to facilitate the establishment and promotion of standardized diagnosis and treatment guidelines, in order to have a more systematic, in-depth, and scientific understanding of related diseases, and better solve or reduce the pain in the vast majority of patients. As early as 20 years ago, we began to collect information on various diseases of cranial and maxillofacial bones, which allows to show a large number of high-quality photographs in this book. In recent decades, with the transformation of medical mode, as well as the rapid development of medical science and technology, especially the vigorous development of microsurgical technology and the increasing maturity of digital medical technology, the diagnosis and treatment of diseases of cranial and maxillofacial bones have been greatly improved. In the diagnosis and treatment of a large number of clinical cases, we have carried out further research, have a deeper understanding of the clinical characteristics, imaging manifestations and pathological characteristics of various diseases of cranial and maxillofacial bones, and accumulated some experience in the diagnosis and treatment of all kinds of difficult and rare cases. On this basis, we organized the compilation of *Inflammatory and Neoplastic Diseases of Cranial and Maxillofacial Bones: Diagnosis and Treatment* as a reference and exchange for fellows of oral and maxillofacial surgery, oncology, E.N.T department, head and neck surgery, radiology, microreconstructive surgery, and oral pathology department in order to accelerate the etiological and basic research of disease of cranial and maxillary bones, promote the development of standardized treatment, and finally serve the patients.

A total of 100 clinical patients with the diseases of cranial and maxillofacial bones have been collected and organized in this book, who used to be treated in the Shanghai Ninth People's Hospital, Shanghai JiaoTong University School of Medicine, Hospital of Stomatology, Guanghua College of Stomatology, Sun Yat-sen University, Hospital of Stomatology Wuhan University in nearly 20 years. It covers common diseases, rare diseases, and intractable diseases. All these collected clinical cases have been designed and organized, with both systematic and clinical practicality. The book consists of 13 parts; the first 6 parts introduce the inflammatory diseases of the jaws, various cystic diseases, giant cell lesions, and fibro-osseous lesions. Parts VII to XII mainly reveal all kinds of benign and malignant odontogenic and non-odontogenic tumors. Part XIII introduces some of the diseases of cranial and maxillofacial bones which are still controversial. Compared with previous similar books which mainly show the initial clinical, imaging, and pathological characteristics of diseases, this book emphasizes the concept of clinical diagnosis and treatment and summarizes the key points of diagnosis and treatment and research progress, so as to help readers better get familiar with and master relevant knowledge.

During writing this book, professor Qiu Weiliu, the honorary dean of the School of Stomatology, Shanghai JiaoTong University, lifetime professor of Shanghai Ninth People's Hospital, Shanghai JiaoTong University School of Medicine, academician of the Chinese Academy of Engineering, gave us careful guidance and help, and wrote a preface to this book. In addition, we also received the encouragement, help, and preface from my mentor, professor Zhang Zhiyuan, the academic leader of Shanghai JiaoTong University School of Stomatology, the director of the National Center for Stomatology, the director of the National Clinical Research Center for Oral Diseases, and the academician of the Chinese Academy of Engineering, so that the book can be successfully completed and published. We hereby would like to extend our most sincere respect and heartfelt thanks to these two masters in the field of oral and maxillofacial surgery! Although we try to standardize and integrate the relevant materials with unified standards as much as possible in the writing process, there are still different comments on the key points of diagnosis and treatment of different diseases. It is also inevitable that there are omissions in the book. Readers are kindly invited to comment in case of republication and supplementary revision.

Yue He

Contents

Part I Inflammatory Diseases of Jaws

1 Pyogenic Osteomyelitis of Jaws 3
Yue He, Hui Shan Ong, Zhen Tian, Lin Zhu, and Weixin Cai

2 Garré's Osteomyelitis of the Jaw 11
Yue He, Hui Shan Ong, Zhen Tian, Lin Zhu, and Jie He

3 Osteoradionecrosis of the Jaws 19
Yue He, Hui Shan Ong, Zhen Tian, Lin Zhu, and Hang Chen

4 Medication-Related Osteonecrosis of Jaw 39
Yue He, Hui Shan Ong, Zhen Tian, Lin Zhu, and Hang Chen

Part II Odontogenic and Non-odontogenic Developmental Cysts

5 Dentigerous Cyst 57
Bing Liu, Hui Shan Ong, Zhen Tian, Lin Zhu, and Bing Guo

6 Odontogenic Keratocyst 63
Bing Liu, Hui Shan Ong, Zhen Tian, Lin Zhu, and Yong Jie Hu

7 Glandular Odontogenic Cyst 83
Bing Liu, Hui Shan Ong, Zhen Tian, Lin Zhu, and Xiao Guang Li

8 Calcifying Odontogenic Cyst 87
Bing Liu, Hui Shan Ong, Zhen Tian, Lin Zhu, and Jian Feng Liang

9 Orthokeratinized Odontogenic Cyst 93
Bing Liu, Hui Shan Ong, Zhen Tian, Lin Zhu, and Shang Hui Zhou

10 Nasopalatine Duct Cyst 97
Bing Liu, Hui Shan Ong, Zhen Tian, Lin Zhu, and Shang Hui Zhou

Part III Odontogenic Cysts of Inflammatory Origin

11 Radicular Cyst 103
Bing Liu, Hui Shan Ong, Zhen Tian, Lin Zhu, and Bing Guo

12 Inflammatory Collateral Cysts 107
Bing Liu, Hui Shan Ong, Zhen Tian, Lin Zhu, and Xiao Mei Zhao

Part IV Pseudocyst

13 Simple Bone Cyst 113
Bing Liu, Hui Shan Ong, Zhen Tian, Lin Zhu, and Yong Jie Hu

14 Aneurysmal Bone Cyst 119
Bing Liu, Hui Shan Ong, Zhen Tian, Lin Zhu, and Qi Wen Man

Part V Giant Cell Diseases

15 Giant Cell Granuloma 127
Bing Liu, Hui Shan Ong, Zhen Tian, Lin Zhu, and Xiao Yen Meng

16 Cherubism 137
Bing Liu, Hui Shan Ong, Zhen Tian, Lin Zhu, and Xiao Tang

Part VI Fibro-osseous Lesions

17 Fibrous Dysplasia 145
Yue He, Hui Shan Ong, Zhen Tian, Lin Zhu, and Yu Han

18 Cemento-osseous Dysplasia 157
Yue He, Hui Shan Ong, Zhen Tian, Lin Zhu, and Qing Long Wu

19 Familial Gigantiform Cementoma 161
Yue He, Hui Shan Ong, Zhen Tian, Lin Zhu, and Li Li Hou

Part VII Benign Epithelial Odontogenic Tumor and Its Evolution

20 Ameloblastoma 167
Jing Song Hou, Hui Shan Ong, Zhen Tian, Lin Zhu, and Xing Zhou Qu

21 Calcifying Epithelial Odontogenic Tumor 187
Jing Song Hou, Hui Shan Ong, Zhen Tian, Lin Zhu, and Min Ruan

22 Adenomatoid Odontogenic Tumor 193
Jing Song Hou, Hui Shan Ong, Zhen Tian, Lin Zhu, and Tian Fu Wu

Part VIII Benign Epithelial Mesenchymal Complex Odontogenic Tumor

23 Ameloblastic Fibroma 199
Jing Song Hou, Hui Shan Ong, Zhen Tian, Lin Zhu, and Yang Wang

24 Odontoma 205
Jing Song Hou, Hui Shan Ong, Zhen Tian, Lin Zhu, and Xing Zhou Qu

25 Ameloblastic Fibro-Odontoma 209
Jing Song Hou, Hui Shan Ong, Zhen Tian, Lin Zhu, and Xiao Mei Zhao

26 Dentinogenic Ghost Cell Tumor 215
Jing Song Hou, Hui Shan Ong, Zhen Tian, Lin Zhu, and Min Ruan

Part IX Benign Mesenchymal Odontogenic Tumor and Its Evolution

27 Odontogenic Myxoma/Myxofibroma 223
Jing Song Hou, Hui Shan Ong, Zhen Tian, Lin Zhu, and Wen Yu Yang

28 Cementoblastoma 237
Jing Song Hou, Hui Shan Ong, Zhen Tian, Lin Zhu, and Ze Hang Zhuang

29 Odontogenic Fibroma 241
Jing Song Hou, Hui Shan Ong, Zhen Tian, Lin Zhu, and Bing Bing Sun

Part X Malignant Odontogenic Tumors

30 Ameloblastic Carcinoma 259
Jing Song Hou, Hui Shan Ong, Zhen Tian, Lin Zhu, and Xing Zhou Qu

31 Odontogenic Ghost Cell Carcinoma 267
Jing Song Hou, Hui Shan Ong, Zhen Tian, Lin Zhu, and Min Ruan

32 Ameloblastic Fibrosarcoma 273
Jing Song Hou, Hui Shan Ong, Zhen Tian, Lin Zhu, and Wen Jun Yang

33 Odontogenic Carcinosarcoma 279
Jing Song Hou, Hui Shan Ong, Zhen Tian, Lin Zhu, and Jie He

Part XI Benign Tumors of Craniomaxillofacial Bones and Cartilage

34 Osteoma 287
Yue He, Hui Shan Ong, Zhen Tian, Lin Zhu, and Wei Wei Deng

35 Chondroma 291
Yue He, Hui Shan Ong, Zhen Tian, Lin Zhu, and Wei Wei Deng

36 Osteoblastoma 295
Yue He, Hui Shan Ong, Zhen Tian, Lin Zhu, and Jin Song Li

37 Osteoid Osteoma 299
Yue He, Hui Shan Ong, Zhen Tian, Lin Zhu, and Wen Jun Yang

38 Chondroblastoma 303
Yue He, Hui Shan Ong, Zhen Tian, Lin Zhu, and Xing Zhou Qu

39 Osteochondroma 309
Yue He, Hui Shan Ong, Zhen Tian, Lin Zhu, and Jun Shi

40 Ossifying Fibroma 313
Yue He, Hui Shan Ong, Zhen Tian, Lin Zhu, and Zhe Shao

41 Chondromyxoid Fibroma 327
Yue He, Hui Shan Ong, Zhen Tian, Lin Zhu, and Wen Jun Yang

42 Desmoplastic Fibroma 331
Yue He, Hui Shan Ong, Zhen Tian, Lin Zhu, and Zheng Wu Liu

43 Melanotic Neuroectodermal Tumor of Infancy 341
Yue He, Hui Shan Ong, Zhen Tian, Lin Zhu, and Wen Jun Yang

Part XII Malignant Tumors of Craniomaxillofacial Bones and Cartilage

44 Osteosarcoma 347
Yue He, Hui Shan Ong, Zhen Tian, Lin Zhu, and Shan Liang Jin

45 Chondrosarcoma 363
Yue He, Hui Shan Ong, Zhen Tian, Lin Zhu, and Zhong Long Liu

46 Mesenchymal Chondrosarcoma 373
Yue He, Hui Shan Ong, Zhen Tian, Lin Zhu, and Min Ruan

47 Postirradiation Sarcoma of Jaws 379
Yue He, Hui Shan Ong, Zhen Tian, Lin Zhu, and Xing Zhou Qu

48 Ewing Sarcoma 387
Yue He, Hui Shan Ong, Zhen Tian, Lin Zhu, and Ji Ping Ding

49 Primary Intraosseous Squamous Cell Carcinoma 393
Yue He, Hui Shan Ong, Zhen Tian, Lin Zhu, and Jun Jian Jiang

50 Primary Intraosseous Mucoepidermoid Carcinoma of Jaws . . . 403
Yue He, Hui Shan Ong, Zhen Tian, Lin Zhu, and Feng Shuo Zhu

51 Primary Intraosseous Adenoid Cystic Carcinoma of Jaws 409
Yue He, Hui Shan Ong, Zhen Tian, Lin Zhu, and Chen Ye

52 Metastatic Malignant Tumor in Jaws 415
Yue He, Hui Shan Ong, Zhen Tian, Lin Zhu, and Zhong Long Liu

53 Solitary Plasmacytoma of Bone 419
Yue He, Hui Shan Ong, Zhen Tian, Lin Zhu, and Xiao Guang Li

Part XIII Miscellaneous

54 Retiform Hemangioendothelioma 427
Yue He, Hui Shan Ong, Zhen Tian, Lin Zhu, and Zhong Long Liu

55 Langerhans Cell Histiocytosis 433
Yue He, Hui Shan Ong, Zhen Tian, Lin Zhu, and Jing Jing Sun

56 Osteopetrosis 441
Yue He, Hui Shan Ong, Zhen Tian, Lin Zhu, and Zhou Zhu

57 Hemophilic Pseudotumor 447
Yue He, Hui Shan Ong, Zhen Tian, Lin Zhu, and Jing Jing Sun

Contributors

Weixin Cai Hospital of Stomatology, Guanghua College of Stomatology, Sun Yat-sen University, Guangdong, China

Hang Chen Department of Oral Maxillofacial-Head & Neck Oncology, Shanghai Ninth People's Hospital, Shanghai Jiao Tong University School of Medicine, Shanghai, China

Wei Wei Deng Hospital of Stomatology Wuhan University, Hubei, China

Ji Ping Ding Department of Oral Maxillofacial-Head & Neck Oncology, Shanghai Ninth People's Hospital, Shanghai Jiao Tong University School of Medicine, Shanghai, China

Bing Guo Department of Oral Maxillofacial-Head & Neck Oncology, Shanghai Ninth People's Hospital, Shanghai Jiao Tong University School of Medicine, Shanghai, China

Yu Han Department of Oral Maxillofacial-Head & Neck Oncology, Shanghai Ninth People's Hospital, Shanghai Jiao Tong University School of Medicine, Shanghai, China

Jie He Department of Oral Maxillofacial-Head & Neck Oncology, Shanghai Ninth People's Hospital, Shanghai Jiao Tong University School of Medicine, Shanghai, China

Yue He Department of Oral Maxillofacial-Head & Neck Oncology, Shanghai Ninth People's Hospital, Shanghai Jiao Tong University School of Medicine, Shanghai, China

Jing Song Hou Hospital of Stomatology, Guanghua College of Stomatology, Sun Yat-sen University, Guangdong, China

Li Li Hou Department of Oral Maxillofacial-Head & Neck Oncology, Shanghai Ninth People's Hospital, Shanghai Jiao Tong University School of Medicine, Shanghai, China

Yong Jie Hu Shanghai Ninth People's Hospital Affiliated, Shanghai Jiao-Tong University School of Medicine, Shanghai, China

Jun Jian Jiang Department of Oral Maxillofacial-Head & Neck Oncology, Shanghai Ninth People's Hospital, Shanghai Jiao Tong University School of Medicine, Shanghai, China

Shan Liang Jin Shanghai Ninth People's Hospital Affiliated, Shanghai Jiao-Tong University School of Medicine, Shanghai, China

Jin Song Li Sun Yat-Sen Memorial Hospital, Sun Yat-Sen University, Guangdong, China

Xiao Guang Li Department of Oral Maxillofacial-Head & Neck Oncology, Shanghai Ninth People's Hospital, Shanghai Jiao Tong University School of Medicine, Shanghai, China

Jian Feng Liang Hospital of Stomatology, Guanghua College of Stomatology, Sun Yat-sen University, Guangdong, China

Bing Liu Hospital of Stomatology Wuhan University, Hubei, China

Zheng Wu Liu The Second Nanning People's Hospital (the Third Affiliated Hospital), Guangxi Medical University, Guangxi, China

Zhong Long Liu Department of Oral Maxillofacial-Head & Neck Oncology, Shanghai Ninth People's Hospital, Shanghai Jiao Tong University School of Medicine, Shanghai, China

Qi Wen Man Hospital of Stomatology Wuhan University, Hubei, China

Xiao Yen Meng Shanghai Ninth People's Hospital Affiliated, Shanghai JiaoTong University School of Medicine, Shanghai, China

Hui Shan Ong Department of Oral Maxillofacial-Head & Neck Oncology, Shanghai Ninth People's Hospital, Shanghai Jiao Tong University School of Medicine, Shanghai, China

Xing Zhou Qu Department of Oral Maxillofacial-Head & Neck Oncology, Shanghai Ninth People's Hospital, Shanghai Jiao Tong University School of Medicine, Shanghai, China

Min Ruan Department of Oral Maxillofacial-Head & Neck Oncology, Shanghai Ninth People's Hospital, Shanghai Jiao Tong University School of Medicine, Shanghai, China

Zhe Shao Hospital of Stomatology Wuhan University, Hubei, China

Jun Shi Department of Oral Maxillofacial-Head & Neck Oncology, Shanghai Ninth People's Hospital, Shanghai Jiao Tong University School of Medicine, Shanghai, China

Bing Bing Sun Shanghai Ninth People's Hospital Affiliated, Shanghai Jiao-Tong University School of Medicine, Shanghai, China

Jing Jing Sun Department of Oral Maxillofacial-Head & Neck Oncology, Shanghai Ninth People's Hospital, Shanghai Jiao Tong University School of Medicine, Shanghai, China

Xiao Tang Shanghai Ninth People's Hospital Affiliated, Shanghai JiaoTong University School of Medicine, Shanghai, China

Zhen Tian Department of Oral Maxillofacial-Head & Neck Oncology, Shanghai Ninth People's Hospital, Shanghai Jiao Tong University School of Medicine, Shanghai, China

Yang Wang Shanghai Ninth People's Hospital Affiliated, Shanghai Jiao-Tong University School of Medicine, Shanghai, China

Qing Long Wu Department of Oral Maxillofacial-Head & Neck Oncology, Shanghai Ninth People's Hospital, Shanghai Jiao Tong University School of Medicine, Shanghai, China

Tian Fu Wu Hospital of Stomatology Wuhan University, Hubei, China

Wen Jun Yang Department of Oral Maxillofacial-Head & Neck Oncology, Shanghai Ninth People's Hospital, Shanghai Jiao Tong University School of Medicine, Shanghai, China

Wen Yu Yang Shanghai Ninth People's Hospital Affiliated, Shanghai Jiao-Tong University School of Medicine, Shanghai, China

Chen Ye Department of Oral Maxillofacial-Head & Neck Oncology, Shanghai Ninth People's Hospital, Shanghai Jiao Tong University School of Medicine, Shanghai, China

Xiao Mei Zhao Shanghai Ninth People's Hospital Affiliated, Shanghai Jiao-Tong University School of Medicine, Shanghai, China

Shang Hui Zhou Department of Oral Maxillofacial-Head & Neck Oncology, Shanghai Ninth People's Hospital, Shanghai Jiao Tong University School of Medicine, Shanghai, China

Feng Shuo Zhu Department of Oral Maxillofacial-Head & Neck Oncology, Shanghai Ninth People's Hospital, Shanghai Jiao Tong University School of Medicine, Shanghai, China

Lin Zhu Department of Radiology, Ninth People's Hospital Affiliated to Shanghai Jiao Tong University, Shanghai, China

Zhou Zhu Department of Oral Maxillofacial-Head & Neck Oncology, Shanghai Ninth People's Hospital, Shanghai Jiao Tong University School of Medicine, Shanghai, China

Ze Hang Zhuang Hospital of Stomatology, Guanghua College of Stomatology, Sun Yat-sen University, Guangdong, China

Part I

Inflammatory Diseases of Jaws

1 Pyogenic Osteomyelitis of Jaws

Yue He, Hui Shan Ong, Zhen Tian, Lin Zhu, and Weixin Cai

1.1 Introduction

Pyogenic osteomyelitis of jaws usually occurs in young adults, with the highest incidence generally between the ages of 16 and 30. It is more common in men than women, with a ratio of 2:1. It is commonly seen in the mandible clinically. However, the maxilla is the most common site in infants and young children. The common pathogen is the staphylococcus aureus, followed by hemolytic streptococcus, diplococcus pneumoniae, escherichia coli and proteus species. The route of infection mainly includes odontogenic infection, damaging infection and blood-borne infection [1–3]. The clinical development process of the osteomyelitis of the jaws can be divided into two stages: acute phase and chronic phase. According to the cause of infection and the characteristics of lesions, purulent osteomyelitis is divided into central osteomyelitis of the jaws and marginal osteomyelitis of the jaws in clinical practice. Correct clinical diagnosis is generally not difficult according to the patient's history, etiology, clinical manifestations and imaging examination. In terms of treatment, sufficient and effective antibiotics should be given in the acute phase to control the development of inflammation. Moreover, targeted antibiotics should be applied according to the results of bacterial culture and drug sensitivity tests, as well as necessary systemic and supportive therapies [2, 4, 5]. The purpose of operation treatment is to drain the pus and remove the lesions. The treatment in the chronic phase is mainly surgical. The patient can be cured by removing the formed dead bones and lesions.

Y. He (✉) · H. S. Ong · Z. Tian
Department of Oral Maxillofacial-Head & Neck Oncology, Shanghai Ninth People's Hospital, Shanghai Jiao Tong University School of Medicine, Shanghai, China

L. Zhu
Department of Radiology, Ninth People's Hospital Affiliated to Shanghai Jiao Tong University, Shanghai, China

W. Cai
Hospital of Stomatology, Guanghua College of Stomatology, Sun Yat-sen University, Guangdong, China

1.1.1 Case 1

The patient, male, 65 years old. The patient has suffered from pain in the left lower posterior teeth with numbness of the lower lip for more than seven months.

[Present medical history] The patient felt pain in the left lower posterior teeth when eating more than 7 months ago, and then developed numbness in the left lower lip. He was treated in another hospital and received the root canal treatment.

Y. He (ed.), *Inflammatory and Neoplastic Diseases of Craniofacial Bones*,
https://doi.org/10.1007/978-981-97-4155-7_1

However, the numbness was not improved. Then the affected tooth was removed, but the numbness was still not relieved. Cranial MRI was performed in another hospital to exclude intracranial lesions. Outpatient panoramic radiographs in our hospital showed the left mandible bone defect involving the neural tube.

[Specialized examination] The face is symmetrical. The proportion of the upper, middle and lower 1/3 face is coordinated. There is no redness or swelling in the skin on the left facial and neck. Both tactile and algesia are decreased in the left lower lip. The degree and type of mouth opening are normal. In the intraoral permanent dentition, tooth 36 is missing, with slight redness and swelling of the local gingiva and no pyorrhea. No ping-pong ball sensation is found in the local mandible. The 34 and 35 were tender to percussion (+) but no sign of mobile. Bilateral submaxillary and cervical lymph nodes are not enlarged.

[Auxiliary examination] Panoramic radiographs show the left mandibular bone defect involving the neural tube (Fig. 1.1).

[Primary diagnosis] Left mandibular osteomyelitis.

[Treatment] "Curettage for the left mandibular osteomyelitis + soft tissue debridement" was performed under general anesthesia. An intraoral incision was made to cut the lesion open and turn the flap over. A small amount of inflammatory granulation tissue and bone sclerosis were seen. The diseased bone was abraded. It was sent to the frozen

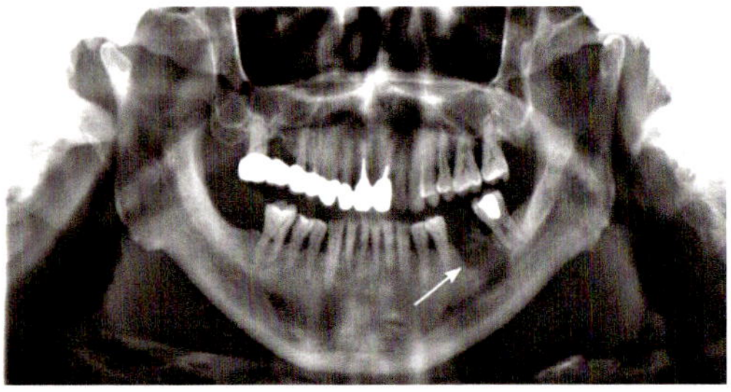

Fig. 1.1 The left mandibular bone defect involving neural tube (preoperative)

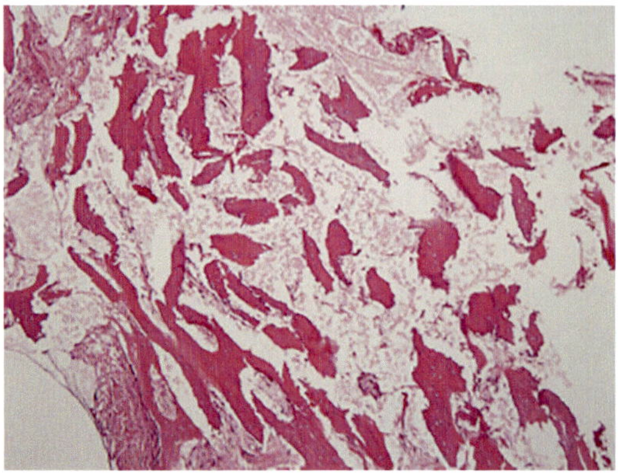

Fig. 1.2 The lamina structure disappears and the bone edge is irregular, indicating a dead bone. Degeneration and necrosis of trabecular tissue

pathological examination with the granulation tissue. The results indicated "the left mandibular" trabecular structure, fibrous connective tissue hyperplasia, scattered inflammatory cell infiltration, and no positive evidence of the tumor. Combined with imaging findings, it can be considered as the chronic osteomyelitis. Thorough hemostasis, rinsing and layered suture were carried out. A piece of tela iodoformum was placed in.

[Pathological examination] A small amount of grayish-yellow broken bone tissue was sent for biopsy. Under the microscope, there is no connection between the trabecular bones into small pieces. The lamina structure disappears, and the bone edge is irregular, showing dead bones. Degeneration and necrosis of trabecular tissue (Fig. 1.2).

[Pathological diagnosis] "Left mandibular" chronic osteomyelitis.

[Follow-up visit] The patient recovered well after the operation. The wound healed well with no obviously abnormal swelling and exudation in the postoperative review.

1.1.2 Case 2

The patient, male, 46 years old. The patient has suffered from repeatedly swelling, pain and discomfort in the left anterior auricular area for more than two months.

[Present medical history] The patient experienced pain and swelling in the left lower posterior teeth region without obvious cause two months ago, secondary to the left facial swelling, especially more significant in the left preauricular region. The patient visited a local hospital and improved after receiving anti-inflammatory and symptomatic treatment. The same symptoms emerged again a month ago, and the pain symptoms were relieved after anti-inflammatory and symptomatic treatment. A mass was found in front of the left ear, without numbness of the lower lip. "Fine needle aspiration biopsy for the left mandibular ascending ramus mass" was performed in our hospital, and the results showed prismatic and epithelioid cells and possible malignant tumor cells. PET/CT examination suggested that the bone destruction was found in the local left mandibular ascending ramus with soft tissue mass formation and peripheral soft tissue swelling, considering possible malignant tumor.

[Specialized examination] The face is asymmetrical. The proportion of the upper, middle and lower 1/3 face is coordinated. The left anterior ear area is swollen. The left mandibular ascending ramus is expanded outward with an ill-defined edge. Tenderness (−). No obvious redness or swelling has been discovered on the surface of the skin. The degree of mouth opening is normal, and the mouth is deviated to the left when opening. The occluding relation of the permanent dentition is normal, with no obvious tooth loosening, pain on percussion (−), and no obvious mucosal redness, swelling and faciocutaneous fistulae. No significantly abnormally enlarged lymph nodes have been found in the bilateral submaxilla and neck.

[Auxiliary examination]

1. Panoramic radiographs show that the osteolytic bone destruction and sclerotin discontinuity of the left mandibular ascending ramus and the neck of the condylar process, with multiple spotted high-density shadows (Fig. 1.3).

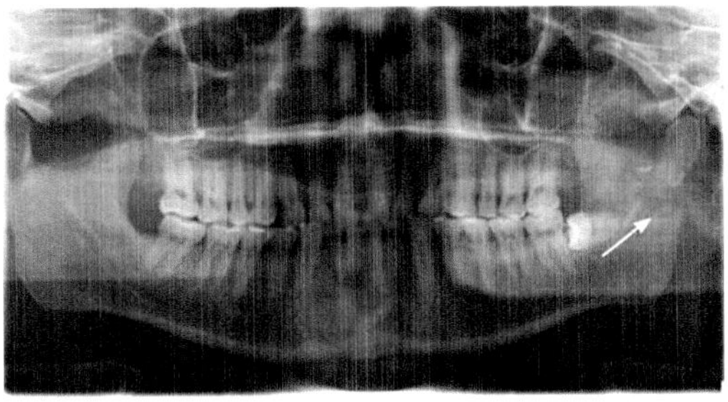

Fig. 1.3 Osteolytic bone destruction and sclerotin discontinuity of the left mandibular ascending ramus and the neck of the condylar process, with multiple spotted high-density shadows

2. Maxillofacial CT enhanced scan: The bone destruction is noted in the left mandibular ascending ramus, showing osteolytic resorption, with multiple spotted high-density shadows, sclerotin interruption, and peripheral periosteal reaction. The adjacent left mouth chewing space is significantly enlarged, with an ill-defined edge. C− 42 Hu, C+ 56 Hu, showing uneven enhancement, with scattered spotted high-density shadows. The adjacent left temporal bone and zygomatic sclerotin are slightly absorbed and rough. No abnormalities have been found in the bilateral foramen ovales and cavernous sinus regions. No obvious enlarged lymph node shadow is observed in the neck. The malignancy in the left mandibular ascending ramus with hypertrophy of masseteric muscle: Possible squamous cell carcinoma of jaws or metastatic tumor. Please combine with clinical findings (Fig. 1.4).
3. PET/CT indication: the bone destruction was found in the local left mandibular ascending ramus with soft tissue mass formation and peripheral soft tissue swelling, considering possible malignant tumor.

[Primary diagnosis] Possible left mandible malignancy

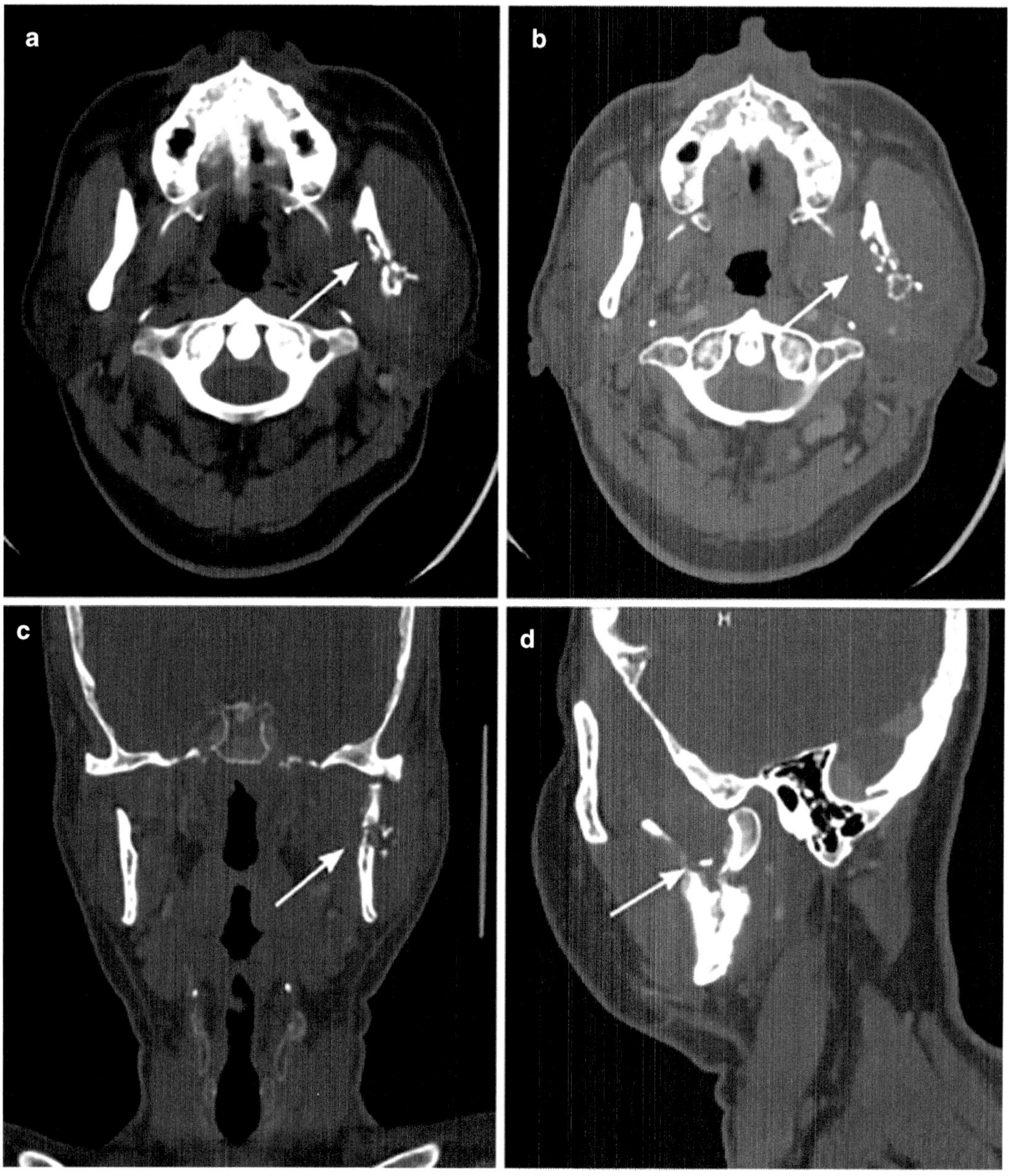

Fig. 1.4 (**a**) Transverse view of CT plain scan: The left mandibular ascending ramus was destroyed, showing osteolytic absorption, with multiple spotted high-density shadows and peripheral periosteal reaction. The adjacent left masticatory space was significantly enlarged, with an ill-defined edge, and a CT value of 42 Hu. (**b**) Transverse view of CT enhanced scan: Inhomogeneous enhancement, a CT value of 56 Hu. (**c**, **d**) Coronary view and sagittal view of CT enhanced scan: The adjacent left temporal bone and zygomatic sclerotin were slightly absorbed and rough

[Treatment] "Mass resected with biopsy" was performed under the general anesthesia. Intraoperative frozen pathology suggested: "the left mandibular mass." A small number of proliferative fat spindle cells were seen in the background of a large number of inflammatory cells, and the cells showed atypia and prone to neoplastic lesions. It was considered the origin of

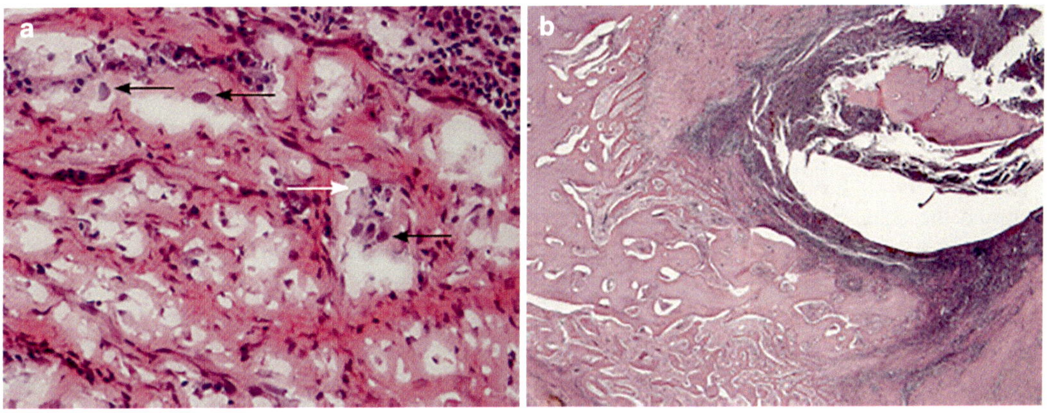

Fig. 1.5 (**a**) Frozen sections showed a small number of fat spindle cells (black arrow) in the background of inflammation, with atypia, and suspicious mitotic figures (white arrow) (400×). (**b**) Fibrous tissue was significantly hyperplastic between bone tissues, with focal inflammatory cell infiltration, vascular proliferation, granulation tissue formation, and small pieces of dead bone tissue (20×)

the interlobes in the first place (Fig. 1.5a). The device was replaced and an "extended resection of the mass" was performed. Intraoperative frozen pathology suggested: "the left mandibular mass." A small number of proliferative spindle cells were seen in the background of a large number of inflammatory cells. The cytoplasm was eosinophilic and the cells showed atypia. Mitotic figures were occasionally seen. Combined with imaging findings, it tends to be malignant, and the origin of the interlobes cannot be excluded (Fig. 1.5a). No obvious tumor cells were found in frozen sections of these submitted margins (−).

[Pathological examination] Partial mandible and the peripheral tissue were sent for biopsy, approximately 12 cm * 10 cm * 6 cm in size, with a tooth attached and the surface covered by skin, approximately 7 cm * 4.5 cm in size. The partial region of the mass was greyish white, approximately 3 cm * 2.5 cm * 2.5 cm in size, and phymatoid. Microscopically, the lesion significantly invaded and destroyed the mandible, with focal abscess formation, a large number of acute and chronic inflammatory cell infiltration, an empty bone lacuna of central residual bone tissue, and irregular margins. Spindle fiber/myofibroblastic proliferation, some cells with atypia, and scar-like tissue formation (Fig. 1.5b).

[Pathological diagnosis] "Left mandible" chronic pyogenic osteomyelitis, ICD code: K10.202, with dead bone formation.

1.2 Key Points of Diagnosis and Treatment

The most common clinical cause of pyogenic osteomyelitis of jaws is the odontogenic infection, accounting for about 90% of pyogenic osteomyelitis of jaws, which is commonly caused by the direct spread of odontogenic infection such as acute apical periodontitis, peridentitis and pericoronitis of the wisdom tooth, etc. It is often divided into two stages: acute phase and chronic phase. In the acute stage, the main manifestations include systemic fever, chills, fatigue, weakness, an increase in the number of white blood cells and neutrophils; local severe pain, cheek soft tissue and oral mucosa swelling and congestion; secondary to the peripheral acute cellulitis. Focal teeth may have significant percussion pain and elongation sensation. The characteristics of the chronic stage mainly consist of mild systemic symptoms, normal body temperature or only a low fever. The body shows chronic toxic consumption manifestations, such as anemia and emaciation. The disease progresses slowly, with local swelling and reddish skin. The mouth or cheek may appear to be a fistula pyorrhea, and the tooth may be loosening in the swelling area.

Classification According to the cause of infection and the characteristics of lesions, suppurative osteomyelitis is divided into two categories: central osteomyelitis of the jaws and marginal osteomyelitis of the jaws. Inflammation of central osteomyelitis of the jaws first develops in the bone marrow cavity and then spreads outward from the center of the jaws, which may involve the compact bone and periosteum. Most suppurative central osteomyelitis of the jaws occurs in the mandible, which is closely related to the local anatomy of the upper and lower jaws. Due to the thick and dense mandible bone plate and the single source of blood supply, it is not easy to puncture and drain when inflammation occurs. Vascular embolism may cause blood supply disorder of large bone tissue, leading to the formation of dead bone. While the maxilla has a sinus cavity, loose bone tissue, thin bone plate, and rich blood vessels. Sometimes the infection easily penetrates the bone wall, thus draining to the low level of the oral cavity, with fewer risks of bone nutrition disorder and bone tissue necrosis, small area of dead bone formation, and not easy to develop into diffuse osteomyelitis. Marginal osteomyelitis of the jaws refers to the inflammatory lesions of the outer plate of the compact bone secondary to periostitis or subperiosteal abscess. It often occurs based on infection in the perimaxillary space and frequently emerges in the mandible, with the mandibular ramus and mandibular angle most. According to the pathological characteristics of bone damage, marginal osteomyelitis of the jaws can be divided into osteoplastic and osteolytic-destructive.

Imaging characteristics The X-ray film shows no bone destruction imaging in the acute phase. The onset of acute pyogenic osteomyelitis of the jaws has entered the chronic stage after 2–4 weeks. X-ray imaging has diagnostic value after obvious bone destruction, which is mainly manifested as bone destruction and bone hyperplasia. CT and MRI examinations have different advantages in the diagnosis of osteomyelitis of the jaws: When the osteomyelitis of the mandible spreads in the myofascial space, a CT scan shows swelling and thickening of masticatory muscles, increased density of intermuscular fat space, and unclear intermyofascial border. The CT enhanced scan shows inhomogeneous enhancement in the diseased muscles and the myofascial spaces, more clearly displaying the extent of the lesion. MRI has a high tissue contrast and is more ideal than CT in displaying the spread of the osteomyelitis of the jaws in the myofascial space [2, 4]. The spread of inflammation on T1WI shows muscle swelling, signal reduction, and uneven band-like low signals in the high signals of inter-muscle fats. T2WI lesion muscles and intramuscular fat show high signals. The enhanced scan shows uneven enhancement of diseased tissue. CT scans are beneficial for showing smaller bone destruction, especially better than MRIs for displaying bone destruction in the bone cortex.

Diagnosis Acute pyogenic osteomyelitis of jaws is based on the obvious systemic and local symptoms, which are similar to fascial space infection in the acute phase. Pathogenic teeth and most adjacent teeth appear percussion pain, loosening, and even alveolar pyorrhea. Numbness of the lower lip on the affected side is strong evidence for diagnosing osteomyelitis of the mandible. Osteomyelitis of maxilla affects the maxillary sinus and may have the symptoms of the maxillary sinusitis. Sometimes the nasal pyorrhea may come from the affected side. The main diagnosis evidence of chronic osteomyelitis of the jaws is based on the fistula formation and pyorrhea. Small pieces of dead bone can be discharged from the fistulous opening after the formation of dead bone.

Differential diagnosis Marginal osteomyelitis of the mandible should be differentiated from osteosarcoma and ossifying fibroma. Central osteomyelitis of the mandible should be differentiated from central cancer of the mandible. In addition, when diagnosing osteomyelitis of the maxilla, the possibility of maxillary sinus cancer should be excluded. Both preoperative imaging examination and puncture report of two patients in this study group suggest the possibility of a malignant tumor. The intraoperative freezing report also reveals that the cells have atypia, with occasional mitotic figures. Combined with the imaging findings, it tends to be malignant and cannot exclude the origin of the interlobes. At the same time, the final postoperative pathological diagnosis is chronic pyogenic osteomyelitis with dead bone formation. Therefore, similar clinical patients should choose the corresponding diagnosis and treatment plan after the pathology is clear to avoid misdiagnosis and overtreatment.

Treatment The principle of treatment for acute osteomyelitis of the jaws is the same as the general acute inflammation. Acute pyogenic osteomyelitis of jaws is generally fast and severe and often causes bloody infection. Therefore, in the course of treatment, systemic supportive and antimicrobial therapies shall be considered first. Meanwhile, it should cooperate with necessary operation treatment. The main purpose of acute surgery is to achieve the drainage for apocenosis and remove the lesions. Chronic surgery mainly involves the removal of the dead bone and the lesion.

References

1. Wang JY, Sa GL, Liu ZK, He SG. Expressions of IL-17, IL-1β, and IL-6 in osteomyelitis of jaw. J Oral Sci Res. 2017;33(10):1082–5.
2. Shin JW, Kim JE, Huh KH, et al. Computed tomography imaging features of osteomyelitis of the jaw: comparison between antiresorptive medication-related conditions and medication-unrelated conditions [J]. Oral Surg Oral Med Oral Pathol Oral Radiol. 2020;129(6):629–34.
3. Jin YZ. Analysis of 86 cases of pyogenic osteomyelitis of the jaws [J]. Chin J Misdiagn. 2008;8(24):156–7.
4. Zhang ZY, Yu KY. Oral and maxillofacial surgery [M]. Beijing: People Health Press; 2012.
5. Krakowiak PA. Alveolar osteitis and osteomyelitis of the jaws [J]. Oral Maxillofac Surg Clin North Am. 2011;23(3):401–13.

2 Garré's Osteomyelitis of the Jaw

Yue He, Hui Shan Ong, Zhen Tian, Lin Zhu, and Jie He

2.1 Introduction

Garré's osteomyelitis of the jaws was first reported and defined by GarréCar in 1891 as a sclerotin disorder and characterized by chronic nonpurulent osteomyelitis with proliferative periostitis, mostly in adolescents with a mean age of 12.3 years [1–4]. Clinical manifestations include local painless swelling. It often involves unilateral mandible, a rare disease of the jaws. Besides, it is rarer with bilateral involvement. The imaging characteristics of Garré's osteomyelitis of the jaws include dense bone sclerosis with periosteal new bone formation. The pathological changes of this disease are active subperiosteal osteogenesis with visible deposition of numerous osteoblasts. The etiology of Garré's osteomyelitis of the jaws is related to odontogenic infection, endocrine and trauma [5–7]. Operation treatment with adjunctive systemic antibiotic therapy is the best regimen for Garré's osteomyelitis of the jaws.

Y. He (✉) · H. S. Ong · Z. Tian · J. He
Department of Oral Maxillofacial-Head & Neck Oncology, Shanghai Ninth People's Hospital, Shanghai Jiao Tong University School of Medicine, Shanghai, China

L. Zhu
Department of Radiology, Ninth People's Hospital Affiliated to Shanghai Jiao Tong University, Shanghai, China

2.1.1 Case 3

The patient, female, aged 27, The patient has suffered from right mandibular swelling and discomfort with the limitation of mouth opening and recurrent attacks for one and a half years.

[Present medical history] The patient has a past history of repeated swelling and pain of the wisdom tooth in the right mandible and once performed "48 extraction surgery" in another hospital. A year and a half ago, the patient consciously felt pain and discomfort in the right mandibular angle area and did not pay attention to it in the early stage. With the right facial swelling and the limitation of mouth opening, the patient came to our hospital for treatment 14 months ago. The pain was relieved after receiving anti-inflammatory and detumescence therapies. The maxillofacial CT suggested the possibility of the right mandibular osteomyelitis. One year ago, "scaling for the right mandibular osteomyelitis" was performed under general anesthesia in our hospital. Postoperative pathology indicated that it was consistent with chronic osteomyelitis. Two months after the surgery, the swelling with the limitation of mouth opening was repeated, with recurrent attacks.

Y. He (ed.), *Inflammatory and Neoplastic Diseases of Craniofacial Bones*,
https://doi.org/10.1007/978-981-97-4155-7_2

[Specialized examination]

1. Acute inflammatory phase: The left and right sides are asymmetric. The right jaw and face are swelling. The surface of the skin is mildly red, with no obvious fluctuation. The mouth opening is about a horizontal finger. The mucosa of the right inferior posterior teeth area is mildly swollen, with no obvious rupture and pyorrhea, no obvious sinus tract and orificium fistulae.
2. Stabilizing period: No obvious mass is discovered in the right mandibular angle area. The skin is not tender. Mouth opening is about three fingers. The oral hygiene is good. 45–47 relative to the buccal oral vestibular groove and gingiva are not obviously swelling and not tender.

[Auxiliary examination]

1. Panoramic radiographs: The bone density of the right mandibular angle is not even, with no obvious bone destruction, periosteal reaction, and soft tissue mass (Fig. 2.1).
2. Maxillofacial CT plain scan: The bone marrow cavity density is unevenly increased in the right mandibular angle. A periosteal reaction is seen on the buccal and lingual sides. The bone cortex is not smooth, and no obvious abnormalities in the surrounding soft tissue (Fig. 2.2).
3. MR-enhanced scan of the maxillofacial region: The signals are inhomogeneous from the right mandible body to the bone pulp cavity of the mandibular ascending ramus. T2WI shows slightly higher signals and T1WI shows low signals, with mild enhancement after enhanced scan. Peripheral medial pterygoid and masseter are slightly swollen. The local fat space is slightly blurred, with patchy T2WI high signal shadows, ill-defined edge and scope, and mild enhancement after an enhanced scan. No bone destruction is observed in the skull base sclerotin. No enlarged lymph node shadows are observed in the neck (Fig. 2.3).

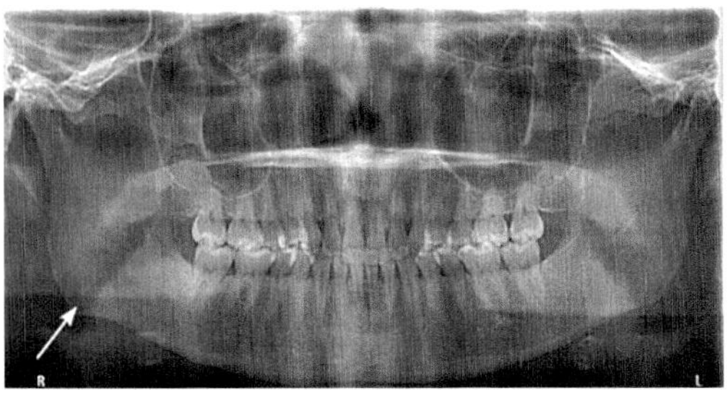

Fig. 2.1 The right mandibular angle bone density is uneven, with no obvious bone destruction, no periosteal reaction and soft tissue mass (preoperative)

[Primary diagnosis] Right mandibular osteomyelitis.

[Treatment]

1. "Curettage for the osteomyelitis of the right mandible" was performed under general anesthesia. An incision was made relative to 45–47 buccal oral vestibular grooves of the right mandible. After cutting open and turning the flap over, the buccal and lingual surfaces of the right mandible were not smooth during the operation. It was scratched with a curette, seeing that a large number of dead bone tissue was formed. The specimen was submitted for routine pathology. The wound was washed, the bleeding was stopped, and the wound was closed.
2. Combined with imaging findings, previous application of antibiotics, and so on symptomatic treatment, the symptoms were relieved, considering functional preservation and reducing trauma. For the patient's wishes, it is suggested that antibiotics in combination with hormone-symptomatic treatment be given in the acute inflammatory stage. Please closely observe and follow up, and record episode intervals and medication. If the acute attacks are significantly frequent or symptoms aggravate, the operation treatment shall be considered.

[Pathological examination] A pile of grayish-yellow broken bone tissue was sent for biopsy, 1.5 cm * 2 cm * 0.4 cm in size. The trabecular

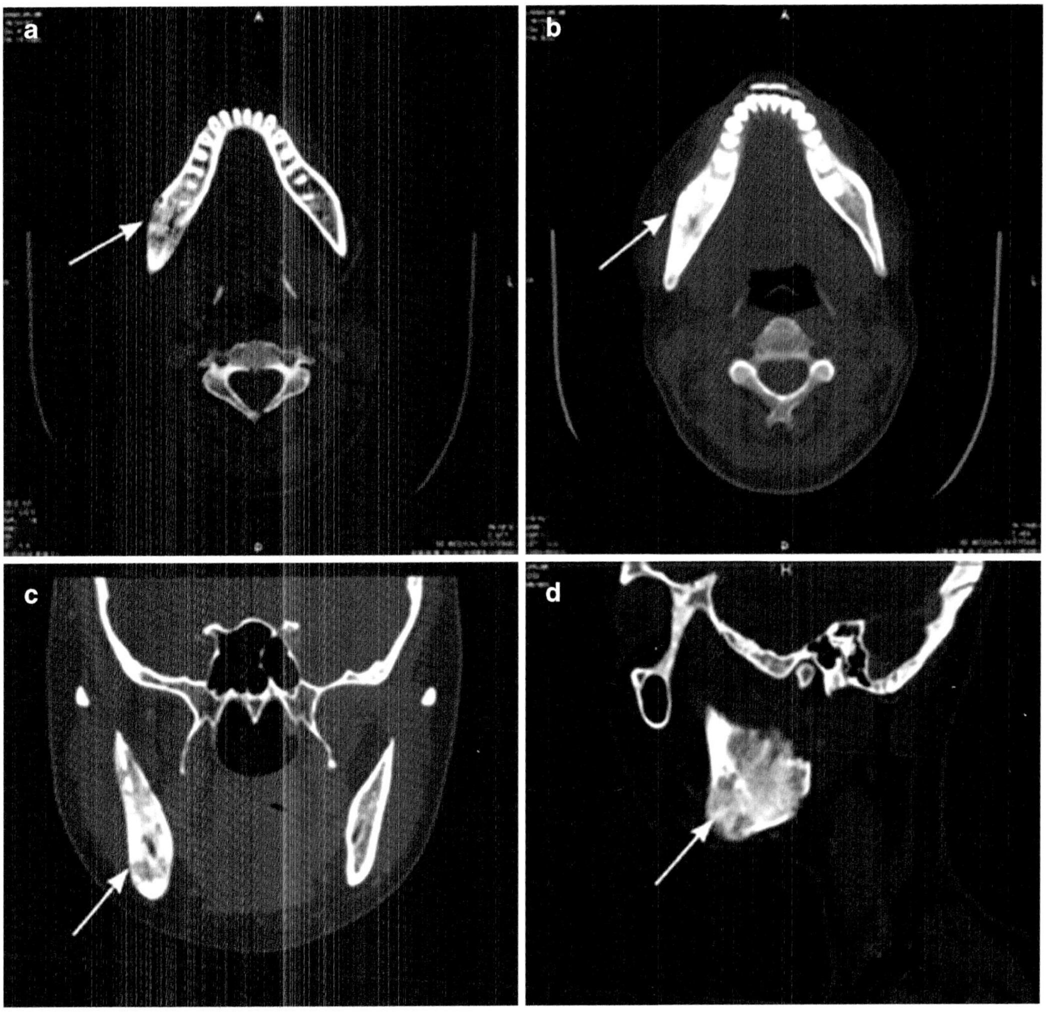

Fig. 2.2 (**a**) Cross section of CT Plain Scan: The bone marrow cavity density of the right mandibular ascending ramus increases unevenly with a ground-glass change. (**b**) Cross section of CT Enhanced Scan: No enhanced soft-tissue mass is seen. (**c**) Coronal view of CT enhanced scan: The bone cortex is still continuous, with no obvious periosteal reaction; (**d**) Coronal view of CT enhanced scan: Temporomandibular joint in place

bone is seen under the microscope. The osteocytes are around by peripheral bone. Loose fibrous tissue is filled in the trabecular space, with rich blood vessels and the infiltration of inflammatory cells (Fig. 2.4).

[Pathological diagnosis] Garré osteomyelitis of right mandible, ICD code: K10.202.

[Follow-up visit] During the follow-up visit period, the patient has one acute symptom in about a month: swelling with limited mouth opening. The symptoms were relieved with intravenous antibiotics in combination with hormonal medication. There was no significant change in the frequency of acute episodes since follow-ups.

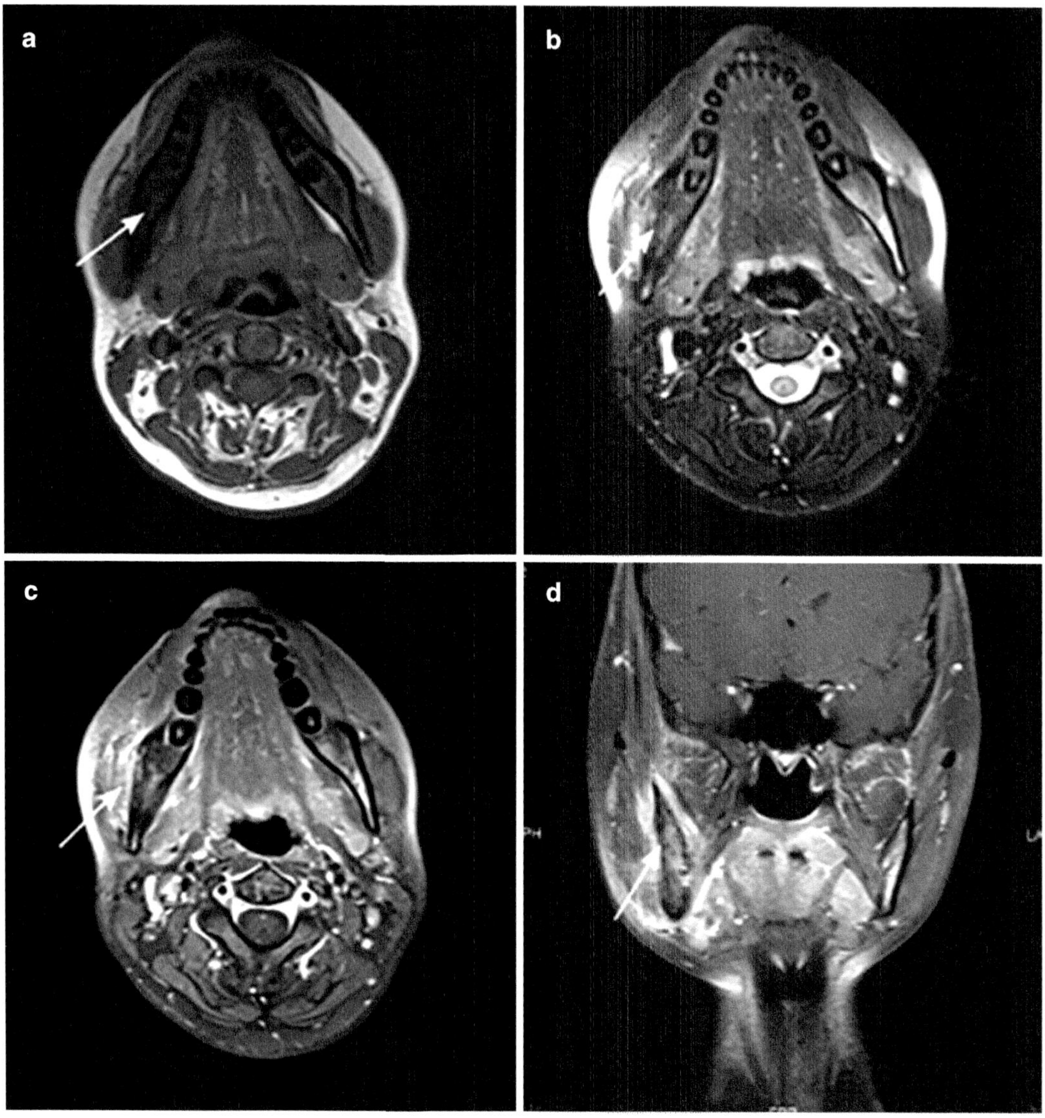

Fig. 2.3 (**a**) Transverse view of MRI T1WI: Low signals are observed in the right mandible body to the bone marrow cavity of the mandibular ascending ramus. (**b**) Transverse section of MRI T2WI: A slightly higher signal. (**c**) Transverse view of enhanced MRI: Mildly inhomogeneous enhancement, external pterygoid muscle and masseter swelling (**d**) Coronal view of enhanced MRI: Mild inhomogeneous enhancement, blurred peripheral fatty space with enhancement, and no enlarged lymph nodes in the neck

2.1.2 Case 4

The patient, male, 25 years old. Left facial swelling repeated for 2 years after tooth extraction.

[Present medical history] The patient went to a community hospital for treatment 2 years ago due to the left lower posterior teeth pain with the left facial swelling and was diagnosed with the left lower eight impacted tooth, which was removed after anti-infection. The left facial swelling was turned up 2 months after tooth extraction. The patient went to the community hospital again and was diagnosed with mumps.

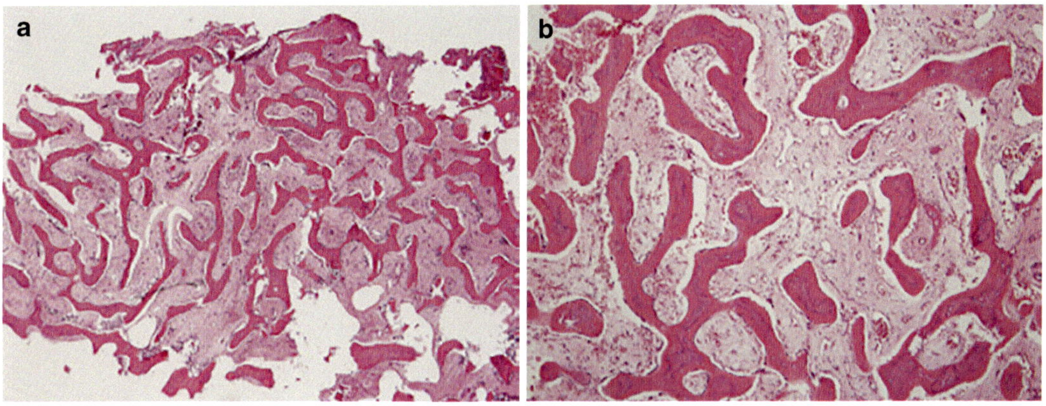

Fig. 2.4 (**a**) Hyperplastic trabecular bone is seen in the background of loose fibrous tissue, with loose fibrous connective tissue between the trabecular bones and scattered infiltration of inflammatory cells (40×). (**b**) Trabecular bone is thin, not surrounded by osteoblasts. The proliferation of fibrous tissue is seen between bone trabecula, with abundant blood vessels (100×)

The anti-inflammatory symptomatic treatment was given (unknown details of specific drug name and dosage). The swelling subsided. After that, the swelling of the left face was repeated, with no fever, no discomfort, and occasional difficulty opening the mouth. The patient was diagnosed with osteomyelitis of the mandible after taking a CT scan in a superior hospital and panoramic radiographs, etc. It was recommended that the patient receive the hyperbaric oxygen treatment and attend a return visit after half a year. Subsequently, the patient experienced repeated left facial swelling, and the frequency gradually increased. The patient was diagnosed with bone abnormality in the left mandible after completing the panoramic radiographs: possible osteomyelitis. Hospitalized operation treatment was recommended to the patient.

[Specialized examination] The left side face and right side face are asymmetric. The proportion of the upper, middle and lower 1/3 face is coordinated. The left masseter area is mildly swelling, without swelling and redness in local skin, no rupture, slight tenderness locally, and without obvious fluctuation. The degree and type of mouth opening are normal. Oral permanent dentition. No local gingival swelling and redness

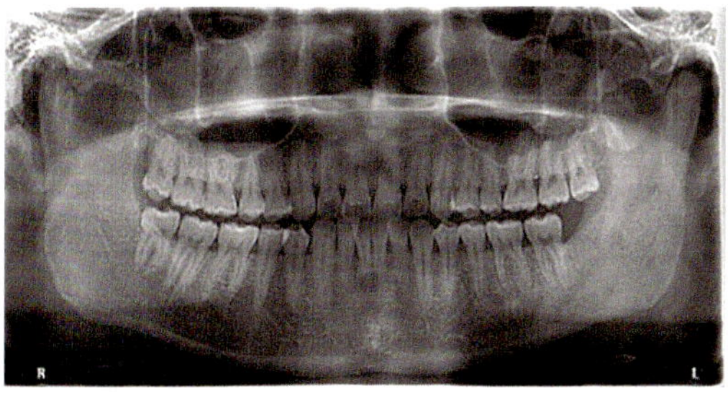

Fig. 2.5 The bone density of the left mandible body and mandibular ramus increases with uneven enhancement compared with the contralateral side (preoperative)

are found in the left lower posterior teeth, no obvious bulging and pyorrhea, no numbness of the face and lips, and no swollen lymph nodes in the face and neck.

[Auxiliary examination]

1. Panoramic radiographs indicated that the bone density of the left mandible body and mandibular ramus increases unevenly compared with the contralateral side (Fig. 2.5).
2. CT enhanced scan of the maxillofacial region indicated that the density of the bone marrow cavity in the left mandible is uneven, showing ground-glass changes, uncontinuous local bone cortex, no obvious periosteal reaction, and no abnormally enhanced soft tissue mass after enhancement (Fig. 2.6).

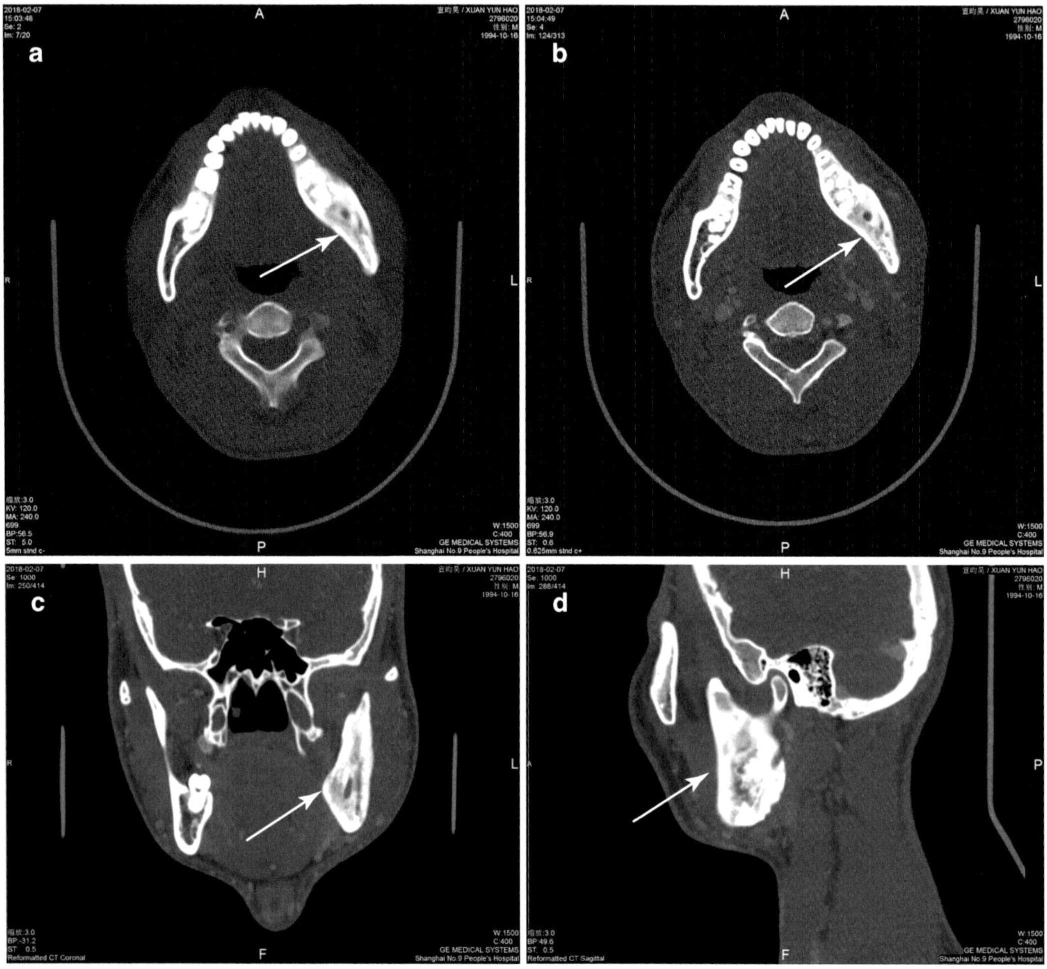

Fig. 2.6 (**a**) Transverse view of CT plain scan: The density of the marrow cavity of the left mandible is uneven with ground-glass changes. (**b**) Cross section of CT Enhanced Scan: No abnormal enhanced soft tissue mass was seen. (**c**) Coronal view of CT enhanced scan: The bone cortex is continuous, with no obvious periosteal reaction; (**d**) Sagittal view of CT enhanced scan: Temporomandibular joint in place

[Primary diagnosis] Marginal osteomyelitis of left mandible.

[Treatment] "Curettage for the osteomyelitis of the left mandible + the left upper tooth 8 extraction" was performed under general anesthesia. A longitudinal incision was made in the left posterior molar area to cut open and turn the flap over to expose the focal bone. The destroyed and softened bones were removed by power grinding. The necrotic tissue and granulation tissue were removed. The necrotic bone in lateral mandibular ramus was abraded. Fast-freezing results revealed that the "left mandible" was submitted for fibers, muscles and bone tissue. The bleeding was completely stopped and washed. An iodiform gauze strip was retained in the local surgical site, and the wound was sutured and closed.

[Pathological examination] The submitted specimen is grayish-yellow broken tissue, approximately 0.7 cm * 0.7 cm * 0.3 cm in size, with hard nature. The proliferation of woven trabecular bone is seen under the microscope, with osteoblasts around the bone margin. The proliferation of blood vessels and fibrous tissue is noted between the trabecular bones, with scattered inflammatory cell infiltration (Fig. 2.7).

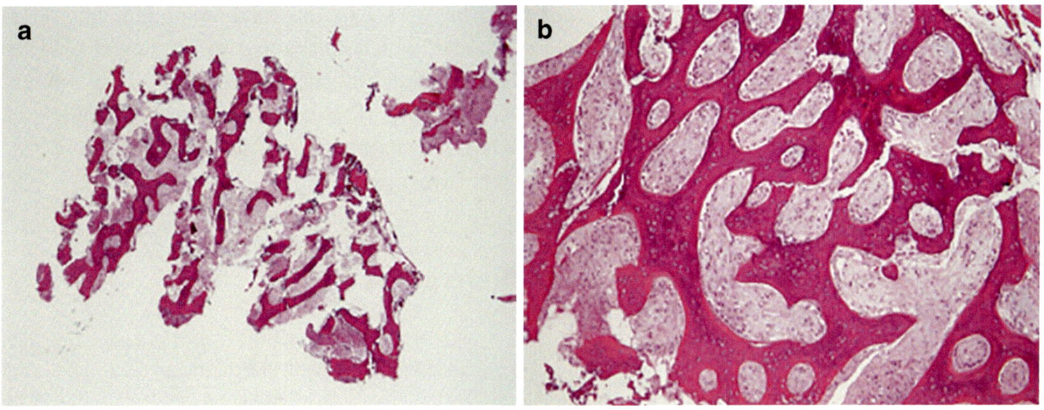

Fig. 2.7 (**a**) Fibrous tissue proliferation was seen between the woven bone trabecula, with scattered inflammatory cell infiltration (4×). (**b**) Bone edge was surrounded by osteoblasts, with proliferation of blood vessels and fibrous tissue between trabecular bones (200×)

[Pathological diagnosis] Garré osteomyelitis of left mandible, ICD code: K10.202.

[Follow-up visit] The patient recovered well after surgery with no progression.

2.2 Key Points of Diagnosis and Treatment

Garré's osteomyelitis was first defined by Garré as a special bone disorder caused by low-virulence infection and stimulation, characterized by chronic non-pyogenic osteomyelitis with hyperplastic periostitis [8–10]. The exact etiology of the disease was unknown. It may be related to odontogenic and non-odontogenic infections. In terms of anatomical structure, the teeth were directly connected to the jaws. The odontogenic pathogens can spread to the root tip, alveolar process and the jaws through the dental pulp and periodontal infection. A large number of related studies had shown that the periapical inflammation of the mandibular first molar was the most common cause of Garré's osteomyelitis of the jaws. Still, infection of impacted third molar may also cause Garré's osteomyelitis of the jaws. Non-odontogenic factors involved endocrine (estrogen and progesterone or the osteogenic differentiation of periodontal membrane stem cells) and external stimuli (mechanical stimulation, trauma stimulation). In addition, Claudia Elera-Fitzcarrald et al. confirmed that salmonella may cause Garré's osteomyelitis of the jaws. Since Garré's osteomyelitis of the jaws is currently considered one of the inflammatory diseases, Garré's osteomyelitis of the jaws may have the expression of inflammatory markers during the inflammatory activity, including C reactive protein and erythrocyte sedimentation rate, etc. However, there was no expression of specific markers of Garré's osteomyelitis of the jaws.

Imaging and pathological characteristics The imaging features of Garré's osteomyelitis of the jaws include dense bone sclerosis with periosteal new bone formation, mainly manifested by the formation of the periosteal membrane. Bone destruction is rare. The external sclerotin of compact bone showed a thin layer. Low-density images of trabecular structures were visible between the thin bone and dense bone. The continuous stimulation of inflammation made the normal bone tissue form the periosteum and stratify. The radiation-resistant layer and transmission layer were alternating, and onions showed skin-like changes. The pathological change of the disease was active subperiosteal osteogenesis, showing the deposition of a large number of new bone and osteoblasts. The fibrous connective tissue was wrapped by a newly developed bone trabecula, with a small amount of plasma cells and lymphocyte infiltration.

Differential diagnosis In addition to Garré's osteomyelitis of the jaws, new bone formation may also occur in many pathological conditions. Therefore, other pathological factors that cause new bone formation should be distinguished clinically from Ewing sarcoma and osteosarcoma. In addition, Garré's osteomyelitis of the jaws must be differentiated from radiation osteomyelitis, medication-related osteomyelitis of the jaws, pyogenic osteomyelitis of jaws, abnormal proliferation of bone fibers, Langerhans cell histiocytosis, and infantile cortical hyperostosis, etc. [8, 9]

Treatment At present, due to the etiology of Garré's osteomyelitis of the jaws being unknown, as well as its low positive rate of bacterial culture, long course of disease and limited effect of medical treatment, the final therapeutic method is still unclear. Extraction of affected teeth in the diseased area, pulp treatment, and surgery under systemic application of antibiotics are widely used to treat the disease. For a limited lesion, a good treatment effect and prognosis can usually be obtained. Studies have shown that NSAID and antibiotic therapy are effective in Garré's osteomyelitis of the jaws. There are also some studies showing that pamidronate may be beneficial for the pain relief of Garré's osteomyelitis of the jaws [8].

Garré's osteomyelitis of the jaws is a subclass of osteomyelitis of the jaws. Currently, a surgical adjuvant anti-inflammatory therapy is relatively effective in the treatment of Garré's osteomyelitis of the jaws. Currently, the reason for the cause and condition of recurrent Garré's osteomyelitis of the jaws and the final treatment method is unclear, which means that the treatment plan for Garré's osteomyelitis of the jaws is extremely challenging. The best therapy and etiology of Garré's osteomyelitis of the jaws need to be further investigated.

References

1. Suei Y, Taguchi A, Tanimoto K. Diagnosis and classificaion of mandibular osteomyelitis [J]. Oral Surg Oral Med Oral Pathol Oral Radiol Endod. 2005;100(2):207–14.
2. Muhetaer Y. Garrè's osteomyelitis research. Xinjiang Medical University; 2020.
3. Muhetaer Y, Abasi K, Hu LL, Gong ZC. Clinical characteristic of 6 patients with Garrè's osteomyelitis. J Sci Res. 2020;7:678–82.
4. Zaidman M, Katzman A, et al. New treatment option for sclerosing osteomyelitis of Garré. J Pediatr Orthop B. 2013;22(6):577–82.
5. Gao P, Wang X, Xuan M, Ma X, Chang Z, Xiong S. Garrè's osteomyelitis with bilateral mandible: a case report. West China J Stomatol. 2015;33(4):436–8.
6. Park J, Myoung H. Chronic suppurative osteomyelitis with proliferative periostitis related to a fully impacted third molar germ: a report of two cases [J]. J Korean Assoc Oral Maxillofac Surg. 2016;42(4):215–20.
7. Elera-Fitzcarrald C, Alfaro-Lozano JL, Pastor-Asurza CA. Garré's sclerosing osteomyelitis caused by salmonella group D in a patient with systemic lupus erythematosus: an unusual complication [J]. Clin Rheumatol. 2015;34(12):2155–8.
8. Urade M, Noguchi K, Takaoka K, et al. Diffuse sclerosing osteomyelitis of the mandible successfully treated with pamidronate: a long-term follow-up report [J]. Oral Surg Oral Med Oral Pathol Oral Radiol. 2012;114(4):E9–E12.
9. Franco-Jimenez S, Romero-Aguilar JF, Bervel-Clemente S, et al. Garré's chronic sclerosing osteomyelitis with sacral involvement in a child [J]. Rev Esp Cir Ortop Traumatol. 2013;57(2):145–9.
10. Schwartz AJ, Jones NF, Seeger LL, et al. Chronic sclerosing osteomyelitis treated with wide resection and vascularized fibular autograft: a case report [J]. Am J Orthop. 2010;39(3):28–32.

Osteoradionecrosis of the Jaws

3

Yue He, Hui Shan Ong, Zhen Tian, Lin Zhu, and Hang Chen

3.1 Introduction

Osteoradionecrosis of the jaws (ORNJ) is a serious complication occurring after radiotherapy of oral, maxillofacial, head and neck tumors, with an incidence ranging from 5% to 15%. ORNJ is often characterized by chronic necrosis and infection [1]. The clinical manifestations consist of local redness, pain, limitation of mouth opening, dysphagia, chewing and language disorders, pyorrhea of facial soft tissue fistula and inability to heal, exposure to dead bones, and even pathological fractures in severe cases. The pathogenesis of ORNJ is still unclear. The basic research and preliminary clinical translational research based on different theoretical hypotheses are in their infancy. Whether antifibrotic therapy can achieve clinical benefits and improve patients' quality of life while reducing the rate of ORNJ progression, the results of prospective clinical studies still need to be confirmed. ORNJ treatment plan should be comprehensively considered according to lesion classification and stages, the patient's age, occupation and compliance, comprehensive hospital conditions, clinical skills of doctors, and other factors to make an individual choice [2–4]. Due to the rich maxillary blood supply, it generally rarely appears to have widespread necrosis [5–10]. Therefore, there are some differences in its clinical manifestations and management methods compared with the necrosis of the jaws. It generally takes conservative treatment, curettage of necrotic jaw and so on, relatively conservative surgical methods [9–22]. For dead bones with clear boundaries, it is also feasible with vascularized bone tissue or soft tissue flap repair [23–34]. As for osteoradionecrosis of the jaws, we recommend the corresponding treatment according to BS classification and staging [2, 11, 23].

3.2 Maxilla Osteoradionecrosis

3.2.1 Case 5

The patient, male, 51 years old. The patient has suffered from the facial pus for a year after radiotherapy for recurrent left maxillary sinus carcinoma.

[Present medical history] The patient underwent "the left nasal mass resection" twice, two and a half years ago and one and a half years ago.

Y. He (✉) · H. S. Ong · Z. Tian · H. Chen
Department of Oral Maxillofacial-Head & Neck Oncology, Shanghai Ninth People's Hospital, Shanghai Jiao Tong University School of Medicine, Shanghai, China

L. Zhu
Department of Radiology, Ninth People's Hospital Affiliated to Shanghai Jiao Tong University, Shanghai, China

Y. He (ed.), *Inflammatory and Neoplastic Diseases of Craniofacial Bones*,
https://doi.org/10.1007/978-981-97-4155-7_3

Postoperative pathology: The left nasal mass, squamous carcinoma with local inverting papilloma. Postoperative PET-CT indicated "residual left upper sinus mass." The patient had two courses of TPF chemotherapy in our hospital. The CT scan was performed 15 months ago and the results indicated that the malignant tumor of the left maxillary sinus invaded the skull base. The radiotherapy was performed 32 times, with an unknown specific dose. One year ago, the left face was repeatedly swollen and purulent. The anti-infection treatment was not significantly improved, and the bone of the infraorbital area was exposed 7 months ago.

[Specialized examination] The patient's skin in the left infraorbital area is slightly red and swollen. The left temporal area is bulging, with a hard nature and an ill-defined edge. It changes after radiotherapy, dead bone exposure in the infraorbital area, little pus, eyeball exposure, and closed teeth. The oral condition was not checked (Fig. 3.1). No obvious enlarged lymph nodes were palpated in the neck.

[Auxiliary examination]

1. Panoramic radiographs: The bone wall sclerotin of the left maxilla and maxillary sinus is destroyed, the bone cortex is discontinuous, no obvious periosteal reaction is seen, and the surrounding soft tissues are swollen (Fig. 3.2).
2. CT enhanced scan of the maxillofacial region: "After chemotherapy for recurrent cancer of left maxillary sinus," the sclerotin of left maxilla, maxillary sinus wall, left orbital floor, lateral wall and zygomatic bone are destroyed and partially lost, and the left maxillary sinus connects with the body surface. Irregular soft tissue density thickening shadow is seen around the left maxillary sinus area, and the boundary is unclear. After enhancement, the lesion enhancement is not obvious, with C− of 49 Hu and C+ of 66 ~ 79 Hu. Increased density is seen in the left frontal sinus, ethmoid sinus and sphenoid sinus. Soft tissue thickening is seen in the left pterygopalatine fossa. No obvious abnormal enhancement focus is seen in the brain. No obvious swollen lymph node shadow is seen in the neck (Fig. 3.3).

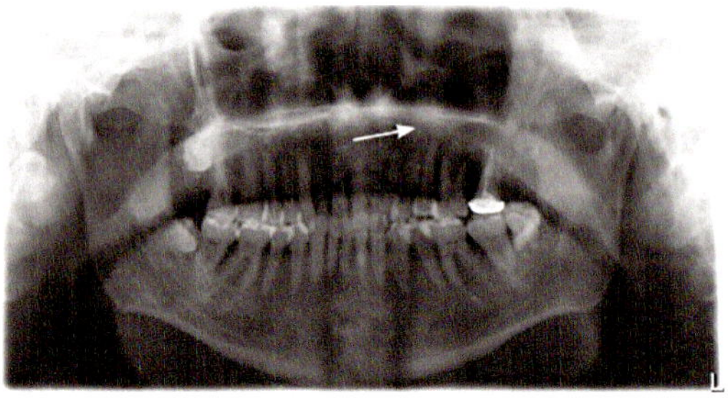

Fig. 3.2 The bone wall sclerotin of the left maxilla and maxillary sinus was destroyed, the bone cortex was discontinuous, no obvious periosteal reaction was seen, and the surrounding soft tissues were swollen

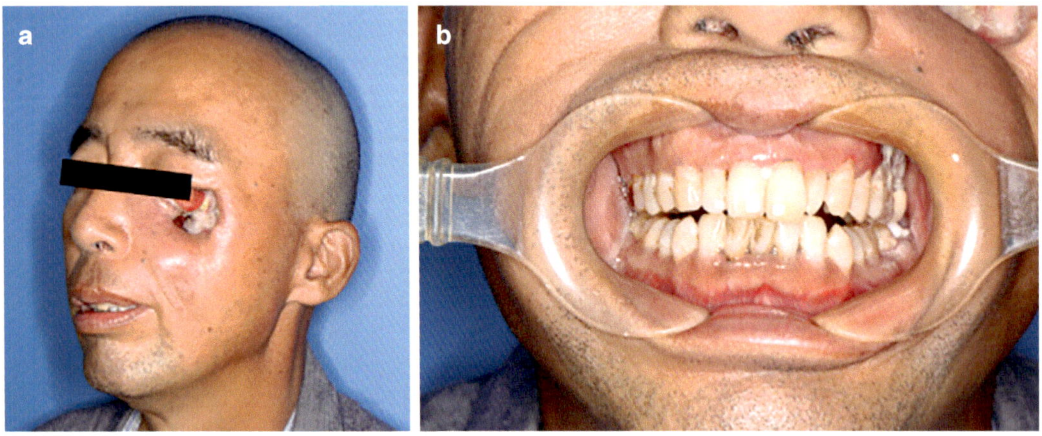

Fig. 3.1 (**a**) Exposed dead bone below left eye socket. (**b**) When the mandibular joint closes, pyorrhea is seen on the gingiva

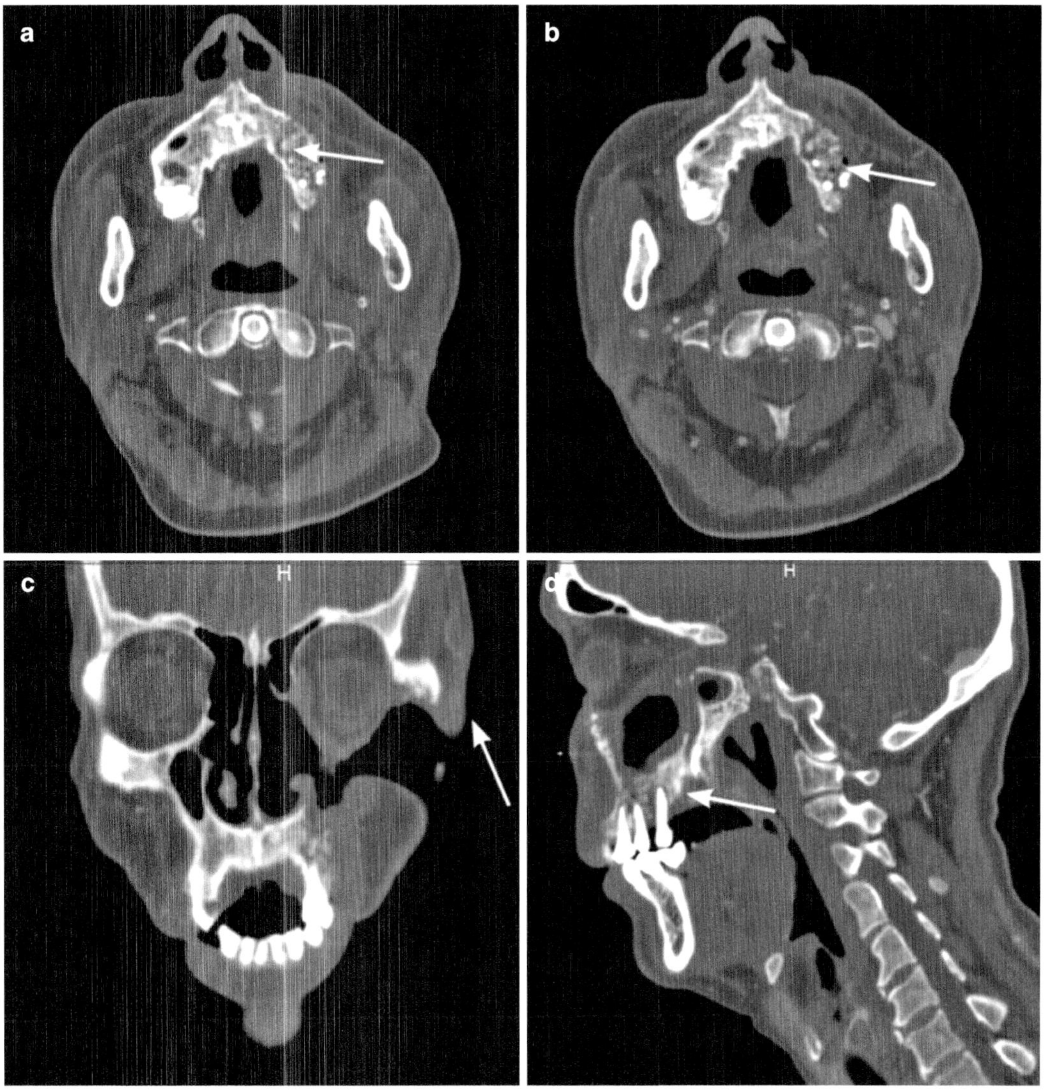

Fig. 3.3 (**a**) Cross-section of CT plain scan: Sclerotin of left maxilla is destroyed. (**b**) Cross-section of CT enhanced scan: No abnormal enhanced soft tissue mass is seen. (**c**) Coronal CT enhanced scan: Bone cortex is discontinuous, and no swollen lymph nodes are seen. (**d**) Coronal CT enhanced scan: Upper alveolar bone is involved

[Primary diagnosis] Left maxilla osteoradionecrosis.

[Treatment] Under general anesthesia, "maxillary extended resection + zygomatic bone amputation + coracoid process amputation + muscle release operation + anterolateral thigh flap repair + tracheotomy" were implemented. During the operation, an incision was made along philtrum to basis nasi, around the ala nasi and along the nose, and extended to the coloboma below the eye socket. Maxilla, zygomatic bone and orbital floor of the lesion area were removed. It was seen that the lesion area connected with the nasal cavity, and there were a lot of inflammatory granulation-like substances on the inner surface of the maxillary sinus, and bone necrosis can be seen at the orbital apex of the orbital floor. After the coracoid process was cut off by a dynamic system, the mouth of the patient was opened with a mouth opener, and there was no obvious improvement in the mouth opening. Therefore, the medial pterygoid muscle, part of lateral pterygoid muscle and temporal muscle were loosened, and the relevant tissues in the lesion were cut and sent to the operation for intraoperative frozen pathology examination. Pathological examination indicated that no obvious evidence of malignancy was seen, and all margins were negative (−). The opening degree was about 2 cm. An incision about 2 cm long was made at the lower edge of the left mandible to prepare the recipient blood vessels. At the same time, the right anterolateral thigh flap was taken and transferred to the wound. After the mandible was supported and the tunnel on the surface of the mandibular ramus was passed through, the flap was anastomosed with facial artery and vein, respectively. The flap was trimmed and shaped, and the wound coloboma was repaired. The operation wound was rinsed, bleeding was stopped strictly, the negative pressure drainage tube was reserved, the suture was performed in layers, and the wound was closed (Fig. 3.4).

[Pathological examination] A piece of bone tissue is sent for pathological examination, 7 cm * 6 cm * 2 cm, grayish yellow, and part of the tissue is necrotic. Microscopically, dead bone is found locally, and the bone tissue around the dead bone shows osteomyelitis, hyperostosis and absorption, with obvious fibrous tissue proliferation between trabeculae and significant infiltration of inflammatory cells in some areas (Fig. 3.5).

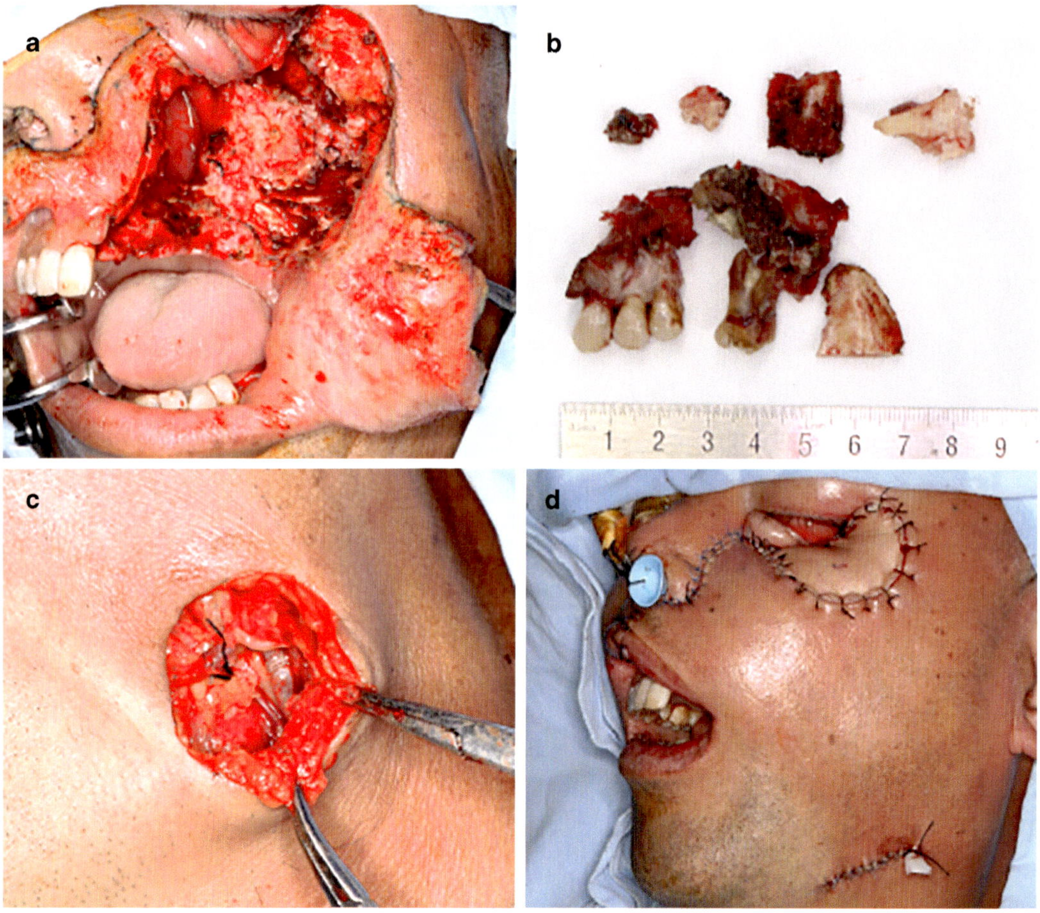

Fig. 3.4 (**a**) Coloboma after removal of dead bone and surrounding soft tissue. (**b**) In-vitro dead bone. (**c**) Vascular anastomosis in submandibular region. (**d**) Postoperative observation of anterolateral thigh flap

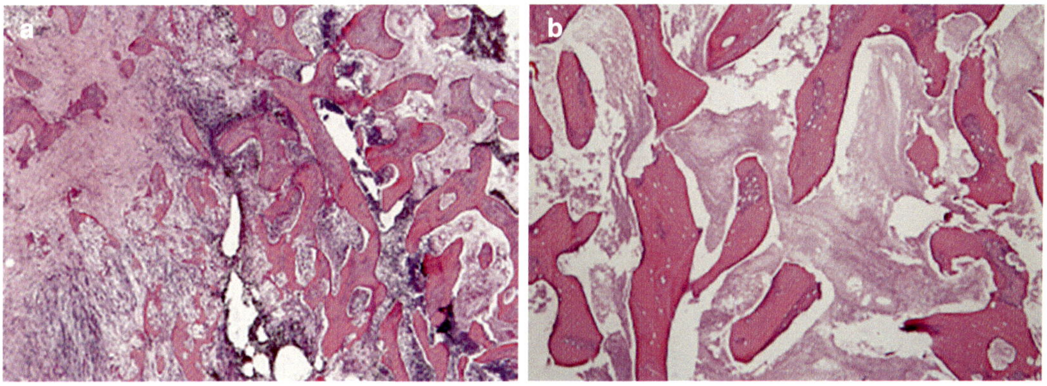

Fig. 3.5 (**a**) Obvious fibrous tissue proliferation between trabecular bones, significant local inflammatory cell infiltration, and coexistence of bone tissue absorption and proliferation. The formation of dead bone was seen on one side (40×). (**b**) The edge of trabecular bone was absorbed and depressed, the lacuna was empty, and the tissue between trabecular bones was degenerated and necrotic, being dead bone tissue (100×)

[Pathological diagnosis] radiation osteomyelitis of "left maxilla," ICD code: K10.201, with formation of dead bone.

[Follow-up visit] Follow-up visit half a year after operation: the color of the skin flap in the operative region was good, there was no obvious exudation in the operative region, the left vision was normal and the eye movement was normal.

3.2.2 Case 6

The patient, male, 62 years old. Repeated swelling and pain in the left face for 6 years.

[Present medical history] The patient received radiotherapy for "fibrous dysplasia of bone of left maxilla" 46 years ago. The exact dose and location were unknown. About 6 years ago, the left face repeatedly swelled, and the anti-infection treatment was effective. The condition was repeated. Three years ago, he suffered from curettage surgery in a local hospital. Postoperative pathology indicated inflammatory tissue (self-report), and after the operation, swelling and pain symptoms recurred.

[Specialized examination] The facial form is asymmetrical, the left face is slightly sunken, the surface skin is pigmented, and there is no obvious fistula, fistula or abnormal exudation. Mouth opening and mouth opening shape are normal, the occluding relation in the mouth is acceptable, the permanent dentition, the left upper vestibular sulcus has a 3 cm * 1 cm fistula, connected with the maxillary sinus, purulent secretions can be seen locally, dead bone is exposed, and the local mucosa is slightly red. No obvious swollen lymph nodes are palpated in the bilateral neck and submandibular region.

[Auxiliary examination]
CT enhanced scan of the maxillofacial region indicated that the bone density on the left side of the maxilla is uneven, with local sclerotin loss and irregular sclerotin margin, moth-eaten. The front wall of the left maxillary sinus is missing. The soft tissue density shadow and irregular cloud-like bone density are seen in the maxillary sinus, and the soft tissue is slightly enhanced after enhancement. No obvious enlarged lymph nodes are seen in the neck (Fig. 3.6).

[Primary diagnosis] Right maxilla osteoradionecrosis.

[Treatment] Under general anesthesia, "subtotal resection of left maxilla + fibula musculocutaneous flap transfer repair" was performed: Webern incision was used conducted, flapling, exposing the anterolateral wall of maxilla, and the sclerotin

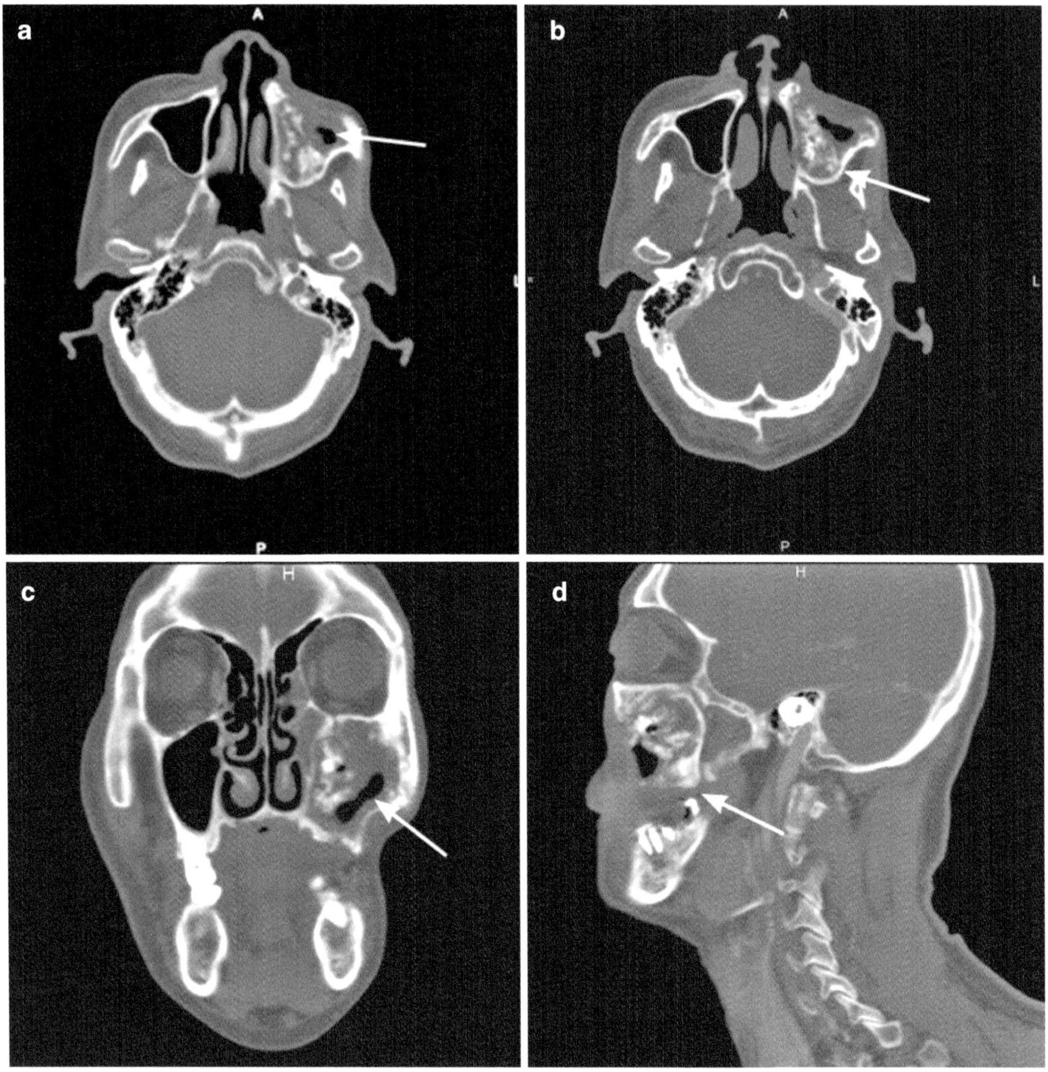

Fig. 3.6 (**a**) Cross-section of CT plain scan: The sclerotin of the left maxilla was destroyed, the front wall of the left maxillary sinus was absent, soft tissue density shadow and irregular cloud-like bone high density were seen in the maxillary sinus. (**b**) Cross-section of CT enhanced scan: No abnormal enhanced soft tissue mass was seen. (**c**) Coronal CT enhanced scan: The left maxillary sinus was invaded and the maxillary sinus cavity disappeared. (**d**) Sagittal position of CT enhanced scan: The sclerotin of the left superior alveolar bone was destroyed

below the eye socket was preserved. The maxillary connection was severed by a dynamic system. From the interior to the turbinate, from the upper boundary to the lower margin of the orbital floor, the maxilla was severed, and the normal mucosa of the palate was preserved. Mucosal tissue sample was sent for frozen section examination and reported as NAD (no abnormality detected). Chronic inflammation of the mucosa and soft tissue of "left maxilla," with small pieces of dead bone. The fibular musculocutaneous flap was cut, the length of the fibula was 10 cm, and the fibula was shaped and divided into two segments. One was from the alveolar ridge to the zygomatic bone, and the other was from the eye socket's lower margin. The peroneal artery and

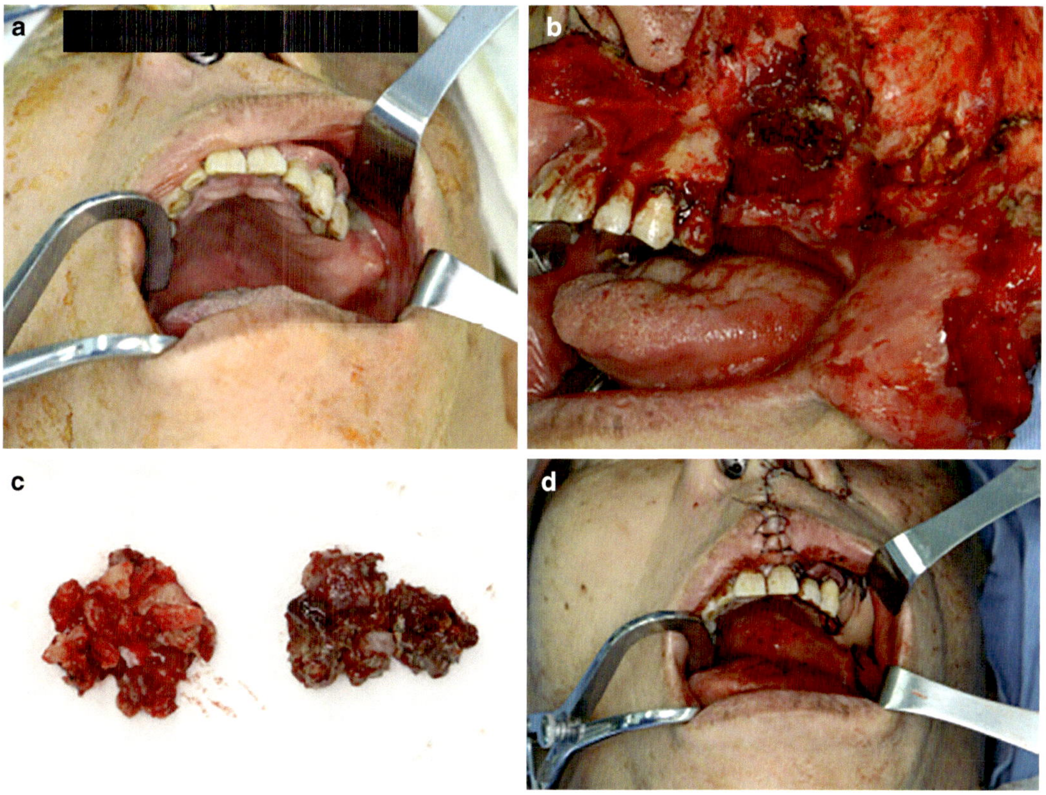

Fig. 3.7 (**a**) The left maxillary gingiva was red, swollen, and with pyorrhea and exposed dead bone. (**b**) The dead bone was removed and the surrounding soft tissue was repaired. (**c**) In-vitro dead bone and inflammatory granulation tissue. (**d**) Postoperative observation of fibular musculocutaneous flap

vein were anastomosed with facial movement. The operation wound was rinsed, bleeding was stopped strictly, a negative pressure drainage tube was reserved, the suture was performed in layers, and the wound was closed (Fig. 3.7).

[Pathological examination] Crushbone tissues were sent for pathological examination, grayish yellow and hard. Microscopically, it was seen that bone tissue was degenerated, lamellar bone structure had disappeared or fractured, some bone cells disappeared, bone lacunae were empty, dead bone was formed, the edges were not covered with osteoblasts, in moth-eaten depressions. Significant and compact proliferation of fibrous tissue between trabeculae was seen, and a small amount of inflammatory cell infiltration was seen (Fig. 3.8).

[Pathological diagnosis] osteoradionecrosis of "left maxilla" ICD code: K10.201.

[Follow-up visit] The patient recovered well after the operation. In the follow-up visit after half a year, the reconstructed shape of maxilla was satisfactory and the right occluding relation was good.

3.3 Osteoradionecrosis of Mandible

3.3.1 Case 7

The patient, female, 61 years old. Left mandibular residual root with gingival hyperplasia and pyorrhea for a half year.

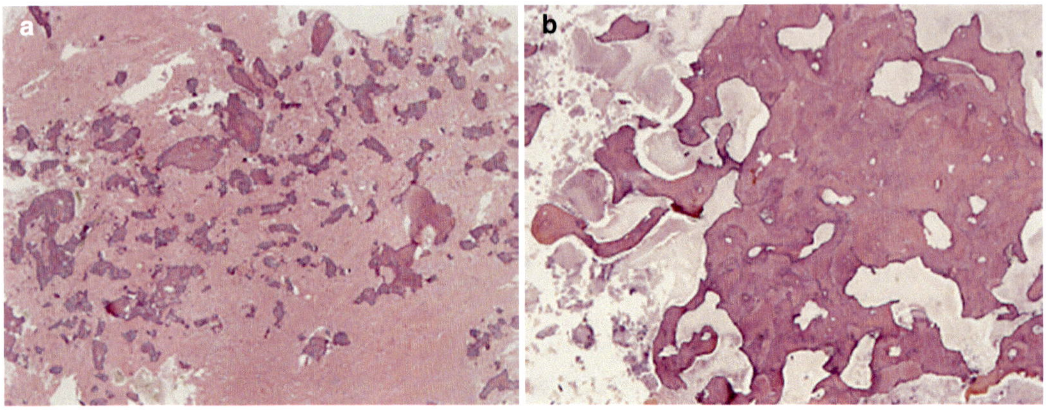

Fig. 3.8 (**a**) Significant proliferation and glassy degeneration of fibrous tissue between trabeculae and disappeared endoskeleton lacunae in bone tissue, showing dead bone (40×). (**b**) Dead Bone tissue, bone lacunae, tissue denaturation and necrosis of bone trabeculae (100×)

[Present medical history] 14 years ago, the patient received radiotherapy for nasopharyngeal carcinoma in the other hospital. The specific dose was unknown, and there were many residual roots in the mouth. Six months ago, there was gingival hyperplasia on the left mandible, chewing discomfort, and a small amount of pyorrhea on the gingival margin. No special treatment was given. Recently, the patient felt a red and swollen gingiva with pain.

[Specialized examination] The maxillofacial region is basically symmetrical on both sides, and the proportion of the upper, middle and lower 1/3 is coordinated. The mouth opening degree and mouth opening type are normal, with poor oral hygiene, unclear speech, tongue movement disorder, limited tongue extension, 33 ~ 37 residual roots, widened alveolar ridge, gingival mucosa proliferation, redness and swelling, a small amount of pyorrhea on gingival margin, no obvious dead bone exposure (Fig. 3.9), 16, 17 and 43 residual roots, maxillary 15 ~ 27 fixed denture restoration, the gingival margin is slightly red and swollen, no obvious abnormality is seen in the remaining mucosa, swollen lymph nodes are not palpated in submandibular region and neck, and the mobility of bilateral submandibular region joints is consistent.

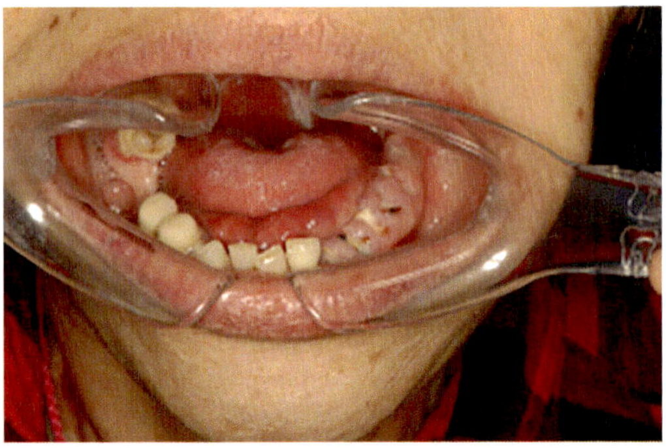

Fig. 3.9 33 ~ 37 residual roots, gingival hyperplasia, and a small amount of pyorrhea on the gingival margin

[Auxiliary examination]
Panoramic radiographs: 33 ~ 37 residual roots, low-density apical shadow, uneven density reduction in the bone marrow cavity at 36 and 37 teeth. 16, 17, 43 residual roots, 43 low-density apical shadows (Fig. 3.10).

[Primary diagnosis] Radiation-induced osteomyelitis of the left mandible.

[Treatment] Under general anesthesia, "debridement and scaling of left mandible + extraction of residual roots" were performed: 33 ~ 37 residual roots were removed, and it was seen that there was no blood supply to the alveo-

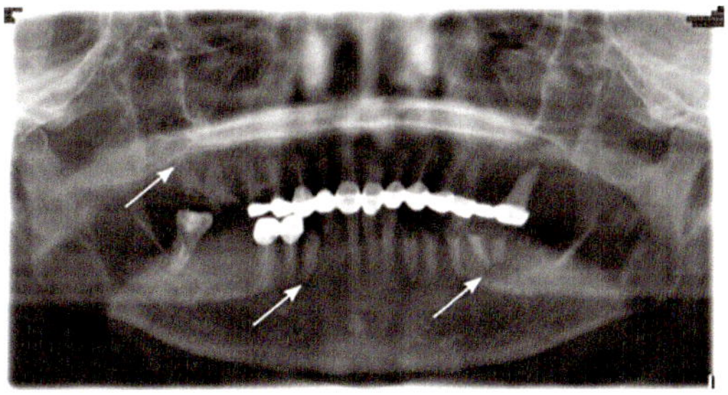

Fig. 3.10 33 ~ 37 residual roots, low-density apical shadow, and uneven decrease of bone marrow cavity density at 36 and 37 teeth. 16, 17, 43 residual roots, 43 apical low-density shadow (preoperative)

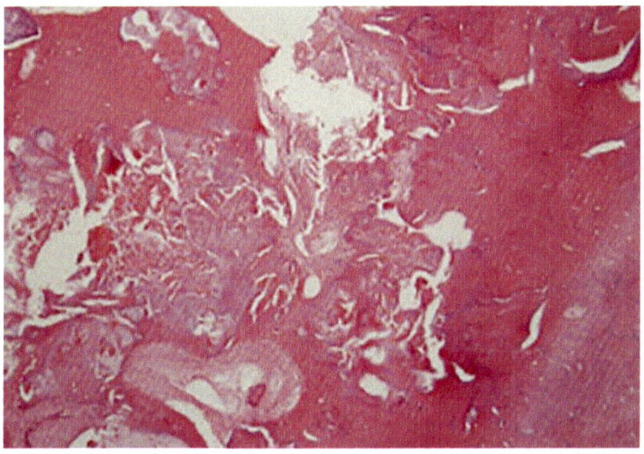

Fig. 3.11 Fibrous tissue proliferation and focal inflammatory cell infiltration between trabecular bones (100×)

lar bone, the dead bone was removed. The dynamic system ground the mandible to a fresh wound. After that, the gingival mucosa was trimmed, 16, 17 and 43 residual roots were removed to remove the dead bone, the sharp bone edge was trimmed, the wound was rinsed, bleeding was stopped completely, and local drawing and suture were performed.

[Pathological examination] A piece of bone tissue was sent for pathological examination, 1.7 cm * 1.5 cm * 0.5 cm, grayish-yellow. Microscopically, there was a significant proliferation of fibrous tissue between bone tissues and inflammatory cell infiltration. Local bone tissue degenerated, a bone lacuna was empty, and dead bone formed (Fig. 3.11).

[Pathological diagnosis] radiation osteomyelitis of "mandible," ICD code: K10.201.

[Follow-up visit] The patient recovered well after operation, and the mucosa in the operative region was intact and there was no obvious ulceration and exudation after a half year.

3.3.2 Case 8

The patient, male, 57 years old. Nine years after radiotherapy and chemotherapy for nasopharyngeal carcinoma, the right mandible was swollen, painful, and purulent for 1 year.

[Present medical history] 9 years ago, the patient was treated with radiotherapy and chemotherapy (radiotherapy 33 times and chemotherapy 4 times) in a local hospital for nasopharyngeal carcinoma. One year ago, he suffered from pain in the lower right posterior teeth and took oral anti-inflammatory drugs, but his symptoms did not improve. After several months, the lower right posterior teeth were repeatedly suppurated, his mouth opening was limited, and his right face was obviously swollen. He went to a local stomatological hospital 11 months ago, considering "infection of masseter space and osteomyelitis of the mandible." Under local anesthesia, "extraoral and intraoral incision and drainage + extraction of the lower right 7" were performed, anti-inflammatory, irrigation and other symptomatic treatments were given, and hyperbaric oxygen therapy was performed (30 times). The submandibular incision was protracted with local pyorrhea. Half a year ago, there was limited mouth opening and numbness of the lower lip. A month ago, the patient went to the outpatient department for CT enhanced scan of the maxillofacial region, indicating osteoradionecrosis of the right mandible, with pathological fracture.

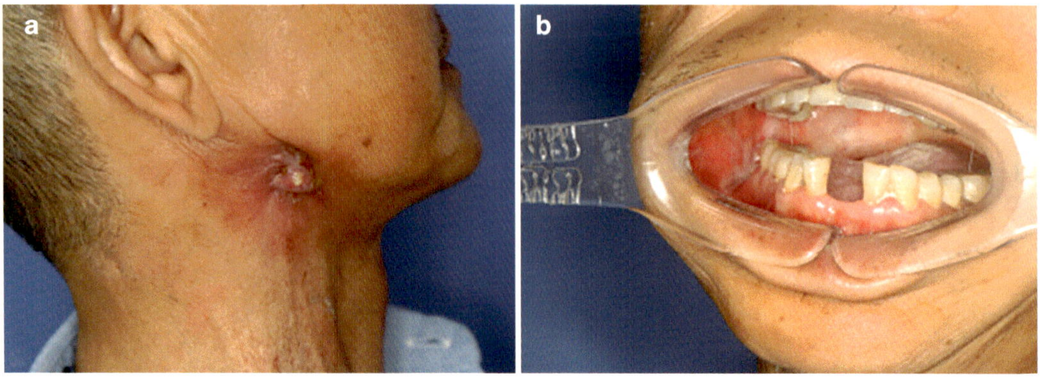

Fig. 3.12 (**a**) After radiotherapy, change of right submandibular region and neck, skin contracture, right submandibular fistula, surrounding skin redness and purulent exudation. (**b**) The mouth opening was about 1.5 cm, and the mucosa of the lower right posterior teeth area was red and swollen with pyorrhea

[Specialized examination] The facial form is basically symmetrical, and a wound about 5 cm long can be seen at the right mandibular angle. The wound margin is uneven, and the surrounding skin is red and swollen, with local pus. The degree of mouth opening is about 1.5 cm, the mouth opening is severely limited, and 47 is missing. The wound has a diameter of about 0.5 cm, purulent secretion, local mucosal swelling and scar formation are seen locally, and no obvious new tumor is seen (Fig. 3.12). The lower right lip is numb. No obvious abnormal swollen lymph nodes are seen in the submandibular region and neck.

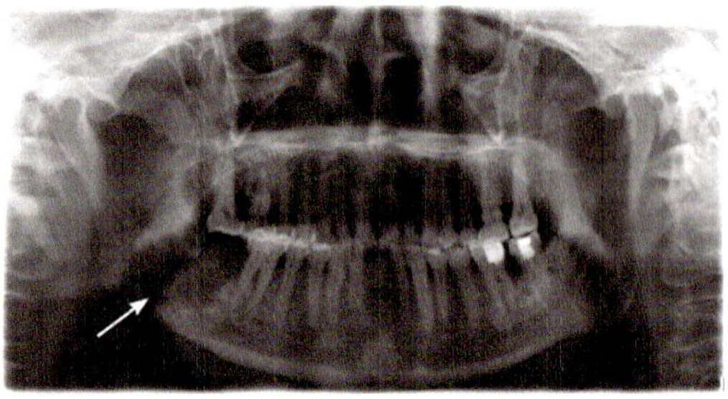

Fig. 3.13 The sclerotin of diaphysis and dertrotheca and ascending ramus part of the right mandible is destroyed, the density in the bone marrow cavity is uneven, the bone cortex is discontinuous, and the periosteal reaction is not obvious

[Auxiliary examination]

1. Panoramic radiographs: The sclerotin of the diaphysis, dertrotheca and ascending ramus part of the right mandible is destroyed, the density in the bone marrow cavity is uneven, the bone cortex is discontinuous, and the periosteal reaction is not obvious (Fig. 3.13).
2. CT-enhanced scan of the maxillofacial region indicated the sclerotin of diaphysis and dertrotheca the ascending ramus part of the right mandible is destroyed, the density in the bone marrow cavity is uneven, and the soft tissue density shadow is seen. The CT value of the plain scan is about 61 Hu, the shadow is enhanced after enhancement, and the C+ is 76 Hu, involving the subcutaneous area. Residual bone is seen in the lesion, and the boundary is unclear. Buccal and lingual bone cortex discontinuation is seen, and no obvious layered periosteum reaction is seen. Surrounding soft tissue is thickened. Dertrotheca sclerotin is close to the epidermis. The soft tissue on the top wall of the nasopharynx is slightly plump, symmetrical in structure and uniform in density. The CT value of the plain scan is about 44 Hu, slight enhancement is seen after enhancement, and the C+ was 57 Hu. There is no obvious destruction of skull base sclerotin. The mucosa of paranasal sinuses and nasopharynx is slightly thickened. Bilateral parotid gland and submandibular gland atrophy. No swollen lymph node shadow is seen in the neck (Fig. 3.14).

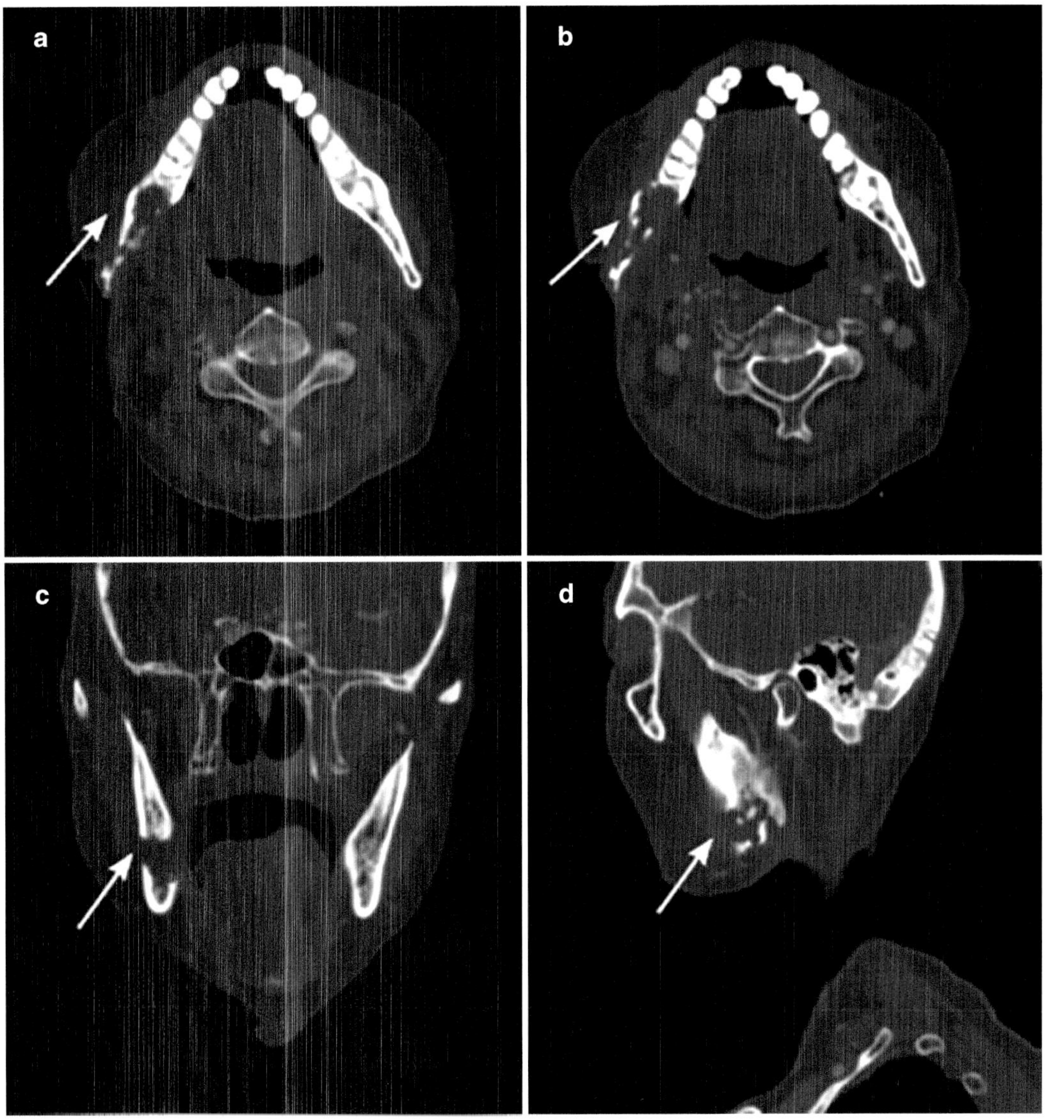

Fig. 3.14 (**a**) Cross section of CT Plain Scan: The sclerotin of the right mandible body is destroyed, the bone cortex is discontinuous, and no obvious layered periosteum reaction is seen. (**b**) Cross section of CT Enhanced Scan: No obvious enhanced soft tissue mass is seen. (**c**) Coronal view of CT enhanced scan: Bone cortex is discontinuous, and the periosteal reaction is not obvious. (**d**) Sagittal view of CT enhanced scan: Temporomandibular joint is in situ

[Primary diagnosis] osteoradionecrosis of the right mandible.

[Treatment] Under general anesthesia, "segmental resection of right mandible + fibula musculocutaneous flap transfer repair + tracheotomy" was performed; Incision was conducted 1 ~ 2 cm along the lower edge of the mandible and around the fistula, and the mandible was cut and flap was turned. The mandible was cut at 45 distal and B-shaped notch, respectively, and the tissues around the lesion were taken for frozen pathology examination during operation, indicating chronic inflammation of the skin and soft tissue of "right mandible 1 and 2," fibrous tissue proliferation. A free fibula musculocutaneous flap with vascular pedicle was prepared on the left side, the fibula with a length of about 13 cm was cut, shaped, and reconstructed, and the continuity and occluding relation of the mandible was restored. The artery and vein of the fibula were anastomosed with the branches of the superior thyroid artery and internal jugular vein, respectively, and the wound was washed, bleeding was tightly stopped, a negative pressure drainage tube was left, and the wound was sutured in layers and closed (Fig. 3.15).

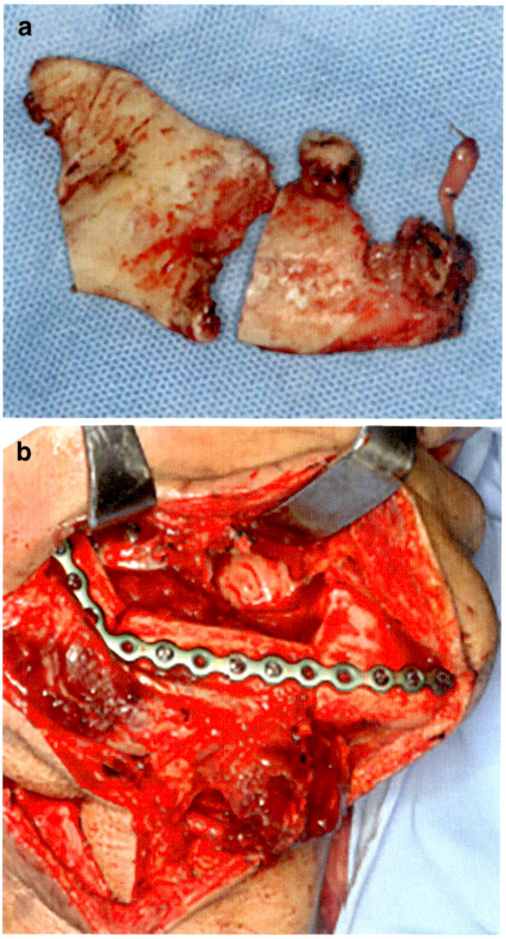

Fig. 3.15 (**a**) In-vitro dead bone. (**b**) Restoring of mandible continuity by reconstruction of fibula musculocutaneous flap

[Pathological examination] 3 pcs of jaw tissues were sent for pathological examination, grayish yellow. Wherein 1 pcs was with skin, the skin surface was broken and ulcerated. Microscopically, fibrous tissue and blood vessel proliferation between trabecular bone, inflammatory cell infiltration, and bone resorption lacunae were seen on the surface of local bone tissue (Fig. 3.16).

[Pathological diagnosis] radiation osteomyelitis of "right mandible," ICD code: K10.201.

[Follow-up visit] The patient recovered well after operation. In the follow-up visit after half a year, the reconstructed shape of mandible was satisfactory and the restoring of the left occluding relation was good.

3.3.3 Case 9

The patient, male, 53 years old. Seven years after radiotherapy for nasopharyngeal carcinoma, the left mandible was swollen, painful and purulent for a half year.

[Present medical history] Seven years ago, the patient received radiotherapy (bilateral) for nasopharyngeal carcinoma, and there was pus in the right posterior teeth area with limited mouth opening, which gradually worsened. Four years ago, the patient underwent "segmental resection of the right mandible + reconstruction and repair of fibular musculocutaneous flap" in our hospital. The operative region recovered well, and the patient had follow-up visits regularly. Six months ago, mouth opening was limited again, accompanied by pain and discomfort on the left face. Two months ago, the skin of the left face was ulcerated and purulent, and the skin fistula was basically healed after debridement in a local hospital. The patient went to the outpatient of our hospital for CT examination, indicating that: Sclerotin destruction of left mandible with swelling and enhancement of surrounding soft tissue. Maybe

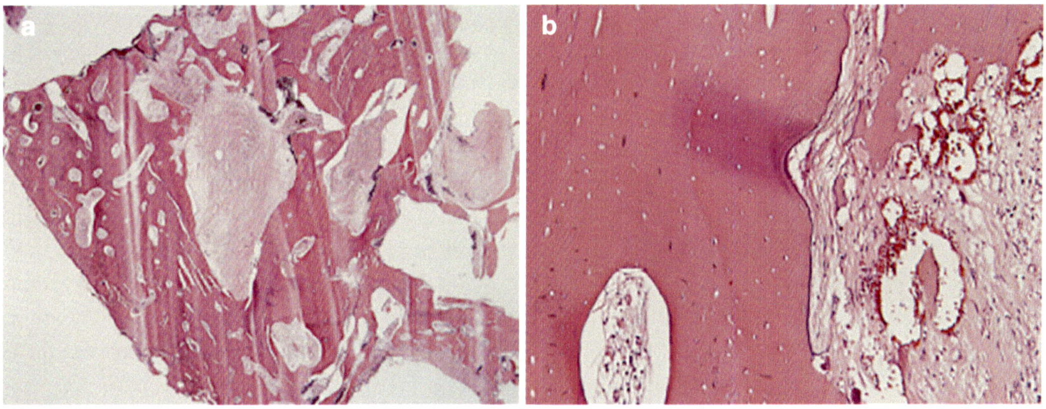

Fig. 3.16 (**a**) The original loose fat and vascular tissue in the bone marrow cavity was replaced by hyperplastic fibrous tissue (20×). (**b**) Fibrous tissue proliferation between bone tissues with abundant blood vessels and bone resorption lacunae were found on the surface of local bone tissues (200×)

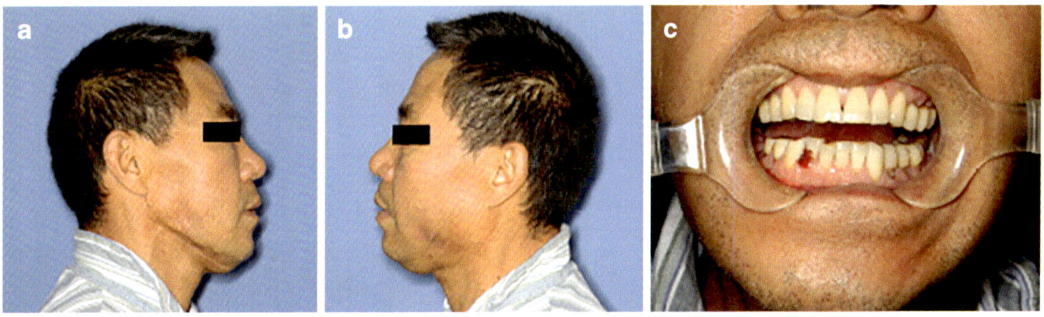

Fig. 3.17 (**a**) Postoperative observation after reconstruction of right mandible fibula. (**b**) A fistula is seen on the left face, which is basically healed. (**c**) Severe limitation of mouth opening

osteomyelitis with soft tissue infection and the possibility of tumor lesions were to be eliminated.

[Specialized examination] The maxillofacial region is developed in symmetry, no obvious deformity is seen, the skin texture of the right face is hard, and the skin fistula of the left cheek has been healed. The mouth opening is limited, and the mouth opening degree is about 1.5 cm. Fistula and pyorrhea are seen in the buccal gingiva 36 and 37, and no obvious abnormality is found in the mucosa in the rest of the mouth (Fig. 3.17). No obvious swollen lymph nodes are seen in bilateral submandibular regions and neck.

[Auxiliary examination]

1. Panoramic radiographs: The bone density of bilateral mandible dertrotheca is uneven and reduced, the bone cortex is still continuous, and no obvious periosteal reaction or soft tissue mass is seen (before the first operation, Fig. 3.18a). During the internal fixation of the right mandible, the bone density of the left mandible body is uneven and reduced, the boundary is blurred, the bone cortex is still continuous, no obvious periosteal reaction is seen, and no obvious soft tissue mass is seen (before this operation, Fig. 3.18b).
2. CT enhanced scan of the maxillofacial region indicates: After "right mandibular surgery," the transplanted bone and metal internal fixa-

tion shadow can be seen, and no obvious abnormal enhancement shadow is seen. The density of the bone marrow cavity in the body, corner and ascending ramus of the left man-

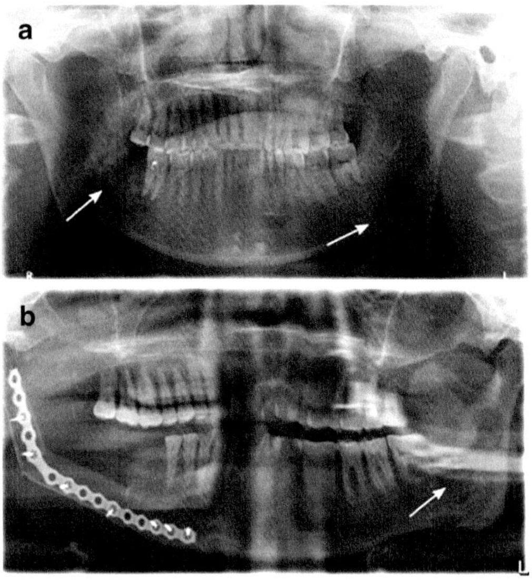

Fig. 3.18 (**a**) The bone density of the bilateral mandibular angle is uneven and reduced, the bone cortex is still continuous, and no obvious periosteal reaction or soft tissue mass is seen (before the first operation). (**b**) During the internal fixation of the right mandible, the bone density of the left mandible body is uneven and reduced, the boundary is blurred, the bone cortex is still continuous, no obvious periosteal reaction is seen, and no obvious soft tissue mass is seen (before this operation)

dible body is uneven, the bone cortex is rough and discontinuous, the soft tissues adjacent to the left masseter muscle, cheek and pterygomandibular space are swollen, and the boundary is unclear, with C− 67 Hu and C+ 127 Hu, enhanced posterior margin. The bone marrow density of the left maxilla is slightly high. Bilateral paranasal sinus mucosa thickened and enhanced. Several 10 mm * 11 mm lymph node shadows are seen under the mentum, obviously enhanced after enhancement (Fig. 3.19).

[Primary diagnosis] osteoradionecrosis of left mandible.

[Treatment] "Segmental mandibulectomy of left mandible + fibula musculocutaneous flap reconstruction + tracheotomy" was performed under general anesthesia. A trancervical incision was performed along the lower edge of the mandible and around the fistula. The mandible was osteotomized and skin flap was elevated to expose the mandible body and ascending ramus. The exposed bone from the mandibular angle of the left mandible to the ascending ramus was rough. Necrotic dead bone and abnormal secretion were seen in the medullary cavity of the bone, and edema and adhesion of the surrounding tissues were seen. The mandible was osteoto-

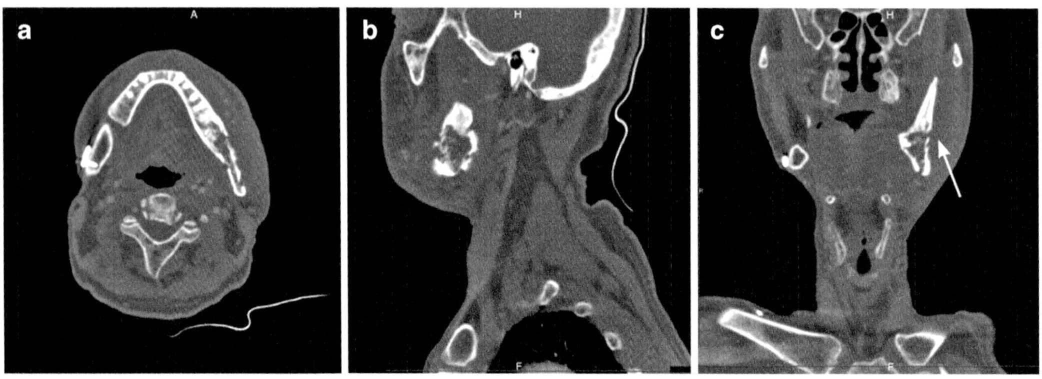

Fig. 3.19 (**a**) After the right mandible operation, bone graft and metal internal fixation can be seen, sclerotin destruction can be seen in the left mandibular angle, the boundary was unclear, the buccal bone cortex was rough, and the surrounding soft tissue was slightly swollen. (**b**, **c**) Sagittal view and coronal view: The density of bone marrow cavity in the body, corner and ascending ramus of the left mandible body was uneven, and the bone cortex was rough and discontinuous

mized at distal 36, and the mandible was completely removed from 36 to condyle. The left peroneal musculocutaneous flap was taken, and the peroneal artery and vein were anastomosed with the superior thyroid artery and external jugular vein, respectively. The fibula was shaped, and the continuity of the mandible and the occlusion was reestablished. The surgical wound was rinsed, bleeding was stopped completely, a negative pressure drainage tube was left, the suture was conducted in layers, and the wound was closed (Fig. 3.20).

[Pathological examination] A piece of bone tissue was sent for pathological examination; partial bone tissue was in grayish yellow and necrotic. Microscopically, dead bone tissue, bone cells disappear, bone lacunae are empty, inflam-

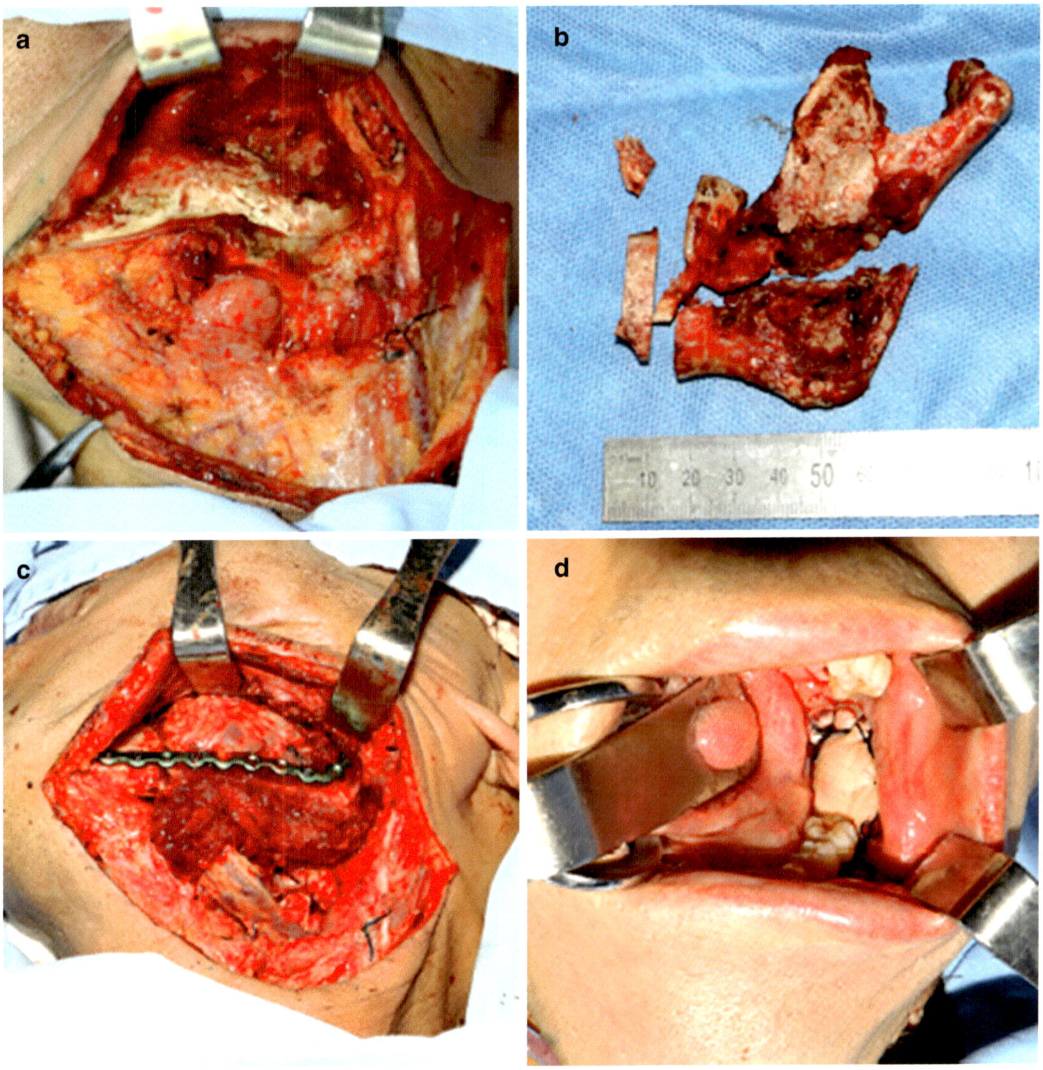

Fig. 3.20 (**a**) The body and ascending ramuses of the mandible were exposed, and dead bone formation and sclerotin destruction were seen in the mandibular angle area. (**b**) In-vitro dead bone. (**c**) Restoring of mandible continuity by reconstruction of fibula musculocutaneous flap. (**d**) Skin paddle was used to repair mucosa coloboma

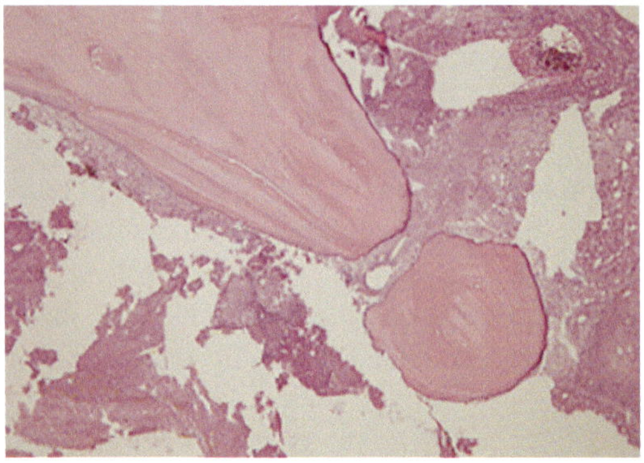

Fig. 3.21 The lamellar structure of bone tissue still existed, but the vitality was reduced, with bone lacuna lacunae, degeneration and necrosis around bone tissue and inflammatory cell infiltration (100×)

matory granulation tissue was around the dead bone, inflammatory cell infiltration, blood vessel proliferation and bleed was seen (Fig. 3.21).

[Pathological diagnosis] osteoradionecrosis of "mandible" ICD code: K10.201, with inflammation.

[Follow-up visit] The patient recovered well after the operation. In the follow-up visit after half a year, the reconstructed shape of the mandible was satisfactory and mouth opening and closing were normal.

3.4 Key Points of Diagnosis and Treatment

Regaud et al. put forward ORNJ for the first time in 1922. They defined ORNJ as a chronic disease and believed that ORNJ was a chronic disease caused by the loss of jaw tissue activity and blood supply disorder caused by radiation [2, 11–16]. In 1970, Meyer proposed that ORNJ was a special type of osteomyelitis [2]. Titterington named ORNJ as "radiation osteomyelitis" in 1971. In 1983, Marx, et al. defined ORNJ as "the bone cortex exposed in the irradiated area, with a diameter of more than 1 cm, lasting for at least 6 months, and having no tendency to heal" [3]. At present, although the definition of ORNJ has not been unified, most scholars agree that ORNJ is a sclerotin lesion based on inflammation and necrosis of jaw tissue with soft tissue injury in the irradiated area, and the course of disease cannot heal itself for more than 3 months [17–22]. At the same time, primary tumor recurrence, medication-related bone lesions and radiation-induced new tumors of jaw tissue are excluded.

Pathogenesis Up to now, the pathogenesis of radiation-induced osteonecrosis of the jaw has not been fully clarified. In 1970, Meyers put forward the theory of "radiotherapy, trauma and infection," assuming that the soft tissue trauma caused by radiotherapy created a channel for bacteria in the oral cavity to enter the jaws and the lack of resistance of the irradiated jaw eventually led to bone infection, being the theoretical basis for antibiotic treatment of radiation-induced osteonecrosis of the jaw. In 1983, Marx put forward the theory of "hypoxia-low cell-low blood vessel," arguing that the main pathological process of radiation-induced osteonecrosis of the jaw was jaw lesions caused by bone tissue metabolism and bone regeneration disorders, and hyperbaric oxygen (HBO) therapy based on this theory had been used as a conservative treatment for radiation-induced osteonecrosis of the jaw for a long time. However, the clinical efficacy of hyperbaric oxygen therapy for ORNJ has not been fully confirmed, and there are still many disputes. There is still no consensus on the effectiveness in different literature studies. In 2004, Delanian et al. put forward a new theory of radiation-induced fibrosis (Rif), arguing that radiotherapy caused damage to local tissues and endothelial cells, released a large number of oxygen free radicals, induced acute inflammatory reaction of vascular endothelium, excessive proliferation and abnormal differentiation of fibroblasts, and secreted a large number of extracellular matrix components. Excessive deposition of extracellular matrix swallowed the surrounding tissues, eventually leading to osteonecrosis of jaw. Based on this theory, Delanian et al. put forward an anti-fibrosis treatment scheme for ORNJ, providing a new direction for its conservative treatment.

Diagnosis At present, the clinical diagnosis of ORNJ is mainly based on the following aspects: ① History of radiotherapy; ② Clinically, there is sclerotin exposure accompanied by mucosal or skin injury; ③ Or, although there is no sclerotin exposure, there is sclerotin change or destruction on imaging (oral panoramic film, CT or MRI); ④ There is no local tumor recurrence. ⑤ Histopathology finds typical manifestations of osteoradionecrosis, such as severe bone destruction, blurred or broken lamellar bone structure, most of the bone cells disappeared, and dead bone formed. In addition, the diagnosis of this disease shall be differentiated from chronic pyogenic osteomyelitis, medication-related osteonecrosis of the jaw, cancer recurrence, radiation osteosarcoma, metastasis, jaw tuberculosis, etc.

Treatment The treatment of ORNJ mainly includes conservative treatment and operation treatment. Commonly used conservative treatment methods are: HBO therapy, drug therapy, ultrasound therapy and nutritional support therapy, etc. Previous studies have shown that 25% ~ 44% ORNJ patients can get certain curative effects by conservative treatment. However, the effects of conservative treatment are not exact, and the curative effects of patients with different total radiotherapy doses and different parts are also significantly different. When the total dose of radiotherapy reaches more than 60 Gy, 65% of ORNJ patients of conservative treatment have poor curative effects. However, conservative treatment has a good therapeutic effect on ORN of the maxilla. Therefore, for patients with severe ORNJ, direct operation treatment is recommended, rather than conservative treatment. Operation treatment is aimed at patients with ineffective conservative treatment or severely limited mouth opening, oral skin fistula, suffering from pain, and osteolysis and pathological fracture of the jaw can be observed by imaging examination. The methods of operation treatment include local tissue flap, free tissue flap or bone flap transplantation, reconstruction of titanium plate, etc., among which vascularized free bone flap transplantation is the most effective treatment method, and the donor site of bone tissue flap can come from ilium, fibula, radius, scapula, etc., among which fibula musculocutaneous flap is the most commonly used. However, the survival rate of free bone transplanted in the operative region is very low, especially in the diseased area of ORN, the blood supply of soft tissue is poor, the free bone usually cannot survive, and the incidence of complications is as high as 80%, so it is not recommended. For patients who are with large soft tissue coloboma and are not suitable for repairing with bone tissue flap, soft tissue flap repair is feasible, and pectoralis major musculocutaneous flap and anterolateral thigh perforator flap are preferred, followed by rectus abdominis flap and latissimus dorsi flap [16, 22, 23, 25, 26].

The operation treatment of ORNJ has made great progress in recent years. In accordance with the classification of "BS," the corresponding treatment strategy has been formulated in *Expert Consensus Statement on Diagnosis and Clinical Management of Osteoradionecrosis of Mandible*, and the experience treatment has entered the standard treatment stage [23]. For early ORNJ which mainly focuses on the alveolar process without involving the lower edge of mandible, scaling of mandibular osteomyelitis, removal of dead bone or marginal resection can be considered, and for more serious patients, segmental resection of diseased jaw with or without free vascularized bone transplantation is suggested. For ORNJ involving both sides, unilateral long fibula repair or bilateral fibula repair in stages can be selected. For "Frozen Neck" after local radiotherapy, digital techniques, such as preoperative Doppler ultrasound, CTA, MRA, etc., are used to evaluate the cervical vessels, select appropriate recipient vessels and match the diameter, reduce vascular crisis and improve the success rate. With the rapid development of digital surgery, computer-aided design and manufacturing (CAD-CAM), rapid prototyping technology, navigation technology and 3D printing technology, etc., have been gradually applied to the repair and reconstruction of ORNJ coloboma, greatly improving the accuracy of jaw reconstruction and condyle position, and restoring the occluding relation and oral physiological function of patients to the maximum extent [25].

Due to the obvious inflammation and fibrosis of local soft tissue in ORNJ patients, often accompanied by infection, there are often different degrees of infection, necrosis, titanium plate exposure and even skin flap or bone flap necrosis after vascularized bone tissue flap or soft tissue flap repair, and it is usually necessary to take local dressing change, debridement and titanium plate removal, etc. to promote wound healing. It has been reported that the failure rate of free tissue flap transplantation reached 9.8%, and the incidence of postoperative complications reached 39.7%. The most common complications were sinus tract formation (8.4%), titanium plate exposure (7.1%) and operative region infection (6.5%). In addition, the common postoperative complications of ORNJ include poor local wound healing, limited mouth opening, occlusal disorder, artery rupture in the operative region, vascular crisis and tissue flap necrosis, a lung infection caused by epiglottis insufficiency, embolism of heart, brain and lung, severe psychological trauma, etc. The medical staff shall fully understand how to prevent and reduce serious complications to the maximum extent, ensure patients' safety, and improve the clinical treatment effects of ORNJ.

With the development of regenerative medicine, scholars generally believe that adult bone marrow mesenchymal stem cells (BMSC) derived from bone marrow can be used for the regenerative treatment of ORNJ. Jose et al. used BMSC and hydroxyapatite/β-tricalcium phosphate complex to treat 3 cases of mandibular ORN, and achieved satisfactory results [31–33]. The research on tissue engineering repair of mandibular osteoradionecrosis by JunjiXu et al. on the constructed ORN pig model of the mandible has achieved remarkable results and successfully induced bone and blood vessel regeneration; Park et al. [34] used mesenchymal cells derived from tonsils in the ORNJ model of rats and observed the regeneration of jaw tissue. Although they are all case studies, they provide a new idea and research direction for the treatment of ORNJ.

References

1. Chronopoulos A, Zarra T, Ehrenfeld M, et al. Osteoradionecrosis of the jaws: definition, epidemiology, staging and clinical and radiological findings. A concise review [J]. Int Dent J. 2018;68(1):22–30.
2. He Y, Li X. Prevention and treatment of osteoradionecrosis of the jaws [J]. J Prev Treat Stomatol Dis. 2019;27(3):143–52.
3. Meyer I. Infectious diseases of the jaws [J]. J Oral Surg. 1970;28(1):17–26.
4. Marx RE. A new concept in the treatment of osteoradionecrosis [J]. J Oral Maxillofac Surg. 1983;41(6):351–7.
5. Ravi P, Vaishnavi D, Gnanam A, et al. The role of hyperbaric oxygen therapy in the prevention and management of radiation-induced complications of the head and neck – a systematic review of literature [J]. J Stomatol Oral Maxillofac Surg. 2017;118(6):359–62.
6. Delanian S, Lefaix JL. The radiation-induced fibroatrophic process: therapeutic perspective via the antioxidant pathway [J]. Radiother Oncol. 2004;73(2):119–31.
7. Han Y, He Y. Research progress of the etiology of osteoradionecrosis of the jaws [J]. Stomatology. 2020;40(4):362–5.
8. Delanian S, Depondt J, Lefaix JL. Major healing of refractory mandible osteoradionecrosis after treatment combining pentoxifylline and tocopherol: a phase II trial [J]. Head Neck. 2005;27(2):114–23.
9. Regaud C. Sur la nécrose des osattente par unprocessuscancéreux et traits par les radiations [J]. Compt Rend Soc Biol. 1922;87:427–9.
10. Wong JK, Wood RE, Mclean M. Conservative management of osteoradionecrosis [J]. Oral Surg Oral Med Oral Pathol Oral Radiol Endod. 1997;84(1):16–21.
11. Marx RE. Osteoradionecrosis: a new concept of its pathophysiology [J]. J Oral Maxillofac Surg. 1983;41(5):283–8.
12. Cheriex KC, Nijhuis TH, Mureau MA. Osteoradionecrosis of the jaws: a review of conservative and surgical treatment options [J]. J Reconstr Microsurg. 2013;29(2):69–75.
13. Kubota H, Miyawaki D, Mukumoto N, et al. Risk factors for osteoradionecrosis of the jaw in patients with head and neck squamous cell carcinoma [J]. Radiat Oncol. 2021;16(1):1.
14. Lajolo C, Gioco G, Rupe C, et al. Tooth extraction before radiotherapy is a risk factor for developing osteoradionecrosis of the jaws: a systematic review [J]. Oral Dis. 2020;27:1595.
15. Acharya S, Pai KM, Acharya S. Risk assessment for osteoradionecrosis of the jaws in patients with head and neck cancer [J]. Med Pharm Rep. 2020;93(2):195–9.
16. He Y, Li JS, Li XG, et al. Expert consensus on clinical diagnosis and treatment of osteoradionecrosis of mandible [J]. China J Oral Maxillofac Surg. 2017;15(5):445–56.

17. Lyons A, Osher J, Warner E, et al. Osteoradionecrosis – a review of current concepts in defining the extent of the disease and a new classification proposal [J]. Br J Oral Maxillofac Surg. 2014;52(5):392–5.
18. He Y, Liu Z, Tian Z, et al. Retrospective analysis of osteoradionecrosis of the mandible: proposing a novel clinical classification and staging system [J]. Int J Oral Maxillofac Surg. 2015;44(12):1547–57.
19. Chiao TB, Lee AJ. Role of pentoxifylline and vitamin E in attenuation of radiation-induced fibrosis [J]. Ann Pharmacother. 2005;39(3):516–22.
20. Lin MC, Shueng PW, Chang WK, et al. Consensus and clinical recommendations for nutritional intervention for head and neck cancer patients undergoing chemoradiotherapy in Taiwan [J]. Oral Oncol. 2018;81:16–21.
21. Alhambra Expósito MR, Herrera-Martínez AD, Manzano García G, et al. Early nutrition support therapy in patients with head-neck cancer [J]. Nutr Hosp. 2018;35(3):505–10.
22. He Y, Dai T, Sun J, et al. Clinical application of free vascularized bone flaps for reconstruction for osteoradionecrosis of the mandible [J]. Chin J Clin Oncol. 2015;42(16):827.
23. He Y, Liu Z, Dai T, et al. Proposed "BS" classification of osteoradionecrosis of the mandible and the corresponding therapeutic strategy [J]. Chin J Clin Oncol. 2015;42(16):817–26.
24. Bender-Heine A, Petrisor D, Wax MK. Advances in oromandibular reconstruction with three-dimensional printing [J]. Facial Plast Surg. 2020;36(6):703–10.
25. Allen RJ Jr, Nelson JA, Polanco TO, et al. Short-term outcomes following virtual surgery-assisted immediate dental implant placement in free fibula flaps for oncologic mandibular reconstruction [J]. Plast Reconstr Surg. 2020;146(6):768e–76e.
26. Dahake S, Kuthe A, Mawale M, et al. Development of customized implant and customized surgical osteotomy guide in ablative tumor surgery for accurate mandibular reconstruction [J]. Int J Med Robot. 2020;16(1):e2046.
27. Wehrhan F, Weber M, Neukam FW, et al. Fluorescence-guided bone resection: a histological analysis in medication-related osteonecrosis of the jaw [J]. J Craniomaxillofac Surg. 2019;47(10):1600–7.
28. Tomo S, Da Cruz TM, Figueira JA, et al. Fluorescence-guided surgical management of medication-related osteonecrosis of the jaws [J]. Photodiagn Photodyn Ther. 2020;32:102003.
29. Lee M, Chin RY, Eslick GD, et al. Outcomes of microvascular free flap reconstruction for mandibular osteoradionecrosis: a systematic review [J]. J Craniomaxillofac Surg. 2015;43(10):2026–33.
30. Hou JS, Zhang YD. Difficulties and prevention and management of serious complications in surgical treatment of osteoradionecrosis of jaw [J]. J Prev Treat Stomatol Dis. 2019;27(7):409–16.
31. Gundestrup AK, Lynggaard CD, Forner L, et al. Mesenchymal stem cell therapy for osteoradionecrosis of the mandible: a systematic review of preclinical and human studies [J]. Stem Cell Rev Rep. 2020;16(6):1208–21.
32. Mendonça JJ, Juiz-Lopez P. Regenerative facial reconstruction of terminal stage osteoradionecrosis and other advanced craniofacial diseases with adult cultured stem and progenitor cells [J]. Plast Reconstr Surg. 2010;126(5):1699–709.
33. Xu J, Zheng Z, Fang D, et al. Mesenchymal stromal cell-based treatment of jaw osteoradionecrosis in swine [J]. Cell Transplant. 2012;21(8):1679–86.
34. Park HS, Lee J, Kim JW, et al. Preventive effects of tonsil-derived mesenchymal stem cells on osteoradionecrosis in a rat model [J]. Head Neck. 2018;40(3):526–35.

Medication-Related Osteonecrosis of Jaw

4

Yue He, Hui Shan Ong, Zhen Tian, Lin Zhu, and Hang Chen

4.1 Introduction

Medication-related osteonecrosis of jaws (MRONJ) is a kind of bone tissue lesion caused by bisphosphonates, RANK-L inhibitors, antiangiogenic drugs or some hormonal drugs, which is different from radiation-induced osteonecrosis of jaws. Bisphosphonate-related osteonecrosis of jaws (BRONJ) was first reported in 2003. Recently, it was found that some other anti-angiogenesis and anti-bone resorption drugs can also cause osteonecrosis of the jaw. Therefore, in 2014, the American Association of Oral and Maxillofacial Surgeons suggested renaming it as "medication-related osteonecrosis of jaws," and it has been used ever since. MRONJ is essentially a jaw metabolic disorder disease, and its pathogenesis and treatment are still in the stage of exploration and discussion [1–7]. The ultimate goal of conservative or surgical intervention is to stabilize the disease and prevent its progress.

Y. He (✉) · H. S. Ong · Z. Tian · H. Chen
Department of Oral Maxillofacial-Head & Neck Oncology, Shanghai Ninth People's Hospital, Shanghai Jiao Tong University School of Medicine, Shanghai, China

L. Zhu
Department of Radiology, Ninth People's Hospital Affiliated to Shanghai Jiao Tong University, Shanghai, China

4.2 Medication-Related Osteonecrosis of Maxilla

4.2.1 Case 10

The patient, male, 81 years old. The swelling and pus in the upper anterior teeth area lasted for 8 months, and the tooth extraction wound did not heal for more than 3 months.

[Present medical history] The patient underwent operation treatment for prostate cancer 4 years ago and began to use bisphosphonates (the details were unknown), ethinyl estradiol tablets (0.05 mg/time, three times/day) and spironolactone tablets (20 mg/day) after the operation. Eight months ago, the anterior teeth were repeatedly swollen, painful and purulent. The Periodontal Department of our hospital gave basic periodontal treatment, and the effect was not good. The patient was recommended to transfer to oral surgery to extract the affected teeth. After tooth extraction, the wound did not heal, and the pain symptoms were not obviously relieved. After anti-inflammatory drug treatment, the symptoms of swelling and pain were slightly relieved, the symptoms were repeated, and tooth extraction caused purulent exudation.

[Specialized examination] The face is basically symmetrical from left to right, the proportion of upper, middle and lower 1/3 is coordinated, the

Y. He (ed.), *Inflammatory and Neoplastic Diseases of Craniofacial Bones*, https://doi.org/10.1007/978-981-97-4155-7_4

mouth opening degree and mouth opening type are normal, the dentition is defective, 11 ~ 12, 17, 21, 27, 28, 36 ~ 38 and 44 ~ 46 are missing, and the gingiva and mucosa around the vestibular groove in the upper anterior teeth area are swollen and ulcerated, the tooth extraction wound from 12 to 21 does not heal, with purulent secretion and tenderness (+), and necrotic bone tissue is exposed in the wound (Fig. 4.1). The tongue is centered, the tongue moves freely, the tip has no obvious numbness and other sensory abnormalities, the skin on both sides of the face and submandibular region is normal, and no abnormal swollen lymph nodes are found in the submandibular region and neck.

[Auxiliary examination]

1. Panoramic radiographs: The bone density of the maxilla is not even, with no obvious bone destruction, and no periosteal reaction and soft tissue mass (Fig. 4.2).

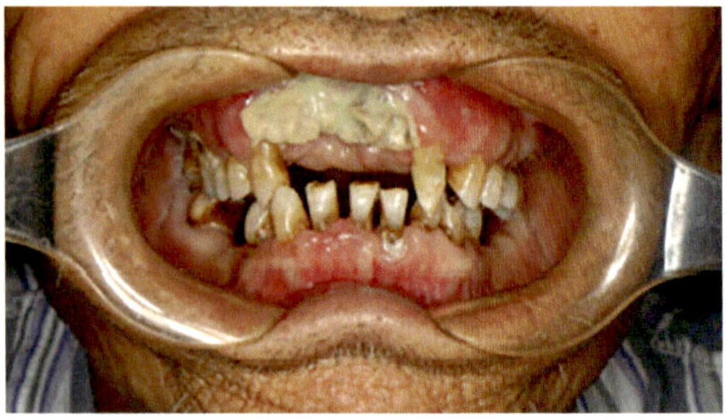

Fig. 4.1 The dead bone in the upper anterior teeth area is exposed, with purulent secretion on the surface (preoperative)

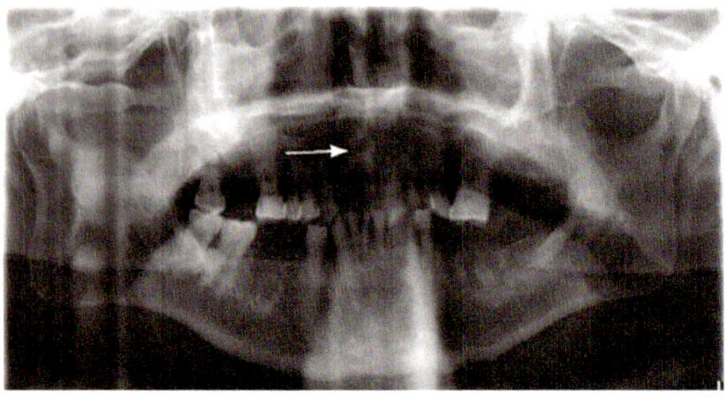

Fig. 4.2 The preoperative radioimages showed that the bone density of the premaxilla teeth area is none homogenous with no obvious bony destruction, no periosteal reaction and no soft tissue mass occupied within the bone. The cortical bone is visible

2. CT enhanced scan of the maxillofacial region: Bone density of maxilla is uneven, with patchy low-density foci, local bone destruction, swelling, thickening and uneven density of soft tissues adjacent to the nose and upper gingiva, uneven enhancement after enhancement, and no abnormal swollen lymph nodes are found in neck (Fig. 4.3).

[Primary diagnosis] medication-related osteonecrosis of maxilla.

[Treatment] "Maxilla lesion debridement" was performed under general anesthesia. Incision of gingiva was performed along the 14 ~ 26 distal gingival margin, the flap was turned, the lesion scope was exposed, gray sclerotin was seen without obvious boundary with normal bone, osteotome was used to remove necrotic bone, grinding head was used to fresh the wound, and the mucosa of the place where pyorrhea persists was removed. Intraoperative frozen pathological examination suggested that most of the "maxilla" sent for pathological examination was necrotic bone tissue, and chronic mucosa and soft tissue inflammation were seen locally. The wound was thoroughly irrigated, bleeding was thoroughly stopped, and iodoform gauze was used in the wound area for suture.

[Pathological examination] A grayish-yellow bone tissue with surface bone necrosis was sent for pathological examination. Microscopically, dead bone tissue was seen, showing that bone cells disappeared, bone lacunae were empty, and there was amorphous necrosis between trabeculae (Fig. 4.4).

[Pathological diagnosis] Medication-related osteonecrosis of "maxilla."

[Follow-up visit] The patient recovered well after the operation. In the reexamination in half a year, the maxillary anterior teeth recovered well, and there was no swelling and exudation of mucosa.

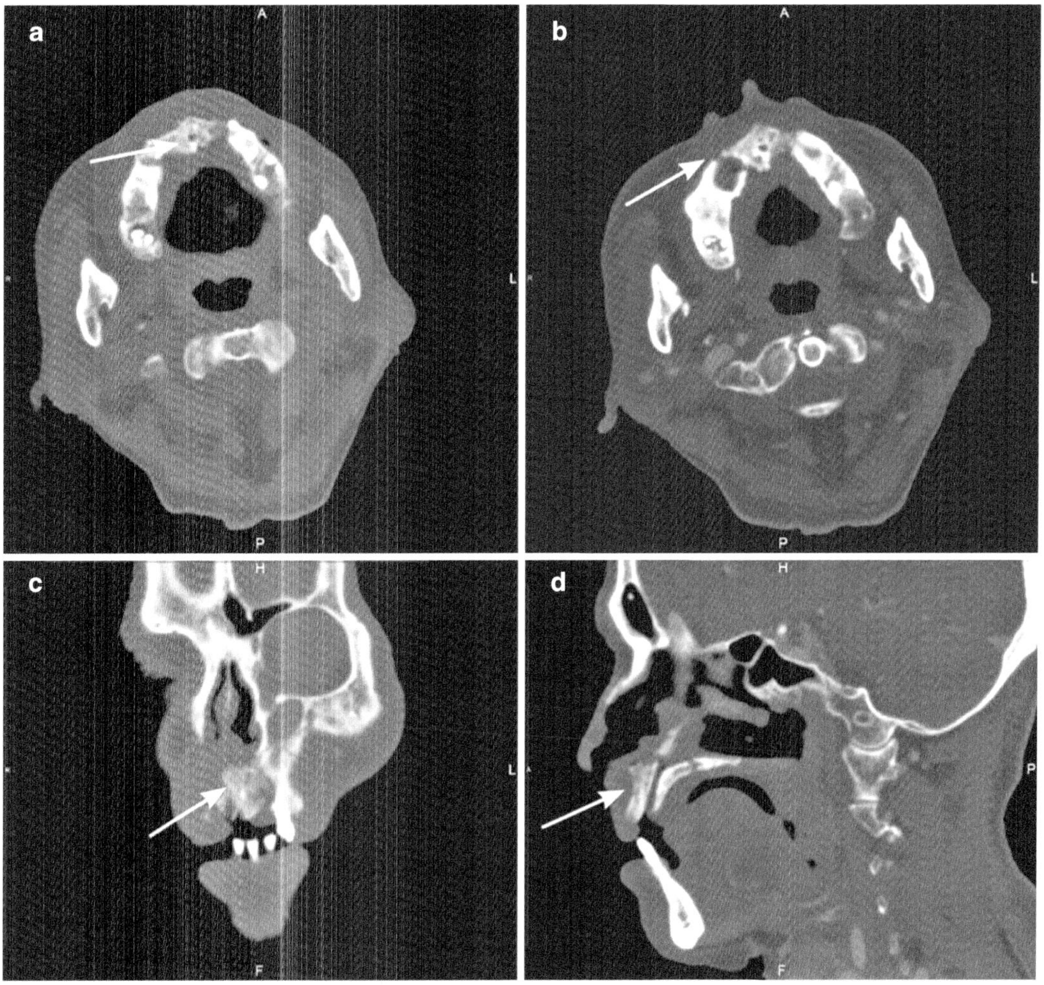

Fig. 4.3 (**a**) Cross section of CT Plain Scan: Maxilla bone destruction and uneven bone density. (**b**) Cross section of CT Enhanced Scan: No obvious enhanced soft tissue mass was seen. (**c**) Coronal view of CT enhanced scan: Left maxillary sinus and orbit were not involved. (**d**) Sagittal view of CT enhanced scan: The soft tissue of the upper gingiva was swollen and thickened with enhancement, and no abnormal swollen lymph nodes were found in the neck

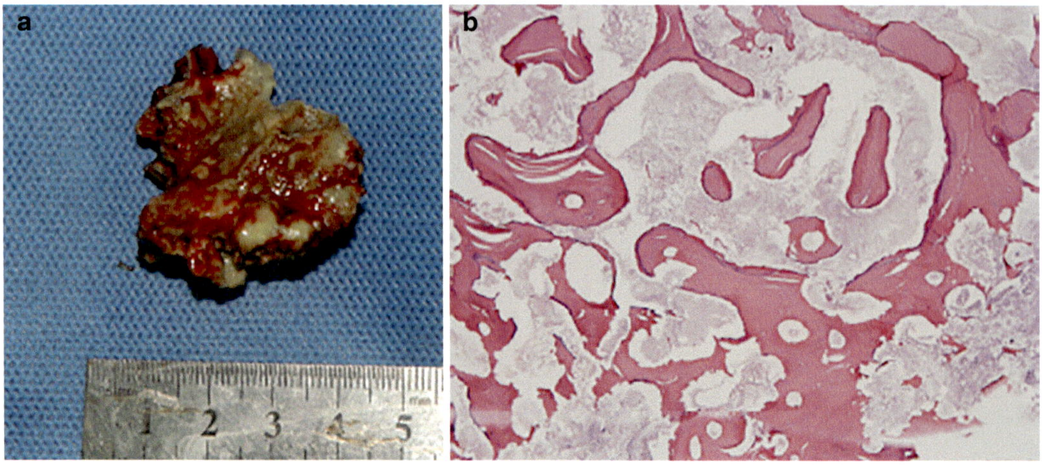

Fig. 4.4 (**a**) In-vitro dead bone. (**b**) The dead bone tissue was sent for pathological examination, with necrosis and fracture, empty bone lacunae, and absorption lacunae on the bone surface (40×)

4.3 Medication-Related Osteonecrosis of the Mandible

4.3.1 Case 11

The patient, female, aged 58, The right mandible was painful for 3 months.

[Present medical history] The patient felt pain and discomfort in the right mandible 3 months ago and went to the outpatient department of our hospital for CT examination, suggesting that local sclerotin discontinuity of the right mandible with abnormal density may be chronic osteomyelitis. Questioning the medical history, the patient suffered from lung cancer 2 years ago and has been undergoing VEGFR targeted therapy yet; zoledronic acid has been injected every month because of bone metastasis, and injection of zoledronic acid has been stopped 1 year ago.

[Specialized examination] Facial symmetry: there is no tenderness or snapping on bilateral temporomandibular joints. The degree and type of mouth opening are normal. Oral permanent dentition and oral hygiene are average. 46 is missing, 47 has lingual mucosa coloboma, dead bone is exposed, there is a small amount of pyorrhea, and there is tenderness (+) (Fig. 4.5a). The protruded tongue is in the middle, moves freely, and tastes normal.

[Auxiliary examination]

1. Panoramic radiographs: The density of medullary cavity in the right mandibular angle, r ascending ramus and condyle is uneven, the local bone cortex is discontinuous, and no obvious periosteal reaction and soft tissue mass are found (Fig. 4.5b).
2. CT enhanced scan of the maxillofacial region: The density of medullary cavity in the right mandibular angle, ascending ramus and condyle are uneven, and the local bone cortex is discontinuous. The right masseter muscle is slightly thickened. No obvious soft tissue mass shadow is found. No obvious swollen lymph node shadow is seen in the neck (Fig. 4.6).

[Primary diagnosis] Medication-related osteonecrosis of the jaw of the right mandible.

[Treatment] "Sequestretomy of right maxilla and mandible dead bone + debridement" was performed under general anesthesia. During the operation, the gray-white dead bone around 47 was exposed, and the mucosa was slightly red.

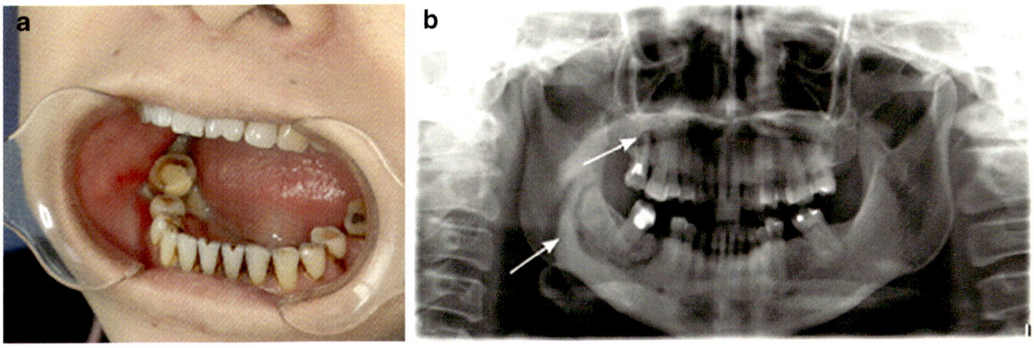

Fig. 4.5 (**a**) Gingiva coloboma surrounding 47, dead bone exposure and a small amount of pyorrhea on the surface. (**b**) The density of medullary cavity in the right mandibular angle, ascending ramus and condyle was uneven, the local bone cortex was discontinuous, and the dead bone was separated

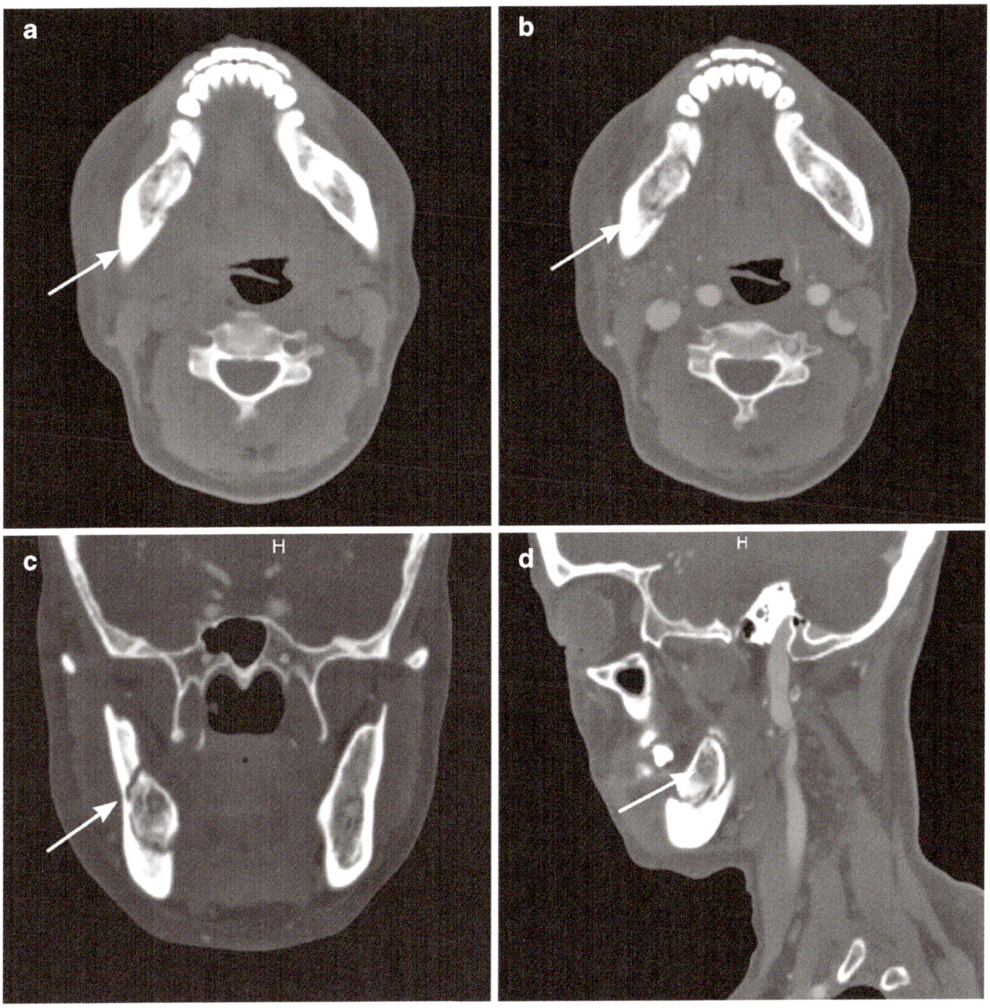

Fig. 4.6 (**a**) Cross section of CT Plain Scan: The bone destruction of the right mandible, and the bone density was uneven, showing ground-glass changes. (**b**) Cross section of CT Enhanced Scan: No obvious enhanced soft tissue mass was seen. (**c**) Coronal view of CT enhanced scan: Discontinuous bone cortex. (**d**) Sagittal view of CT enhanced scan: Formation of dead bone

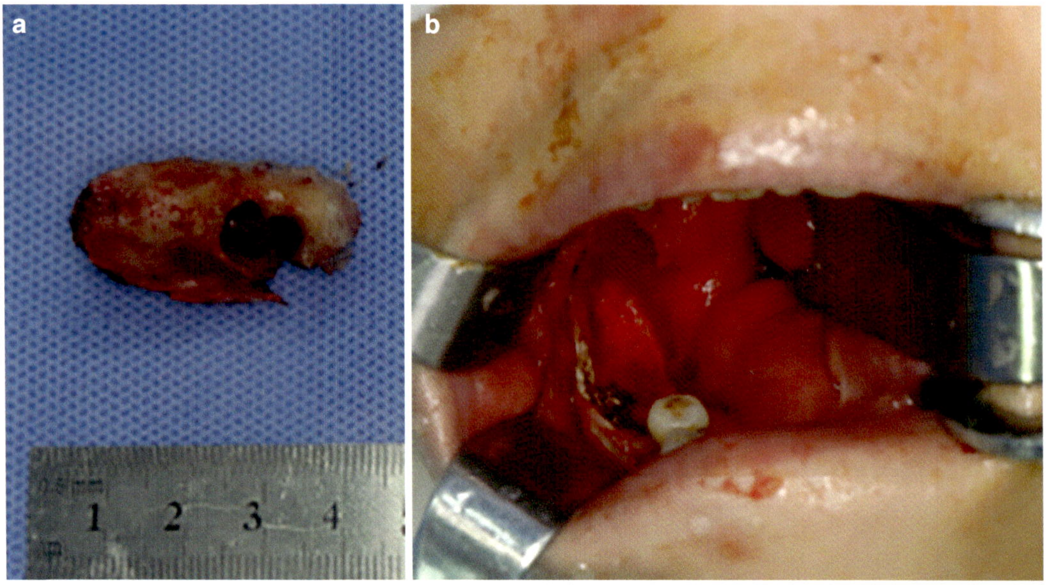

Fig. 4.7 (**a**) In-vitro dead bone. (**b**) Dead bones were separated during the operation, and the boundary was clear. After the dead bones were removed, fresh and bloody exudation was seen on the bone surface, repaired by the dynamic system

After 47 was removed, the flap was turned over, and a clear demarcation line could be seen between the dead bone and the normal jaw. Free dead bone was completely removed, and a little inflammatory proliferation tissue was seen in the wound cavity, completely scraped off and sent for frozen section pathology. The results suggested that the inflammatory fibrous tissue and a small amount of bone tissue of the "right mandible" were sent for pathological examination. Part of the mandible was removed until a fresh bleeding wound. In the same way, 16 and 17 were removed, the dead bone around the roots was removed, and the dynamic system ground to fresh wounds. The wound was thoroughly irrigated, bleeding was thoroughly stopped, iodoform gauze on the right mandible was packed, apposition suture was conducted for the mucosa, the wound was closed, and the wound on the upper maxilla operative region was closed (Fig. 4.7).

[Pathological examination] A pile of grayish-yellow bone tissue of the right maxilla lesion was sent for biopsy, 1.5 cm * 1 cm * 0.8 cm in size. A pile of grayish-yellow bone tissue of the right mandible lesion was sent for biopsy, partially necrotic, 4 cm * 2.5 cm * 2 cm in size. Microscopically, the bone edge was irregular, with wormlike depression, the bone lacuna was empty, there were no bone cells in, blood vessels and fibrous tissue between trabeculae of bone proliferated, and inflammatory cells infiltrated (Fig. 4.8).

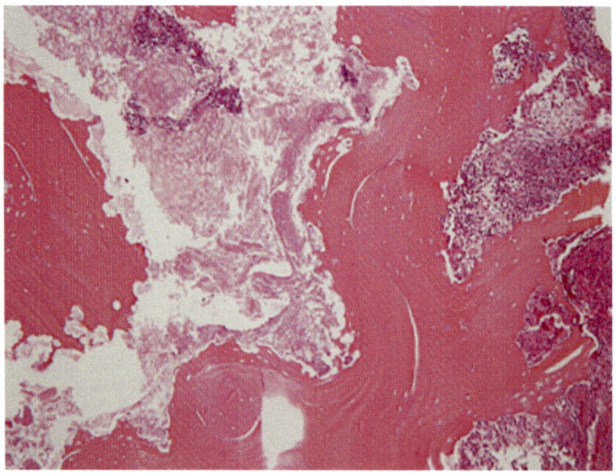

Fig. 4.8 Large dead bone tissue was sent for pathologic examination, the bone margin was moth-eaten depression, and chronic suppurative inflammation was found in the bone marrow cavity (100×)

[Pathological diagnosis] medication-related osteonecrosis of "right maxilla and mandible."

[Follow-up visit] The patient recovered well after the operation, the operative region recovered well, and the mucosa had no redness, swelling or exudation after a half year.

4.3.2 Case 12

The patient, female, 68 years old. The left lower posterior teeth area was painful and purulent for 4 months.

[Present medical history] Four months ago, the patient had spontaneous pain in the left lower posterior teeth area without obvious inducement, and there were no symptoms of cold and hot stimulation pain and nocturnal pain. The symptoms were not significantly improved when the left lower residual crown was removed at a local dental clinic. Half a month ago, the patient sought a doctor in a superior hospital and had a CT examination of the jaw, suggesting that there was an abnormal signal of the left mandible, maybe metastasis. After a local biopsy, inflammatory tissue was revealed, and no cancer cells were found (no pathological report was found). After a puncture, the sinus tract appeared in the left submandibular region, and there was repeated pus, so local radiotherapy was performed 13 times, and the symptoms of local pain and pus did not improve significantly. The outpatient department of our hospital inquired about the medical history. Four years ago, the patient took gefitinib [1 tablet per day] for a total of 11 months because of "right upper lung cancer," and then changed the drug to Osimertinib [1 tablet per day] and started zoledronic acid injection 4 years ago, once a month, and stopped 4 months ago.

[Specialized examination] The facial appearance is symmetrical. A sinus tract with an area of about 1.0 cm^2 can be seen in the left mandible body. The local skin is crusted, tender (+), slightly red and swollen, and a little inflammatory secretion flows out when pressed. The left lower lip is numb on the cheek. The mouth opening is normal, the alveolar bone in the left lower posterior teeth area is exposed, there are a lot of necrotic substances in the alveolar fossa, the oral odor is serious, and there is local tenderness (+) (Fig. 4.9). There are many residual roots and crowns in the mouth, with fracturing and coloboma. Tongue extension and movement are normal, and there is no obvious numbness. Swollen lymph nodes can be palpated in the left submandibular region, with good mobility, no obvious adhesion with surrounding tissues or tenderness or seen (−).

[Auxiliary examination]

1. Panoramic radiographs: The bone density of the left mandible body is unevenly increased, the bone cortex is discontinuous, and no obvi-

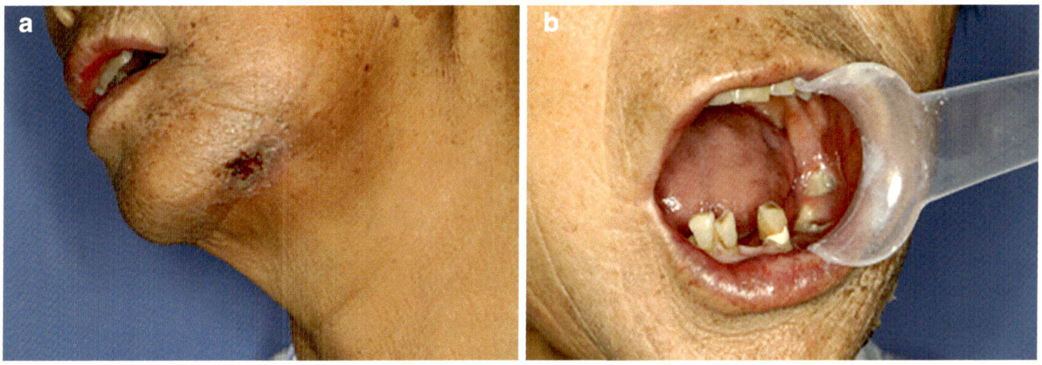

Fig. 4.9 (**a**) Left submandibular region fistula with scab. (**b**) The mouth opening was normal, and the dead bone in the left lower posterior teeth area was exposed

ous periosteal reaction and soft tissue mass are found (Fig. 4.10).
2. CT plain scan of the maxillofacial region: On the left mandible body, there are localized sclerotin swelling changes, uneven density, local periosteal reaction, thickening of surrounding soft tissue and loss of corresponding dentition. No abnormal enlarged lymph nodes are seen in the neck (Fig. 4.11).

[Primary diagnosis] medication-related osteonecrosis of the jaw of the lower left mandible.

[Treatment] "segmental resection of left mandible" was performed under general anesthesia: Incision was conducted 1 ~ 2 cm along the lower edge of the mandible, flapling, exposing the anterolateral wall of maxilla. The mandible was resected from the middle of the mandible to the left mandibular angle, and the necrotic gingiva and skin tissue were resected and sent to the frozen pathological examination. Chronic inflammation of skin in "left submandibular region," local surface ulcer formation. The wound was rinsed, bleeding was stopped completely, the anterior abdomen of genioglossus muscle and digastric muscle were suspended on the broken end of the mandible, and the wound area in layers was closed (Fig. 4.12).

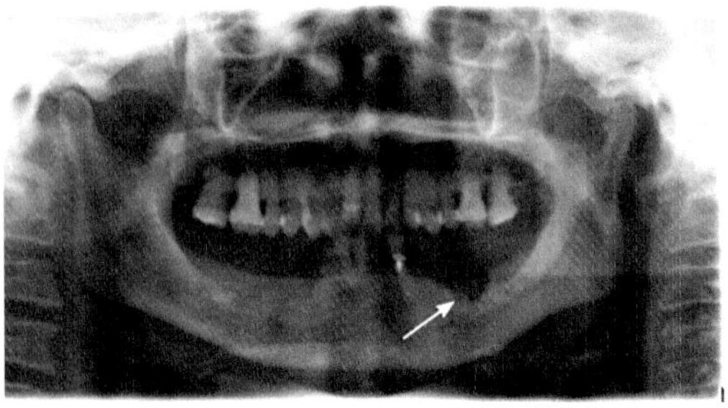

Fig. 4.10 The bone density of the left mandible body was uneven and increased, the bone cortex was not continuous, and no obvious periosteal reaction or soft tissue mass was seen (before the operation)

[Pathological diagnosis] A piece of bone tissue was sent for pathological diagnosis, 7 cm * 3 cm * 2 cm, grayish yellow. Microscopically, fibrous tissue hyperplasia, inflammatory cell infiltration, empty bone lacuna, lack of osteoblasts around, and irregular bone edge were seen in the bone marrow cavity (Fig. 4.13).

[Pathological diagnosis] Chronic osteomyelitis of the "left mandible" with dead bone formation, combined with medical history, complying with medication-related osteonecrosis of jaws.

[Follow-up visit] The patient recovered well after operation, the operative region recovered well, the mucosa had no redness, swelling or exudation after a half year. The mandible is slightly left, and the occluding relation of the right posterior teeth was OK.

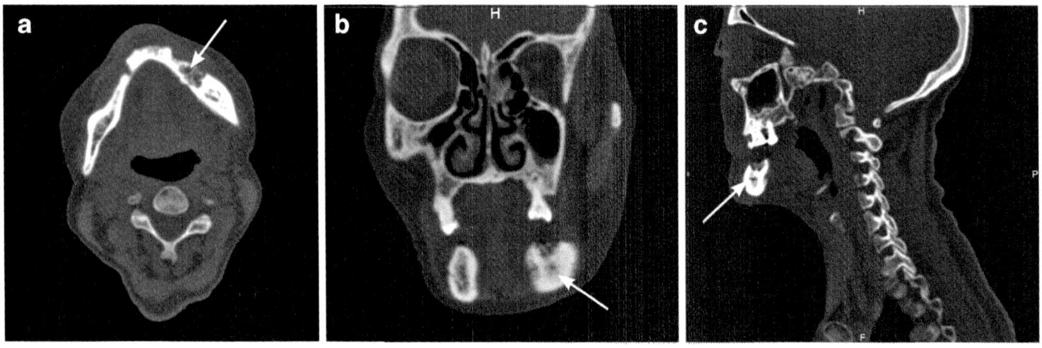

Fig. 4.11 (**a**) Cross section of CT Plain Scan: The left mandible body showed localized sclerotin swelling, uneven density and ground glass-like changes. (**b**) Coronary view of CT plain scan: Periosteal reaction can be seen locally. (**c**) Sagittal view of CT plain scan: The bone cortex was discontinuous, and no abnormal swollen lymph nodes were found in the neck

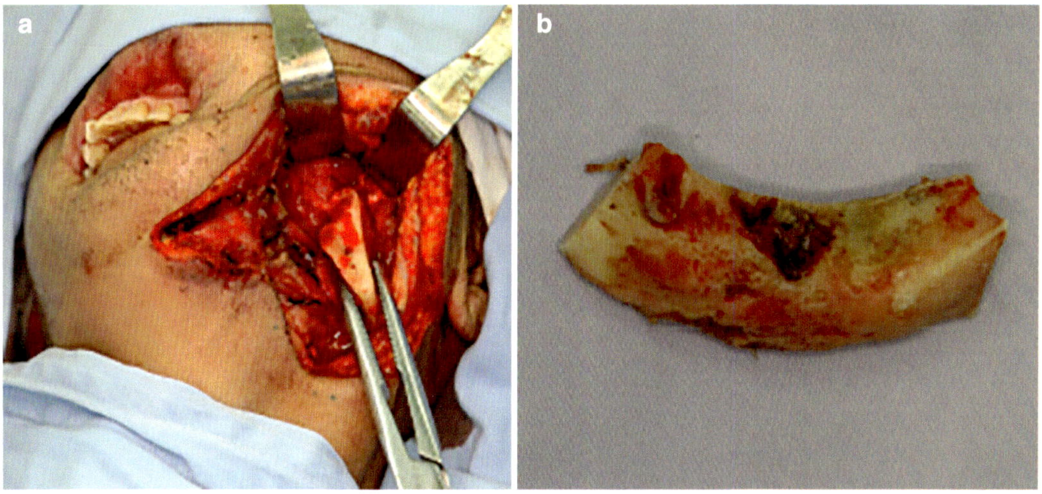

Fig. 4.12 (**a**) The mandible was amputated, and fresh blood oozed from the broken end. (**b**) In-vitro necrosis

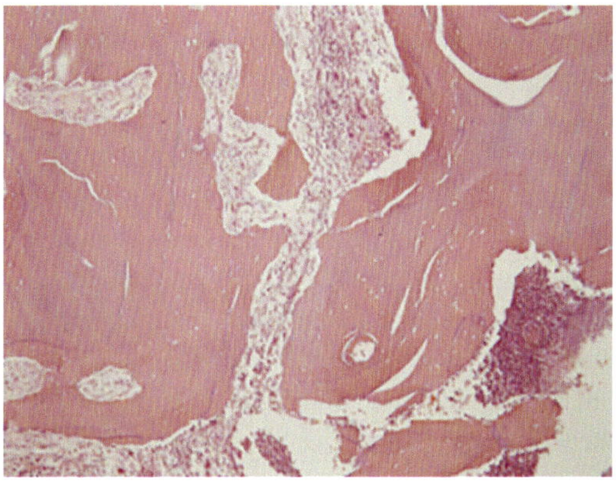

Fig. 4.13 The lamellar structure of bone tissue was unclear, and there were no bone cells in the empty bone lacuna, being dead bone tissue, with fibrous tissue hyperplasia in the bone marrow cavity and chronic suppurative inflammation (100×) locally

4.3.3 Case 13

The patient, female, 62 years old. Pain and pus in the right mandible for more than 1 year.

[Present medical history] Six years ago, the patient underwent chemotherapy in another hospital for "lung adenocarcinoma with bone metastasis" and then underwent "lumbar bone cement surgery/" She injected zoledronate sodium once a month until she stopped taking the drug 4 months ago. She continued to take Iressa once a day 5 years ago. More than a year ago, she developed pain, discomfort and pus in the right lower posterior teeth area and was given anti-inflammatory symptomatic treatment, having no obvious effect. Eight months ago, she underwent "left lower back tooth extraction + dead bone removal" in our hospital. The wound was not healed, there was repeated pus, and there was a fistula in the facial skin.

[Past history] History of diabetes for more than 10 years.

[Specialized examination] Maxillofacial development is symmetrical and there is no obvious deformity. The skin on the right cheek is locally red and swollen, ulcerated with pus, and the palpation is mild. The mouth opening degree is about 2 fingers, and the oral hygiene is poor. 12 ~ 16 porcelain crowns are continuous, 25 crown is residual, and 44 is missing. In the 44 missing area, the gingiva is red and swollen, ulcerated and purulent, and the local pain is obvious. The buccal alveolar bone is destroyed, and a fistula is formed between the buccal mucosa and the mouth, with more local exudate (Fig. 4.14). The secretion of the three salivary glands in the mouth is normal, and there is no abnormal swelling.

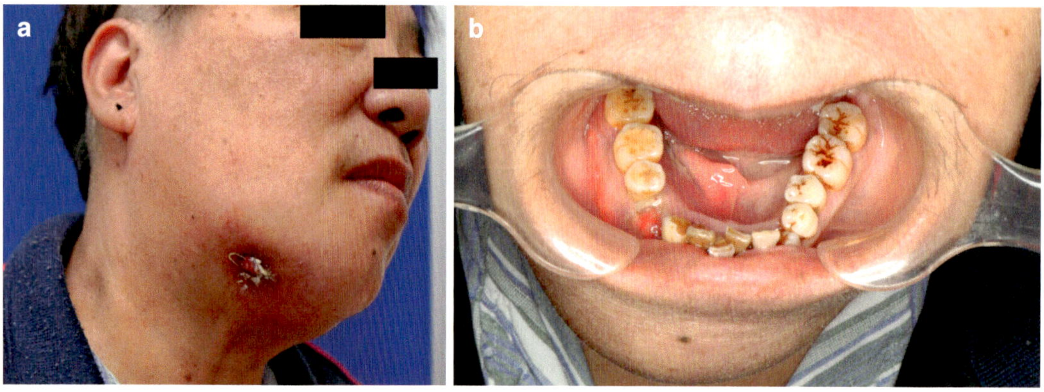

Fig. 4.14 (**a**) Skin fistula of right submandibular region (**b**) The degree and type of mouth opening are normal. Gingival granuloma proliferation and pyorrhea in the right lower premolar area

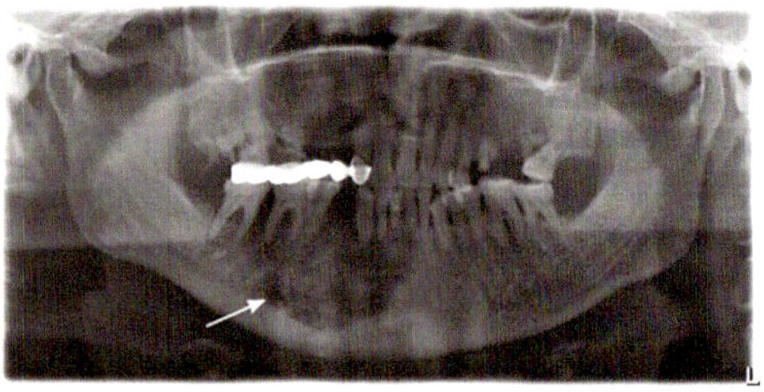

Fig. 4.15 The density of bone marrow in the chin and the body of the right mandible is unevenly increased, the continuity of local bone cortex is poor, the periosteal reaction is not obvious, and the surrounding soft tissue is swollen

[Auxiliary examination]

1. Panoramic radiographs: The density of bone marrow in the chin and the body of the right mandible is unevenly increased, the continuity of local bone cortex is poor, the periosteal reaction is not obvious, and the surrounding soft tissue is swollen (Fig. 4.15).
2. CT enhanced scan of the maxillofacial region: The density of bone marrow in the chin and the body of the right mandible is unevenly increased, the labial bone cortex is continuously interrupted, the periosteal reaction is observed, and the surrounding soft tissues are swollen, enhanced after enhancement, and lymph nodes with short diameter of 1.0 ~ 1.1 cm are seen in areas Ib and II of the right neck. T the structure of the lymphatic portal is visible (Fig. 4.16).

[Primary diagnosis] Medication-related osteonecrosis of the jaw of the lower right mandible.

[Treatment] Under general anesthesia, "segmental resection of lower mandible + fibula musculocutaneous flap transfer repair + tracheotomy" was performed. The broken skin in the right submandibular region was completed, cut, and sent for intraoperative frozen pathology. Pathological examination indicated that "right face" has local multifocal tissue infiltration, xanthoma to be discharged, chronic suppurative inflammation of skin and local granulation tissue formation. At present, there is insufficient evidence of metastatic malignant tumor (−). An incision in the submandibular region was made to cut open and turn the flap over. The dynamic system cut segment diseased mandibles of 34 ~ 47. It was observed that both sides of the broken ends had obvious bleeding and the blood supply was good. The left fibula musculocutaneous flap was taken, and the fibula was about 10 cm long. It was shaped to restore the continuity of mandible. The occluding relation of the left posterior teeth recovered well, and the blood vessels were anastomosed with the facial artery and vein, respectively. The wound was rinsed, bleeding was stopped completely, the negative pressure drainage tube was reserved, a suture was conducted in layers, and the wound was closed (Fig. 4.17).

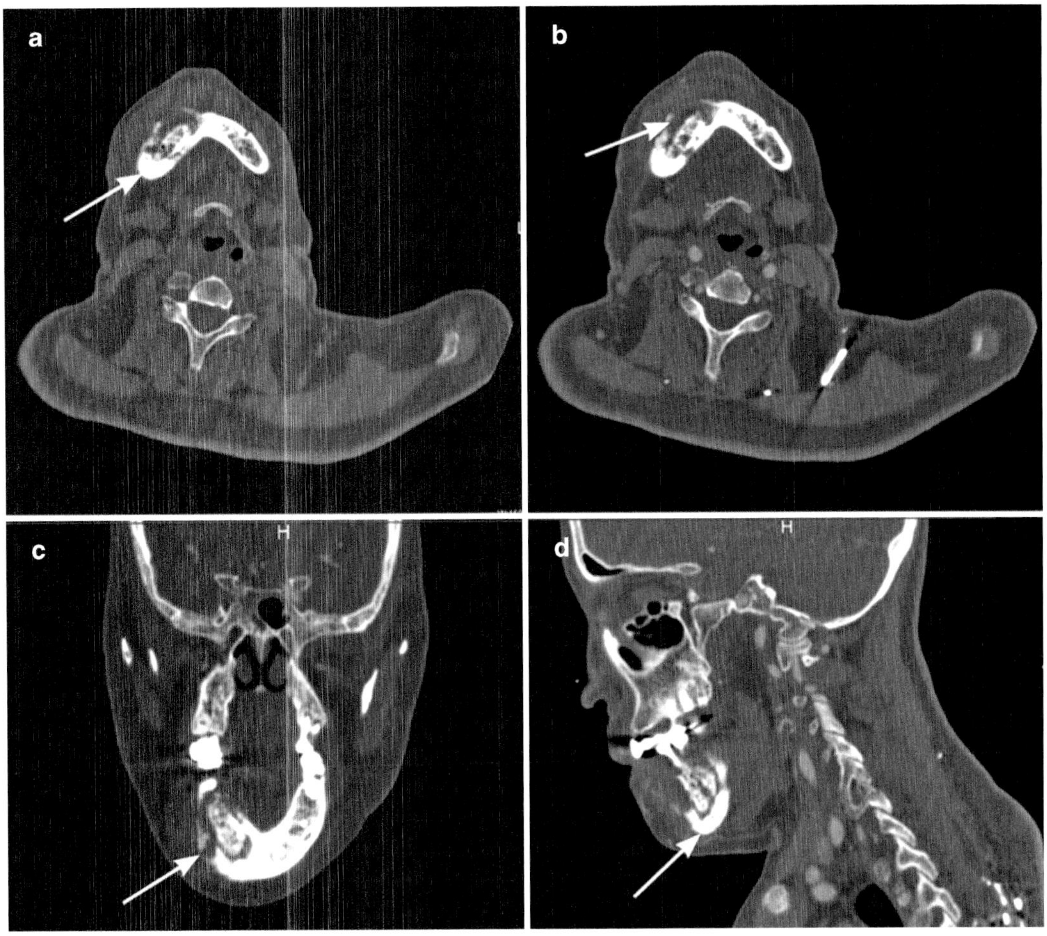

Fig. 4.16 (**a**) Cross section of CT Plain Scan: Right mandible body bone destruction and uneven bone density. (**b**) Cross section of CT Enhanced Scan: No obvious enhanced soft tissue mass was seen. (**c**) Coronal view of CT enhanced scan: Discontinuous bone cortex. (**d**) Sagittal view of CT enhanced scan: Lower alveolar bone is involved

[Pathological examination] The part sent for pathological examination was mandible tissue. The surface was necrotic, grayish yellow and grayish black. Microscopically, fibrous tissue hyperplasia, fibroblast and capillary hyperplasia were found in the bone marrow cavity, accompanied by different degrees of infiltration of lymphocytes, plasma cells and neutrophils. Dead bone tissue was seen locally, with bone cells disappearing, bone lacunae empty, osteoblasts lacking around the trabecular bone, and inflammatory granulation tissue forming around the dead bone (Fig. 4.18).

[Pathological diagnosis] Medication-related osteonecrosis of "mandible."

[Follow-up visit] The patient recovered well after the operation, the operative region recovered well, and the mucosa had no redness, swelling or exudation after a half year. The appearance of the mandible recovered well, and the occluding relation of the left posterior teeth was good.

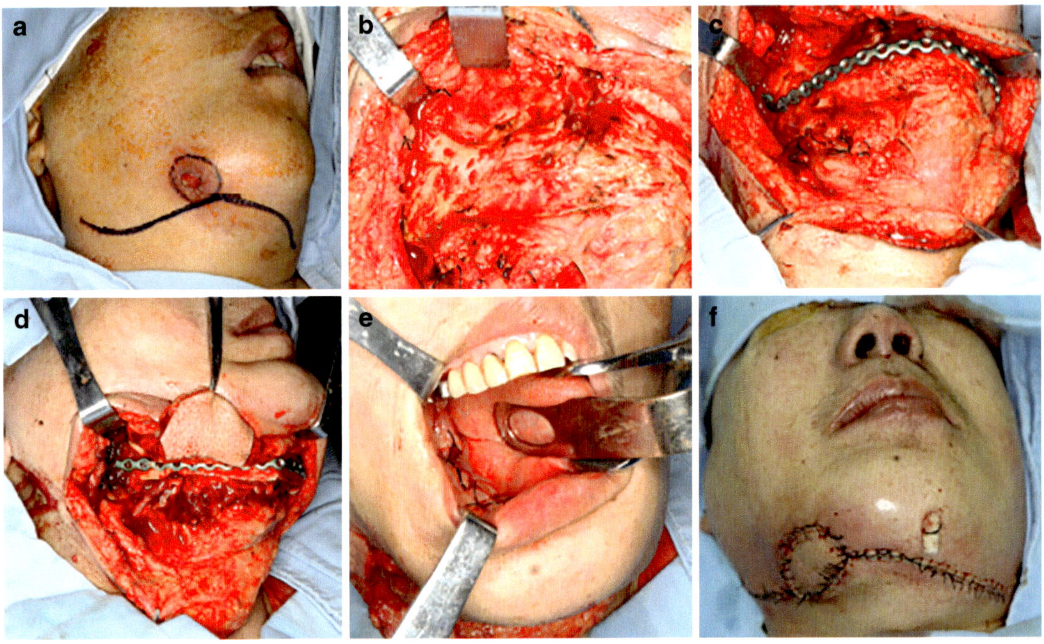

Fig. 4.17 (**a**) Design of incision. (**b**) Exposed mandible lesion. (**c**) Reconstructed pre-bent titanium plate. (**d**) Reconstructed and recovered fibula mandible continuity. (**e**) Intraoral mucosa was tightly sutured in alignment. (**f**) Repair of submandibular region coloboma with skin paddle

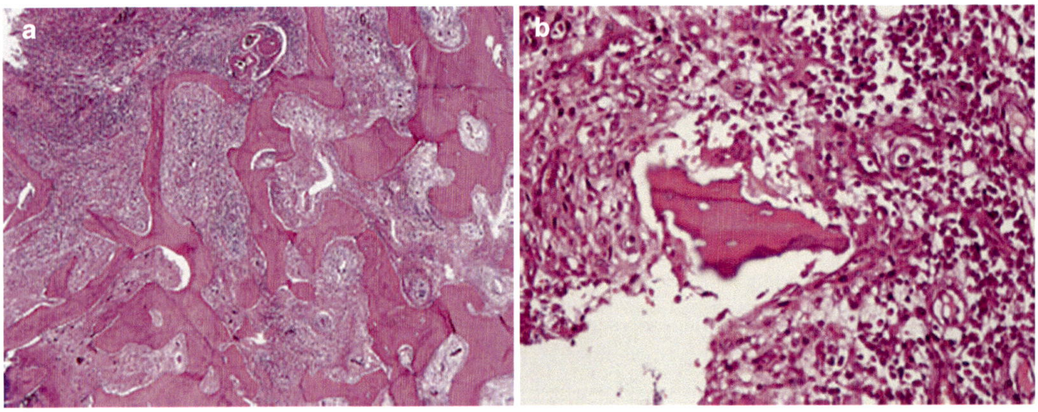

Fig. 4.18 (**a**) Fibrous tissue between trabeculae of bone proliferated significantly, blood vessels were abundant, lymphocytes, neutrophils and plasma cells infiltrated, and inflammation was obvious (40×). (**b**) A small piece of dead bone tissue surrounded by inflammatory granulation tissues (400×)

4.4 Key Points of Diagnosis and Treatment

The occurrence of MRONJ is closely related to the use of bisphosphonates, Rank-L inhibitors, antiangiogenic drugs or some hormonal drugs, and it is essentially a metabolic disorder of the jaws. In 2003, Marx reported for the first time 36 cases of bone lesions caused by taking bisphosphonates, which were different from radiation osteonecrosis of jaws, and defined them as "bisphosphonate-related osteonecrosis of the jaws (BRONJ)" [1, 3]. Subsequently, more and more clinical reports showed that the use of some non-bisphosphonate drugs, such as tyrosine kinase inhibitors, VEGF monoclonal antibodies, mTOR inhibitors, and some hormonal drugs, can also cause the same jaw lesions. In view of this important discovery, the American Association of Oral and Maxillofacial Surgeons renamed it " medication-related osteonecrosis of jaw" in 2014, and the name has been used ever since [5–8].

Pathogenesis The pathogenesis of MRONJ is not clear; it may be related to cell physiological changes, such as osteoclast activity inhibition, angiogenesis inhibition, inflammation and infection, etc. The target cells, cell physiology, signal pathways and key factors of different drugs are different, making the study of pathogenesis still in the exploratory stage and needing to be further revealed by a large number of basic and clinical transformation studies.

Diagnosis In 2014, the opinion of American Association of Oral and Maxillofacial Surgeons on MRONJ recommended three conditions for diagnosing MRONJ: ① being receiving or have received anti-bone resorption and anti-angiogenesis therapy; ② exposed dead bone in maxillofacial region, or the dead bone can be explored through the oral or extraoral fistula, and not improving for 8 weeks. ③ Jaw has not been irradiated and there is no definite metastatic disease of jaw. Patients need to meet the above three points at the same time to be diagnosed as MRONJ.

Differential diagnosis MRONJ is often differentiated from osteoradionecrosis of the jaws (ORNJ), pyogenic osteomyelitis of jaws and some idiopathic osteomyelitis of the jaws. The pathological features of MRONJ are bone lacunae, the disappearance of osteogenic ring, the absence of Hafersian system and Volkmann Canals. The bone marrow cavity lacks blood vessels and inflammatory cells, showing a state of lack of cells and collagen. There is a small amount of bacteria on the surface of bone necrosis. The vitality of periosteum still exists. The pathology of ORNJ shows that the bone lacunae are empty, and the osteogenic ring, Hafersian system and Volkmann Canals disappear. The cells, tissues and structures of the bone marrow cavity disappear and are replaced by collagen fibers with few cells; The same microbes only exist on the surface of necrotic bone. On the basis of bone destruction, suppurative osteomyelitis is mainly characterized by inflammatory changes in the bone marrow cavity, infiltration of neutrophils and lymphocytes, obvious enhancement of osteoclast activity, and microbial infiltration in some biological samples. If the patients of MRONJ have a special history of drug use and have not received radiotherapy, the main inducement is that the infection of the tooth extraction wound is not healed after the tooth in the mouth is extracted, characterized by grayish brown dead bone exposure and local pus. If the patients of ORNJ have a clear history of radiotherapy. The inflammation of residual teeth in the mouth can induce and promote the inflammation and necrosis of the jaws, and bone exposure, skin fistula formation, radiation caries in the mouth and changes in the skin of the face and neck after radiotherapy are often seen. Suppurative osteomyelitis is closely related to the inflammation of patients in the mouth and can be divided into central osteomyelitis and marginal osteomyelitis in accordance with the location of the lesion.

Treatment At present, there is no symptomatic treatment based on etiological research. Hyperbaric oxygen (HBO) can promote the proliferation of capillaries, increase the effective oxygen content of tissues, improve the hypoxic microenvironment, and improve the vitality of immune cells and bone cells. It has been reported that HBO treatment can completely heal early MRONJ, accelerate the healing, and at the same time relieve the pain and improve the quality of life of patients. The anti-fibrosis scheme of pentoxifylline combined with vitamin E has been used in the conservative treatment of ORNJ and has achieved good results. Some scholars tried to treat MRONJ with this scheme and found that the broken mucosa healed again, and the imaging showed new bone formation. However, this clinical effect is contingent and needs to be verified by prospective trials. In addition, there are also successful cases of using ozone, parathyroid hormone analogues-teriparatide and platelet concentrated products, etc., to treat MRONJ. Generally speaking, the conservative treatment of MRONJ is still in the exploratory stage.

In accordance with the different severity of the lesions, MRONJ can be classified into clinical stages to guide the choice of clinical diagnosis and treatment. The team of He Yue summarized the panoramic radiograph and CT image data of the patient's mouth and combined with the intraoperative experience, the connection level of the inferior alveolar neural tube and bilateral mental holes was used as a longitudinal symbol to divide the severity of MRONJ. At the same time, further sub-classification is set in accordance with whether there is a clear boundary of jaw lesions. Correspondingly, the gradual treatment scheme of MRONJ is put forward, including conservative observation (antibiotics, oral hygiene, tooth extraction, etc.), debridement (dead bone removal + inflammatory tissue removal), marginal mandibular resection, segmental mandibular resection with or without repair and reconstruction, hemimandibular resection, partial maxillary resection with or without maxillary sinus radical operation, maxillary enlarged resection, etc. (Table 4.1). MRONJ is an unbalanced disease of jaw tissue metabolism, and the influence of drugs on the jaw microenvironment is persistent and diffuse. The ultimate goal of conservative or surgical intervention is to stabilize the disease and prevent its progress.

Table 4.1 New clinical stages and treatment strategies of MRONJ [9]

Classification and staging	Specific interpretation	Treatment strategy
Phase 0	There is no obvious bone abnormality in imaging, but the clinical manifestations are unhealed tooth extraction wound or even pus, tooth loosening or bone exposure (excluding periodontal disease)	Conservative treatment or local debridement
Phase I	Imaging changes of mandible sclerotin are located in the area above the neural tube or bilateral mental foramen line Maxilla sclerotin changes do not break through maxillary sinus floor or nasal floor	
Phase Ia	There is a certain boundary between dead bone and normal sclerotin (limited type)	Phase Ia debridement
Phase Ib	There is no obvious boundary between dead bone and normal sclerotin (diffuse type)	Phase Ib Resection of mandible margin; Resection of maxilla
Phase II	Imaging changes of mandible sclerotin spread to the area below the neural tube or bilateral mental foramen line Does not involve the lower edge of the left mandible; maxilla sclerotin changes and breaks through the maxillary sinus or basis nasi and does not reach foramina infraorbitale	
Phase IIa	Limited dead bone of maxilla and mandible; Maxillary lesions without maxillary sinusitis syndrome	IIa local treatment or debridement can be considered

Table 4.1 (continued)

Classification and staging	Specific interpretation	Treatment strategy
Phase IIb	Diffuse dead bone of maxilla and mandible; Maxillary lesions with obvious maxillary sinus inflammation	Phase IIb segmental resection + titanium plate reconstruction or bone tissue/soft tissue flap repair; Partial maxilla resection + maxillary sinus radical operation
Phase III	In imaging, changes in mandibular sclerotin involve the lower edge of the mandible; Maxillary bone changes break through the suborbital foramen or do not involve the orbital floor or skull base, with or without maxillary sinus inflammation	Phase III segmental resection of mandible or hemimandibular resection + titanium plate reconstruction or bone tissue/soft tissue flap repair; Partial, subtotal or total maxillary resection + maxillary sinus radical operation

References

1. Marx RE. Pamidronate (Aredia) and zoledronate (Zometa) induced avascular necrosis of the jaws: a growing epidemic [J]. J Oral Maxillofac Surg. 2003;61(9):1115–7.
2. Ruggiero SL, Dodson TB, Fantasia J, et al. American Association of Oral and Maxillofacial Surgeons position paper on medication-related osteonecrosis of the jaw – 2014 update [J]. J Oral Maxillofac Surg. 2014;72(10):1938–56.
3. Marx RE, Tursun R. Suppurative osteomyelitis, bisphosphonate induced osteonecrosis, osteoradionecrosis: a blinded histopathologic comparison and its implications for the mechanism of each disease [J]. Int J Oral Maxillofac Surg. 2012;41(3):283–9.
4. Freiberger JJ, Padilla-Burgos R, McGraw T, et al. What is the role of hyperbaric oxygen in the management of bisphosphonate-related osteonecrosis of the jaw: a randomized controlled trial of hyperbaric oxygen as an adjunct to surgery and antibiotics [J]. J Oral Maxillofac Surg. 2012;70(7):1573–83.
5. Owosho AA, Estilo CL, Huryn JM, et al. Pentoxifylline and tocopherol in the management of cancer patients with medication-related osteonecrosis of the jaw: an observational retrospective study of initial case series [J]. Oral Surg Oral Med Oral Pathol Oral Radiol. 2016;122(4):455–9.
6. Agrillo A, Filiaci F, Ramieri V, et al. Bisphosphonate-related osteonecrosis of the jaw (BRONJ): 5 year experience in the treatment of 131 cases with ozone therapy [J]. Eur Rev Med Pharmacol Sci. 2012;16(12):1741–7.
7. Kim KM, Park W, Oh SY, et al. Distinctive role of 6-month teriparatide treatment on intractable bisphosphonate-related osteonecrosis of the jaw [J]. Osteoporos Int. 2014;25(5):1625–32.
8. Adornato MC, Morcos I, Rozanski J. The treatment of bisphosphonate associated osteonecrosis of the jaws with bone resection and autologous platelet derived growth factors [J]. J Am Dent Assoc. 2007;138(7):971–7.
9. Liu Z, Jiang J, Li X, et al. Osteoradionecrosis of the jaws and proposed new classification [J]. China J Oral Maxillofac Surg. 2020;18(6):501–7.

Part II

Odontogenic and Non-odontogenic Developmental Cysts

5 Dentigerous Cyst

Bing Liu, Hui Shan Ong, Zhen Tian, Lin Zhu, and Bing Guo

5.1 Introduction

A dentigerous cyst is a common developmental odontogenic cyst, accounting for about 20% of odontogenic cysts. It is also called a follicular cyst by the World Health Organization, and its prevalence rate is second only to that of an apical cyst. About 60% are odontogenic cysts in mixed dentition, with the predilection age ranging from 10 to 39 years old, more males than females, and the predilection sites are as follows: third mandibular molar area, maxillary canine area, third maxillary molar area and mandibular premolar area [1–8].

5.1.1 Case 14

The patient, female, aged 38; a space-occupying lesion of the left mandible was found for 2 weeks.

B. Liu (✉)
Hospital of Stomatology Wuhan University, Hubei, China
e-mail: liubing9909@wuhan.edu.cn

H. S. Ong · Z. Tian · B. Guo
Department of Oral Maxillofacial-Head & Neck Oncology, Shanghai Ninth People's Hospital, Shanghai Jiao Tong University School of Medicine, Shanghai, China

L. Zhu
Department of Radiology, Ninth People's Hospital Affiliated to Shanghai Jiao Tong University, Shanghai, China

[Present medical history] Two weeks ago, the patient took an oral X-ray film in another hospital and found a low-density space-occupying shadow on the left mandible. The patient denied a history of swelling and pain, bleeding, trauma and mouth opening limitation. The patient went to the outpatient of our hospital for a maxillofacial region CT examination, indicating that left mandible 8 embedded with a cystic space-occupying lesion.

[Specialized examination] Para-oral: The patient's bilateral maxillofacial regions are basically symmetrical, the left mandible has good continuity, and no obvious bone cortex swelling is palpated. The degree of mouth opening is three horizontal fingers, the mouth opening type is vertically downward, and the bilateral temporomandibular joints have no snapping or tenderness. No obvious swollen lymph nodes are seen in bilateral submandibular regions and neck. Intraoral: In the mouth, 26 and 27 are missing, 36 and 37 crowns are elongated, 45 is defective to 1 mm above the gum, and 38 and 48 are missing.

[Auxiliary examination]

1. Panoramic radiographs: A cystic low-density focus was found in the mandibular angle, with irregular shape and clear boundary, and a crown was enclosed in it (Fig. 5.1).
2. CT enhanced scan of the maxillofacial region: A round low-density shadow was seen in the alveolar bone of the left lower 8 area, with

Y. He (ed.), *Inflammatory and Neoplastic Diseases of Craniofacial Bones*, https://doi.org/10.1007/978-981-97-4155-7_5

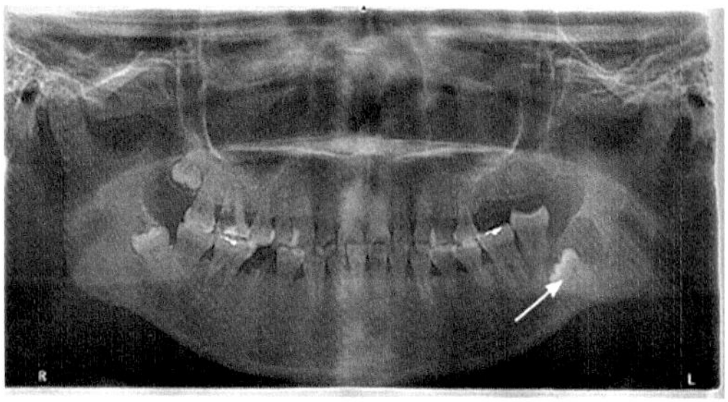

Fig. 5.1 A cystic low-density focus was found in the mandibular angle, with irregular shape and clear boundary, and a crown was enclosed in it

swollen bone and clear boundary, with the size of about 21 mm * 16 mm, C− 10 Hu and C+ 11 Hu, without obvious enhancement, and the alveolar and lingual cortical bone cortex is discontinuous. No abnormality is found in the surrounding soft tissues. The left lower 8 is impacted and the crown is located in the lesion. No abnormal enlarged lymph node shadow is seen in the neck (Fig. 5.2).

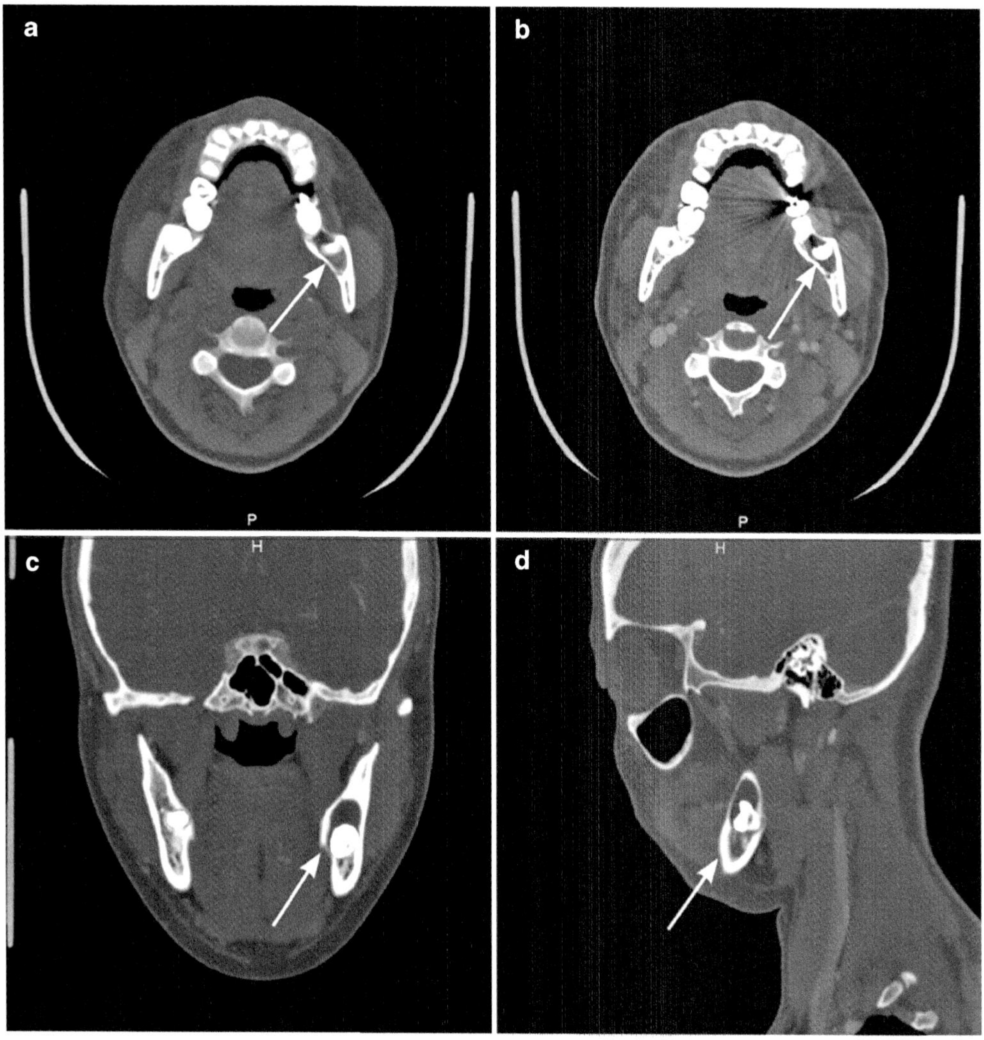

Fig. 5.2 (**a**) Cross section of CT Plain Scan: A round-like low-density shadow is seen in the alveolar bone of the left lower 8 area, with sclerotin swelling and clear boundary. (**b**) Cross section of CT Enhanced Scan: No significant enhancement was seen. (**c**) Coronal view of CT enhanced scan: Alveolar and lingual bone cortex discontinuity. (**d**) Sagittal view of CT enhanced scan: The left lower 8 is impacted and the crown is located in the lesion

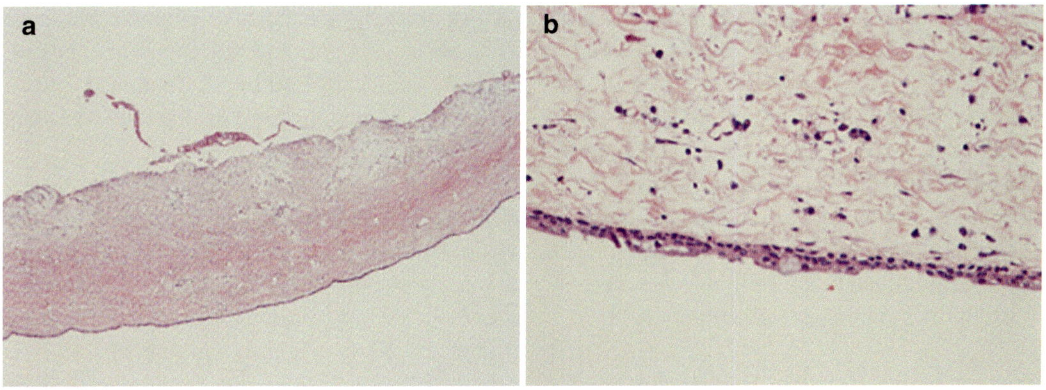

Fig. 5.3 (**a**) The loose fibrous connective tissue capsule wall is lined with a thin layer of epithelium similar to the residual enamel epithelium, and the inflammation is not obvious (40×). (**b**) The lining epithelium is thin, containing a small amount of mucous cells, without keratinization and epithelial spikes, and the junction with the cyst wall is flat. The cyst wall is loose, and a small amount of inflammatory cells infiltrates (400×)

[Primary diagnosis] Dentigerous Cyst at the left mandible.

[Treatment] "left mandibular cyst extraction + left lower mandible impacted tooth extraction" were performed under general anesthesia; Incision of gingiva from 36 distal ends to turn the flap over, removal of 37, grinding off part of the bone to expose cyst wall tissue and embedding of 38; 38 was removed, the cyst wall tissue was scraped off completely close to the bone surface, and send to frozen pathological examination during operation, indicating that the fibrous capsule wall-like tissue and thin lining epithelium of "left mandible" contained individual mucous cells, combined with imaging findings, a dentigerous cyst was complied with, and iodoform gauze was filled in the capsule cavity.

[Pathological examination] One molar was submitted for pathological examination, with cyst-wall-like tissue attached to the dental neck, about 1.8 cm * 1.2 cm * 0.3 cm in size and grayish red. Microscopically, fibrous capsule wall-like tissue was seen, a small amount of inflammatory cells infiltrated, the lining epithelium was thin, similar to the residual enamel epithelium, composed of 2 ~ 4 layers of cubic or flat non-keratinized cells, and the epithelium has no spikes. The junction with connective tissue is flat (Fig. 5.3).

[Pathological diagnosis] Dentigerous cyst of "left mandible," ICD code: K09.001.

[Data of follow-up visit] The patient recovered well after the operation, and the cyst did not recur after half a year.

5.2 Key Points of Diagnosis and Treatment

The most common odontogenic oral disease cysts are apical and dentigerous cysts. In 1908, Paget put forward the term "dentigerous cysts" for the first time. Among the patients with dentigerous cysts, males account for the majority, male to female ratio is about 1.84:1.2, and patients with dentigerous cysts account for about 24% of jaw cyst diseases [3]. A dentigerous cyst is a tooth eruption obstacle caused by fluid accumulation between the residual enamel epithelium and the crown surface during tooth eruption. The normal follicular gap is about 3 ~ 4 mm, but when the gap is greater than 5 mm, it can be suspected as a dentigerous cyst, which can contain the crown of one or more teeth.

Clinical manifestation The same as other jaw cysts, dentigerous cysts are asymptomatic and grow slowly in the early stage. When the cysts are large, jaw swelling, bone thinning and ping-pong sensation may occur, most of which are accompanied by the loss of the corresponding tooth position. Grass yellow or green cystic fluid becomes yellow cystic fluid after secondary infection, and symptoms of pain and discomfort may occur. Dentigerous cysts are usually found by accident during oral examination, mostly due to delayed eruption of teeth, loss of permanent teeth, maxillofacial deformities, etc., and are found during imaging examination.

Imaging characteristics The imaging performance is a clear round or oval low-density shadow with neat and clear edges and white bone lines around it. The capsule cavity contains a crown, which faces into the cavity. Because of the different stages of tooth development, the crown shapes are also different. Therefore, the teeth can be at all stages. Dentigerous cysts are mostly single-chamber images, and sometimes multi-chamber images can also be seen. Dentigerous cysts can be divided into three types in accordance with the light-transmitting parts around the crown of unexplored teeth: central, lateral, and annular.

Pathological feature Histologic findings of dentigerous cysts: Macroscopically, it can be seen that the cyst contains a crown, and the cyst's wall is thin and attached to the enamel cementum. Microscopically, there is a multi-layered squamous epithelial lining, and the epithelial layer is thin, without keratinization and epithelial spikes, and consists of 2 ~ 4 layers of flat cells or short cubic cells. The wall of the fibrous capsule is rich in glycoprotein and mucopolysaccharide; the epithelial connective tissue interface is flat. When the cysts lead to infection or inflammation, epithelial hyperplasia and nail process are obvious. Sometimes, odontogenic epithelial islands, sebaceous cells and lymphatic follicles can be seen in the wall of the fibrous capsule. Sometimes, mucous cells or ciliated columnar cells can appear in some dentigerous cysts. According to the clinical manifestations, cholesterol crystals are found in puncture cyst fluid examination, X-ray films show circular or elliptical transmission areas with clear and tidy edges, and the cyst cavity contains dental crowns. Combined with its pathological examination, dentigerous cysts can be diagnosed.

Differential diagnosis The differential diagnosis of dentigerous cysts includes ameloblastoma, odontogenic keratocyst, odontogenic fibroma, odontogenic myxoma, cementoma, Pindborg tumor, etc. Early diagnosis and resection are necessary because dentigerous cysts may develop into odontogenic tumors, such as ameloblastoma, and malignant tumors, such as squamous cell carcinoma and mucoepidermoid carcinoma.

Treatment At present, operation is the main method of treating dentigerous cysts. In order to reduce the probability of recurrence, removing the whole cyst and the impacted teeth is generally recommended, but this will lead to the loss of teeth and affect the quality of life of patients. In recent years, decompression has been increasingly applied to treating dentigerous cysts [6–11]. Decompression was first proposed by Partsch in 1892. This operation can preserve the affected teeth to the maximum extent, promote the self-repair of the jaws, and improve the prognosis of patients. Bagging has been widely used in the treatment of various jaw cysts [9–11].

References

1. Meningaud J, Oprean N, Pitak-Arnnop P, et al. Odontogenic cysts: a clinical study of 695 cases [J]. J Oral Sci. 2006;48(2):59–62.
2. Mervyn S, Paul S. Cysts of the oral and maxillofacial regions [M]. Oxford: Blackwell Munksgaard; 2007.
3. Wardbooth P. Cysts of the oral regions [M]. Cambridge University Press; 1992.
4. Kasat VO, Karjodkar FR, Laddha RS. Dentigerous cyst associated with an ectopic third molar in the maxillary sinus: a case report and review of literature [J]. Contemp Clin Dent. 2012;3(3):373–6.
5. Sannomiya E, Nogueira MQ, Diniz MC, et al. Trauma-induced dentigerous cyst involving the anterior maxilla [J]. J Dent Child (Chic). 2007;74(2):161–4.

6. Li N, Gao X, Xu Z, et al. Prevalence of developmental odontogenic cysts in children and adolescents with emphasis on dentigerous cyst and odontogenic keratocyst (keratocystic odontogenic tumor) [J]. Acta Odontol Scand. 2014;72(8):795–800.
7. Patil A, Jathar P, Panse A, et al. Infected dentigerous cyst and its conservative management: a report of two cases [J]. Int J Clin Pediatr Dentist. 2019;12(1):68–72.
8. Sha XC. Clinical presentation and pathology of dentigerous cyst [J]. J Oral Sci Res. 1986;2(1):11–2.
9. Ramakrishna A, Lambade P. Dentigerous cyst associated with ectopic canine and a supernumerary tooth: a rare occurrence [J]. J Surg Tech Case Rep. 2013;5(2):85–8.
10. Guo ZZ, Wang ZJ, Yang XW. Marsupialization and orthodontology in promoting eruption of impacted tooth with dentigerous cyst [J]. Chin J Pract Stomatol. 2020;13(10):582–5.
11. Zhao YF, Liu B, Jiang BQ. Marsupialiazation of jaw cyst [J]. Shanghai J Stomatol. 2005;4:325–9.

Odontogenic Keratocyst

6

Bing Liu, Hui Shan Ong, Zhen Tian, Lin Zhu, and Yong Jie Hu

6.1 Introduction

Odontogenic keratocyst (OKC) is a benign odontogenic lesion of the jaws, which is derived from the remains of upper and lower jaws or primitive tooth germs. It is one of the four most common odontogenic cysts, accounting for about 10% of jaw cysts. It has the characteristics of a high recurrence rate and strong clinical invasion and can occur at any age. Young and middle-aged men are prone to it, and the mandible is the most easily affected part [1–6].

6.1.1 Case 15

The patient, male, 14 years old. Swelling of the right mandible with pain for 6 months.

[Present medical history] Six months ago, the patient had no obvious cause for swelling of the right mandible, which was occasionally accompanied by pain. Panoramic radiographs were performed and a low-density shadow of the right mandible was found. There was no swelling, pyorrhea or bleeding in the gingival area, and no obvious numbness of the lower lip or limited mouth opening. Without further treatment, the symptoms of swelling and discomfort were obviously aggravated in the past 3 months.

[Specialized examination] The patient's maxillofacial region was basically symmetric. The degree and type of mouth opening were normal. The lingual jaw in the oral cavity was not obviously prominent, and the buccal jaw at the front edge of the ascending ramus of the right mandibular posterior teeth area was slightly swollen, with obvious ping-pong sensation and no obvious pain. No obvious loosening was found in the whole mouth.

[Auxiliary examination]
Panoramic radiographs: The bone density of the right mandibular angle and ramus is reduced, with irregular morphology, clear boundary, continuous bone cortex,

There was no obvious periosteal reaction and no abnormal swelling of soft tissue (Fig. 6.1a).

B. Liu (✉)
Hospital of Stomatology Wuhan University, Hubei, China
e-mail: liubing9909@wuhan.edu.cn

H. S. Ong · Z. Tian · Y. J. Hu
Department of Oral Maxillofacial-Head & Neck Oncology, Shanghai Ninth People's Hospital, Shanghai Jiao Tong University School of Medicine, Shanghai, China

L. Zhu
Department of Radiology, Ninth People's Hospital Affiliated to Shanghai Jiao Tong University, Shanghai, China

Y. He (ed.), *Inflammatory and Neoplastic Diseases of Craniofacial Bones*,
https://doi.org/10.1007/978-981-97-4155-7_6

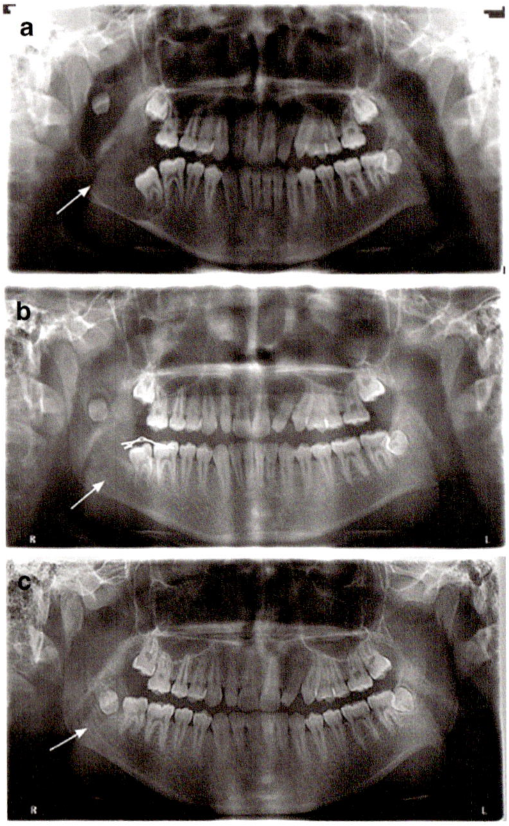

Fig. 6.1 (**a**) The bone density of the right mandibular angle and ramus is reduced, with irregular morphology, clear boundary, continuous bone cortex, no obvious periosteal reaction and abnormal swelling of soft tissue (before fenestration). (**b**) After the right mandibular fenestration, the linear dense shadows are noted, the scope of the low-density area is decreased, the density is slightly higher than before, and the bone cortex is continuous. (**c**) After the right mandibular fenestration, the scope of the low-density area is further reduced, and the density is slightly higher than before

[Primary diagnosis] Cyst at the right mandible.

[Treatment] "Right lower mandible jaw cyst fenestration" was performed under general anesthesia: A circular incision was made at the 46 tooth root, approximately 1.5 cm in diameter. The mucosa was removed to expose the cystic mass. Part of the cystic wall was removed and sent for rapid frozen pathology during the surgery: "The right mandible" lesion tends to be the odontogenic keratocyst. The cystic fluid was light yellow and clear. The cystic fluid was completely absorbed and the cystic cavity was rinsed. The wound was bandaged and fixed with the iodoform gauze. An obturator was prepared after the operation and the wound was irrigated. Please follow up on the schedule.

[Pathological examination] A small amount of grayish-white biopsy tissue is sent for pathology after the fenestration, approximately 0.8 cm * 0.6 cm * 0.3 cm in size. The hyperplastic fibrous cystic wall-like tissue was seen under the microscope, lined by multi-layer squamous epithelium, with hyperparakeratosis on the surface, well-arranged fence-like basal layer cells, and epithelial rete peg hyperplasia (Fig. 6.2).

[Pathological diagnosis] "Right mandible" odontogenic keratocyst. ICD code: K09.002. Mild dysplasia of the lining epithelium.

[Follow-up visit] The mouth window drainage was kept unobstructed, local irrigation was strengthened, and panoramic radiographs were regularly followed up. The lesion range was gradually narrowed.

Three years after fenestration, the cyst was significantly reduced (Fig. 6.1b, c). "Removal of

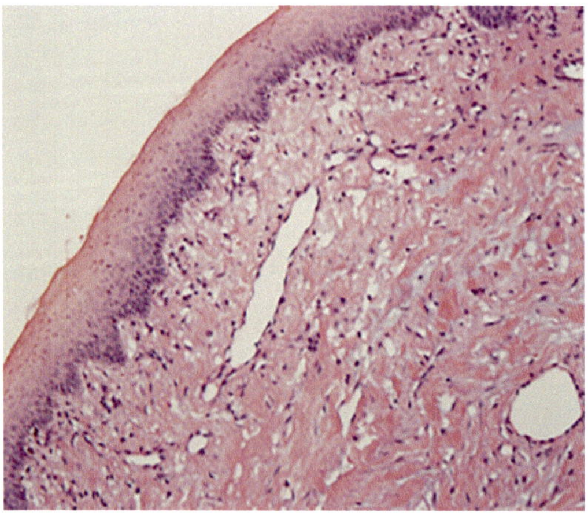

Fig. 6.2 Hyperplastic fibrous connective tissue is lined with keratinized multi-layer squamous epithelium. Fence-like basal layer cells are well arranged. The epithelial hyperplasia forms small epithelial rete pegs, with epithelial surface parakeratosis (200×)

the right mandibular cyst + 48 extraction" was performed under the general anesthesia again. The postoperative recovery was good.

6.1.2 Case 16

The patient, female, aged 23, The patient has suffered from gingival swelling in the right upper posterior teeth area for more than 2 months.

[Present medical history] Two months ago, the patient found the gingival swelling in the right upper posterior teeth area without obvious inducement, with no obvious spontaneous or stimulating pain. The patient went to a local hospital for treatment, considering the possibility of "the right maxillary bone cyst." The swelling gradually worsened during that period, with no obvious growth or decline history. The patient denied a history of trauma and toothache and denied numbness symptoms. The patient went to our hospital's outpatient for a CT examination, indicating a cystic mass of the right maxilla.

[Specialized examination] The face is bilaterally asymmetric. The proportion of the upper, middle and lower 1/3 face is coordinated. The degree and shape of mouth opening are normal. From 15 to 17, the gingival swelling is palpated on the buccal side. The upper side is close to the gingival-buccal groove, with an obvious sense of fluctuation, and the underlying bone is absent, with interrupted continuity, no rupture and exudation, and no obvious swelling on the palatal side. 18 is not seen, and 17 are loosening for II°. No obvious swollen lymph nodes are seen in bilateral submandibular regions and neck.

[Auxiliary examination]

1. Panoramic radiographs: A density-decreased area was seen in the right maxilla, with irregular morphology but still clear boundary, continuous bone cortex, and no obvious periosteal reaction and soft tissue mass. An impacted tooth was seen (Fig. 6.3a).
2. CT enhanced scan of the maxillofacial region indicated an impacted tooth was seen in the upper right 7 root and the dental crown was towards the buccal side. A quasi-circular low-density shadow was noted on the crown side and wrapped around the neck of the tooth. C− 32 Hu, C+ 38 Hu. No obvious enhancement was observed after the enhanced scan, and the lesion was about 34 mm * 28 mm in size and expanded to the buccal side and maxillary sinus cavity. The buccal bone cortex became thin and interrupted. No obvious abnormalities were discovered in the surrounding soft tissue (Fig. 6.4).

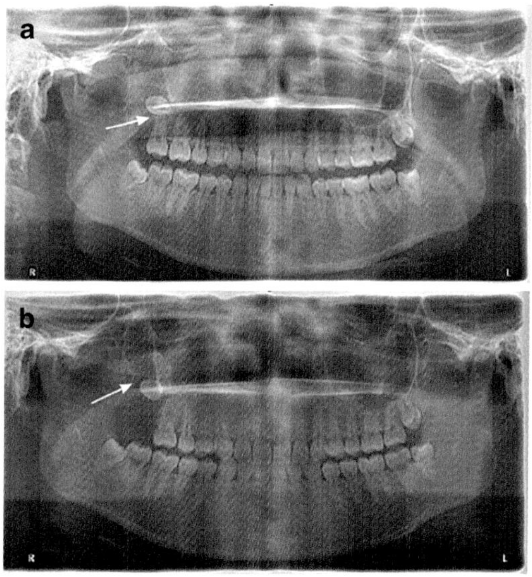

Fig. 6.3 (**a**) There is a cystic density-decreased area in the right maxilla, with irregular morphology but still clear boundary, continuous bone cortex, no obvious periosteal reaction and soft tissue mass. An impacted tooth was seen (before fenestration). (**b**) After the right maxilla fenestration, a density-decreased area is seen and the scope is slightly smaller than that of previous images

[Primary diagnosis] Cyst at the right maxilla.

[Treatment] "Fenestration for the right maxillary cyst + 17 extraction" was performed under general anesthesia. The gingiva was cut open at 17 distal sites, and the flap was turned over. After removing partial bone, a cystic mass was seen below, with a large amount of yellow-brown tofu residue-like secretion discharged. Partial maxillary bone was removed and part of the cyst wall tissue was cut off and sent for frozen biopsy, indicating "right maxil-

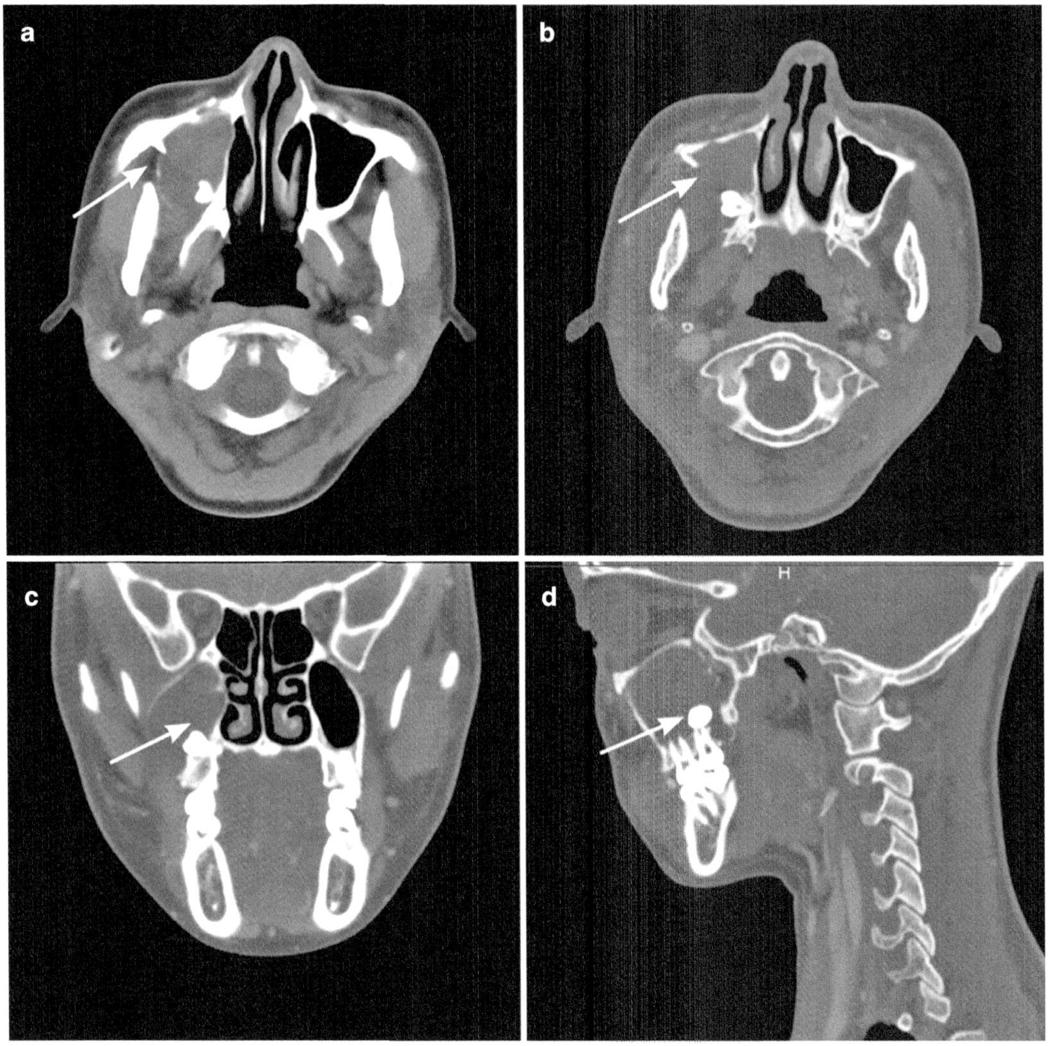

Fig. 6.4 (**a**, **b**) An impacted tooth is seen in the upper right 7 root and the dental crown is towards the buccal side. A quasi-circular low-density shadow is noted on the crown side and wrapped around the neck of the tooth, without significant enhancement after an enhanced scan. (**c**, **d**) It has expanded into the cavity of the maxillary sinus. The buccal bone cortex becomes thin and interrupted. No obvious abnormalities are found in the surrounding soft tissue

lary" odontogenic keratocyst. Strict hemostasis, rinsing and tela iodoformum packing suture were carried out. The plug applicator was prepared after the operation with local rinsing. Regular follow-up visit shall be carried out.

[Pathological examination] Cystic wall-like tissue was sent for biopsy. 1 cm * 1.5 cm * 0.2 cm, grayish yellow. Fibrous cystic wall-like tissue was seen under the microscope, lined with multilayer squamous epithelium. The lining epithelium was thin, with hyperparakeratosis on the surface, and wavy, with well-arranged fence-like basal layer cells. No rete pegs were seen in the epithelium. The junction with fibrous connective tissue was flat. The local lining epithelium was separated from the cystic wall of the underlying connective tissue (Fig. 6.5).

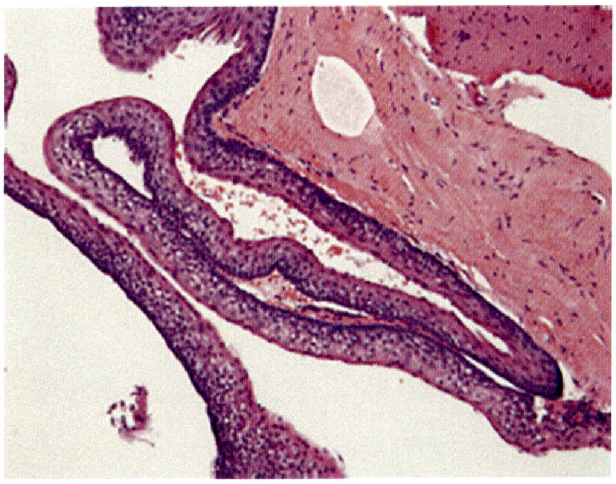

Fig. 6.5 The lining epithelium becomes thin, with hyperparakeratosis on the surface, wavy, with well-arranged fence-like basal layer cells, inverted nuclear polarity, and no epithelial rete pegs. The local epithelium is separated from the fibrous cystic wall, and the inflammation in the cystic wall is not obvious (200×)

[Pathological diagnosis] odontogenic keratocyst of "right maxilla," ICD code: K09.002.

[Follow-up visit] Keep the window drainage unobstructed, strengthen the local irrigation, and regularly follow up the panoramic radiographs. The scope of the was gradually narrowed (Fig. 6.3b).

6.1.3 Case 17

The patient, male, 24 years old. The patient has discovered a mass in the left mandible for more than a year.

[Present medical history] One year ago, a left mandibular mass was discovered on the X-ray film during the extraction of the impacted tooth, with no obvious spontaneous or stimulating pain. No further examination and treatment were carried out in that period. There was no special change in the area of the lesion. The patient felt pain in the left mandibular angle area a week ago, which was more severe when eating or touching and improved significantly after anti-inflammatory treatment. The patient went to our hospital's outpatient for a CT examination, indicating that it is likely a benign cystic mass in the left mandible.

[Specialized examination] The bilateral face was symmetrical. No obvious bone swelling was found in the left mandible body, angle and ramus. The degree and shape of mouth opening were normal. Intraoral examination: 38 not seen. The retromolar pad area was slightly swollen. The mucosa was red and swollen, with no orificium fistulae tenderness (+). The mandibular angle, ramus and buccal bone were not bulged. No obvious swollen lymph nodes are seen in bilateral submandibular regions and neck.

[Auxiliary examination]

1. Panoramic radiographs: A cystic low-density lesion was discovered in the junction of the left mandible body and angle, with irregular morphology, unclear boundary, continuous bone cortex, no periosteal reaction and soft tissue mass (Fig. 6.6)
2. CT enhanced scan of the maxillofacial region: A cystic low-density shadow was seen in the left mandible, approximately 31 mm * 14 mm in size, with a clear boundary, not bulging obviously, no obvious peripheral periosteal reaction and no soft tissue mass (Fig. 6.7).

[Primary diagnosis] Cyst at the right maxilla.

[Treatment] "Left mandibular cyst extraction" was performed under general anesthesia: The gingiva was cut open from the 37 to the buccal side of the retromolar pad area, and the flap was turned over. Partial bone was abraded by a power

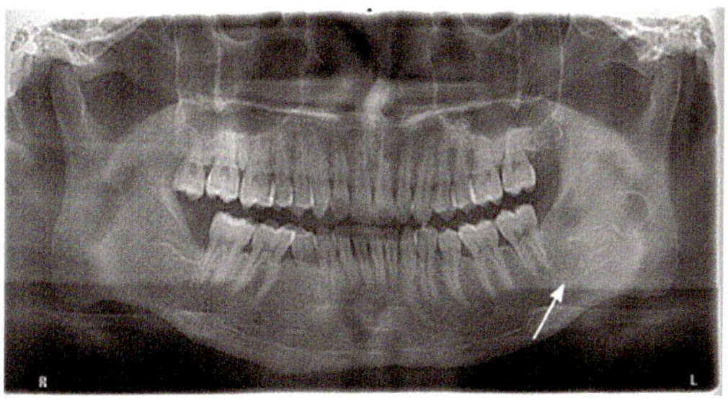

Fig. 6.6 A Cystic low-density lesion is discovered in the junction of the left mandible body and angle, with irregular morphology, unclear boundary, continuous bone cortex, no periosteal reaction and soft tissue mass (preoperative)

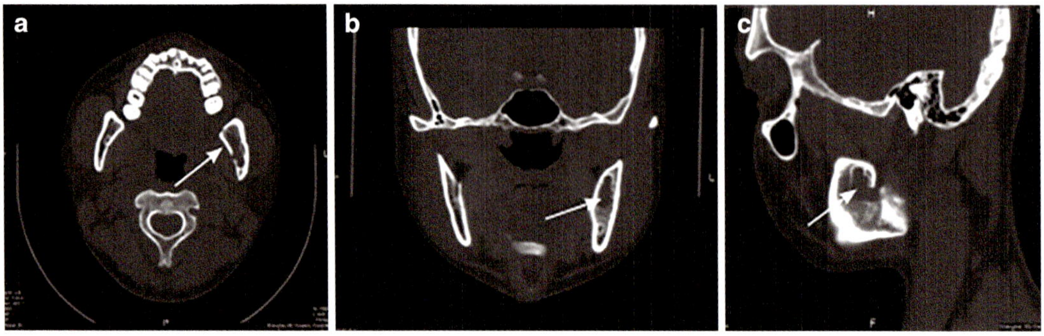

Fig. 6.7 (**a**) Cross-section of CT plain scan: A cystic low-density lesion with irregular morphology is discovered in the junction of the left mandible body and angle. (**b**) Coronary view of CT plain scan: Continuous bone cortex. (**c**) Sagittal view of CT plain scan: No periosteal reaction and soft tissue mass (preoperative)

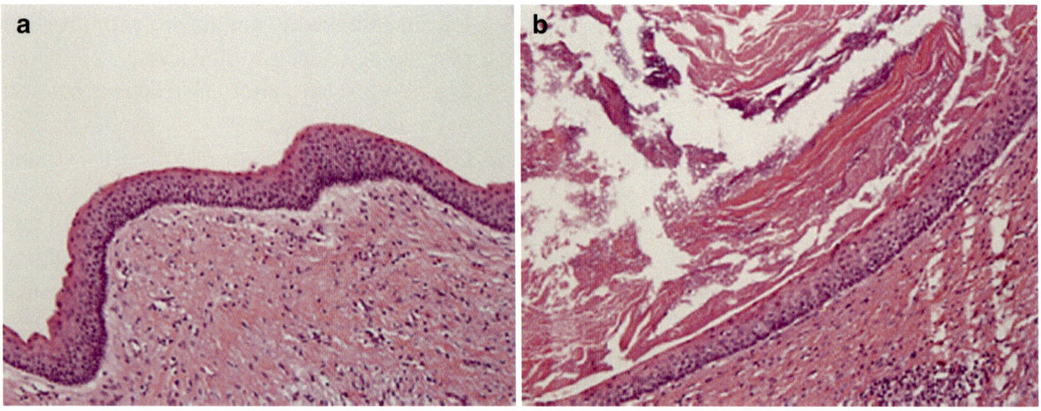

Fig. 6.8 (**a**) The lining epithelium is the squamous epithelium with parakeratosis, wavy surface, and fence-like arranged basal layer cells (200×). (**b**) A large amount of cyclic lamellar keratin is seen in the cystic cavity, as well as local inflammatory cell infiltration in the cystic wall (200×)

system, up to 1 cm deep. The cystic-occupied tissue was noted inside and the ascus was bulged backward and upward. It was completely removed and sent for frozen pathology during the operation, indicating "left mandibular" odontogenic keratocyst with secondary infection. Strict hemostasis, rinsing and suture were carried out.

[Pathological examination] One cystic tissue was sent for pathological examination, 2.5 cm * 2 cm * 0.3 cm in size, and gray red. Fibrous cystic wall-like tissue was seen under the microscope, with inflammatory cell infiltration, and lined with uniformly multi-layer squamous epithelium. The lining epithelium was thin, with parakeratosis on the surface, wavy. A large amount of cyclic lamellar keratin was found in the cystic cavity. The basal layer cells were well arranged and the epithelial rete pegs were not obvious. The junction with the connective tissue was flat (Fig. 6.8).

[Pathological diagnosis] odontogenic keratocyst of "left mandible," ICD code: K09.002, with secondary infection. [Follow-ups] The operative area recovered well, and the patient was reviewed 3 months after surgery, with no obvious abnormalities in the operative area.

6.1.4 Case 18

The patient, male, 43 years old. The patient has suffered from multiple postoperative recurrences of the right mandibular cyst for 10 years.

[Present medical history] Ten years ago, the patient repeatedly underwent "the fenestration for the right mandibular cyst" in other hospital and our hospital due to "the right mandibular cyst." The patient still had recurrent swelling and suppurating and underwent "the curettage for the right mandibular lesion" under general anesthesia in our hospital 8 and 6 years ago, respectively. Postoperative pathology indicated: "It is consistent with odontogenic keratocyst." Coronoidectomy was performed in ensuring the recurrence OKC was en bloc resected, followed by ex vivo curretage and liquid nitrogen freezed before reimplanted under general anesthesia. Pathological results showed a keratocystic odontogenic tumor of the right mandible with infection. The patient reviewed this year. The panoramic radiographs were conducted in the outpatient department and indicated the cystic mass in the mandibular ascending ramus.

[Specialized examination] The face was basically symmetrical, with no obvious bulging in the right mandible. An old scar was visible in the local skin of the right anterior ear, approximately 3 cm in length. Facial nerve function was normal, with no numbness of the lower lip. The tongue movement was fair. The shape of the mouth opening was normal and the degree of mouth opening was about three horizontal fingers, with fair occlusal relationship. The lower right 7 and 8 teeth were missing. There was no swelling of the gingiva. A surgical scar was seen in the mucosa of the right posterior molar region to the lateral mucosa of the pterygomandibular ligament, with no abnormal exudation (Fig. 6.9a, b).

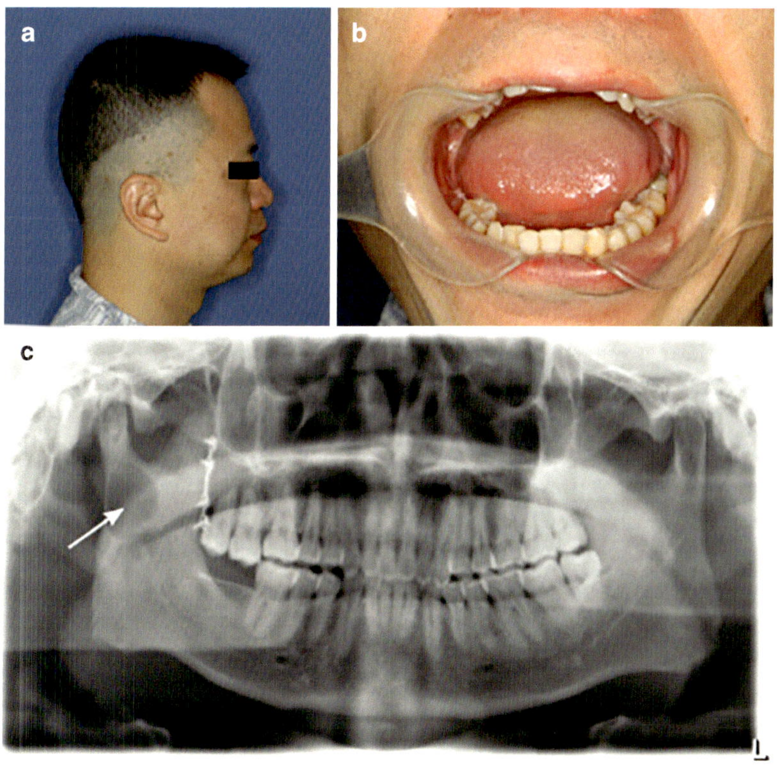

Fig. 6.9 (**a**) Postoperative changes of the right face and the jaws, with no obvious bulge. (**b**) The degree and type of mouth opening are normal. (**c**) A quasi-circular low-density shadow was noted in the right mandibular ascending ramus, with a clear boundary, showing a dilatancy change. The buccal bone cortex became thin, with no obvious periosteal reaction (before this operation)

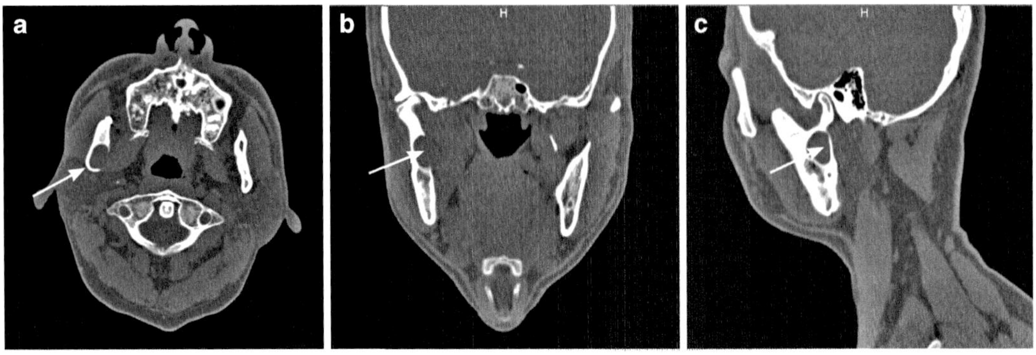

Fig. 6.10 (**a**) Cross section of CT Plain Scan: The quasi-circular low-density shadow was observed in the ascending ramus of the right mandible with a clear boundary. (**b**) Coronary view of CT plain scan: The bone cortex was discontinuous and the buccal bone cortex became thinner. (**c**) Sagittal view of CT plain scan: No periosteal reaction and soft tissue mass (pre-operation this time)

[Auxiliary examination]

1. Panoramic radiographs: A quasi-circular low-density shadow was noted in the right mandibular ascending ramus, with a clear boundary, showing a dilatancy change. The buccal bone cortex became thin, with no obvious periosteal reaction (Fig. 6.9c).
2. CT plain scan of the maxillofacial region: A quasi-circular low-density shadow was noted in the right mandibular ascending ramus, with even density, approximately 1.2 cm * 0.6 cm in size, with a clear boundary, showing a dilatancy change. The buccal bone cortex becomes thin, with no obvious periosteal reaction and soft tissue mass shadow (Fig. 6.10).

[Primary diagnosis] multiple postoperative recurrences for odontogenic keratocyst of the right mandible.

[Treatment] Coronoidectomy with ex vivo curretage and liquid nitrogen cryotherapy. The cryotherapy treated condyle was then reimplanted to the native mandible. An incision of 1~2cm was made along the inferior margin of the mandible, and the flap was turned over to fully expose the right angle of the mandible to the condyle. The neurovascular bundle of the right mandibular angle and the inferior alveolar were cut off. The cyst at the ascending ramus of the right mandible was observed, and the buccal bone cortex was broken through into soft tissue with scar tissues around. The soft tissues were severed. The tissue above the ascending ramus of the mandible was taken out and replanted after being frozen with liquid nitrogen, and the internal fixation was enhanced. Frozen pathology in operation indicated: For the "right mandible," the muscle, nerve and tumor-like proliferative fibrous tissue with hyaline change were sent for pathological examination; The resection margins sent were negative (I). The operation wound was rinsed, bleeding was stopped strictly, a negative pressure drainage tube was reserved, the suture was conducted in layers, and the wound was closed (Fig. 6.11).

[Pathological examination] One tissue was submitted: 4 cm * 2 cm * 0.5 cm, dark red. The elongated fibrous cystic wall-like tissues were observed under the microscope, and few inflammatory cells were infiltrated. The lining epithelium was thin and uniform stratified squamous epithelium without epithelial spike. The epithelial surface was not fully keratinized and it was wavy. The polarity of the basal layer cells was inverted and was arranged in a palisade-like manner (Fig. 6.12a).

[Pathological diagnosis] Odontogenic Keratocyst at the "right mandible," ICD code: K09.002

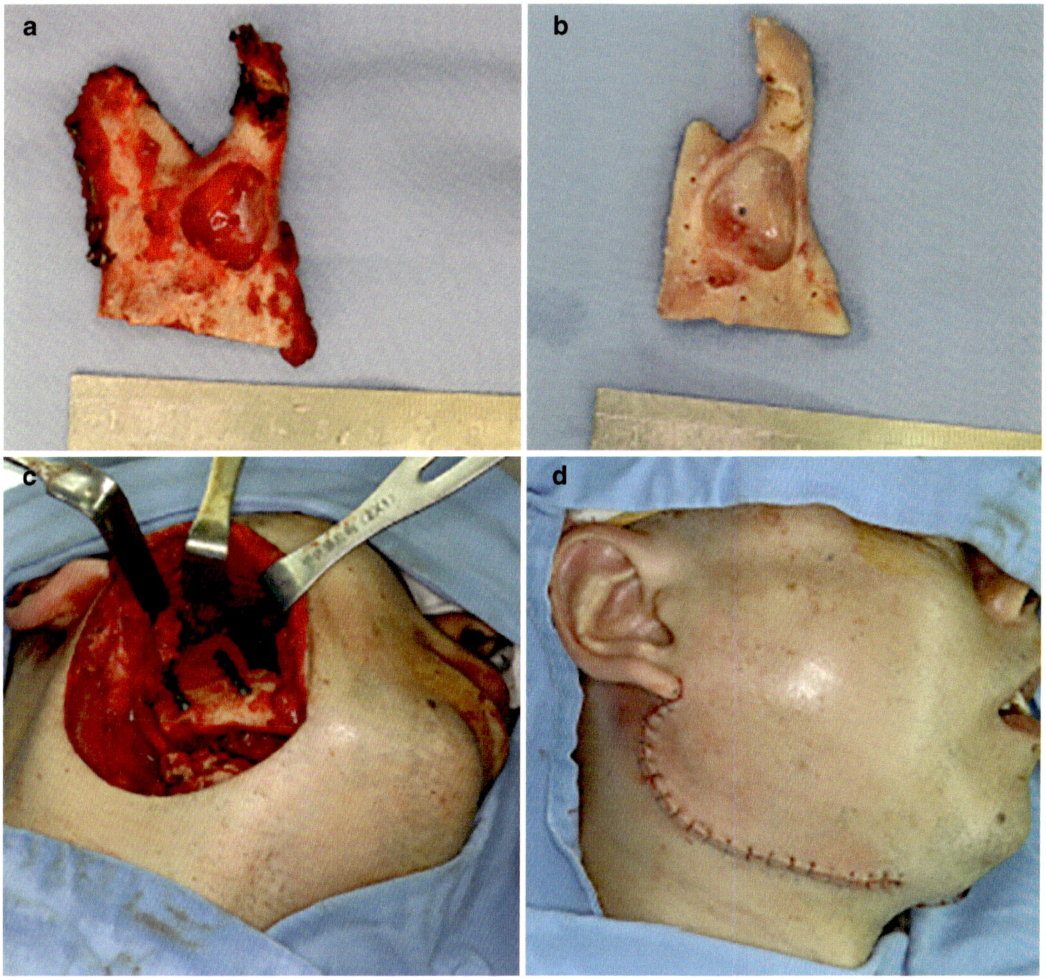

Fig. 6.11 (**a**) The condyle toegtehr with coronoid and lesion was resected in a bloc, and OKC curretage was performed ex-vivo. (**b**) Mandible after freezing with liquid nitrogen. (**c**) The mandible was replanted and fixed. (**d**) Observation after replantation surgery of the mandible

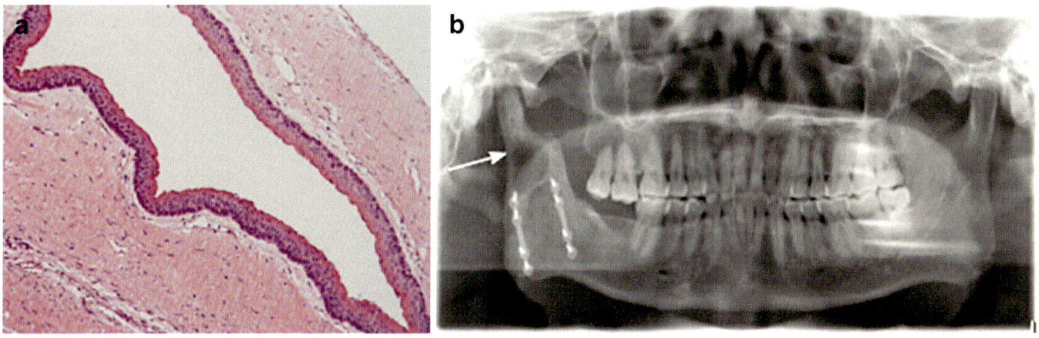

Fig. 6.12 (**a**) Stratified squamous epithelium with incomplete keratinization on the wall of fibrous connective tissue capsule, hyperchromatic cell nucleus of basal layer cells, away from the basement membrane, namely, reversed polarity and not obvious inflammation within the capsule wall (200×). (**b**) Internal fixation after operation of ascending ramus of the right mandible. High-density of metal was seen

[Follow-up visit] The patient recovered well after the operation. In the re-examination after the operation, the cysts were recurred, the shape of the mandible recovered well and the occluding relation was normal (Fig. 6.12b).

6.1.5 Case 19

The patient, male, 35 years old. The left mandible was swollen over half a month.

[Present medical history] About half a month before, the patient suffered from swelling and pain in the left mandible and saw a doctor in the local hospital. The pus was extracted in puncture and the panoramic radiographs showed: The low-density shadow was observed for multiple interatrial septum in the ascending ramus of the left mandible, and the lower mandibular edge was swollen. The CT examination showed a low-density lesion in the ascending ramus of the left mandible and the patient was diagnosed to suffer from the left mandibular tumor with infection. The anti-inflammatory symptomatic treatment was given (the specific medication was known). One week ago, the patient underwent "incision and drainage of intraoral abscess + 38 tooth extraction surgery" under general anesthesia. After the operation, the patient continued to receive the anti-inflammatory treatment and the swelling and pain were relieved.

[Specialized examination] There is facial asymmetry, the ascending ramus of the left mandible is distended, the surface skin is complete, the color and skin temperature are normal, there is no obvious ping-pong-like sensation when palpated and there is no tenderness. The mouth opening is restricted to about 2.0 cm. The occluding relation is normal, there is no loosening of teeth, the sclerotin is distended at the buccal side of the mandibular molar area, there is no obvious ping-pong-like sensation, there is no tenderness, there is no obvious protrusion for the lingual bone and there is no numbness for the lower lip (Fig. 6.13). No significantly abnormally enlarged lymph nodes have been found in the bilateral submaxilla and neck.

[Auxiliary examination]

1. Panoramic radiographs: The cystic density reduction area is observed in the left mandible body, dertrotheca and ascending ramus. The morphology is irregular with a relatively clear boundary. Its continuous spine and bone cortex are observed inside, no obvious periosteal reaction is found and no abnormal soft tissue mass is observed (Fig. 6.14a).
2. CT plain scan of the maxillofacial region: The low-density foci are observed in the ascending ramus of the left mandible, the local bone cortex is discontinuous and the surrounding soft tissue is swollen (Fig. 6.14b, c).

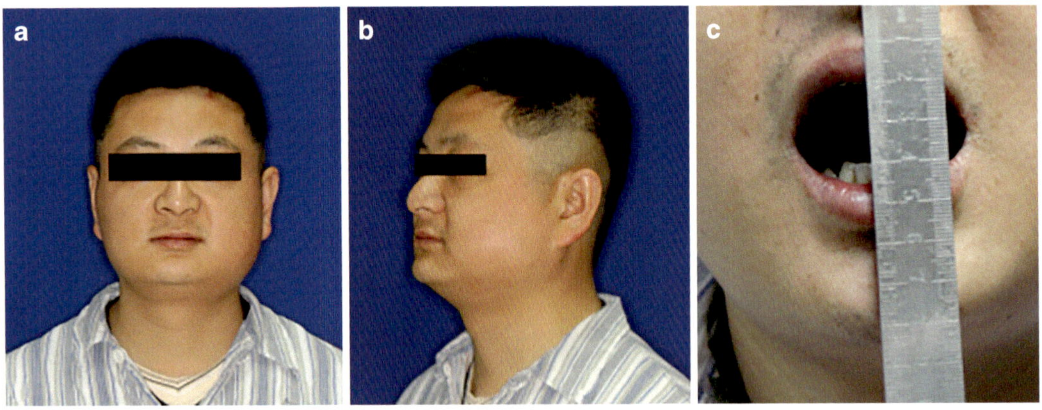

Fig. 6.13 (**a**, **b**) The facial form was asymmetrical and the left face was slightly swollen and distended. (**c**) The mouth opening was restricted to about 2.0 cm

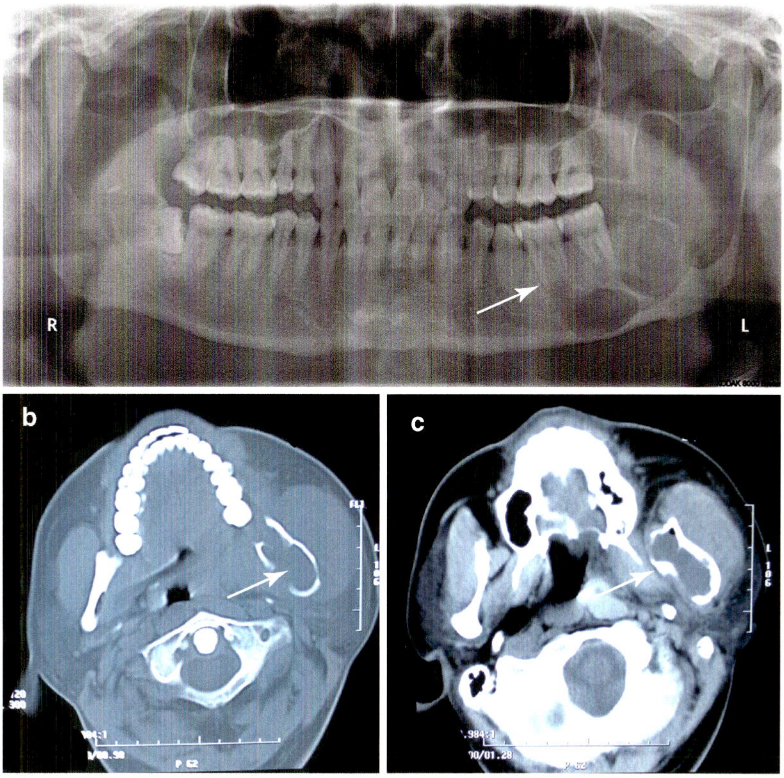

Fig. 6.14 (**a**) The cystic density reduction area was observed in the left mandible body, dertrotheca and ascending ramus, the morphology was irregular with relatively clear boundary. It was multilocular, the bone ridge was found, the bone cortex was continuous, no obvious periosteal reaction was observed and there was no abnormal soft tissue lump. (**b**, **c**) The low density foci were observed in ascending ramus of the left mandible, the local bone cortex was discontinuous and the surrounding soft tissues were swollen

[Primary diagnosis] Lump at the left mandible.

[Treatment] Under general anesthesia, "left lower jaw segmental resection + vascularized iliac muscle flap transfer repair" were performed: An incision was made at 1–2 cm along the inferior margin of the mandible, the flap was turned over to expose the mandible body and ascending ramus. The lump at the ramus of the mandible with bone destruction was observed, the condyle process and other mandibles was cut at the 35 distal segment, the lump was fully resected and the lump was submitted for freezing for pathological examination. indicated: Odontogenic keratocyst of "left mandible." The left vascularized iliac muscle flap was conventionally prepared, shaped, and reconstructed to recover the mandible continuity and occluding relation. The blood vessels anastomosed with the facial arteries and veins. The operation wound was rinsed, bleeding was stopped strictly, the negative pressure drainage tube was reserved, a suture was conducted in layers, and the wound was closed (Fig. 6.15).

[Pathological examination] For some tissues of the left mandible, its size was 9.5 cm * 3.7 cm * 1.9 cm and it was attached with two teeth above. The angle of the mandible and the ascending ramus showed expansive changes and its scope was about 3.4 cm * 2.6 cm * 1.7 cm. The local sclerotin was not continuous. The infiltrated fibrocyst-like tissues were found under the microscope, few inflammatory cells were infiltrated. There was laminated squamous epithelium with incomplete keratinization lining, the lining epithelium was thin, and the thickness was uniform. There were no epithelial spikes. The boundary was clear for the basal-layer cells, which were composed of columnar or cubic cells. The nuclei were deeply stained and far away from the Basement membrane in a palisade arrangement (Fig. 6.16).

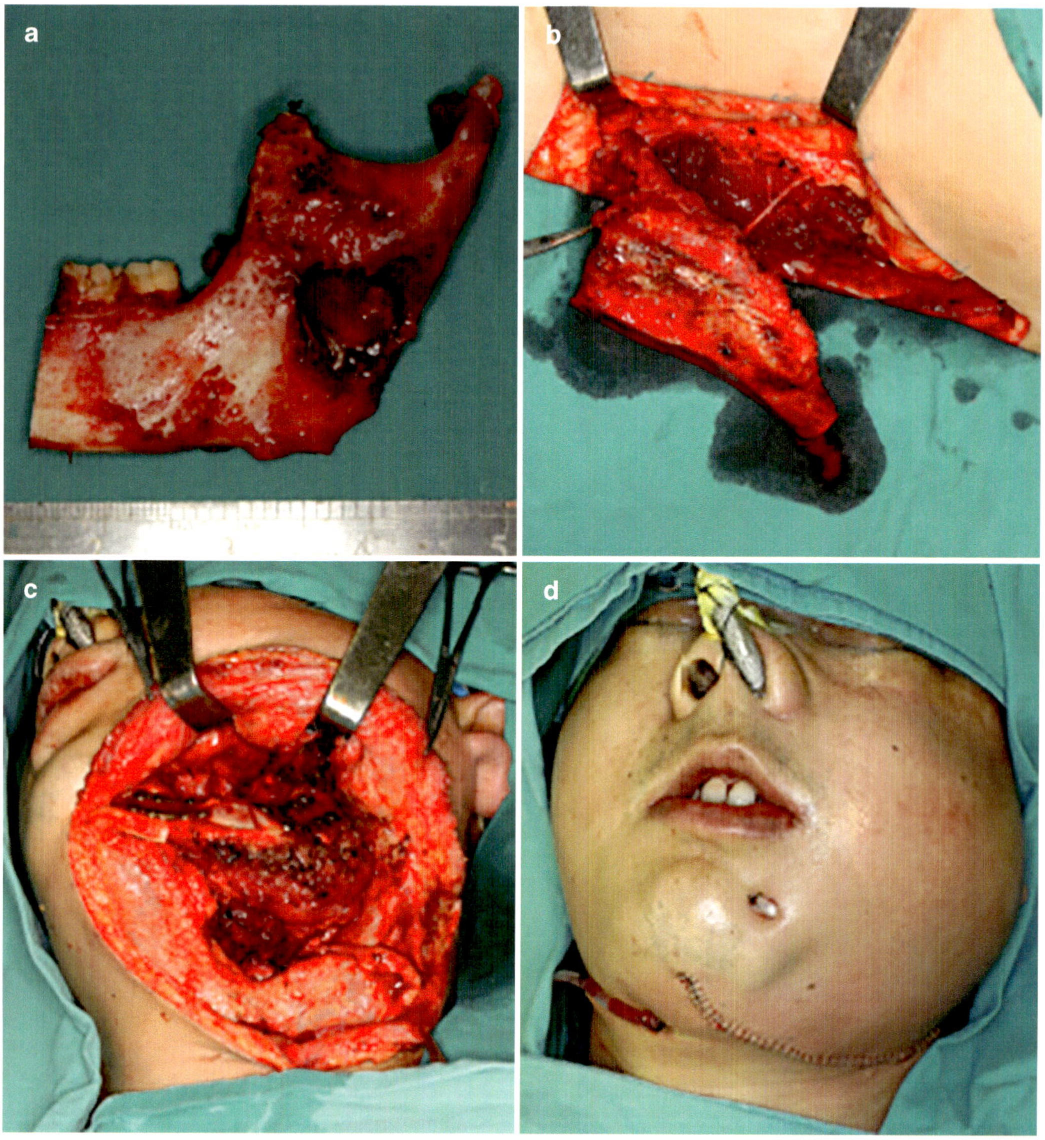

Fig. 6.15 (**a**) Segmental mandibulectomy with radical resection of the lesion was performed. (**b**) A vascularized iliac muscle flap was prepared. (**c**) The mandible continuity was reconstructed and recovered. (**d**) Observation after reconstruction surgery of the mandible

[Pathological diagnosis] Odontogenic keratocyst of "left mandible," ICD code: K09.002. It was locally accompanied by a secondary infection.

[Follow-up visit] The patient recovered well after the operation. In the follow-up visit after half a year, the cyst did not recur, the reconstructed shape of the mandible was satisfactory and restoring the occluding relation was good.

6.1.6 Case 20

The patient, female, aged 42, The image showed the multiple low-density shadow occupations of the maxilla and mandible over half an hour.

[Present medical history] The patient suffered from tooth pain without any cause and took the CT scans at the local dental clinic, which showed multiple low-density shadow occupations at the

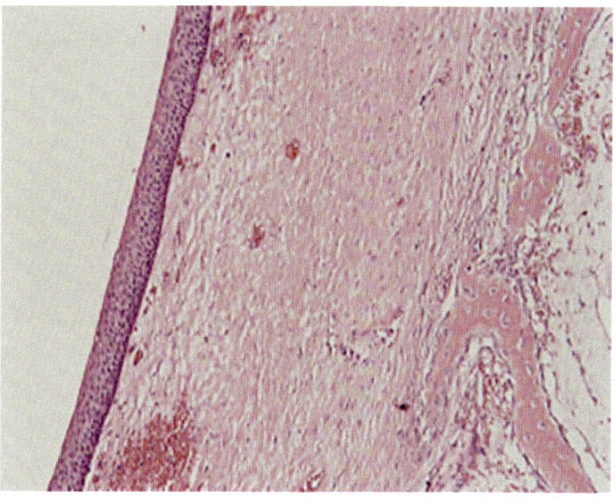

Fig. 6.16 The lining epithelium was a stratified squamous epithelium with incomplete keratinization, and the capsule wall was the fibrous connective tissue. There were abundant blood vessels and the inflammation was significant. The reactive proliferative bone tissues are shown as below (200×)

bilateral maxilla and mandible. It is suggested to undergo further examination and treatment in the superior hospital. The patient underwent the CT examination at the clinic 1 week before, which showed multiple space-occupied lesions at the bilateral maxilla and mandible. Odontogenic keratocyst with calcification in the skull base, consistent with naevoid basal cell carcinoma syndrome.

[Specialized examination] The facial proportions are coordinated and symmetrical on both sides. There is no deformity for the mouth and lip, and the mouth could be opened to a three-finger degree. Permanent dentition: 17 and 27 are lost, 16 has a residual root, 31 has a residual crown and 37 has a residual tooth root. The left mandible is slightly distended, the ping-pong sensation is perceived, and there is no pressing discomfort. The tongue body is centered with flexible movement. The oral mucosa was complete without ulceration.

[Auxiliary examination]

1. Panoramic radiographs: There are multiple low-density shadow occupations at the bilateral maxilla and mandible. The boundary is clear and the epiphyseal white line was found (Fig. 6.17).

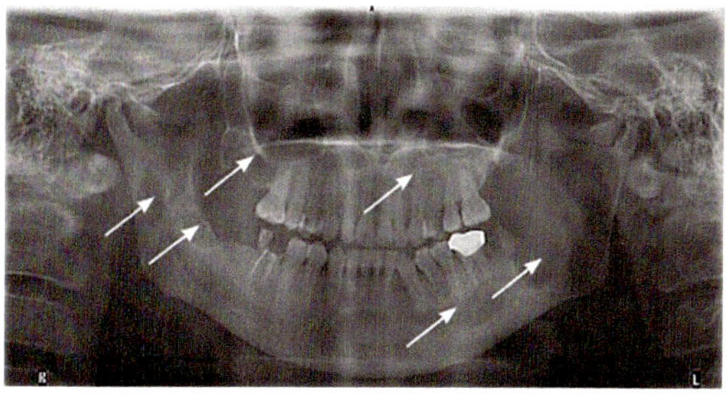

Fig. 6.17 There are multiple low-density shadow occupations at the bilateral maxilla and mandible; the boundary is clear and the epiphyseal white line is found (before operation)

2. CT enhanced scan of the maxillofacial region indicated multiple space-occupied lesions at the bilateral maxilla and mandible. Odontogenic keratocyst with calcification in the skull base, consistent with nevoid basal cell tumor syndrome (Fig. 6.18).

[Primary diagnosis] Multiple cysts at bilateral maxilla and mandible.

[Treatment] "Jaw cyst fenestration (bilateral maxilla and left mandible) + curettage (right mandible)" were performed under general anesthesia: A circular incision about 1.0 cm was taken from 32 to 33, the mucosa was cut and the cystic neoplasm was observed. Some capsule walls were taken for pathological examination, and a light yellow liquid in the lumen was observed. The sac fluid was aspirated, and the sac cavity was rinsed, the iodoform yarn bag was applied to wrap, and the wound was fixed; 37 was extracted, the alveolar bone was repaired, the mucosa and part of the cyst wall was resected, and sent for pathological examination; 46 was extracted, the alveolar bone was repaired, the cyst in the molar area of right mandible was scraped and the incision in place was sutured after stopping bleeding; The cystic neoplasm was handled at the bilateral maxilla, the lesion tissue was taken and sent for pathological examination. The findings showed consistent with odontogenic keratocyst. The iodoform oil yarn was used to wrap, suture and fix the wounds successively. The plug applicator was prepared after the operation with local rinsing. Regular follow-up visits shall be carried out.

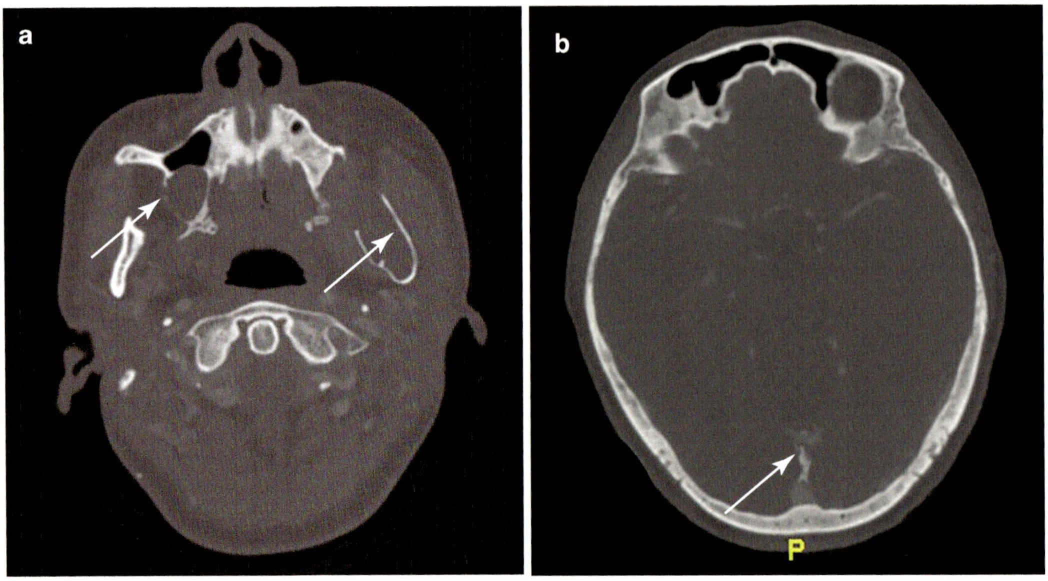

Fig. 6.18 (**a**) Cross-section of CT enhanced scan (bone window): There are multiple cystic low-density lesions at the bilateral maxilla and mandible. The morphology is less regular, the boundary is clear, and no obvious periosteal reaction or soft tissue mass is observed. (**b**) Calcified foci is found in intracranial cerebellar falx

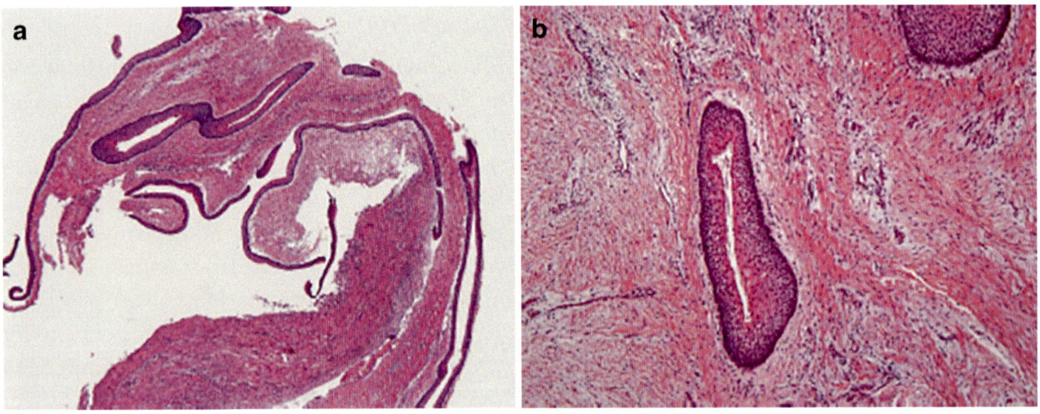

Fig. 6.19 (**a**) The lining epithelium referred to the keratinized stratified squamous epithelium, which was relatively thin without epithelial spikes and local detachment from the fibrous capsule wall (40×). (**b**) The submitted tissues in some regions were the significantly proliferated fibrous tissue, and a small amount of keratinized squamous epithelial mass was found inside, whose features were consistent with odontogenic keratocyst lining epithelium (100×)

[Pathological examination] Selected and submitted the broken tissues from 5 parts of the maxilla and mandible with its size of 0.6 cm * 0.3 cm * 0.3 cm, 1.5 cm * 1 cm * 0.5 cm and others. The infiltrated fibrocyst-like tissues were found under the microscope and it was lined with keratinized stratified squamous epithelium. Its surface was wavy and hyperkeratotic with a palisade-like arrangement of basal layer cells and inverted nuclear polarity. The junction between the lining epithelium and fibrocystic wall was flat (Fig. 6.19).

[Pathological diagnosis] The odontogenic keratocyst could be observed at the bilateral maxilla and mandible. In combination with the clinical imaging findings, it could be confirmed as the naevoid basal cell carcinoma syndrome.

[Follow-up visit] Maintained unobstructed drainage through open windows, strengthened local irrigation, and regularly followed up with panoramic radiographs to gradually reduce the lesion area.

6.1.7 Case 21

The patient, male, 57 years old. He suffered from the right mandibular keratocyst for 4 years and it recurred multiple times with carcinogenesis for 3 years.

[Present medical history] Four years ago, the patient was admitted to the local hospital for operation treatment due to a "right mandibular cystic mass." The pathology indicated the odontogenic keratocyst. The patient's face was swollen, the wounds were not cured, and the pus continued to discharge after the operation. After the multiple debridement and curettage surgeries, the patient did not improve well. Two years ago, the patient under the 4th surgery in the superior hospital, i.e., enlarged resection of the right mandible + repair with right fibular musculocutaneous flap + neck lymph node dissection. "After the operation, the postoperative pathology indicated: "Keratinocyst of right mandible" with local concertation (squamous carcinoma). There was continuous external drainage after the operation; the extraoral wound was cured. Within 2 years, the patient underwent surgical probing and debridement multiple times with recurrent discharge of pus on no surface. 2 months ago, the patient felt the neonatal tumor in the right oral cavity without obvious discomfort and underwent the smear of fistula discharge at the external hospital, which indicated that: squamous carcinoma. PET/CT findings: The sclerotin at the right skull base was destroyed, and the right submaxillary mass infiltrated into surrounding tissues; it was considered a malignant tumor recurrence. There were multiple lymph nodes in bilateral deep cervical space, posterior cervical space, submental and bilateral supraclavicular space, so it was possibly to be transferred. CT enhanced radioimages showed that postoperative changed of the right mandible (in referring to surgical history), neverthess the malignant lesion around the previous surgical flap had invaded the skull base, so do extedned into themandibular region, submandibular region, masticatory space, right temporal bone, the external auditory canal and middle ear with a possibility of the bilateral cervical lymph node metastasis. It was suggested that the MRI enhancement be undertaken to exclude the intracranial invasion. The biopsy of intraoral tumors in our hospital indicated there was severely abnormal hyperplasia in the mucosal squamous epithelium with the local tumor hyperplasia, so it was considered as carcinogenesis.

[Specialized examination] The facial form is not symmetric and the facial proportion is not coordinated. The lower right lip is tilted and there is a postoperative scar on the right jaw chin. The ascending ramus of the right mandible and the mandibular angle are absent, and the face is collapsed. One lump is observed in the right face, which is about 4 cm * 4 cm and is irregular. The skin surface is ulcerated and purulent, accompanied by a foul odor and a feeling of infiltration. Its mouth opening is about 1.5 cm, and one lump with a size of about 4 cm * 4 cm is observed in the right posterior buccal mucosa. Its hardness is close to normal tissue with a cauliflower-like surface. The postoperative changes in the biopsy are involved in the pterygomandibular ligament, soft palate and lower gingiva. The patient suffered from infiltration and tenderness. The extended tongue is centered, and the movement is appropriate. The multiple enlarged lymph nodes are palpated at the right submandibular region, neck and left mentum. The larger one is about 1.5 cm in diameter, and it was hard without obvious adhesion with tissues around it. The ROM is appropriate with tenderness (I) (Fig. 6.20a–d).

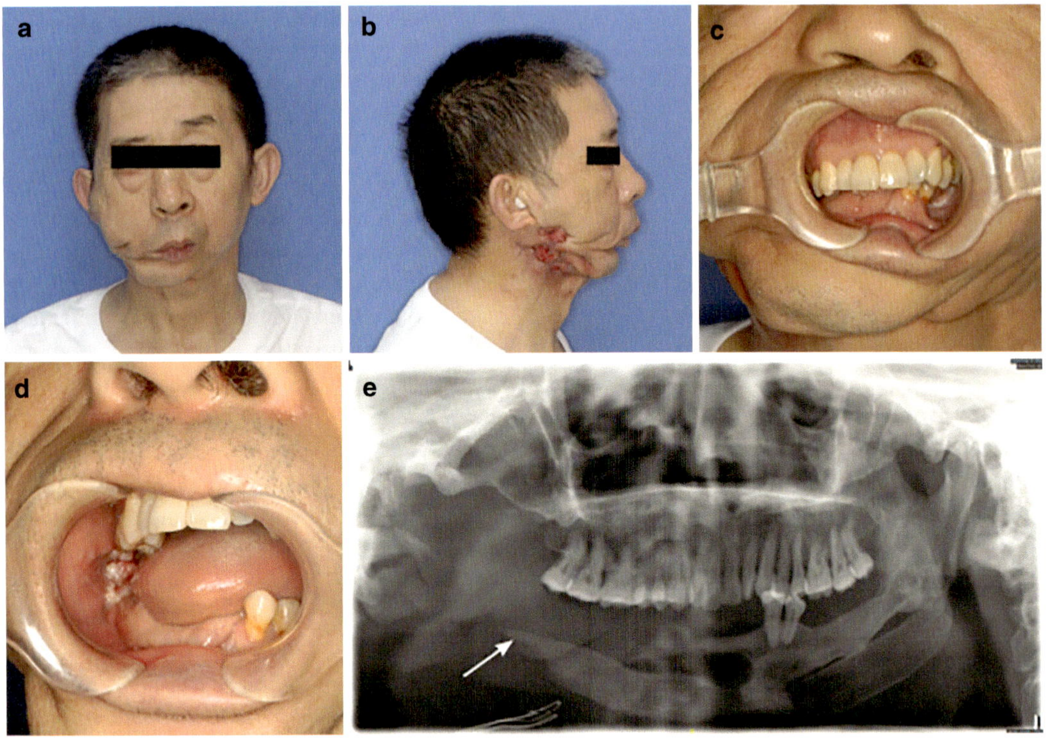

Fig. 6.20 (**a**, **b**) The facial form is asymmetrical, the facial proportion is incompatible, the right face is collapsed, and multiple cauliflower-like neoplasms are found in the facial and submandibular region. It is involved in the scope of about 4 cm * 4 cm; it is irregular and the surface skin is ulcerated with pus discharge. (**c**, **d**) The occlusion is disordered, the mouth opening is restricted, and the cauliflower-like neoplasm is observed in the right mandibular posterior teeth area and buccal mucosa. (**e**) The partial sclerotin and ascending ramuses are absent for the right mandible; the sclerotin is destroyed with the postoperative change of the left mandibular reconstruction surgery

[Auxiliary examination]

1. Panoramic radiographs: The partial sclerotin and ascending ramuses were absent for the right mandible. The sclerotin was destroyed with the postoperative change of the left mandibular reconstruction surgery (Fig. 6.20e).
2. CT enhanced scan of the maxillofacial region: "After the right mandible ossification cyst surgery," the tissues in the operative region are absent, and the soft tissue thickening is observed around the flap and at the right mandible, submandibular region, masticator space, right external auditory canal and the middle ear. The right jugular foramen area may be involved and the lesion boundary was unclear. The plain scan CT value is about 49 Hu and the enhanced CT value was about 78 Hu. The boundary is unclear, the morphology is irregular, the point-shaped gas shadow is observed inside, the adjacent skin is thickened and subcutaneous fat spaces become blurred. The sclerotin at the right mandibular stump is destroyed and the bone cortex is discontinuous. Multiple osteolytic bone destructions are observed in the right temporal bone, and the soft tissue ground-glass opacity is found inside and around. The superior bone cortex became thinner and discontinuous. It protruded to the temporal lobe's bottom and thickened the adjacent meninges. The lesion is involved in the right parapharyngeal space inward. The modular shadow, which is about 9 mm, is found in the mandible mentum with

a clear boundary. The plain scan CT value is about 60 Hu and the enhanced CT value is about 64 Hu. The multiple uneven enhanced lymph node shadows are found at the right deep upper, middle, and right posterior necks. The largest one is located on the left submentum, with a diameter of about 11 mm (Fig. 6.21).

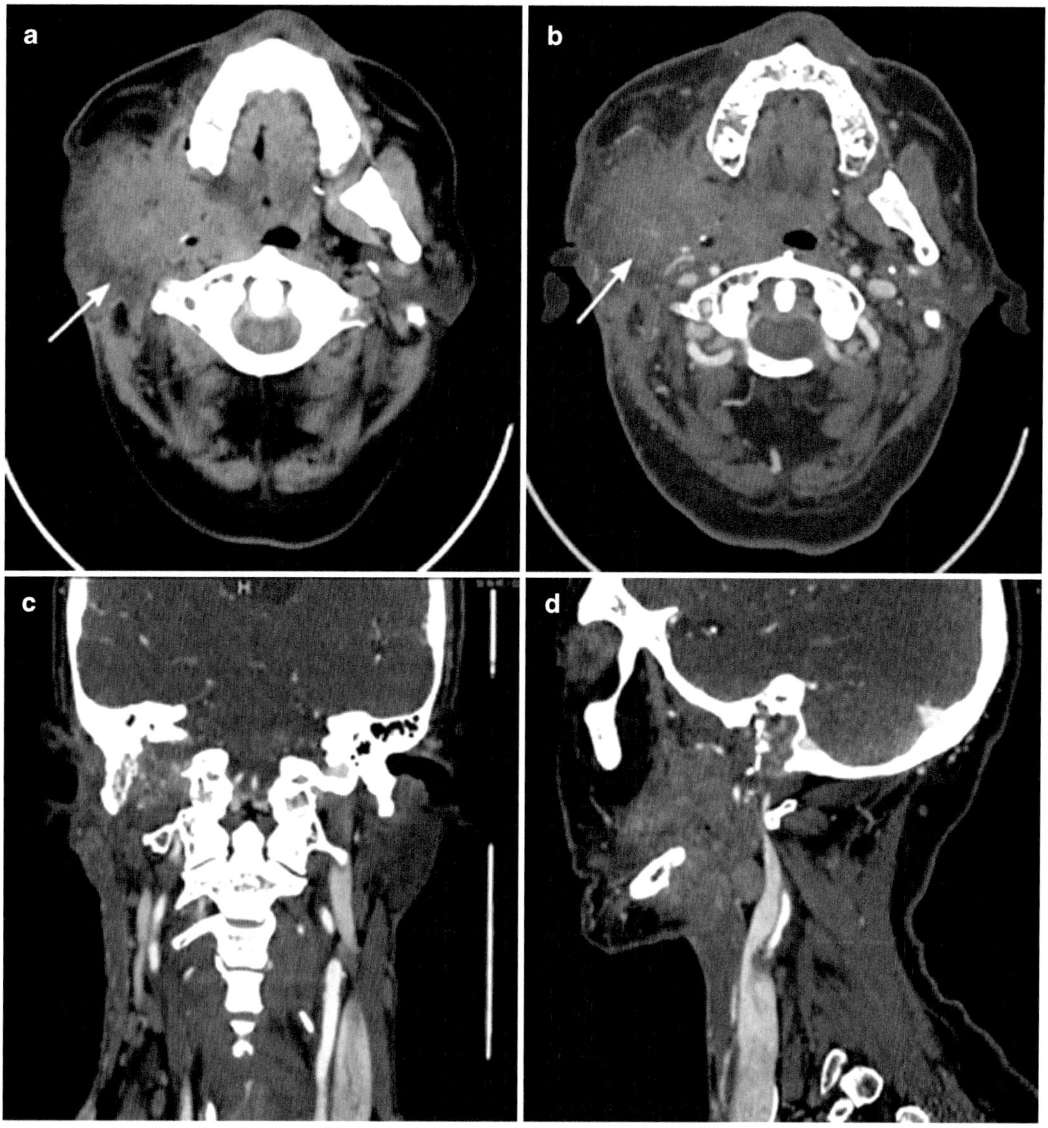

Fig. 6.21 (**a**) Cross section of CT plain scan: "After the right mandible ossification cyst surgery," the tissues in the operative region were absent, and the soft tissue thickening was observed around the flap and at the right mandible, submandibular region, masticator space, right external auditory canal and the middle ear. The lesion boundary was unclear, the morphology was irregular, the point-shaped gas shadow was observed inside and the CT value in scan plain was about 49 Hu. (**b**) Cross section of CT Enhanced Scan: The lesion was uneven and enhanced, and the CT value was 78 Hu. (**c**, **d**) Coronary view and sagittal view of CT enhanced scan: The sclerotin at the right mandibular stump was destroyed. Multiple osteolytic bone destructions were observed in the right temporal bone, and the soft tissue ground-glass opacity was found inside and around. The superior bone cortex became thinner and discontinuous. It protruded to the bottom of the temporal lobe and the adjacent meninges were thickened. The lesion involved in the right parapharyngeal space inward

3. PET/CT findings: The sclerotin at the right skull base is destroyed, the right submaxillary mass infiltrated in surrounding tissues, and it is considered a malignant tumor recurrence. There are multiple lymph nodes in bilateral deep cervical space, posterior cervical space, submental and bilateral supraclavicular space, so it is possible to be transferred.

[Primary diagnosis] Malignant transformation of odontogenic keratocyst in the right mandible accompanied by possible transfer of the lymphonodi cervicales.

[Treatment]

1. After further completing the MR examination, the patient complied with surgical indications after MDT discussion and evaluation in the hospital and underwent the "right skull base, jaw neck combined radical operation + anterolateral thigh flap repair + tracheotomy" under general anesthesia: Designed the incision 3 cm below the inferior margin of right mandible and designed the "T-shaped" incision at the neck, cut and turned the flap over to conduct the modified radical neck lymph node dissection on the right side and a lymph node dissection on the left scapular hyoid bone. Intercepted the mandible in the center, cut the right mandible, masseter muscle, parotid gland, pterygoid muscle and right facial skin tissue (reserved the right earlobe), including the lump, and submitted the intraoperative frozen pathology indicating that the submitted resection margins were negative (I). The dynamical system was applied to repair the skull base sclerotin, and the anterolateral thigh flap was prepared with a size of about 30 cm * 7 cm. To trim and shape the skin flap, the blood vessels anastomosed with the branches of the superior thyroid artery and the internal jugular vein, respectively, repair the tissue coloboma of the mandible, gingiva, mouth floor and facial skin. The operation wound was rinsed, bleeding was stopped completely, a negative pressure drainage tube was reserved, a suture was conducted in layers, and the wound was closed (Fig. 6.22).
2. Postoperative radiotherapy: ① Intensity-modulated radiation therapy: Skull base DT 66 Gy/30 Fx; ② operative region + right total neck lymphatic drainage area DT60 Gy/30 Fx.

[Pathological examination] What is submitted was particle mandible and surrounding tissue with its size of 13 cm * 11 cm * 6 cm. The surface was covered with skin and one gray-white lump was observed in the Chapter. Its size was 7 cm * 5 cm * 4.5 cm with an unclear boundary. There were squamous cell clusters with tumor-like proliferation in the background of fibrous tissues under the microscope, the cellular plasm was rich, and it was eosinophilic. The intercellular bridge could be found, the nucleus was vacuolate, the nucleolus was significant and the mitotic figure was visible. Formation of keratinized beads in the center of tumor nests (Fig. 6.23).

[Pathological diagnosis] Combined with the medical history, the lesion on the "right mandible" was observed, and it was considered to be the recurrence and malignant transformation of odontogenic keratocysts. It was squamous cell carcinoma grade I. ICD code: C41.101.

[Follow-up visit] The patient recovered well after the operation and received a re-examination half a year after the operation. There was tumor recurrence and no rupture and discharge of pus were found locally.

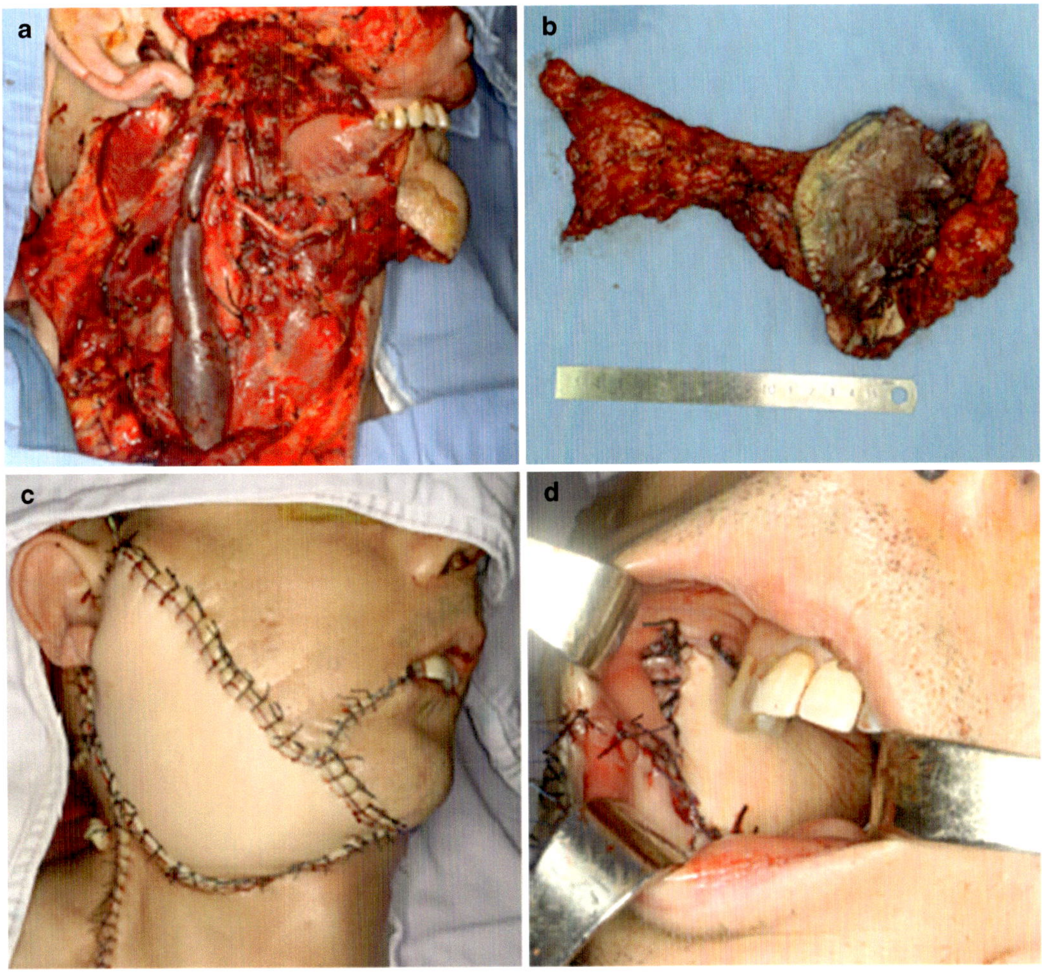

Fig. 6.22 (**a**) The lump was resected completely and the wound in the operative region was largely defected. (**b**) Overall view of detached right mandibular mass and surrounding affected tissue. (**c**, **d**) Prepared the flap at the anterolateral thigh with its size of about 30 cm * 8 cm and the skin paddle to repair the tissue coloboma inside and outside the mouth

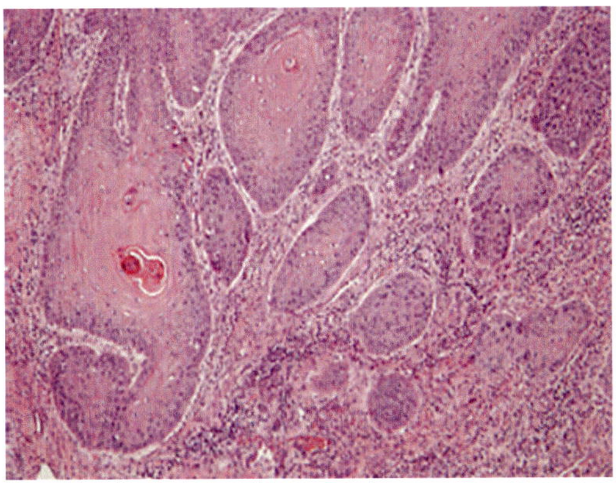

Fig. 6.23 There was invasive growth of squamous cell nests, and the keratin pearl was formed inside (100×)

6.2 Key Points of Diagnosis and Treatment

In 1956, Philipsen first described OKC for the first time and it was the benign odontogenic lesion that was prone to occur in the mandible [1–3]. Mitosis activity was higher than that of other odontogenic cysts, and it was classified by the WHO as a primordial cyst. Due to the histological characteristics and clinical Invasiveness, many lesions were associated with the mutation or inactivation of the tumor suppressor gene (also known as PTCH) in the 3rd version of the WHO

Classification of Head and Neck Tumors, so it was classified as the odontogenic tumor group and was named as keratocystic odontogenic tumor (KCOT). In the latest (version 4) WHO Classification of Head and Neck Tumors in Jan. 2017, there was no sufficient evidence to support the tumor origin, so OKC was re-classified as odontogenic cysts.

Clinical manifestation The OKC developed slowly. It generally had no subjective symptoms and grew along the long axis of the jaw. Sometimes, it develops into the buccal tongue and causes facial deformity. The secondary infection may occur, leading to the skin or mucous membrane rupture, pain, numbness or tissue swelling and other symptoms. In the later stage, if the cyst is too large, the palpable sheepskin-like cracking sound may be heard and pathological fractures may occur.

Pathological characteristics In the histopathology, it featured a thin layered squamous epithelial lining in OKC. It was composed of 5–10 cellular layers, its thickness was uniform, and there were epithelial spikes. The boundary of the basal cell layer was clear. It was cubic or columnar, with deeply colored nuclei arranged in a palisade-like manner. The spinous layer was relatively thin and the cells showed intracellular edema. The keratinization layer was often incomplete keratinization, and sometimes, different parts were keratinized differently. The fibrocyst-like tissues were relatively thin and it generally had no inflammatory infiltration. The skin paddle was observed in the capsule walls and it contained micro vesicles.

Imaging characteristics In iconography, OKC refers to the unilocular or multilocular radiative shadows with clear boundaries. The epiphyseal white line was observed, the root displacement was visible and the adjacent tooth root resorption was rare. OKC was diagnosed according to the medical history and the clinical manifestations and in combination with the radiological and histopathological examination. The differential diagnosis was carried out with other odontogenic cysts, such as dentigerous cysts, root cysts and ameloblastoma.

Treatment The appropriate therapeutic methods were selected according to the cyst size, surrounding bone condition, presence of secondary infection and adjacent tissue structure. The curettage, marsupialization or fenestration decompression and Osteotomy was available [7]. In recent years, the extensively-applied pouch surgery or fenestration decompression surgery had less trauma. In the case of the small lesions, the curettage was preferred. For large lesions, window decompression or selective curettage surgery was available. OKC's recurrence rate ranged from 0% to 62% and it generally occurred within 5 years, so the cyst should be carefully and completely removed and regularly followed up for examination.

References

1. Borghesi A, Nardi C, Giannitto C, et al. Odontogenic keratocyst: imaging features of a benign lesion with an aggressive behaviour [J]. Insights Imaging. 2018;9(5):883–97.
2. Aragaki T, Michi Y, Katsube K, et al. Comprehensive keratin profiling reveals different histopathogenesis of keratocystic odontogenic tumor and orthokeratinized odontogenic cyst [J]. Hum Pathol. 2010;41(12):1718–25.
3. Antonoglou G, Sándor G, Koidou V, et al. Non-syndromic and syndromic keratocystic odontogenic tumors: systematic review and meta-analysis of recurrences [J]. J Craniomaxillofac Surg. 2014;42(7):e364–71.
4. Kinard B, Hansen G, Newman M, et al. How well do we manage the odontogenic keratocyst? A multicenter study [J]. Oral Surg Oral Med Oral Pathol Oral Radiol. 2019;127(4):282–8.
5. Bilodeau E, Collins B. Odontogenic cysts and neoplasms [J]. Surg Pathol Clin. 2017;10(1):177–222.
6. Rajendra Santosh A. Odontogenic cysts [J]. Dent Clin N Am. 2020;64(1):105–19.
7. Zhao Y, Liu B. Clinical application of marsupialization device in mandibular cyst [J]. Chin J Pract Stomatol. 2020;13(10):577–81.

7 Glandular Odontogenic Cyst

Bing Liu, Hui Shan Ong, Zhen Tian, Lin Zhu, and Xiao Guang Li

7.1 Introduction

The glandular odontogenic cyst (GOC) is a relatively rare odontogenic cyst that is often involved in the mandible [1, 2]. It could be manifested as slow growth, painless and transparent cystic masses. In iconography, it was often manifested as a single or multi-locular radiative transparent shadow, which may be invasive. The onset age of adenoodontogenic cysts was relatively scattered, with no predilection of gender. The average onset age was 50 years old, and the recurrence rate was about 30% [3–6].

7.1.1 Case 22

The patient, male, 37 years old. In the X-ray examination, it was found that the low-density shadow of the left mandible was occupied for half a month.

[Present medical history] Half a month ago, the patient took an X-ray while filling teeth in an external hospital. It was found that the low-density shadow of the left mandible occupied the space, and one odontoid shadow was observed without obvious pain or discomfort.

[Specialized examination] The patient's face is symmetric. The degree and type of mouth opening are normal. In the intraoral permanent dentition, the maxilla is 7-7, 25 is the residual root. The mandible is 7-7 and 46 is the residual root. No obvious redness and swelling are found on gingiva and mucosa. No obvious abnormality is observed at the left mandibular molar posterior area.

[Auxiliary examination] Panoramic radiographs: The density-decreased area is found in the left mandible with an obscure boundary. The bone cortex is continuous, with no significant periosteal reaction (Fig. 7.1).

[Primary diagnosis] ① dentigerous cyst at the left mandible; ② 38, 48 impacted teeth; ③ 25, 46 residual root.

[Treatment] "curettage of left mandibular cyst +38, 48, 25, 46 tooth extraction" under general

B. Liu (✉)
Hospital of Stomatology Wuhan University, Hubei, China
e-mail: liubing9909@wuhan.edu.cn

H. S. Ong · Z. Tian · X. G. Li
Department of Oral Maxillofacial-Head & Neck Oncology, Shanghai Ninth People's Hospital, Shanghai Jiao Tong University School of Medicine, Shanghai, China

L. Zhu
Department of Radiology, Ninth People's Hospital Affiliated to Shanghai Jiao Tong University, Shanghai, China

Y. He (ed.), *Inflammatory and Neoplastic Diseases of Craniofacial Bones*,
https://doi.org/10.1007/978-981-97-4155-7_7

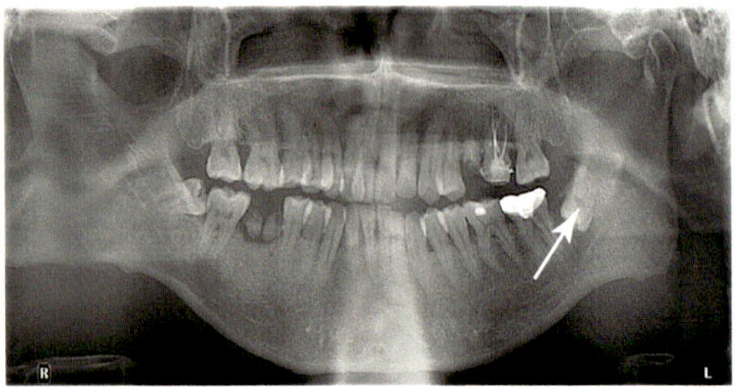

Fig. 7.1 The density-decreased area is found in the left mandible with the obscure boundary. The bone cortex is continuous and there is no significant periosteal reaction

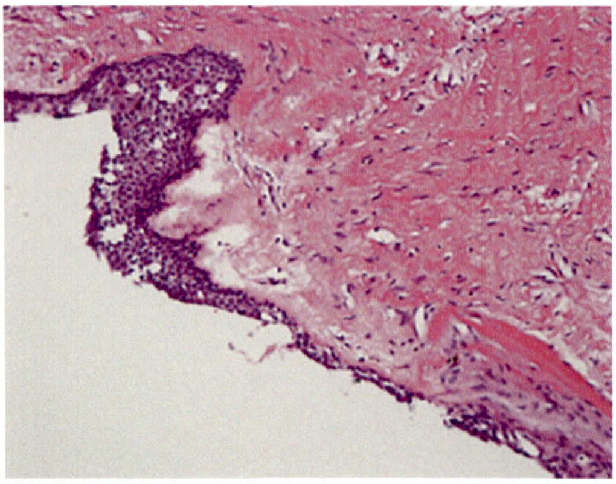

Fig. 7.2 The lining epithelium was locally thickened to form the epithelial spot. The glandular tubular structure was observed and the epithelial spikes were not significant (200×)

anesthesia: With 37 distal incisions, turned the flap to expose the cystic lump. The capsule wall surrounded 38 crowns, with 38 horizontal impactions. After a small amount of bone removal, 38 was removed, the cyst wall was completely peeled off, and a pathological biopsy was submitted. 48 was removed in the same method. The residual roots 25 and 46 were removed. Fully stopped bleeding, rinsed, and sutured the wounds.

[Pathological examination] One cystic tissue was submitted. Its size was 1.5 cm * 1 cm * 0.7 cm, grayish yellow. The fibrocystic-like tissues were observed under the microscope. It was lined with stratified squamous epithelium and ciliated columnar epithelium. The lining epithelium was not uniform in thickness, and the epithelial spikes were not significant. The surface cells were cubic or columnar, with an uneven surface and a papillary shape. The local patchy thickness was found in the lining epithelium, and the glandular tubular structure, which contained a small number of mucus cells, was seen. The proliferative odontogenic epithelial mass was observed in the fibrous cystic wall tissues, and a few inflammatory cells infiltrated them (Fig. 7.2).

[Pathological diagnosis] Glandular odontogenic cyst at the "left mandible," ICD code: K09.203.

[Follow-up visit] The operative region recovered well. The patient underwent the re-examination 3 months after the operation and there was no obvious abnormality in the operative region.

7.2 Key Points of Diagnosis and Treatment

In 1987, Paday Achee and van Wy first described the adenogenic odontogenic cyst as the "salivary odontogenic cyst." Later, Gardner et al. renamed it "Glandular Odontogenic Cyst (GOC)." Such a name has been accepted by WHO and is still applied to this day. GOC was a rare odontogenic cyst and it was featured as high recurrence and potential invasiveness. Its high recurrence was associated with sub-capsules, microcapsules and treatment methods [5–8].

Clinical characteristics The lesion was located in the jaws, and the onset was more likely to occur at the anterior part of the mandible. It was manifested as a painless mass with slow growth, a few of which were accompanied by pain, abnormal sensation, and other symptoms. It had no characteristic imaging manifestations and often consisted of single or multi-chamber transmission shadows. Sometimes, the bone destruction was found. In the histopathology, its manifestation was different from other cysts of the jaw, and it was lined with the layered squamous epithelium at varying thicknesses. The deep connective tissue presented a flat interface, and there was no inflammatory infiltration in the connective tissue. It was featured as the eosinophilic cubic cells forming the superficial layer of the epithelium and the presence of a pool of myxoamine-positive substances within the epithelium.

Diagnosis GOC's incidence rate was low and there were obvious characteristics in the clinical and X-ray manifestation, so the final diagnosis depended on the histological examination. Fowler et al. believed that 7 or more of the following 10 characteristics are met under the endoscopy, and it facilitated the diagnosis: Eosinophilic "spike" cells, metaplasia of sweat glands, intraepithelial microcapsules, variable thickness of epithelial lining, transparent cells in the basal layer, papillary protrusions, cilia, multiple cystic septa, epithelial plaque-like thickening and mucinous cells. According to the clinical and imaging manifestations, the differential diagnosis was carried out between GOC and Ameloblastoma, odontogenic myxoma, central giant cell Granuloma, odontogenic keratocyst and aneurysmal Bone cyst and metastatic jaw bone tumor. The histopathological characteristics of GOC were similar to those of other odontogenic cysts, such as paradental cysts, dentigerous cysts, and central mucoepidermoid carcinoma. Clinically, it was prone to misdiagnosis. No consensus is reached on how many histopathological characteristics are needed to confirm the glandular odontogenic cyst. It is necessary to understand the clear standard definition and specific markers that support a diagnosis to facilitate the diagnosis.

Treatment Clinically, the main therapeutic methods include removal, Carnoy liquid chemical cautery, edge or segmental resection, and the follow-up observation shall last at least 3 years. GOC is a rare odontogenic cyst. Clinically, it was manifested as strong invasiveness and a high recurrence rate. There is no typical specificity clinically and the misdiagnosis may occur, so it is necessary to conduct a precise histopathological examination clinically, which is important for the final diagnosis and long-term follow-up visit to remove the recurrence.

References

1. Jones A, Craig G, Franklin C. Range and demographics of odontogenic cysts diagnosed in a UK population over a 30-year period [J]. J Oral Pathol Med. 2006;35(8):500–7.
2. Fowler C, Brannon R, Kessler H, et al. Glandular odontogenic cyst: analysis of 46 cases with special emphasis on microscopic criteria for diagnosis [J]. Head Neck Pathol. 2011;5(4):364–75.
3. Kaplan I, Anavi Y, Hirshberg A. Glandular odontogenic cyst: a challenge in diagnosis and treatment [J]. Oral Dis. 2008;14(7):575–81.
4. Padayachee A, Van Wyk C. Two cystic lesions with features of both the botryoid odontogenic cyst and the central mucoepidermoid tumour: sialo-odontogenic cyst? [J]. J Oral Pathol. 1987;16(10):499–504.
5. Gardner D, Kessler H, Morency R, et al. The glandular odontogenic cyst: an apparent entity [J]. J Oral Pathol. 1988;17(8):359–66.
6. Chrcanovic B, Gomez R. Glandular odontogenic cyst: an updated analysis of 169 cases reported in the literature [J]. Oral Dis. 2018;24(5):717–24.
7. Martins-Chaves R, Granucci M, Gomez R, et al. Glandular odontogenic cyst-A case series [J]. J Oral Maxillofac Surg. 2020;79:1062–8.
8. Poudel P, Srii R, Chaurasia N, et al. Glandular odontogenic cyst-Report of a rare case [J]. Clin Case Reports. 2020;8(2):351–4.

8 Calcifying Odontogenic Cyst

Bing Liu, Hui Shan Ong, Zhen Tian, Lin Zhu, and Jian Feng Liang

8.1 Introduction

The calcifying odontogenic cyst (COC) refers to an odontogenic benign lesion, and it was first proposed by Gorlin in 1962 as an independent jaw cyst [1–6]. Its incidence rate accounts for less than 2% of total odontogenic cysts and tumors, and there is still controversy about their tissue origin: reduced enamel epithelium, residual dental plate epithelium and others. In the previous WHO classification, it was named a "calcifying cystic odontogenic tumor." In the new classification of head and neck solid tumors in 2017, WHO recovered its name to the calcifying odontogenic cyst. The patient's age peak ranges from 10 to 19 and there is no obvious gender difference. The predilection site is the maxillary premolar area, mostly observed in bone. Sometimes, it was found in the extraosseous soft tissue and was mainly seen in the soft tissue of the dental region. The most common clinical symptom is progressive, painless and facial asymmetric swelling, and it may be manifested as tongue protrusion, tooth displacement, tooth root absorption and cortical bone resorption. In the imaging, it is manifested as the single chamber radiolucent shadow with clear boundaries and sometimes shows the multilocular manifestation. There are some reports of cases where the cyst wall surrounds the neck of impacted canines and molars. Typical histologic findings: Epithelial structures similar to ameloblastoma and epithelial lining composed of shadow cells (calcified tendency) [7–11]. It may be accompanied by other odontogenic tumors, such as ameloblastoma, ameloblastoma Fibroma, odontogenic adenoid tumor, and odontogenic keratocyst. The most common one is odontoma. Most lesions are cystic changes, some cases present as solid lesions, and a few cases have a tendency toward malignancy. At present, there is no specific treatment guidance on COC. The cyst removal combined with scaling is the top priority for treatment. There was less postoperative recurrence, and there was no recurrence report for the peripheral type [12–18].

B. Liu (✉)
Hospital of Stomatology Wuhan University, Hubei, China
e-mail: liubing9909@wuhan.edu.cn

H. S. Ong · Z. Tian
Department of Oral Maxillofacial-Head & Neck Oncology, Shanghai Ninth People's Hospital, Shanghai Jiao Tong University School of Medicine, Shanghai, China

L. Zhu
Department of Radiology, Ninth People's Hospital Affiliated to Shanghai Jiao Tong University, Shanghai, China

J. F. Liang
Hospital of Stomatology, Guanghua College of Stomatology, Sun Yat-sen University, Guangdong, China

Y. He (ed.), *Inflammatory and Neoplastic Diseases of Craniofacial Bones*, https://doi.org/10.1007/978-981-97-4155-7_8

8.1.1 Case 23

The patient, female, aged 8, found a painless mass at the left mandible for 5 days.

[Present medical history] Five days ago, the patient underwent CT imaging of paranasal sinuses at the local hospital and one cystic low-density shadow was observed in the left mandible. Then, the patient underwent the CBCT of the maxillofacial region and one cystic lesion was found at the left mandible, which was adjacent to molars. The patient complained of no special pain, numbness of the lower lip and other obvious discomfort, so no measures were taken.

[Specialized examination] The maxillofacial region is asymmetric, the left mandible protrudes and there is mild palpable sclerotin swelling with its size about 2 cm. The cutaneous sensation is normal and the patient complains of no pain or numbness. The degree and type of mouth opening are normal, and mixed dentition is observed. 75 distal buccal bone is slightly distended, and the mucosa is complete without redness, swelling or exudation. The patient is not painful under compression. The neck was soft, and it was not involved in the swollen lymph node.

[Auxiliary examination]
Jaw CBCT: In 36 buccal mandibles, the cystic reduced bone density area, which is about 1.5 cm * 1.0 cm * 1.7 cm, could be observed with clear boundaries. There was no epiphyseal white line, and the buccal area was slightly distended. 84 residual root, 44 dental follicle was less continuous and no other obvious abnormality was found.

[Primary diagnosis] Cystic lesion in the left mandible.

[Treatment] Under general anesthesia, "scaling of cystic lesions of left mandible + tooth extraction" was performed: A gingival margin incision was made along the left mandible, followed by flap reflection. 75 was extracted, and the lesion was located at the root of 75 and 36, presenting a cystic structure. The cyst wall was completely cured. Frozen pathology in operation indicated "the left mandible" lesion complied with the calcifying odontogenic cyst. The wound was washed, the bleeding was stopped, and the wound was closed.

[Pathological examination] The specimen submitted for examination was a molar with a cystic mass attached to the root, and the cyst wall appeared thick. Fibrous cyst wall-like tissue lining with odontogenic stratified epithelium could be observed under the microscope, and circular calcifications and shadow cells were seen within the epithelium (Fig. 8.1).

[Pathological diagnosis] Calcifying odontogenic cyst at " left mandible," ICD—O code: 9301/0.

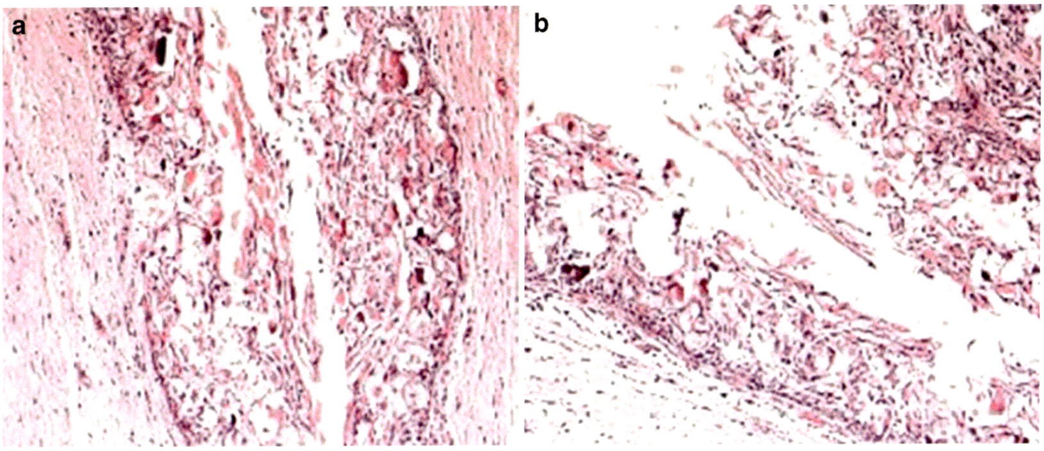

Fig. 8.1 (**a**) Fibrous cyst wall-like tissue lining with odontogenic stratified epithelium could be observed under the microscope. (**b**) Circular calcifications and shadow cells were seen within the epithelium

8.2 Key Points of Diagnosis and Treatment

Since its first report by Gorlin in 1962, the biological behavior of calcifying odontogenic cysts (COC) has been controversial due to the lack of clear understanding and recognition of its nature. Insufficient knowledge of etiology may affect clinicians' diagnosis and appropriate treatment of COC. Some scholars speculated that its pathogenesis may be associated with the downregulation of the Wnt/β-catenin signaling pathway. The transcription mediated by β-catenin/TGF played an important role in the occurrence of human cancer and may also be involved in the development of COC.

According to the latest classification of odontogenic tumors by the World Health Organization (WHO), COC was previously referred to as an odontogenic calcifying cystic tumor and has now been reclassified as a type of odontogenic cyst. Although COC was a benign lesion, which primarily occurred in the young population, delayed diagnosis and treatment could result in significant jaw bone defects, affecting facial aesthetics. In rare cases, COC could exhibit malignant transformation characterized by rapid growth and cortical bone resorption. Therefore, clinicians' proper understanding of COC will facilitate early diagnosis and treatment.

Diagnosis COC presented as a slowly growing painless facial swelling, often causing facial asymmetry, and there were usually no obvious subjective symptoms before, making early diagnosis and treatment challenging. The most diagnostically significant examination in clinical practice was X-ray imaging, with the most common imaging findings being well-defined unilocular (occasionally multilocular) radiolucent shadows, with a few cases showing radiopaque shadows and mixed images. Reports on CBCT examinations showed an impacted wisdom tooth on the right mandible, with small calcifications around the inferior alveolar nerve. The macroscopical appearance of the lesion: The soft tissue and mineralized white structures could be seen within the cystic cavity. HE staining revealed that the cyst wall was composed of columnar basal layer cells of varying thickness, with overlying stellate reticulum cells and calcified shadow cells. In COC coexisting with odontoma, dentin, dental pulp-like structures, cementum, and pericementum could be observed within the cyst. In cases associated with ameloblastoma, typical proliferative cell patterns could be seen.

Differential diagnosis Based on its clinical and pathological characteristics, it needed to be differentiated from the following diseases:

1. Dental sac: Cystic tissue surrounding an impacted tooth crown. Some scholars pointed out that all impacted teeth should be extracted, regardless of the presence or absence of disease symptoms, and histopathological examination of the dental sac around the crown should be routinely performed. The author reported two cases in which the imaging examination showed radiolucent shadows with a thickness of less than 2.5 mm in the crown circumference of an impacted wisdom tooth on the left mandible. Histopathological examination revealed typical shadow cells within the epithelium, consistent with the presentation of COC. Some other scholars proposed that the ratio of the thickness of the crown circumference tissue and the mesiodistal width of the impacted teeth could not be used as a diagnostic criterion, and Bcl-2 and Ki-67 should be tested to differentiate between normal tissues and proliferating cells.
2. Odontogenic Keratocyst (OKC): ① X-rays: Similar to COC, OKC often appeared as a unilocular radiographic image but could also presented as a multilocular lesion, with a clear border and an irregular shape, which was commonly found in the mandibular third molar region and mandibular ramus. It grew slowly and was usually asymptomatic in the early stages. ② Histological features: The cyst wall of OKC was lined by a thin fibrous capsule. The inner layer of the epithelium exhibited a non-keratinized corrugated surface and cylindrical cell basal layer. Some scholars proposed that in individual cases, COC may show incompletely keratinized epithelium on the cyst wall, leading to the designation of OKC-like COC. ③ Differential points: OKC mostly occurred in the mandibular angle and mandibular ramus, progressing along the longitudinal axis of the jaws. The multiple types belonged to the associated basal cell nevus syndrome.
3. Ameloblastoma (AM): ① Histologically: In some cases of COC, the cyst wall epithelium consisted of columnar basal cells and ameloblast-like epithelial cells, resembling ameloblastoma. The ameloblastoma typically occurs in the mandible in clinical presentation, with the mandible body and mandibular angle being the most common sites, and most cases presented as solid lesions. ② Typical imaging features of AM include: Early lesions appeared as honeycomb-like structures, later forming multilocular cystic shadows, with fewer unilocular lesions. Due to the multilocular nature and some degree of local infiltrative growth, the periphery of the cyst wall in ameloblastoma was often irregular, showing a crescent-shaped defect, and the root apices within the cyst were resorbed, presenting a serrated appearance. Based on the typical clinical features of ameloblastoma, it could be differentiated from COC.

Treatment Regarding the treatment of COC, there were currently no internationally unified standards. Traditional treatment methods involved a two-stage approach: Decompression surgery + complete cyst removal. This approach could effectively promote a reduction in lesion volume and sclerotin repair. Moreover, it could significantly reduce the recurrence rate and treatment costs. As the lesion volume decreased before the second surgery, repair and reconstruction were generally not required. The overall effect was favorable, with no reports of recurrence during a 5- to 10-year follow-up period after surgery. However, some scholars pointed out that for confirmed COC patients, the standard treatment strategy aimed at optimal prognosis should involve a combination of cyst removal surgery and scaling, followed by long-term postoperative follow-up. Recently, a new treatment strategy has been introduced by Castro-Núñez: ADDS (active decompression and distraction sugosteogenesis), which utilizes a novel device called the Evacuator, which resembles a vacuum cleaner, to provide negative pressure and induce bone formation. The results of the observation showed the application of ADDS could lead to a 50% reduction in lesion volume as early as 11 days postoperatively, along with reorganization of the epithelium and accelerated bone formation in the lesion area. However, in case reports, chronic inflammatory cell infiltration in the epithelium was observed after ADDS surgery, while the exact mechanism remained unknown.

In summary, the diagnosis of calcifying odontogenic cysts primarily relied on X-ray imaging, and the standard treatment approach involved decompression surgery + cyst removal. The overall effect was favorable, with rare cases of recurrence. However, further research on the etiology of COC required collaborative efforts from scholars to achieve a comprehensive understanding and enable early diagnosis and treatment.

References

1. Mahdavi N, Kardooni Khoozestani N, Hasheminasab M, et al. Hybrid odontogenic tumor of calcifying odontogenic cyst and ameloblastic fibroma: a case report and review of literature [J]. J Dent (Shiraz, Iran). 2020;21(2):153–7.
2. Sarode G, Sarode S, Prajapati G, et al. Calcifying cystic odontogenic tumor in radiologically normal dental follicular space of mandibular third molars: report of two cases [J]. Clin Pract. 2017;7(1):933.
3. Irani S, Foroughi F. Histologic variants of calcifying odontogenic cyst: a study of 52 cases [J]. J Contemp Dent Pract. 2017;18(8):688–94.
4. Speight P, Takata T. New tumour entities in the 4th edition of the World Health Organization Classification of Head and Neck tumours: odontogenic and maxillofacial bone tumours [J]. Virchows Arch. 2018;472(3):331–9.
5. Uzun T, Çinpolat E. Calcifying odontogenic cyst associated with the impacted third molar: a case report [J]. Pan Afr Med J. 2019;33:151.
6. Costa L, Neto J, de-Assis E, et al. Peripheral calcifying odontogenic cyst: a rare case report [J]. J Clin Exp Dent. 2018;10(11):e1140–4.
7. Santos H, de Morais E, Moreira D, et al. Calcifying odontogenic cyst with extensive areas of dentinoid: uncommon case report and update of main findings [J]. Case Rep Pathol. 2018;2018:8323215.
8. Ide F, Muramatsu T, Miyazaki Y, et al. Calcifying odontogenic cyst showing a varied epithelial lining: an additional case with implications for the divergent differentiation capacity of the cyst epithelium [J]. Head Neck Pathol. 2019;13(2):251–4.
9. de Moraes A, Soares H, Viana Pinheiro J, et al. Marsupialization before enucleation as a treatment strategy for a large calcifying odontogenic cyst: case report [J]. Int J Surg Case Rep. 2020;67:239–44.
10. Ahn S, Kim S, Kim S, et al. Beta-catenin gene alterations in a variety of so-called calcifying odontogenic cysts [J]. APMIS. 2008;116(3):206–11.
11. Sekine S, Sato S, Takata T, et al. Beta-catenin mutations are frequent in calcifying odontogenic cysts, but rare in ameloblastomas [J]. Am J Pathol. 2003;163(5):1707–12.
12. Polakis P. Wnt signaling in cancer [J]. Cold Spring Harb Perspect Biol. 2012;4(5):a008052.
13. Basile J, Klene C, Lin Y. Calcifying odontogenic cyst with odontogenic keratocyst: a case report and review of the literature [J]. Oral Surg Oral Med Oral Pathol Oral Radiol Endod. 2010;109(4):e40–5.
14. Haghanifar S, Moudi E, Seyedmajidi M, et al. Can the follicle-crown ratio of the impacted third molars be a reliable indicator of pathologic problem? [J]. J Dent (Shiraz, Iran). 2014;15(4):187–91.
15. Jiang W, Yang G, Chen F, et al. Disruption of Smad4 in odontoblasts and dental epithelial cells influences the phenotype of multiple keratocystic odontogenic tumors [J]. Biochem Biophys Res Commun. 2015;463(3):280–4.
16. Bilodeau E, Collins B. Odontogenic cysts and neoplasms [J]. Surg Pathol Clin. 2017;10(1):177–222.
17. Moreno-Rodríguez P, Guerrero L, Gómez-Delgado A, et al. Active decompression and distraction sugosteogenesis for the treatment of calcifying odontogenic cyst [J]. Oral Maxillofac Surg. 2021;25(1):89–97.
18. Zhang ZY, Yu GY. Oral maxillofacial surgery [M]. Beijing: People's Medical Publishing House; 2012.

9 Orthokeratinized Odontogenic Cyst

Bing Liu, Hui Shan Ong, Zhen Tian, Lin Zhu, and Shang Hui Zhou

9.1 Introduction

Orthokeratinized odontogenic cyst (OOC) is a relatively rare developmental cyst of odontogenic origin, accounting for approximately 1% of all odontogenic cysts. It predominantly occurs in the posterior region of the mandible, and literature reports suggest that OOC primarily affects individuals of white ethnicity aged 21–40 years. It is more common in males, with a ratio of incidence between males and females (2–2.59) to 1 [1–5]. OOC typically presents as an isolated, well-defined unilocular radiolucency in imaging examination, with approximately half of the cases exhibiting an association with an unerupted tooth. The cyst wall is composed entirely or predominantly of orthokeratinized stratified squamous epithelium in histology, accompanied by a prominent granular cell layer. No reports on the OOC related to the nevoid basal cell carcinoma syndrome have been found. Although OOC shares clinical and imaging similarities with odontogenic keratocyst (OKC), the differences in histological features and biological behavior could distinguish the two [4–8]. In accordance with literature reports, the recurrence rate of OOC was less than 2%. A close postoperative follow-up visit is still necessary.

9.1.1 Case 24

The patient, female, aged 36, 6 years after scaling of a maxillary bone cyst, recurrence was observed 4 years ago.

[Present medical history] Six years ago, the patient received "scaling of a cyst in the anterior maxillary region" at our hospital. Postoperative recovery was satisfactory, and the specific pathological diagnosis was unknown.

Four years ago, the patient returned to our hospital for a follow-up visit, which suggested the possibility of local recurrence and recommended surgery. The patient opted for observation. Over the past year, the patient has experienced obvious swelling and pain in the affected area. The patient went to the outpatient for CT examination, indicating that there was a cystic space occupying a lesion in the maxillary bone after surgery.

B. Liu (✉)
Hospital of Stomatology Wuhan University, Hubei, China
e-mail: liubing9909@wuhan.edu.cn

H. S. Ong · Z. Tian · S. H. Zhou
Department of Oral Maxillofacial-Head & Neck Oncology, Shanghai Ninth People's Hospital, Shanghai Jiao Tong University School of Medicine, Shanghai, China

L. Zhu
Department of Radiology, Ninth People's Hospital Affiliated to Shanghai Jiao Tong University, Shanghai, China

Y. He (ed.), *Inflammatory and Neoplastic Diseases of Craniofacial Bones*, https://doi.org/10.1007/978-981-97-4155-7_9

[Specialized examination] The patient's bilateral maxillofacial region is basically symmetric. The degree and type of mouth opening are normal. The permanent teeth in the maxillary anterior region (13–23) are missing, with significant sclerotin bulging on the root positions of the teeth on the buccal side in the corresponding area, extending upward to the nasal floor. The local sclerotin continuity is interrupted, while no significant palatal bulging is observed. The mucosa is intact, and there is no significant pyorrhea discharge.

[Auxiliary examination]

1. Panoramic radiographs: In the anterior maxillary region, there is a region of decreased density with irregular morphology, relatively clear borders, discontinuity of the bone cortex, and no significant periosteal reaction (Fig. 9.1a).
2. Maxillofacial CT plain scan: After the surgery of the maxilla, a circular area of sclerotin destruction is seen in the middle part of the maxilla, measuring approximately 1.8 cm * 1.3 cm. C-measured at 23 Hounsfield units (HU), and no significant abnormalities are observed in the surrounding soft tissues (Fig. 9.1b, c).

[Primary diagnosis] Recurrence of a maxillary bone cyst after previous surgery.

[Treatment] Under general anesthesia, "excision of the maxillary bone cyst" was performed: An incision was made on the gingiva near the central incisors (teeth 13–23), and a flap was reflected to expose the bone surface. The cyst was observed protruding beyond the bone surface, with local sclerotin loss. The local sclerotin was removed, and the lesion was completely excised. Upon incision, the cyst was found to be filled with keratinous material. Frozen section analysis indicated that there was a benign cystic lesion in the "maxillary bone," lined by orthokeratinized stratified squamous epithelium, suggesting a pos-

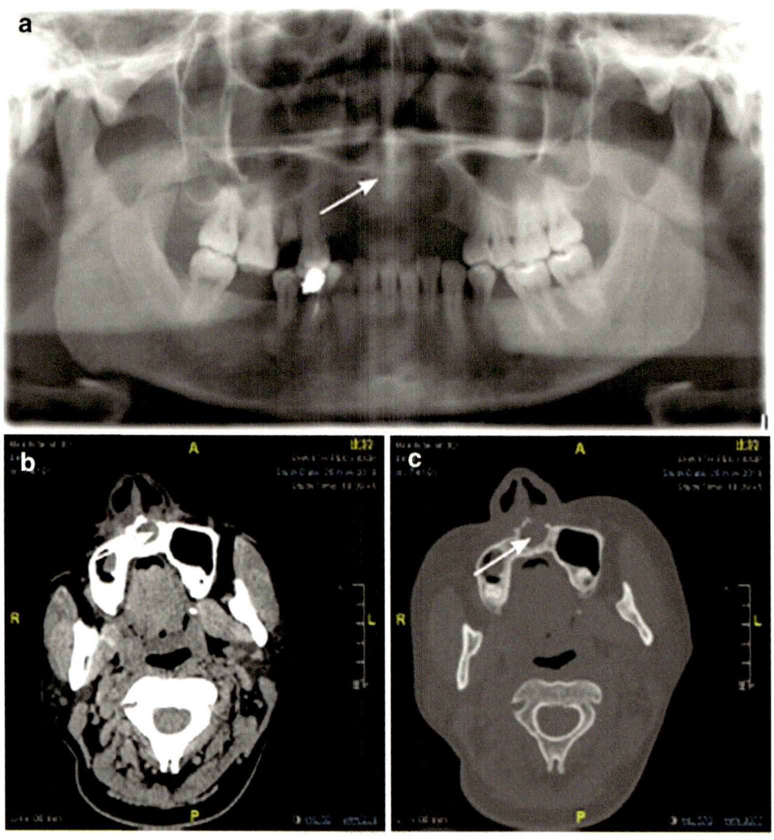

Fig. 9.1 (**a**) The region of decreased density with irregular morphology, relatively clear borders, discontinuity of the bone cortex, and no evident periosteal reaction was observed in the anterior maxillary region. (**b**, **c**) Cystic low-density lesion with expansile changes, regular morphology, relatively clear borders, discontinuity of the bone cortex, and no evident periosteal reaction or soft tissue mass was observed in the anterior maxillary region (preoperative)

sibility of orthokeratinized odontogenic cyst or odontogenic keratocyst, and pending formalin-fixed paraffin-embedded pathology. Irrigation, hemostasis, and placement of iodoform gauze strip were performed, followed by gingival apposition suture.

[Pathological examination] The specimen received for examination was a cystic tissue measuring 2.7 cm * 1.9 cm * 0.5 cm, with a gritty and grayish-white content. Microscopic examination revealed proliferative fibrous cystic wall-like tissue lined by stratified squamous epithelium. The lining epithelium was relatively thin, with surface orthokeratinization resembling the appearance of onion skin. The granular layer was evident within the epithelium, and the junction between the epithelium and connective tissue was flat, without epithelial pegs. The basal layer cells showed no polarity inversion and exhibited a palisaded arrangement. The cyst cavity contained numerous concentrically arranged keratinized materials. There was no infiltration of inflammatory cells in the cyst wall tissue (Fig. 9.2a).

[Pathological diagnosis] Orthokeratinized odontogenic cyst (OOC) of the "maxilla," ICD code: K09.005.

[Follow-up visit] The patient had a satisfactory postoperative recovery. At the 6-month follow-up, there was no recurrence of the cyst (Fig. 9.2b).

9.1.2 Key Points of Diagnosis and Treatment

OOC was first described as a dermoid cyst by Schultz in 1927 and later recognized as a variant type of OKC in 1981. It was first included in the fourth edition of the new classification of head and neck tumors in 2017 by the WHO. The diversity in classification and nomenclature reflected the unclear understanding of its pathogenesis.

Pathogenesis Since the emergence of OOC, researchers have been continuously exploring its pathogenesis. The current research findings could be summarized as follows:

1. The proliferative potential and self-renewal ability of the lining epithelial cells in OOC were inferior to those in OKC, and there were significant differences in the fibrous components of the cystic wall between the two entities, which may account for their different biological behaviors.
2. PTCH was a tumor suppressor gene closely associated with the SHH signaling pathway, which played a crucial role in embryonic development. Previous studies showed frequent PTCH loss of heterozygosity (LOH) in odontogenic cysts and tumors such as calcifying odontogenic cysts, odontogenic keratocyst, ameloblastoma, dentigerous cysts, and periapical cysts [9–13].

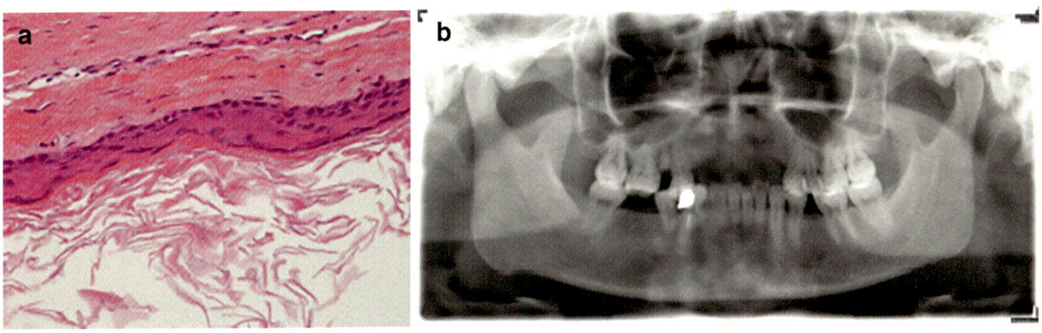

Fig. 9.2 (**a**) The lining epithelium showed an excessive Orthokeratinized stratified squamous epithelium with an obvious granular layer. The basal layer cells showed no polarity inversion and exhibited a palisaded arrangement, and the junction between the epithelium and connective tissue was flat, without epithelial pegs (400×). (**b**) Postoperative change occurred in the anterior maxillary region with an increase in bone density

3. BRAFV600E mutation was occasionally observed in OOC [13].
4. Downregulation of P73 and TRAIL expression.

Diagnosis OOC predominantly occurred in the diaphysis of the mandible, but there were literature reports of OOC occurring in the mandible condyle of a 41-year-old male. Initially, he was diagnosed with temporomandibular joint disorder (TMD) based on clinical symptoms, but imaging examination revealed osteolysis of the right condylar head. After condylectomy, a histopathological examination of the specimen suggested OOC. Imaging findings typically showed isolated, unilocular radiolucent lesions with clear borders, occasionally with multiple lesions. Literature reports have also indicated an association between OOC and impacted teeth. Typical histological features included an onion skin-like keratinized layer, a prominent granular cell layer beneath the keratinized layer, and a flat basal cell layer arranged by low cuboidal cells.

Differential Diagnosis The main differential diagnosis for OOC is with OKC, with the following key points: OKC consisted of a uniform, corrugated, incompletely keratinized lining epithelium, while the basal cell layer of OOC consisted of low cuboidal cells arranged in a flatter manner. In OKC, there was high expression of Ki-67, Bcl-2, and P63, while the expression levels were lower in OOC, indicating lower proliferative potential and higher apoptotic index. There was no evidence linking multiple OOC cases to nevoid basal cell carcinoma syndrome. Additionally, differentiation from dentigerous cysts should be considered.

Treatment The current treatment approach for OOC primarily involved enucleation of the cyst + peripheral bone resection. The choice of treatment should be based on a comprehensive evaluation of factors such as cyst size, infection status, etc. Different treatment methods may include cyst enucleation, cyst enucleation + scaling, marsupialization + cyst enucleation, and cyst enucleation + peripheral bone resection. A long-term close follow-up visit, regular imaging, and clinical examinations were necessary postoperatively.

References

1. Jain K, Bodhankar K, Desai R, et al. Absence of BRAFV600E immunohistochemical expression in sporadic odontogenic keratocyst, syndromic odontogenic keratocyst and orthokeratinized odontogenic cyst [J]. J Oral Pathol Med. 2020;49(10):1061–7.
2. Chien C, Wu Y, Kuo Y, et al. Orthokeratinized odontogenic cyst in the right maxilla [J]. J Formos Med Assoc. 2019;118(9):1375–7.
3. Carvalho C, Aquino A, Nonaka C, et al. Infected orthokeratinized odontogenic cyst: a rare cause of facial cellulitis [J]. Braz Dent J. 2012;23(5):612–6.
4. Li T, Kitano M, Chen X, et al. Orthokeratinized odontogenic cyst: a clinicopathological and immunocytochemical study of 15 cases [J]. Histopathology. 1998;32(3):242–51.
5. Dong Q, Pan S, Sun L, et al. Orthokeratinized odontogenic cyst: a clinicopathologic study of 61 cases [J]. Arch Pathol Lab Med. 2010;134(2):271–5.
6. Speight P, Takata T. New tumour entities in the 4th edition of the World Health Organization Classification of Head and Neck tumours: odontogenic and maxillofacial bone tumours [J]. Virchows Arch. 2018;472(3):331–9.
7. Managutti A, Managutti S, Patel H, et al. Orthokeratinized odontogenic cyst (OOC) of condylar head: a rare entity [J]. J Maxillofac Oral Surg. 2016;15:315–9.
8. Crane H, Da Forno P, Kyriakidou E, et al. Multiple orthokeratinized odontogenic cysts: a report of two cases and review of the literature [J]. Head Neck Pathol. 2020;14(2):381–5.
9. Diniz M, Galvão C, Macedo P, et al. Evidence of loss of heterozygosity of the PTCH gene in orthokeratinized odontogenic cyst [J]. J Oral Pathol Med. 2011;40(3):277–80.
10. Peacock Z, Cox D, Schmidt B. Involvement of PTCH1 mutations in the calcifying epithelial odontogenic tumor [J]. Oral Oncol. 2010;46(5):387–92.
11. Vered M, Peleg O, Taicher S, et al. The immunoprofile of odontogenic keratocyst (keratocystic odontogenic tumor) that includes expression of PTCH, SMO, GLI – 1 and bcl – 2 is similar to ameloblastoma but different from odontogenic cysts [J]. J Oral Pathol Med. 2009;38(7):597–604.
12. Mascitti M, Santarelli A, Zizzi A, et al. Expression of p73 and TRAIL in odontogenic cysts and tumors [J]. J Oral Sci. 2016;58(4):459–64.
13. Rangiani A, Motahhary P. Evaluation of bax and bcl – 2 expression in odontogenic keratocysts and orthokeratinized odontogenic cysts: a comparison of two cysts [J]. Oral Oncol. 2009;45(7):e41–4.

10 Nasopalatine Duct Cyst

Bing Liu, Hui Shan Ong, Zhen Tian,
Lin Zhu, and Shang Hui Zhou

10.1 Introduction

Nasopalatine duct cyst (NPDC), also known as incisive couldal cyst, was the maxilla's most common non-odontogenic developmental cyst. It originates from the remnants of the nasopalatine duct epithelium, which could spontaneously activate during the individual's lifespan or be stimulated by various factors such as infection. NPDC occurred most frequently between the ages of 4 and 60, with a slightly higher prevalence in males than females [1, 2]. The cysts typically occurred near the midline of the anterior maxilla, which were often asymptomatic, and a definitive diagnosis should be based on clinical, imaging, and histopathological examinations [3, 4]. The surgical removal of the cystic tissue was the primary treatment approach.

B. Liu (✉)
Hospital of Stomatology Wuhan University, Hubei, China
e-mail: liubing9909@wuhan.edu.cn

H. S. Ong · Z. Tian · S. H. Zhou
Department of Oral Maxillofacial-Head & Neck Oncology, Shanghai Ninth People's Hospital, Shanghai Jiao Tong University School of Medicine, Shanghai, China

L. Zhu
Department of Radiology, Ninth People's Hospital Affiliated to Shanghai Jiao Tong University, Shanghai, China

10.1.1 Case 25

The patient, male, 31 years old. Swelling in the anterior maxillary region for over a month.

[Present Medical History] The patient experienced anterior tooth pain without an apparent cause over a month ago. The pain was notably aggravated by cold stimuli. Swelling was observed 2 days later, and the pain improved with loose anterior teeth. The patient denied any other discomfort and sought medical attention at another hospital, where a cyst (to be confirmed) was suspected. After receiving anti-inflammatory treatment, there was no significant improvement, and the swelling has slightly increased. Further questioning revealed that the patient had occasional anterior tooth pain for the past 2 years, which did not improve with anti-inflammatory treatment and resolved spontaneously. He denied a medical history of swelling.

[Specialized examination] The maxillofacial region is symmetrical on both sides, and the proportion of the upper, middle and lower 1/3 is coordinated. A slight elevation of the upper lip is observed, with normal mouth opening and jaw movements. A soft, fluctuant mass is palpable in the upper anterior teeth region (teeth 13–22). Bulging is also noted on the buccal and palatal sides. There is no significant upper anterior teeth mobility, percussion (−) tenderness, mucosal

Y. He (ed.), *Inflammatory and Neoplastic Diseases of Craniofacial Bones*,
https://doi.org/10.1007/978-981-97-4155-7_10

ulceration or pyorrhea. No obvious swollen lymph nodes are seen in submandibular regions and neck.

[Auxiliary examination]
Panoramic radiographs: A cystic low-density area with a regular shape and clear boundary is observed in the hard palate. The bone cortex is continuous, and no periosteal reaction is observed (Fig. 10.1a).

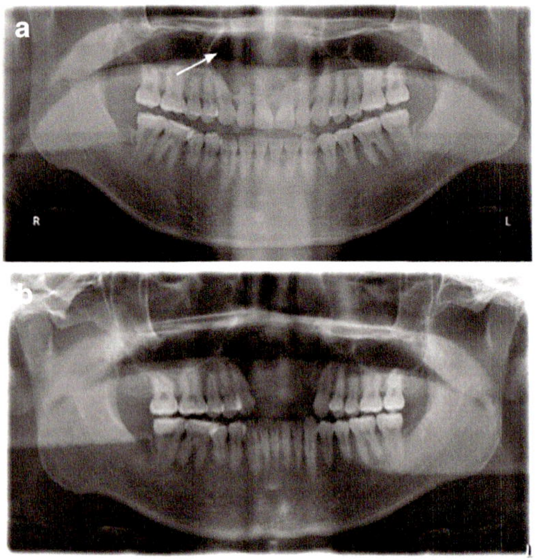

Fig. 10.1 (**a**) Preoperative panoramic images showed a cystic low-density area (arrow) with a regular shape and clear boundary was observed in the maxilla. The bony cortex was continuous, and no periosteal reaction was observed. (**b**) After the surgery on the hard palate, there were partial sclerotin defects with multiple small dot-like high-density shadows

[Primary diagnosis] Swelling in the anterior maxillary region (possible cyst).

[Treatment] Under general anesthesia, "excision of the maxillary bone cyst of anterior teeth area" was performed: An incision was made on the gingiva near the central incisors (teeth 15–24), and a trapezoidal flap was reflected to expose the bone surface. A cystic mass with local sclerotin loss was observed, and the cyst wall protruded beyond the bone surface. The local sclerotin was removed, and the cyst was completely cured. Frozen pathology in operation indicated: The lesion in the "maxilla" was consistent with a nasopalatine cyst. Irrigation, hemostasis, and placement of iodoform gauze strip were performed, followed by gingival apposition suture.

[Pathological examination] The submitted specimen was fragmented cystic wall-like tissue. Microscopic examination revealed a fibrous cystic wall lined by stratified squamous epithelium and pseudostratified ciliated columnar epithelium with goblet cells. There was minimal infiltration of inflammatory cells within the cystic wall (Fig. 10.2).

[Pathological diagnosis] The combined imaging findings of the "maxilla" were consistent with a nasopalatine duct cyst. ICD code: K09.202. [Follow-up visit] The patient had a satisfactory postoperative recovery. At the six-month follow-up, there was no recurrence of the cyst (Fig. 10.1b).

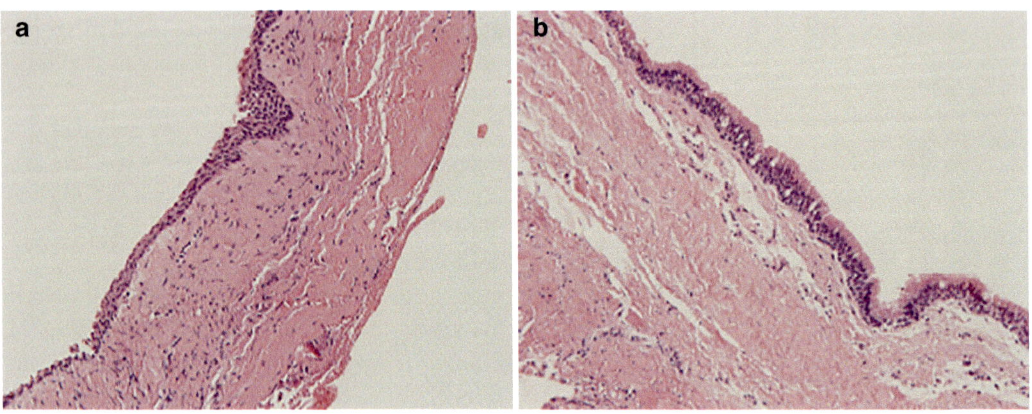

Fig. 10.2 (**a**) The cyst was located near the oral side, and the lining epithelium of the cyst wall was composed of stratified squamous epithelium. Mild inflammation was observed in the cyst wall (200×). (**b**) The cyst was located near the nasal side, and the lining epithelium of the cyst wall was composed of pseudostratified ciliated columnar epithelium with goblet cells. Mild inflammation was observed in the cyst wall (200×)

10.2 Key Points of Diagnosis and Treatment

A nasopalatine cyst (NPDC), first described by Meyer in 1914, was the most common developmental, non-neoplastic, non-odontogenic cyst of the oral cavity, with an incidence rate of approximately 1%. They were believed to originate from remnants of the paired embryonic nasopalatine ducts. It could occur at any age but was more commonly seen in patients aged 30–60. The pathogenesis typically involved progressive regression; however, residual epithelial cells may give rise to NPDC, either by spontaneous proliferation of epithelial cells or as a result of trauma (e.g., removable dentures) or bacterial infection. Genetic factors have also been proposed [1–3].

Diagnosis These cysts were generally asymptomatic and could be detected on routine X-rays. The most common symptoms included swelling, drainage, and pain in the anterior palate. There were a few large cysts that could cause "transillumination" fluctuation, affecting the anterior palate and lip mucosa. If the cyst is close to the surface, the swelling may exhibit a bluish fluctuation. Deep-seated cysts were covered by normal mucosa unless ulceration occurred. Compression of the nasopalatine nerve may cause burning and numbness. Intermittent fluid discharge with a salty taste could occur occasionally. Tooth displacement was rare.

X-ray findings showed circular or oval radiolucent areas between the roots of the central incisors. A heart-shaped appearance could be observed due to the overlap of the nasal spine. Most lesions had well-defined sclerotic borders.

NPDC was composed of stratified squamous epithelium alone or in combination with pseudostratified columnar epithelium (with or without cilia and/or goblet cells), simple columnar epithelium, and simple cuboidal epithelium in histology. The cyst wall typically contains nerves, arteries, and veins. Additionally, salivary gland parenchyma and small islands of cartilage could also be observed. Inflammation reactions ranging from mild to severe were often observed.

Differential diagnosis Differential diagnoses included odontogenic cysts (such as radicular cysts, odontogenic keratocysts), odontogenic tumors (such as ameloblastoma, odontogenic myxoma), and non-odontogenic tumors (such as central giant cell tumor, central hemangioma).

Treatment Squamous cell carcinoma originating from the maxilla was mainly due to metaplasia of the cystic epithelial lining or remnants of epithelial components involved in tooth formation [4]. Therefore, cases of squamous cell carcinoma arising from NPDC in the maxilla have been reported. The standard surgical approach was to completely remove the cyst, with generally low recurrence rates.

References

1. Elliott K, Franzese C, Pitman K. Diagnosis and surgical management of nasopalatine duct cysts [J]. Laryngoscope. 2004;114(8):1336–40.
2. Escoda Francolí J, Almendros Marqués N, Berini Aytés L, et al. Nasopalatine duct cyst: report of 22 cases and review of the literature [J]. Med Oral Patol Oral Cir Bucal. 2008;13(7):E438–43.
3. Gnanasekhar J, Walvekar S, al-Kandari A, et al. Misdiagnosis and mismanagement of a nasopalatine duct cyst and its corrective therapy. A case report [J]. Oral Surg Oral Med Oral Pathol Oral Radiol Endod. 1995;80(4):465–70.
4. Takagi R, Ohashi Y, Suzuki M. Squamous cell carcinoma in the maxilla probably originating from a nasopalatine duct cyst: report of case [J]. J Oral Maxillofac Surg. 1996;54(1):112–5.

Part III

Odontogenic Cysts of Inflammatory Origin

11 Radicular Cyst

Bing Liu, Hui Shan Ong, Zhen Tian, Lin Zhu, and Bing Guo

11.1 Introduction

Radicular cyst is the most common cyst in the jaw, accounting for 7%~54% of all permanent dentition cysts. Most radicular cysts have no obvious clinical symptoms, and most are accidentally found during radiological examinations for other reasons. Radicular cysts originate from the hyperplasia of the Hertwig epithelial root sheath (also known as Malassez-ERM epithelial cells) [1–3]. There are inflammation, migration and infiltration of inflammatory cells, such as leukocytes and monocytes, so it is suggested that caries may be the most important cause of this disease. In the case of symptomatic inflammation in the pulp of deciduous teeth, endodontic therapy shall be used as much as possible to preserve teeth, preferably until they are naturally replaced by permanent teeth. Complications of this treatment may include cyst formation, delayed absorption of deciduous teeth or permanent enamel coloboma [4, 5]. Developing cysts can lead to permanent tooth germ displacement, eruption disorder and even partial destruction. The developing cyst is not easy to detect and can reach a considerable size. The general method of operation is complete cyst wall excision.

11.2 Case 26

The patient, female, 68 years old. The right upper posterior teeth area was swollen and painful for more than 2 months.

[Present Medical History] The patient had no obvious cause of swelling and discomfort in the upper right posterior teeth area for more than 2 months ago, and the X-ray film taken in the other hospital found a cystic space-occupying lesion shadow of the upper right maxilla.

[Specialized Examination] The patient's bilateral maxillofacial region is basically symmetric. The degree and type of mouth opening are normal. Intraoral permanent dentition, 14 root changes after canal treatment, probing (−), knocking (+), loosening (−), there was no local orificium fistulae, no obvious bone swelling on the right maxilla, and there was slight tenderness in 14 buccal mandibles No obvious swollen lymph nodes are seen in bilateral submandibular regions and neck.

B. Liu (✉)
Hospital of Stomatology Wuhan University, Wuhan, Hubei, China
e-mail: liubing9909@wuhan.edu.cn

H. S. Ong · Z. Tian · L. Zhu · B. Guo
Department of Oral Maxillofacial-Head & Neck Oncology, Shanghai Ninth People's Hospital, Shanghai Jiao Tong University School of Medicine, Shanghai, China

Y. He (ed.), *Inflammatory and Neoplastic Diseases of Craniofacial Bones*, https://doi.org/10.1007/978-981-97-4155-7_11

[Auxiliary Examination]
Panoramic radiographs: The suspected hypodensity area of the right maxilla is blurred, the continuity of the bone cortex is acceptable, and no periosteal reaction is found. The alveolar bone absorption of the maxilla and mandible is obvious, and the local bone absorption exceeds 2/3 of the root (Fig. 11.1).

[Primary Diagnosis] ① Radicular cyst of the right maxilla; ② Chronic periodontitis.

[Treatment] "Right maxilla cyst extraction + tooth extraction" were performed under general anesthesia; local bones of 14 were ground and removed by the dynamic system, and the cyst of 14 root was completely removed. The removed part was sent for frozen pathology during the operation. Indicated: Inflammatory fibrous capsule wall-like tissue of the "right maxilla," with a layer of stratified squamous epithelium attached to one side and infiltration of histiocytes. After the bleeding was stopped completely, an apposition suture was conducted for the mucosa.

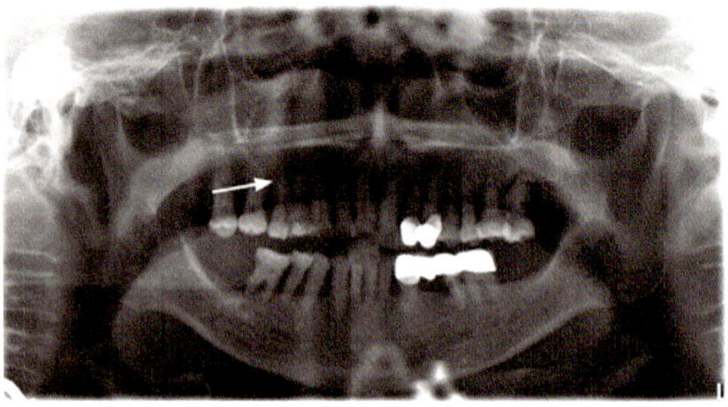

Fig. 11.1 The suspected hypodensity area of the right maxilla is blurred, the continuity of the bone cortex is acceptable, and no periosteal reaction is found. The alveolar bone absorption of the maxilla and mandible is obvious, and the local bone absorption exceeds 2/3 of the root

[Pathological Examination] Two broken tissues were sent for biopsy, 0.5 cm*0.5 cm*0.5 cm in size, grayish yellow. Microscopically, cyst wall-like granulation tissue hyperplasia was seen, a large number of histiocytes and inflammatory cells infiltrated in the cyst wall, and the cyst wall was lined with proliferating stratified squamous epithelium (Fig. 11.2).

[Pathological Diagnosis] radicular cyst of "right maxilla," ICD code: K04.802.

[Follow-Up Visit] The patient recovered well after the operation, there was nothing special, and the cyst did not recur after half a year.

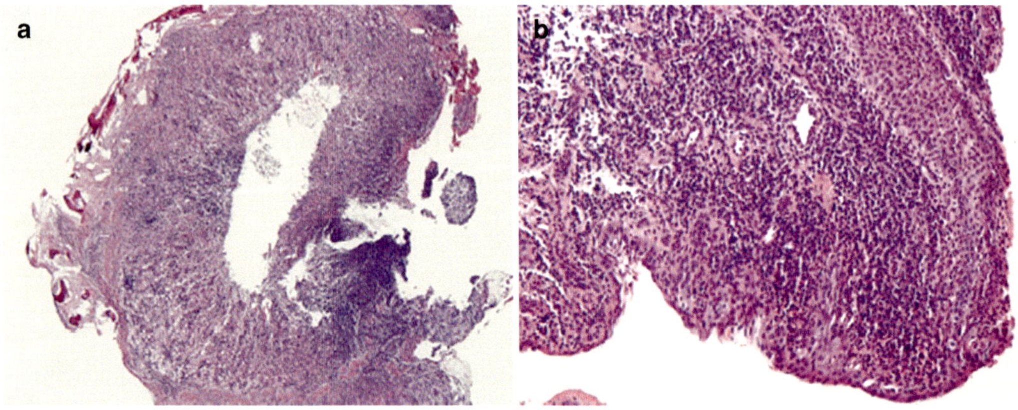

Fig. 11.2 (**a**) Under the low-power microscope, a cystic cavity-like structure surrounded by inflammatory granulation tissue is seen, with a thick wall and peripheral fibrous tissue (40×). (**b**) The cyst wall is lined with hyperplastic stratified squamous epithelium, and a large number of lymphocytes, neutrophils and plasma cells infiltration in the cyst wall, and small blood vessels hyperplasia, with severe inflammation (200×)

11.3 Key Points of Diagnosis and Treatment

Radicular cysts are usually associated with dental caries and lifeless or broken teeth. Generally speaking, the development of radicular cysts is gradual and asymptomatic, and finally, it shows displacement and dislocation of adjacent teeth or bone destruction. Early diagnosis shall be conducted for this kind of pathological damage to ensure proper treatment, which is extremely important for protecting the normal growth of jaws and teeth. A radicular cyst is an inflammatory odontogenic cyst. X-ray shows that the apical part of the tooth is a circular or elliptical unilocular transmission shadow with a radiopaque edge, and fuzzy sclerotic focus can be seen in the cyst with high growth dynamics. A radicular cyst is round or oval, and its edge is sclerosing. In a cyst with high growth kinetics, the fuzzy edge can be seen, and it can be round or oval. The differential diagnosis of radicular cyst shall include ameloblastoma, odontogenic keratocyst, odontogenic fibroma, and odontogenic myxoma. Histologically, the radicular cyst is lined with layered squamous epithelium. The capsule wall is composed of dense fibrous connective tissue, and inflammatory infiltration contains lymphocytes, neutrophils, plasma cells and histiocytes. Although radicular cysts are common, multilocular radicular cysts are not common, and radicular cysts with tooth structures have not been reported. It sometimes develops in the deciduous teeth area. The incidence of radicular cysts in deciduous teeth is very low (0.5%~3.3%), caused by the natural process of deciduous teeth falling off. [1–3] If the lesions are found early, conservative treatment can be used, which is very important for young patients. Therefore, periapical films shall be taken regularly, and the disease shall be diagnosed early to avoid adverse effects on permanent teeth.

References

1. Mahesh BS, Shastry SP, Murthy PS, et al. Role of cone beam computed tomography in evaluation of radicular cyst mimicking dentigerous cyst in a 7-year-old child: a case report and literature review [J]. International. J Clin Pediatr Dent. 2017;10(2):213–6.
2. Toomarian L, Moshref M, Mirkarimi M, et al. Radicular cyst associated with a primary first molar: a case report [J]. J Dent (Tehran, Iran). 2011;8(4):213–7.
3. Spin-Neto R, Wenzel A. Patient movement and motion artefacts in cone beam computed tomography of the dentomaxillofacial region: a systematic literature review [J]. Oral Surg Oral Med Oral Pathol Oral Radiol. 2016;121(4):425–33.
4. Johnson N, Gannon O, Savage N, et al. Frequency of odontogenic cysts and tumors: a systematic review [J]. J Investig Clin Dent. 2014;5(1):9–14.
5. Joshi N, Sujan S, Rachappa M. An unusual case report of bilateral mandibular radicular cysts [J]. Contemp Clin Dent. 2011;2(1):59–62.

Inflammatory Collateral Cysts 12

Bing Liu, Hui Shan Ong, Zhen Tian, Lin Zhu,
and Xiao Mei Zhao

12.1 Introduction

Inflammatory collateral cysts refer to odontogenic cysts of inflammatory origin occurring on the lateral surface of roots (usually mandibular molar) and related to inflammatory reactions, less common than periapical cysts, which are also inflammatory odontogenic cysts. Some scholars call these cysts paradental cysts, mandibular infection cysts, inflammatory adnexal cysts and inflammatory pseudocysts [1].

12.2 Case 27

The patient, male, 20 years old. In the X-ray examination, it was found that the low-density shadow of the left mandible was occupied for two weeks.

B. Liu (✉)
Hospital of Stomatology Wuhan University,
Wuhan, Hubei, China
e-mail: liubing9909@wuhan.edu.cn

H. S. Ong · Z. Tian · X. M. Zhao
Department of Oral Maxillofacial-Head &
Neck Oncology, Shanghai Ninth People's Hospital,
Shanghai Jiao Tong University School of Medicine,
Shanghai, China

L. Zhu
Department of Radiology, Ninth People's Hospital
Affiliated to Shanghai Jiao Tong University,
Shanghai, China

[Present Medical History] Two weeks ago, when the patient was undergoing dental treatment in our hospital, panoramic radiographs found a low-density space-occupying lesion shadow on the left mandible. The patient denied a history of swelling and pain, bleeding and trauma and was transferred to our department for CBCT examination. 35, 36 root had low-density space-occupying lesion shadow.

[Specialized Examination] The patient's bilateral maxillofacial region is basically symmetric. The degree and type of mouth opening are normal. Oral permanent dentition, oral hygiene is acceptable, tooth 46 is defective, teeth 35 and 36 are intact, loose (−), 35 has discomfort for percussion, 36 is knocked (−), and the gingival mucosa has no obvious swelling or no obvious exudation.

[Auxiliary Examination]

1. Panoramic radiographs: The cystic low-density lesions near roots 35 and 36 have a round shape, clear boundary and continuous bone cortex (Figure 12.1).
2. CBCT: A cystic low-density focus is found near roots 35 and 36, with a round shape, clear boundary and continuous bone cortex, and no periosteal reaction or soft tissue mass is found (Figure 12.2).

   [Primary diagnosis] Cyst at the left mandible.

Y. He (ed.), *Inflammatory and Neoplastic Diseases of Craniofacial Bones*,
https://doi.org/10.1007/978-981-97-4155-7_12

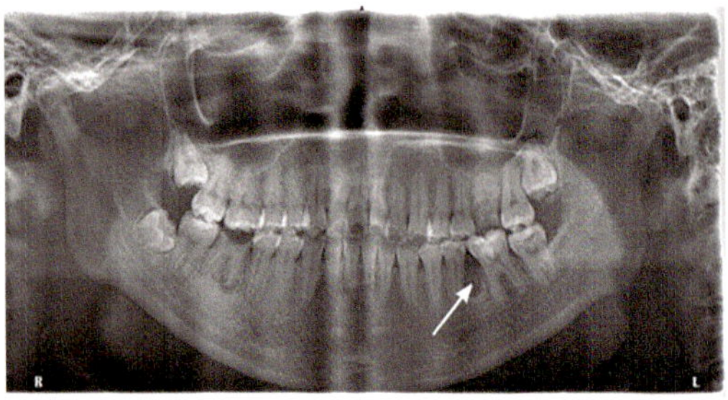

Figure 12.1 There is a cystic low-density lesion near roots 35 and 36, with a round shape, clear boundary and continuous bone cortex

[Treatment] "Left mandibular cyst extraction" was performed under local anesthesia: Combined with CBCT, the lesion involved the distal surface of root 35. Root 35 was removed, and the cyst wall was completely scraped and sent for pathological examination. The alveolar bone was trimmed, bleeding was stopped, and a suture was performed.

[Pathological Examination] A cystic wall-like broken tissue was sent for pathological examination, 1.5 cm*1 cm*0.7 cm in size, grayish yellow.

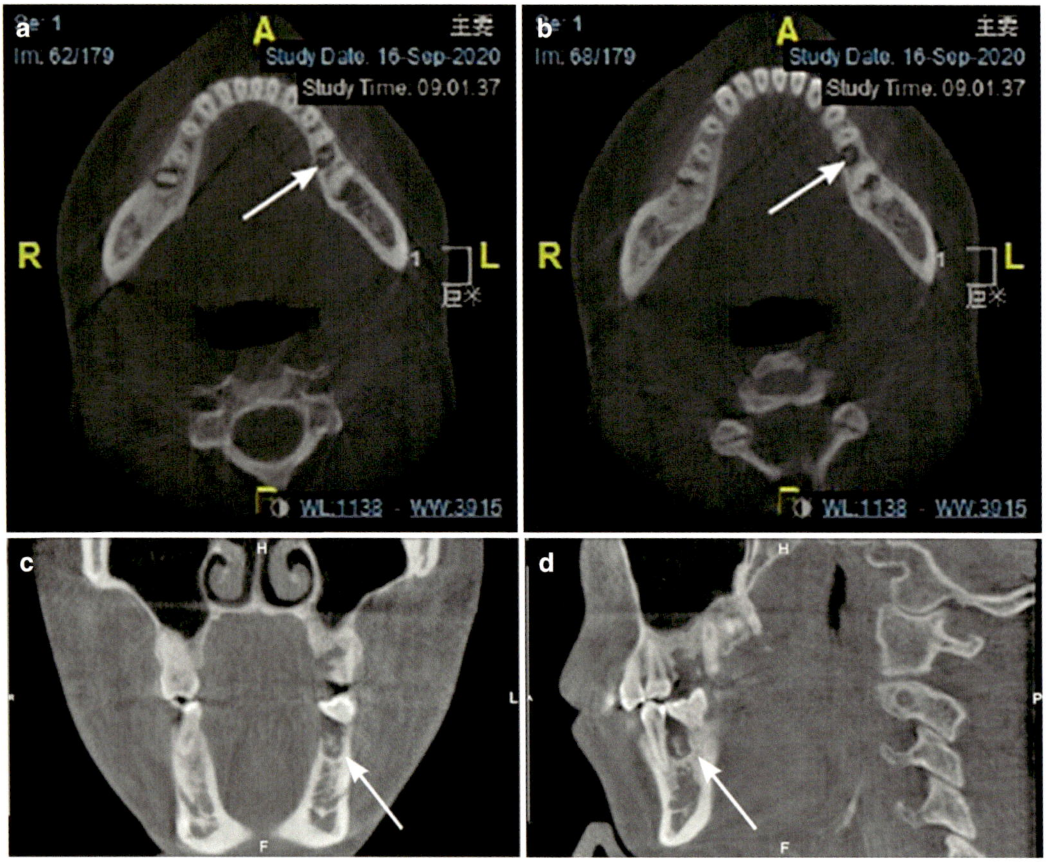

Figure 12.2 (**a, b**) CBCT transverse view: There are cystic low-density lesions near roots 35 and 36, it is round in shape with clear boundary. (**c**) CBCT coronal view: The bone cortex becomes thinner, and no periosteal reaction and soft tissue mass are found. (**d**) CBCT sagittal view: The lesion is located near the root tip of the tooth, and no periapical wrapping is found

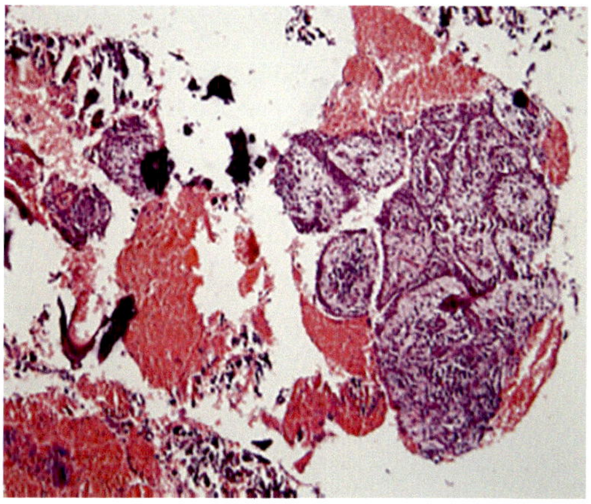

Fig. 12.3 The part sent for pathologic examination is fibrous cystic wall-like tissue, lined with reticular hyperplasia of stratified squamous epithelium, inflammatory cells infiltrate in the cystic wall, with broken bone tissue and bleeding (100×)

Microscopically, inflammatory fibrous tissue and broken bone tissue were seen, lined with reticular hyperplasia of stratified squamous epithelium, accompanied by bleeding (Figure 12.3).

[Pathological Diagnosis] inflammatory lateral cyst of "left mandible," ICD code: K09.005.

[Follow-Up Visit] The patient recovered well after the operation. Nothing special was found by re-examination.

12.3 Key Points of Diagnosis and Treatment

An inflammatory collateral cyst is a unique adhesive cyst, and it was first reported in August 1970. Craig first put forward the term "paradental cyst" in 1976, which was used to classify cysts related to pericoronitis of molars. Stoneman and Worth first described a clinical and imaging entity called mandibular infectious buccal cyst or mandibular infectious cheekbone cyst. According to the World Health Organization (WHO) definition, a paradental cyst refers to a cyst that occurs near the lateral neck of the root due to inflammation in the periodontal pocket, usually on the buccal side of the mandibular molar [1, 2]. Inflammatory collateral cysts and periapical cysts have similar microscopic characteristics, so they are classified as inflammatory cysts by the World Health Organization.

The common type of inflammatory collateral cyst is a paradental cyst, usually occurring in persons of 20~40 years old and involving the buccal or distal buccal side of the third mandibular molar. The other type is a mandibular buccal root bifurcation cyst, usually occurring in persons younger than 20 years old and involving the buccal side of the mandibular first or second molar. Inflammatory collateral cyst rarely affects pulp vitality, mostly asymptomatic development, leading to swelling and pain by infection or accidentally found during a routine examination. In imagining, the manifestations are mostly low-density shadow in the buccal root bifurcation area or near the root, normal periodontal membrane space, periosteal reaction on root side, shadow covering root canal system to varying degrees, and observation of root to varying degrees [3, 4]. The pathological manifestations are not specific, similar to radicular cysts, and the lining epithelium is a stratified squamous epithelium with hyperplasia and no keratinization. Inflammatory infiltration, such as mononuclear cells and polymorphonuclear cells, etc., can be seen in the wall of connective tissue, and sometimes foam cells and hemosiderin can be seen [5, 6]. The epithelial lining can be continuous with the periodontal pocket epithelium or attached to the root surface to form a cavity. Because the clinical and pathological manifestations are not characteristic, we need to pay attention to differential diagnosis with radicular cyst, odontogenic keratocyst, gingival cyst, dental cyst, dentigerous cyst, etc., during diagnosis and treatment to adopt correct treatment strategies.

References

1. Silva T, Batista A, Camarini E, et al. Paradental cyst mimicking a radicular cyst on the adjacent tooth: case report and review of terminology [J]. J Endod. 2003;29(1):73–6.
2. Stanback J. The management of bilateral cysts of the mandible [J]. Oral Surg Oral Med Oral Pathol. 1970;30(5):587–91.

3. Craig G. The paradental cyst. A specific inflammatory odontogenic cyst [J]. Br Dent J. 1976;141(1):9–14.
4. Stoneman D, Worth H. The mandibular infected buccal cyst – molar area [J]. Dent Radiogr Photogr. 1983;56(1):1–14.
5. Chrcanovic B, Gomez R. Gingival cyst of the adult, lateral periodontal cyst and botryoid odontogenic cyst: an updated systematic review [J]. Oral Dis. 2019;25(1):26–33.
6. Zhang YH. Clinical analysis of the differential diagnosis of root cysts [J]. Chin J Postgrad Med. 2007;30:29.

Part IV

Pseudocyst

Simple Bone Cyst

13

Bing Liu, Hui Shan Ong, Zhen Tian, Lin Zhu, and Yong Jie Hu

13.1 Introduction

A simple bone cyst (SBC) is a bone cyst without lining epithelium, first reported by Lucas in 1929. There are different names for traumatic bone cyst, solitary bone cyst, hemorrhagic bone cyst, exosmotic bone cyst, idiopathic bone cyst, idiopathic bone cavity and progressive bone cavity. The diversity of naming reflects the uncertainty of pathogenesis. SBC is common in long bones but rare in jaws. Its incidence accounts for about 1% of bone cysts, mostly in young people, and 75% of patients are between 10 and 20 years old, mostly in men. The most common part of the maxillofacial region is the body of the mandible, mainly involving bicuspids and molars, and the maxilla is extremely rare [1–6]. Most cysts are single and can also occur on both sides of the jaw. Clinically, most of the simple bone cyst is asymptomatic, and it are often found by chance during X-ray examination. Sometimes, the patient may suffer from jaw swelling and pain [6–11]. The teeth adjacent to the lesion part are vital teeth that may cause sensory abnormalities when invading the inferior alveolar nerve. X-ray shows a clear-cut single-locular transmission zone and a thin edge hardening zone. Root resorption and tooth displacement are rare, and the periodontal membrane and lamina dura in the lesion area are intact [12–20].

13.2 Case 28

The patient, female, 11 years old. The space-occupying lesion in the left mandible was found for over a month.

[Present Medical History] The patient checked teeth in another hospital 1 month ago. The radiograph showed that there was a low-density space-occupying lesion shadow on the left mandible, and there was no obvious pain or looseness in the left mandibular teeth. The patient went to our hospital's outpatient for a maxillofacial region CT examination, indicating a Possible bone cyst in the left mandible.

[Specialized Examination] The facial appearance is basically symmetrical. The mouth opening degree and opening type are normal, and the mixed dentition and oral hygiene are average.

B. Liu (✉)
Hospital of Stomatology Wuhan University, Wuhan, Hubei, China
e-mail: liubing9909@wuhan.edu.cn

H. S. Ong · Z. Tian · Y. J. Hu
Department of Oral Maxillofacial-Head & Neck Oncology, Shanghai Ninth People's Hospital, Shanghai Jiao Tong University School of Medicine, Shanghai, China

L. Zhu
Department of Radiology, Ninth People's Hospital Affiliated to Shanghai Jiao Tong University, Shanghai, China

Y. He (ed.), *Inflammatory and Neoplastic Diseases of Craniofacial Bones*, https://doi.org/10.1007/978-981-97-4155-7_13

There is no obvious swelling, ulceration, or exudation of the left mandibular gingiva or no obvious swelling or tenderness. Residual root 35 is in place, and there is no obvious looseness or pain. Root 36 is in position with no obvious looseness or percussion pain.

[Auxiliary Examination]

1. Panoramic radiographs show that dental germ 35 is not found, the cystic shadow of 35 toot is found, mesio-root apical of 36 is located in the cysts, and the epiphyseal white line can be seen nearby (Fig. 13.1).
2. Maxillofacial CT enhanced scan: A cystic low-density focus is found in the left mandible body, with regular shape, clear boundary, and continuous bone cortex. No obvious periosteal reaction is seen, and no soft tissue mass is seen nearby (Fig. 13.2).

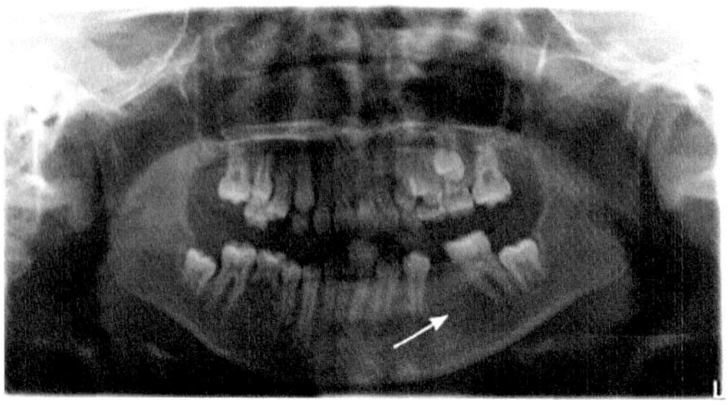

Fig. 13.1 Dental germ 35 is not found, a cystic shadow of 35 toot is found, mesio-root apical of 36 is located in the cysts, and epiphyseal white line can be seen nearby

[Primary Diagnosis] bone cyst at the left mandible.

[Treatment] "left mandibular cyst extraction + tooth extraction" were performed under general anesthesia; Incision of gingiva, flap turning over, and partial removal of alveolar bone were performed to expose the cyst. The cyst wall was completely scraped and sent for pathological examination. The wound was washed, bleeding was stopped, and the wound was repaired and sewn tightly.

[Pathological Examination] The part sent for pathological examination was long tissue, 0.5 cm*0.2 cm*0.2 cm in size, grayish yellow. Microscopically, long bone wall tissue was seen; one side was lined with thin fibrous connective tissue, with abundant blood vessels and no lining epithelium (Fig. 13.3).

[Pathological Diagnosis] simple bone cyst of left mandible," ICD code: K09.203.

[Follow-Up Visit] The patient recovered well after the operation; there was nothing special, and the cyst did not recur after half a year.

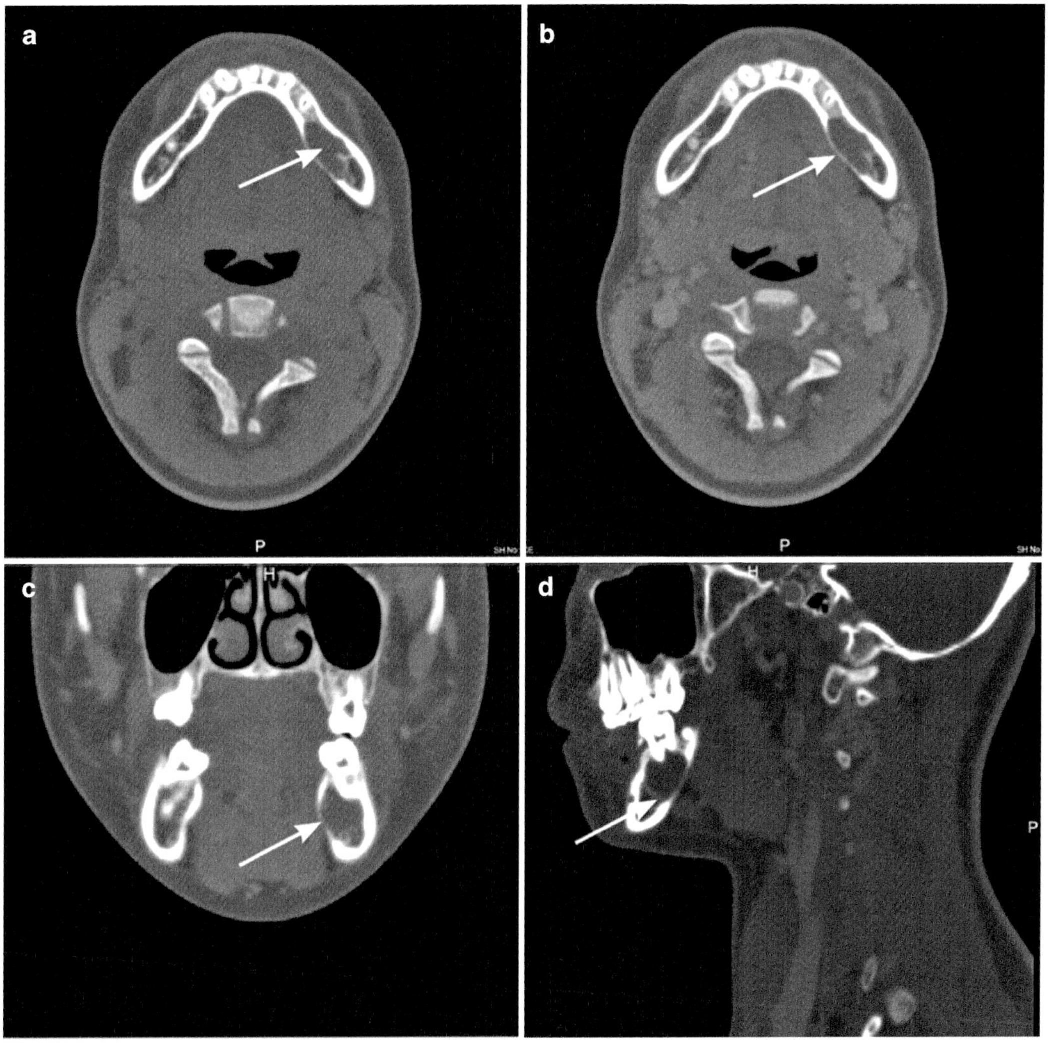

Fig. 13.2 (**a**) Transverse view of CT plain scan: A cystic low-density focus is found in the left mandible body, with regular shape and clear boundary. (**b**) Transverse view of CT enhanced scan: No significant enhancement is seen. (**c**) Coronal view of CT enhanced scan: The bone cortex becomes thinner, and the bone cortex is continuous. (**d**) Sagittal view of CT enhanced scan: The left inferior alveolar nerve canal is still intact

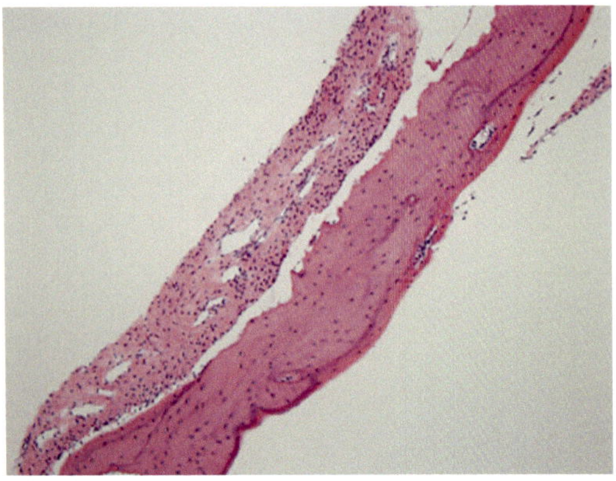

Fig. 13.3 Fibrous connective tissue of vessels rich in thin layers, without lining epithelium (100x)

13.3 Key Points of Diagnosis and Treatment

Lucas and Blum first reported a simple bone cyst (SBC) as an isolated bone cyst in 1929. However, to some extent, this is a misnomer, because SBC lacks epithelial lining. Therefore, it is not a real cyst.

Pathogenesis The pathogenesis of SBC is still unclear. Harnet et al. summarized three popular theories: ① Abnormal growth of jaw; ② The process of tumor degeneration; ③ Trauma-bleeding theory. The most widely accepted theory is the third theory. It relies on the formation of intramedullary hemorrhage and then produces post-traumatic hematoma. The pressure of hematoma causes venous obstruction, leading to bone marrow necrosis and osteoclastic bone absorption due to the decrease of tissue pH. This theory is applicable to the jaw, because teeth and alveolar processes are vulnerable to minor trauma. However, some scholars have questioned this mechanism because more than 50% of the reported cases had no history of trauma. The cases herein also have no obvious history of trauma. Ogasawara et al. thought that occlusal trauma may be an influencing factor of SBC. It cannot be ruled out for the cases herein that chronic occlusal trauma may have certain influences on the pathogenesis of SBC. At present, most cases are considered to have multifactorial etiology. Some scholars also believe that SBC will disappear with the increase of age, so the incidence rate in the elderly population is low. Generally, there is no obvious gender difference in SBC, but Cortell-Ballester et al. reported that women were more common. This may be because the pathogenesis of SBC is related to the levels of estrogen and progesterone [9–14].

There are two possible explanations for the low incidence of the maxilla: ① Maxillary lesions are easily concealed by transmission images of the maxillary sinus; ② Compared with the mandible, the blood supply of the maxilla is richer, and the quality and quantity of bone marrow are better. The mandible has more bone cortexes, and its self-repair speed is slower than that of the maxillary bone.

Imaging Characteristics The most commonly used examination method is X-ray film, but there are artifacts in the chin of panoramic film. Therefore, some scholars suggest that CBCT examination should be carried out when a simple jaw cyst is highly suspected to avoid unnecessary mandibular resection, especially for young patients [15].

Typical image performance: unilocular, transparent images with clear boundaries with fan-shaped or irregular edges. Although these manifestations highly suggest SBC, they cannot be used as a clear diagnostic basis because many cases are not typical in the clinic. It has been reported that SBC can be multilocular and related to impacted teeth. The same individual occurs many times at different sites, causing inner and outer cortical bone swelling. Cases of secondary pathological fractures caused by SBC have also been reported.

Examination by centesis of fine needle: No contents. Visible liquid can be seen occasionally. The formation of hollow bone may be related to the insufficient formation of osteoblasts. The demand for bone mineral deposition cannot be met. During normal remodeling, the number of osteoblasts may be insufficient because of the constant changes in the development of young people's bones, especially middle-aged women.

Differential Diagnosis In accordance with the imaging manifestations, it is necessary to distinguish this disease from some aggressive jaw lesions, such as ameloblastoma, odontogenic keratocyst, myxoma, central giant cell tumor, etc.

Treatment the treatment strategies of SBC have been controversial:

1. Simply scraping the bone wall is also an effective treatment for simple bone cysts [16, 17].
2. Bone wall scaling + surgical exploration is the most commonly used treatment method. Surgical exploration can be used as a diagnostic strategy, and at the same time, it can cause bone wall bleeding to replace sclerotin and fill the cavity, assisting wound healing and bone remodeling. Whether scaling is performed or not, surgical intervention can accelerate bone formation and promote wound occlusion. Even for large jaw lesions, normal imaging manifestations can be observed within 3~12 months after operation [18–20].
3. Other treatments include steroid corticosteroid injection, autologous bone marrow injection, autologous bone transplantation, open scaling, various decompression, calcium phosphate, calcium sulfate and hollow screw application.

Recurrence is rare after adequate sclerotin scaling, and most occur within 5 months after operation. Therefore, scholars suggest that postoperative clinical and imaging examinations should be carried out for at least 3 years to detect the signs of recurrence.

References

1. Cortell-Ballester I, Figueiredo R, Berini-Aytés L, et al. Traumatic bone cyst: a retrospective study of 21 cases [J]. Med Oral Patol Oral Cir Bucal. 2009;14(5):E239–43.
2. Brunet-Llobet L, Lahor-Soler E, Mashala E, et al. Continuous surgical decompression for solitary bone cyst of the jaw in a teenage patient [J]. Case Rep Dent. 2019;2019:9137507.
3. Ahlers E, Setabutr D, Garritano F, et al. Pathologic fracture of the mandible secondary to traumatic bone cyst [J]. Craniomaxillofac Trauma Reconstr. 2013;6(3):201–4.
4. Harnet J, Lombardi T, Klewansky P, et al. Solitary bone cyst of the jaws: a review of the etiopathogenic hypotheses [J]. J Oral Maxillofac Surg. 2008;66(11):2345–8.
5. Ogasawara T, Kitagawa Y, Ogawa T, et al. Simple bone cyst of the mandibular condyle with severe osteoarthritis: report of a case [J]. J Oral Pathol Med. 1999;28(8):377–80.
6. Kim K, Koh K. Recurrent simple bone cyst of the mandibular condyle: a case report [J]. Imaging Sci Dent. 2013;43(1):49–53.
7. Saito Y, Hoshina Y, Nagamine T, et al. Simple bone cyst. A clinical and histopathologic study of fifteen cases [J]. Oral Surg Oral Med Oral Pathol. 1992;74(4):487–91.
8. Kaugars G, Cale A. Traumatic bone cyst [J]. Oral Surg Oral Med Oral Pathol. 1987;63(3):318–24.
9. Kahn M. Clinicopathologic correlation quiz: unilocular periapical radiolucencies. Traumatic bone cyst [J]. J Tenn Dent Assoc. 1997;77(1):24, 35–26.
10. An S, Lee J, Benavides E, et al. Multiple simple bone cysts of the jaws: review of the literature and report of three cases [J]. Oral Surg Oral Med Oral Pathol Oral Radiol. 2014;117(6):e458–69.
11. Xindi J, Gang L, Xinhong W, et al. Simple bone cyst of the jaw: a retrospective study of 11 cases [J]. Hua Xi Kou Qiang Yi Xue Za Zhi. 2016;34(3):272–6.
12. de Souza NV, Sette-Dias A, Abdo E, et al. Asynchronous idiopathic bone cavity: a case report [J]. J Craniomaxillofac Surg. 2012;40(8):e328–30.
13. Forssell K, Forssell H, Happonen R, et al. Simple bone cyst: review of the literature and analysis of 23 cases [J]. Int J Oral Maxillofac Surg. 1988;17(1):21–4.
14. Suomalainen A, Apajalahti S, Kuhlefelt M, et al. Simple bone cyst: a radiological dilemma [J]. Dentomaxillofac Radiol. 2009;38(3):174–7.
15. Sabino-Bezerra J, Santos-Silva A, Jorge J, et al. Atypical presentations of simple bone cysts of the mandible: a case series and review of literature [J]. J Craniomaxillofac Surg. 2013;41(5):391–6.
16. Shirai T, Tsuchiya H, Terauchi R, et al. Treatment of a simple bone cyst using a cannulated hydroxyapatite Pin [J]. Medicine. 2015;94(25):e1027.
17. Saia G, Fusetti S, Emanuelli E, et al. Intraoral endoscopic enucleation of a solitary bone cyst of the mandibular condyle [J]. Int J Oral Maxillofac Surg. 2012;41(3):317–20.
18. Lima L, de Freitas FS, Barbosa de Paulo L, et al. Simple bone cyst: description of 60 cases seen at a Brazilian School of Dentistry and review of international literature [J]. Med Oral Patol Oral Cir Bucal. 2020;25(5):e616–25.
19. Banda N, Nayak U, Vishwanath K, et al. Management of traumatic bone cyst in a 3-year-old child: a rare case report [J]. Int J Clin Pediatr Dent. 2012;5(3):213–6.
20. Suei Y, Taguchi A, Tanimoto K. Simple bone cyst of the jaws: evaluation of treatment outcome by review of 132 cases [J]. J Oral Maxillofac Surg. 2007;65(5):918–23.

Aneurysmal Bone Cyst

14

Bing Liu, Hui Shan Ong, Zhen Tian, Lin Zhu, and Qi Wen Man

14.1 Introduction

The aneurysmal bone cyst (ABC) was first reported as an ossifying hematoma by Van Arsdale in 1893. In 1942, Jaffe and Lichenstein renamed it in accordance with its intraosseous and expandable properties. ABC is a benign, locally invasive tumor in children and early adulthood [1–6]. It usually affects the metaphysis of long bones and may also occur in the spine or pelvis. Patients usually complain of pain in the affected area, and sometimes, pathological fractures can be observed. Osteolytic lesions can be found in plain films; magnetic resonance imaging (MRI) shows that a typical liquid-level cystic structure is formed due to blood deposition. The main treatment of ABC is sclerotherapy. Sclerosing agents, such as polysaccharide alcohol or doxycycline, can be injected into cysts, thus reducing cystic lesions and progressive sclerosis [6–11]. Another treatment (if sclerotherapy fails or pathological fracture is imminent) is scaling with adjuvant. Adjuvants can be hydrogen peroxide, phenol and polymethylmethacrylate to fill lesions [7].

B. Liu (✉) · Q. W. Man
Hospital of Stomatology Wuhan University, Wuhan, Hubei, China
e-mail: liubing9909@wuhan.edu.cn

H. S. Ong · Z. Tian · L. Zhu
Department of Oral Maxillofacial-Head & Neck Oncology, Shanghai Ninth People's Hospital, Shanghai Jiao Tong University School of Medicine, Shanghai, China

14.2 Case 29

The patient, female, 33 years old. The left mandible swelled for more than a month.

[Present Medical History] More than 1 month ago, the patient had swelling of the left face and mandible of no obvious cause. There was no obvious pain or numbness of the lower lip. The patient went to the local hospital for treatment, which was considered "pericoronitis of wisdom teeth," and anti-infection treatment was given; however, there was no obvious improvement. Panoramic radiographs show a low-density change in the left mandible body. A Maxillofacial CT enhancement examination was performed in the outpatient department of our hospital, considering the possibility of an odontogenic tumor.

[Specialized Examination] The facial shape is asymmetrical, the left face and mandible are obviously swollen, the skin of the face and neck is normal, the mouth opening degree and mouth opening type are normal, the midline is half a tooth position to the left, and the occlusion is deeply covered. The buccal and lingual body of teeth 35~38 of the left mandible is swollen, and tooth 37 is loose III°. The diagnosis shows a ping-pong sensation and tenderness (−), no obvious abnormal swelling and exudation of mucosa, and no numbness of the lower lip (Fig. 14.1a). No

Y. He (ed.), *Inflammatory and Neoplastic Diseases of Craniofacial Bones*,
https://doi.org/10.1007/978-981-97-4155-7_14

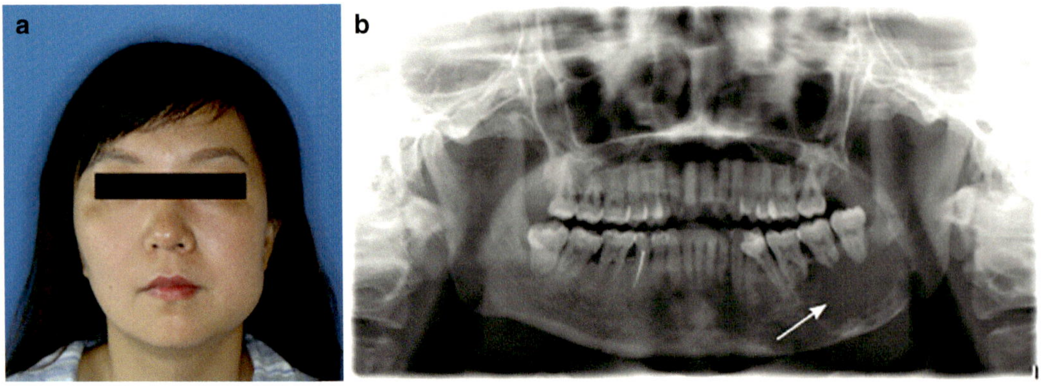

Fig. 14.1 (**a**) The left face and mandible are swollen, the skin is intact, and there is no noticeable swelling and exudation. (**b**) Low-density shadow of the left mandible body and mandibular angle, unclear boundary, involving 36~38, no evident root absorption

obvious swollen lymph nodes are seen in bilateral submandibular regions and neck.

[Auxiliary Examination] panoramic radiographs: There is a low-density shadow of the left mandible body and mandibular angle, with unclear boundary, involving 36~38, and no obvious absorption of the root (Fig. 14.1b).

CT enhanced scan of maxillofacial region: Bone swelling is found in the left mandible body, angle and ascending ramus, bulging to the buccal and lingual sides, and multiple bony divisions are found. Soft tissue density shadow with uneven density is found, with C- of 26, 71 Hu and C+ of 26, and 154 Hu, showing uneven enhancement. The bone cortex around the lesion becomes thinner, local continuity is interrupted, the boundary with surrounding soft tissues is clear, and the left inferior alveolar nerve canal is destroyed. There is no abnormality in the skull base structure. No abnormal enlarged lymph node shadow is seen in the bilateral neck (Fig. 14.2).

[Primary Diagnosis] Mass of left mandible (maybe adamantoblastoma).

[Treatment] Under general anesthesia, "left mandible segmental resection + vascularized fibula musculocutaneous flap transfer repair" were performed: An incision 1~2 cm was designed, cut and flapped over along the lower edge of the mandible. After that, the bone in the mandible body and body was found to be swollen and lavender, and the left mandible was removed from the left mental foramen to the sigmoid notch. The removed parts were sent for pathological examination during the operation, indicating an aneurysmal bone cyst of the left mandible. The left fibula muscle flap was taken and shaped. The continuity and occluding relation of the mandible were reconstructed and restored, and the peroneal artery and vein were anastomosed with the facial artery and vein. The operation wound was rinsed, bleeding was stopped completely, a negative pressure drainage tube was reserved, a suture was performed in layers, and the wound was closed (Fig. 14.3).

[Pathological Examination] The part sent for pathological examination was mandible tissue, 6 cm*6 cm*2 cm in size, attached with 4 teeth. Cystic cavity was found in the mandible body ascending ramus, with a range of about 4 cm*2.5 cm*2 cm, containing a small amount of blood, blood clots were formed, and the cyst wall was dark red. Microscopically, fibrous cyst wall tissue was found, without obvious lining epithelium, and a small amount of residual host bone and reactive new bone was found in the cyst wall, with local multinucleated giant cell infiltra-

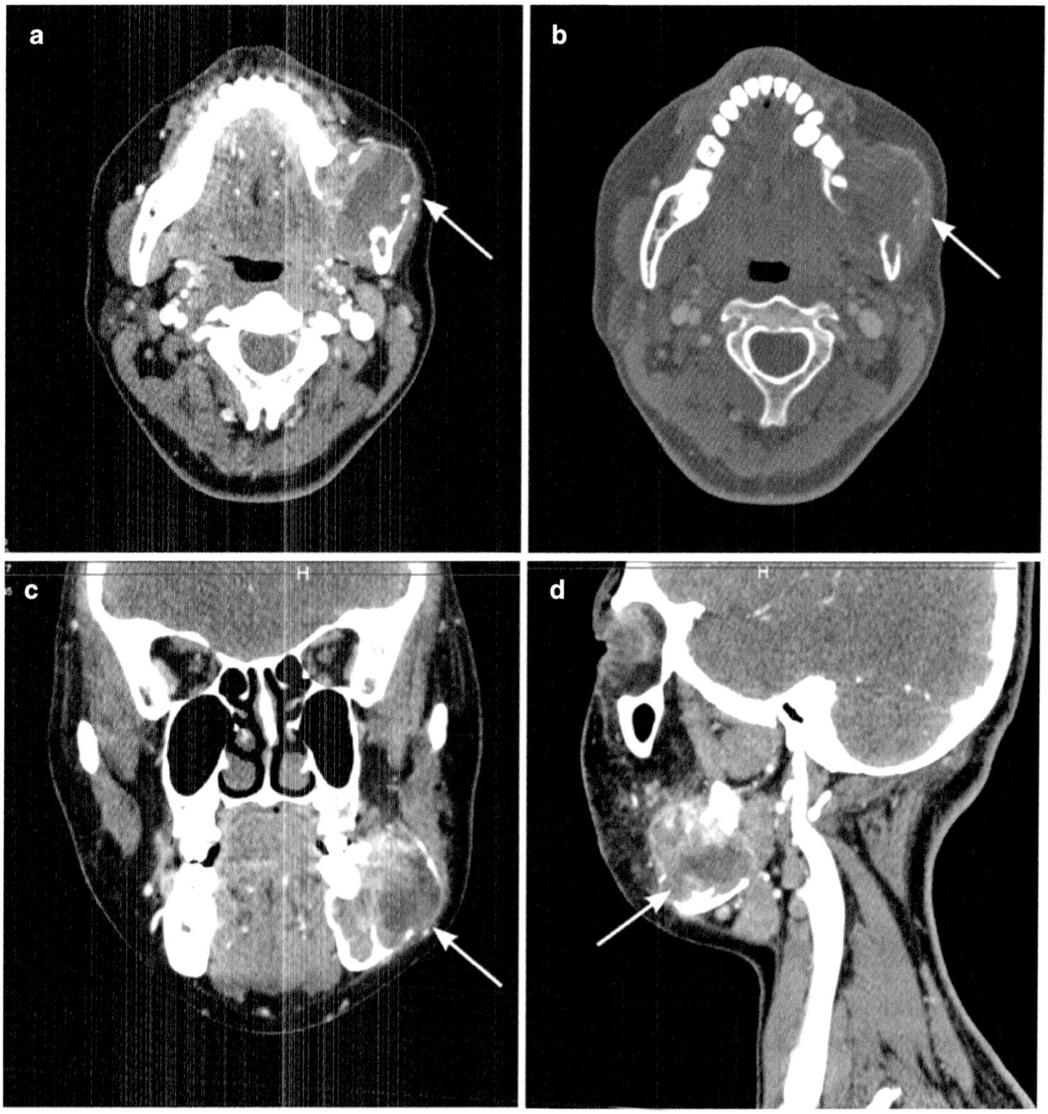

Fig. 14.2 (**a**) Transverse view of CT enhanced scan: Bone destruction of left mandible body and corner with soft tissue mass. The sclerotin shows swelling changes and slight enhancement. (**b**) Transverse view of CT enhanced scan (bone window): The middle part of the bone cortex, seeming to see the bone ridge. (**c**) Coronal view of CT enhanced scan: The bone cortex became thin, and local continuity is interrupted. (**d**) Sagittal view of CT enhanced scan: The left inferior alveolar nerve canal is destroyed

tion, accompanied by bleeding and hemosiderin deposition (Fig. 14.4).

[Pathological Diagnosis] aneurysmal bone cyst of "left mandible," ICD-O code: 9260/0.

[Follow-Up Visit] The patient recovered well after the operation. In the follow-up visit after half a year, the reconstructed shape of the mandible was satisfactory and the restoration of the occluding relation was good.

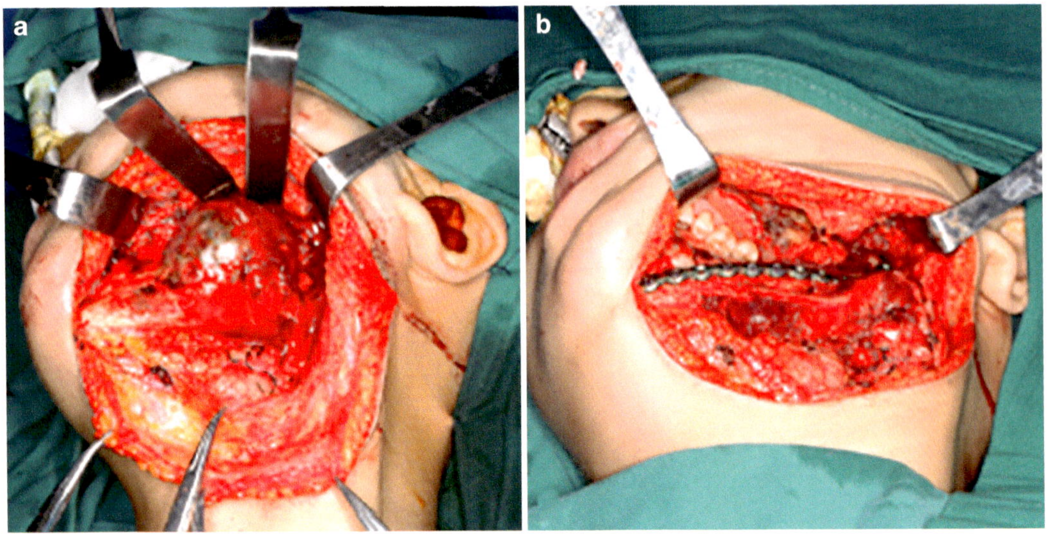

Fig. 14.3 (**a**) The mandible body and mandibular ramus are exposed, and the local bone is swollen and lavender. (**b**) Restoring of mandible continuity by reconstruction

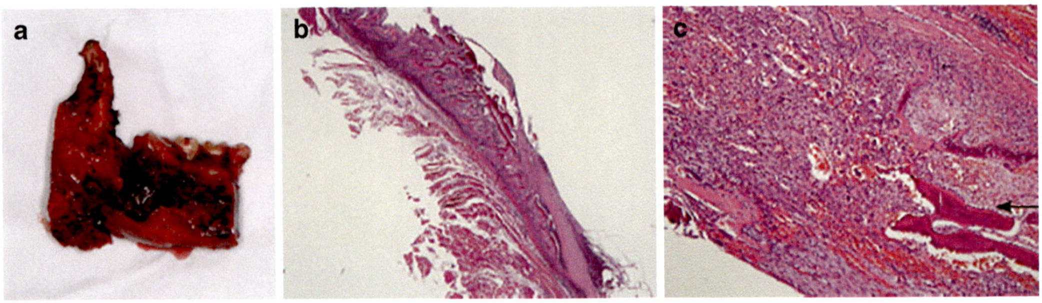

Fig. 14.4 (**a**) Gross view of segmental resection of the mandible (lingual side). (**b**) Under a low-power microscope, fibrous capsule wall-like tissue can be seen, with bone tissue and more bleeding in the capsule wall and normal muscle tissue on the outside (20×). (**c**) There were abundant blood vessels in the fibrous capsule wall, accompanied by bleeding, multinucleated giant cells were scattered and infiltrated, reactive new bone was formed (indicated by the upper arrow), and a small amount of residual host bone (indicated by the lower arrow) was seen, without obvious lining epithelium (100×)

14.3 Key Points of Diagnosis and Treatment

ABC is a benign, osteolytic, fast-growing and expansive bone disease, mainly occurring in the metaphysis of long bones, such as femur, tibia and spine. The most relevant differential diagnosis is osteotelangiectasia and giant giant-cell tumor of bone. More than 80% of patients are younger than 20 years old. About 70% of ABC cases are primary and 30% are secondary. Radiologically, ABC is characterized by balloon-like cortical expansion from unilocular radiotransparent lesions to multilocular radiotransparent lesions. Histopathologically, ABC is characterized by a hyperemia gap, separated by a fibrous septum containing osteoclast-like giant cells. The formation of ABC can be attributed to the disorder of local circulation, leading to the significant increase of venous pressure and the expansion of vascular space in the affected bone. This hemodynamic disorder may be secondary to local trauma or the existence of original lesions in the affected bone. Generally, ABC grows rapidly and is accompanied by pain. Cytogenetic abnormalities were found in primary ABC in 1999. There are three other reports showing that giant cell lesions of the mandible have USP6 gene rearrangement [8–10]. Mankin et al. reported that the anatomical site seemed to have some influences on the local recurrence rate. The recurrence rates of the clavicle and distal femur were 50% and 46%, respectively, and the recurrence rates of other parts were very low or no recurrence.

References

1. Van Arsdale WII. Ossifying haematoma [J]. Ann Surg. 1893;18(1):8–17.
2. Sayama C, MacDonald J. Aneurysmal bone cyst of the petrous bone: case presentation and review of the literature [J]. Pediatr Neurosurg. 2010;46(4):308–12.
3. Tsagozis P, Brosjö O. Current strategies for the treatment of aneurysmal bone cysts [J]. Orthop Rev. 2015;7(4):6182.
4. Struthers P, Shear M. Aneurysmal bone cyst of the jaws. (I). Clinicopathological features [J]. International. J Oral Surg. 1984;13(2):85–91.
5. Motamedi M, Behroozian A, Azizi T, et al. Assessment of 120 maxillofacial aneurysmal bone cysts: a nationwide quest to understand this enigma [J]. J Oral Maxillofac Surg. 2014;72(8):1523–30.
6. Motamedi M, Yazdi E. Aneurysmal bone cyst of the jaws: analysis of 11 cases [J]. J Oral Maxillofac Surg. 1994;52(5):471–5.
7. Cottalorda J, Bourelle S. Modern concepts of primary aneurysmal bone cyst [J]. Arch Orthop Trauma Surg. 2007;127(2):105–14.
8. Dal Cin P, Kozakewich H, Goumnerova L, et al. Variant translocations involving 16q22 and 17p13 in solid variant and extraosseous forms of aneurysmal bone cyst [J]. Genes Chromosomes Cancer. 2000;28(2):233–4.
9. Oliveira A, Hsi B, Weremowicz S, et al. USP6 (Tre2) fusion oncogenes in aneurysmal bone cyst[J]. Cancer Res. 2004;64(6):1920–3.
10. Oliveira A, Perez-Atayde A, Inwards C, et al. USP6 and CDH11 oncogenes identify the neoplastic cell in primary aneurysmal bone cysts and are absent in so-called secondary aneurysmal bone cysts [J]. Am J Pathol. 2004;165(5):1773–80.
11. Jacomacci W, Veloso Perdigão J, Veltrini V, et al. Associated aneurysmal bone cyst and cemento-osseous dysplasia: a case report and review of the literature [J]. Gen Dent. 2017;65(1):28–32.

Part V

Giant Cell Diseases

15 Giant Cell Granuloma

Bing Liu, Hui Shan Ong, Zhen Tian, Lin Zhu, and Xiao Yen Meng

15.1 Introduction

Giant cell granuloma (GCG) is also called giant cell reparation granuloma (GCRG). The incidence of GCG is very low, accounting for about 7% of benign bone lesions. GCG in the head and neck is rarely reported. In 1953, Jaffe first introduced giant cell granuloma of the mandible, including sphenoid bone, ethmoid bone, skull base, temporal bone, orbital bone and craniofacial bone [1–4]. There are also case reports of GCG in ossicles of hands and feet and long bones of limbs, etc. GCG usually occurs in front of the maxillary first molar and can occur in all ages. It often occurs in teenagers, with an average age of 15 years. There is no significant difference in incidence between men and women, and most of the patients have a history of traumatic infection. It is generally believed that GCG is a rare non-neoplastic benign lesion, a proliferative repair reaction caused by traumatic intraosseous hemorrhage and having local invasion [5]. Overall, the understanding of this disease is not comprehensive enough; further study is required.

B. Liu (✉)
Hospital of Stomatology Wuhan University, Wuhan, Hubei, China
e-mail: liubing9909@wuhan.edu.cn

H. S. Ong · Z. Tian · L. Zhu · X. Y. Meng
Department of Oral Maxillofacial-Head & Neck Oncology, Shanghai Ninth People's Hospital, Shanghai Jiao Tong University School of Medicine, Shanghai, China

15.2 Central-Type Giant Cell Granuloma

15.2.1 Case 30

The patient, male, 43 years old. The left upper posterior teeth area is unwell for more than half a year.

[Present Medical History] Six months ago, the patient suffered from general weakness without obvious inducement and went to the local hospital for treatment. After relevant examination, he found that the bone cortex of the left upper alveolar bone was slightly swollen, so he was advised to observe it. PET/CT examination was performed 1 month ago and the results indicated that the posterior margin of the left upper alveolar bone was slightly swollen and its metabolic activity was increased. The patient went to the outpatient of our hospital for a maxillofacial CT enhanced scan, indicating a space-occupying lesion of the left maxilla. The upper left teeth had no obvious pain symptoms, and the upper and lower lips had no numbness and other symptoms.

Y. He (ed.), *Inflammatory and Neoplastic Diseases of Craniofacial Bones*,
https://doi.org/10.1007/978-981-97-4155-7_15

[Specialized Examination] The maxillofacial region is symmetrical on both sides, and the proportion of the upper, middle and lower 1/3 is coordinated. The skin of the maxilla and mandible is intact and the color is normal. The degree and type of mouth opening are normal. No bone swelling is palpated in the permanent dentition in the mouth and the buccal and lingual side of the left maxilla, the surface mucosa is intact, there is no obvious ulceration or fistula, the tongue is in the middle, and the tongue has no obvious sensory or motor disorder. No significantly abnormally enlarged lymph nodes have been found in the bilateral submaxilla and neck.

[Auxiliary Examination]

1. PET/CT: The posterior margin of the left alveolar bone is slightly swollen locally, and its metabolic activity is increased (Fig. 15.1).
2. CT enhanced scan of the maxillofacial region: Space occupying lesion of left maxilla, and whether it is malignant is to be eliminated. Bone destruction can be seen in alveolar bone corresponding to 28, with a slight swelling change, the size is about 17 mm*10 mm, CT- is 64 Hu, CT+ is 107 Hu, the bone cortex becomes thinner, no obvious continuous interruption and periosteal reaction are found, and no obvious swelling is found in surrounding soft tissues. No abnormal enlarged lymph node shadow is seen in the bilateral neck (Fig. 15.2).

[Primary Diagnosis] mass of left maxilla.

[Treatment] "Lesion resection of left maxilla and complicated tooth extraction" was performed under general anesthesia: Incision along the gingival margin was performed, the flap was turned over, and 26 and 27 were removed. Apical of 27 and distal lesions of about 2.0 cm*2.0 cm were found, and some diseased tissues were taken and sent for frozen pathological examination, indicating that "left maxilla tumor" is a giant cell-rich lesion, and giant cell granuloma was considered first. The resection part of the maxilla was enlarged, the sharp bone tip and bone edge were trimmed with the dynamic system, the wound was fully flushed, bleeding was stopped strictly, and the iodoform gauze was used for packing and fixing (Fig. 15.3).

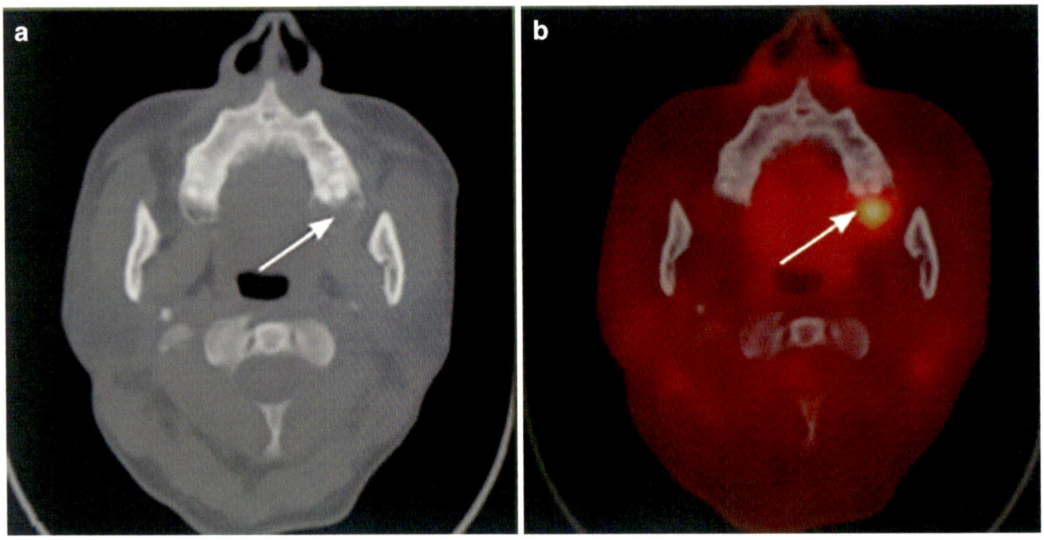

Fig. 15.1 (**a**) The posterior margin of the left upper alveolar bone is slightly swollen and the density is abnormal. (**b**) Increased local metabolic activity

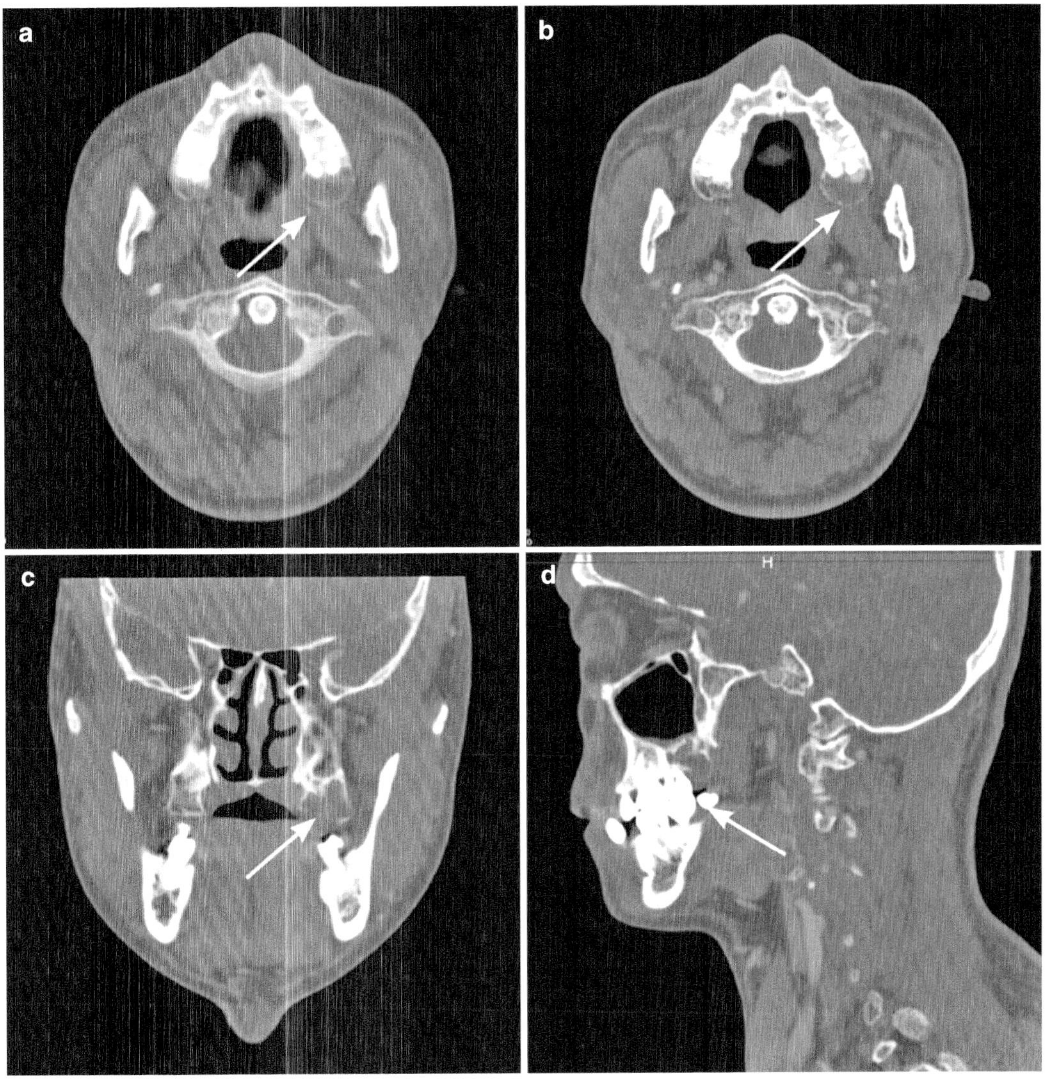

Fig. 15.2 (**a**) Transverse view of CT plain scan: A cystic low-density lesion with an irregular shape and clear boundary is seen at the posterior margin of the left maxilla. (**b**) Transverse view of CT enhanced scan: No significant enhancement is seen. (**c**) Coronal view of CT enhanced scan: There is no interruption of bone cortex and no obvious periosteum. (**d**) Sagittal view of CT enhanced scan: The boundary with maxillary sinus is clear

[Pathological Examination] The part sent for pathologic examination was broken tissue, 3 cm*2 cm*1 cm in size, reddish brown, partially hard. Microscopically, bone tissue was destroyed. In the background of proliferating fibrous connective tissue, multinucleated giant cells were scattered and infiltrated, with small size and uneven distribution. Fibrous tissue around the lesion proliferated, reactive bone formed, histiocytes infiltrated and blood vessels were abundant (Fig. 15.4).

[Pathological Diagnosis] central-type giant cell granuloma of "left maxilla," ICD code: K10.100. Bone tissue was involved locally

[Follow-Up Visit] The patient recovered well after the operation. Nothing special was found by re-examination in a half year.

15.2.2 Case 31

The patient, female, 46 years old. Mandibular tumor gradually enlarged for 10 months, and 4 months after fenestration in other hospitals.

[Present Medical History] Ten months ago, the patient accidentally found a tumor in front of the mandible and was diagnosed as abscess in a local hospital. At the same time, the patient was treated with anti-inflammatory therapy for one week, and the effect was not obvious. The tumor grew slowly. Four months ago, the patient was examined by X-ray to diagnose "mandibular tumor" and underwent "fenestrated drainage of tumor + biopsy." Postoperative pathology: Giant-cell tumor of bone of the mandible was washed daily after the operation, and there was no obvious improvement.

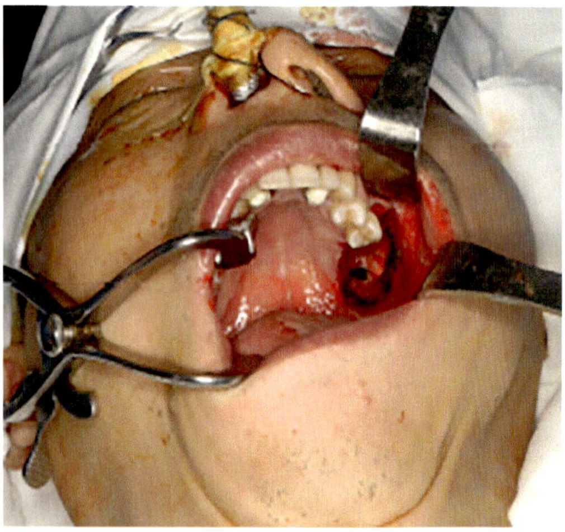

Fig. 15.3 The resection of the lesion was enlarged, and the sharp bone tip and bone edge were ground until becoming smooth

[Specialized Examination] The facial form is basically symmetrical, the degree and type of mouth opening are normal, the anterior mandible is swollen on the buccal and lingual side, ranging from 36 to 48, the mass is medium in texture, with hyperemia on the surface mucosa, and lymph nodes of 1 cm*1 cm in size can be reached under bilateral submandibular regions. The hardness is close to normal tissue, with a clear boundary, and is movable (Fig. 15.5a).

[Auxiliary Examination]

1. Panoramic radiographs: A cystic density reduction area was seen in the anterior part of the mandible with irregular morphology, relatively clear borders, continuity of the bone cortex, and no significant periosteal reaction (Fig. 15.5b).
2. CT enhanced scan of the maxillofacial region indicated bone destruction of the mandible chin with soft tissue mass, bone swelling, irregular shape, unclear boundary, discontinuous bone cortex, residual bone locally, no obvious periosteal reaction (Fig. 15.6).

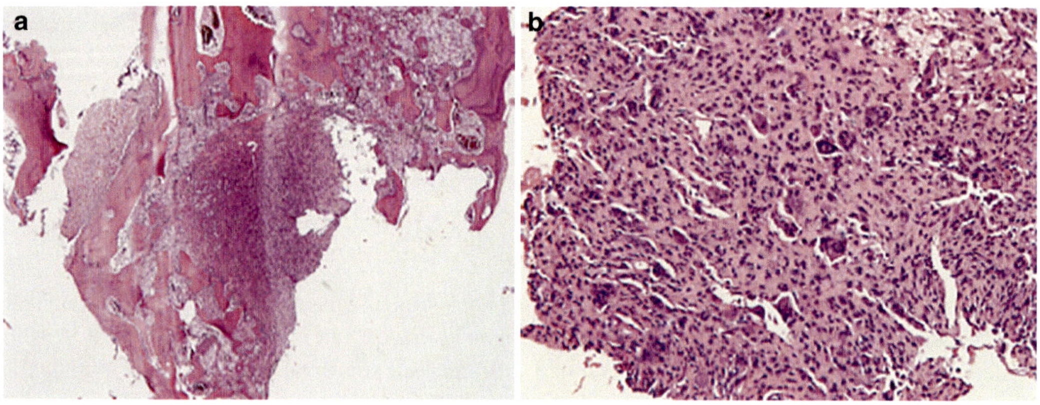

Fig. 15.4 (**a**) The lesion involved bone tissue, the surrounding fibrous tissue proliferated, and reactive bone formation occurred (40×). (**b**) The hyperplasia of fat spindle cells showed multinucleated giant cell infiltration, the size of giant cells varied, and the number of nuclei varied (200×)

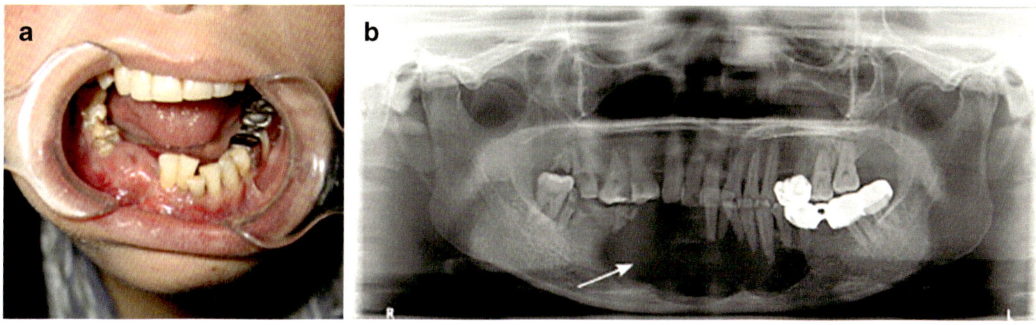

Fig. 15.5 (**a**) The anterior mandible is swollen on the buccal and lingual side, ranging from 36 to 48. The mass is medium in texture, with hyperemia on the surface mucosa. (**b**) A cystic density reduction area was seen in the anterior part of the mandible with irregular morphology, relatively clear borders, continuity of the bone cortex, and no significant periosteal reaction

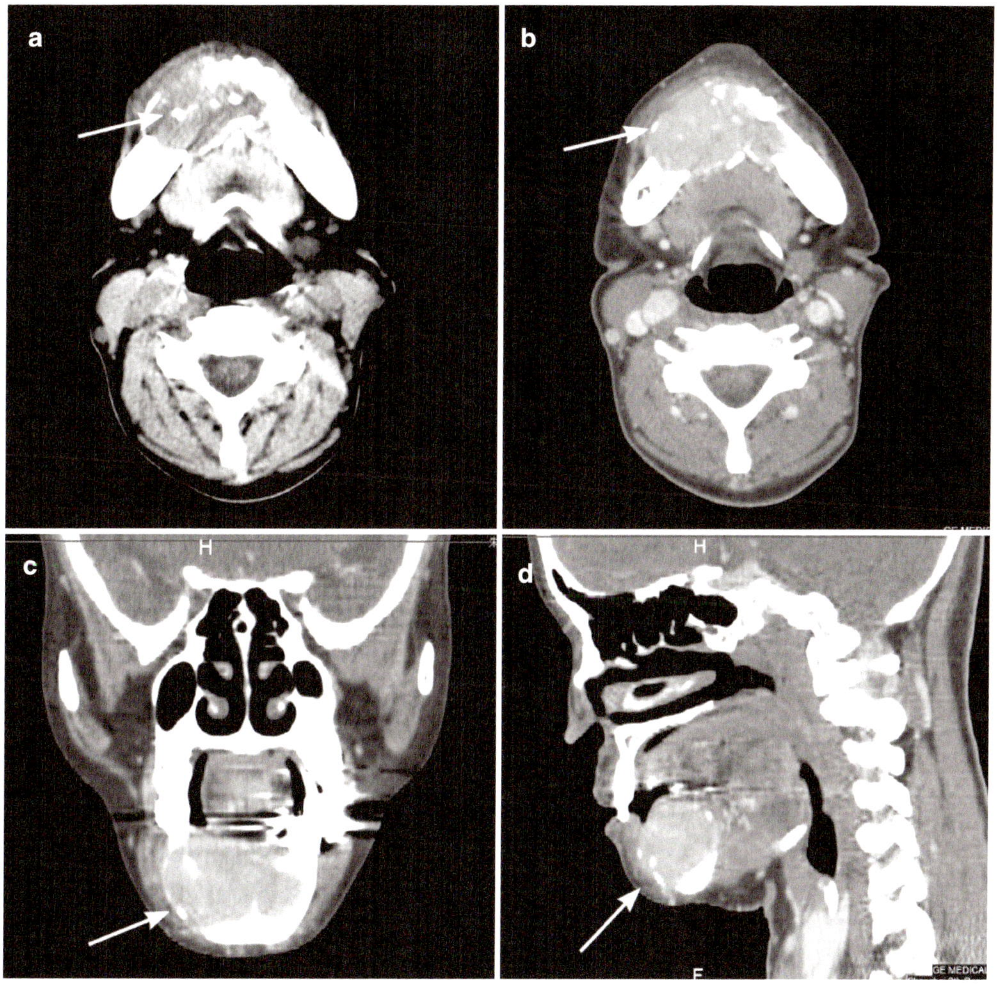

Fig. 15.6 (**a**) Transverse view of CT plain scan: Bone destruction of mandible chin with soft tissue mass, sclerotin shows swelling changes, irregular shape and unclear boundary. (**b**) Transverse view of CT enhanced scan: mild enhancement. (**c**) Coronal view of CT enhanced scan: The bone cortex became thin, and local continuity is interrupted. (**d**) Sagittal view of CT enhanced scan: Tumor compression involves surrounding soft tissue

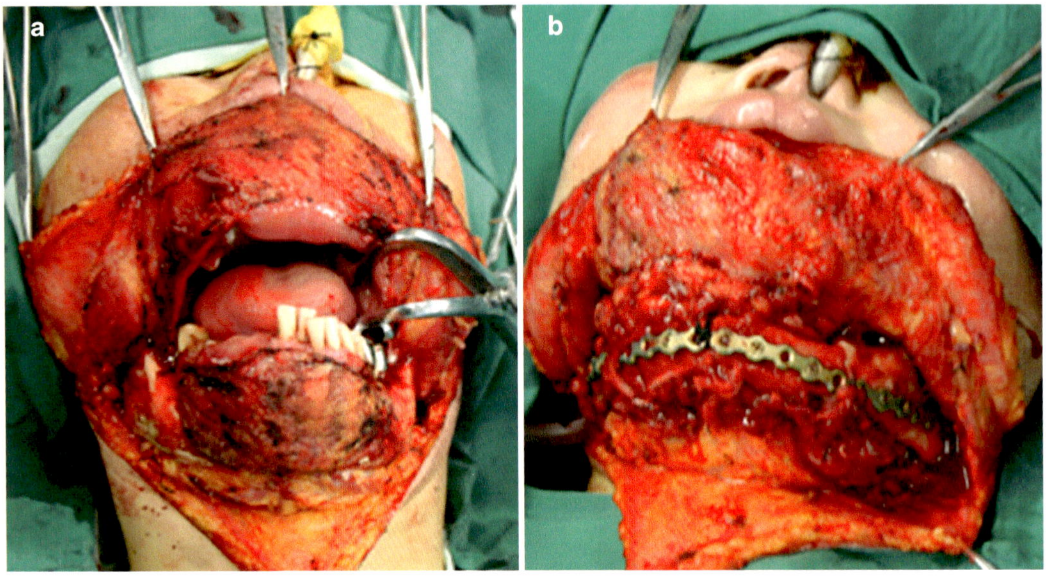

Fig. 15.7 (**a**) When the mandibular tumor was exposed, obvious bone swelling was seen, and the bone cortex was still continuous. (**b**) Restoring of mandible continuity by reconstruction of fibula musculocutaneous flap

[Primary Diagnosis] fenestration of tumor for mandible in other hospitals.

[Treatment] Under general anesthesia, "extended resection of mandible + fibula musculocutaneous flap transfer repair + tracheotomy" was performed. An incision was designed along the lower edge of bilateral mandibles by 1~2 cm, and the mandible was cut, the flap was turned over, the mandible was cut at 36~46, and mucosa adhered to the tumor in the mouth was removed and sent for freezing for pathological examination. Giant cell-rich lesion of "mandible," complying with giant cell reparation granuloma. The left fibula musculocutaneous flap was prepared routinely, and the continuity of the mandible was restored by reconstruction. The peroneal artery and vein were anastomosed with the facial artery and external jugular vein, respectively, and the skin paddle was used to repair the oral mucosal coloboma. The operation wound was rinsed, bleeding was stopped strictly, the negative pressure drainage tube was reserved, a suture was performed in layers, and the wound was closed (Fig. 15.7).

[Pathological Examination] The part sent for pathological examination was the mandible body, 6.5 cm*4.5 cm*3.5 cm in size, attached with six teeth. A gray-red tumor was seen in the section, 4.5 cm*3 cm*2.8 cm in size, quite soft. Microscopically, there are multinucleated giant cells in the background of hyperplastic fibrous connective tissue, mostly concentrated in hemorrhagic foci. The size and number of multinucleated giant cells were different, and small vessels were abundant, resulting in reactive new bone formation (Fig. 15.8).

[Pathological Diagnosis] central-type giant cell granuloma of "mandible," ICD code: K10.100.

[Follow-Up Visit] The patient recovered well after the operation. The mandibular contour recovered satisfactorily, and there was no recurrence after half a year.

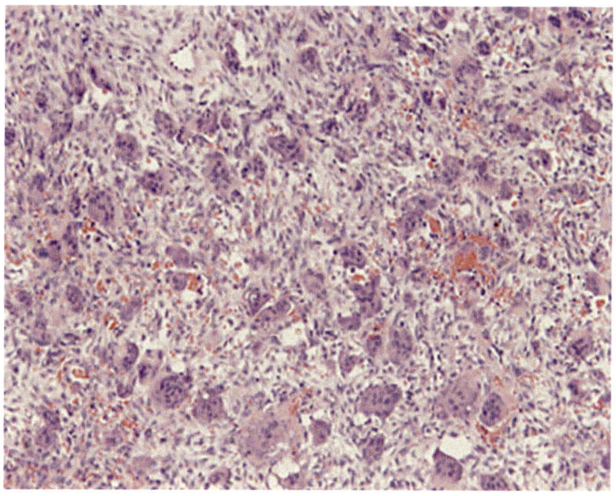

Fig. 15.8 There were many multinucleated giant cells around the hemorrhagic foci, and the background is proliferating spindle cells. The size of multinucleated giant cells and the number of nuclei were different (200×)

15.3 Peripheral-Type Giant Cell Granuloma

15.3.1 Case 32

The patient, female, 79 years old. The painless mass of the lower gingiva grew for 1 month.

[Present Medical History] The patient removed the residual roots of the lower anterior teeth one month ago. Then, there was a tumor in the gingival tissue around the posterior alveolar fossa, growing slowly outward and enlarging to this day.

[Specialized Examination] The maxillofacial region is basically symmetrical on both sides, and the proportion of the upper, middle and lower 1/3 is coordinated. The degree and type of mouth opening are normal. Intraoral permanent dentition 31 is defective; the tumor on the labial side of the alveolar fossa is oval and pedicled, about 2.0 cm*1.5 cm in size and soft in texture. Uneven surface color, no tenderness, no looseness of adjacent teeth. The swollen lymph node does not involve the bilateral submandibular region or neck.

[Auxiliary Examination]
CBCT: Bone destruction of mandible chin, discontinuous bone cortex, with no obvious periosteal reaction, adjacent soft tissue swelling (Fig. 15.9).

[Primary Diagnosis] gingiva lump of lower anterior teeth area.

[Treatment] "Extended resection of the mass of mandible gingiva + mandible edge resection + tooth extraction" was performed under general anesthesia. During the operation, the pedicle of the tumor was between 42 and 31, involving the labial side, and the gingival tumor was completely removed. Freezing pathological examination indicated: There were a lot of fat spindle cells scattered in multinucleated giant cells in "mandibular gingiva," with easy karyokinesis, pathological karyokinesis, undetermined nature and mesenchymal malignant tumor to be eliminated, and the diagnosis required for paraffin and enzyme labeling. Marginal resection was performed for the mandible, about 3.5 cm*1.5 cm in size. The bone margin was trimmed to be smooth. The resection margins sent: "Left, right, inside, outside and bottom" are all negative (−). Fully stopped bleeding, rinsed and sutured the wounds.

[Pathological Examination] The part sent for pathological examination was a tumor-like tissue, 3.3 cm*2.3 cm*2 cm in size, with a surface ulcer, dark red section, and local gray. Microscopically, a large number of multinucleated giant cells proliferated under the background of submucosal spindle cells. The multinucleated giant cells varied in size, with only a few or dozens of nuclei. The lesion was rich in blood vessels with bleeding. Surface mucosal epithelial ulcer formation, acute and chronic inflammatory cell infiltration (Fig. 15.10).

[Pathological Diagnosis] peripheral-type giant cell granuloma of "lower gingiva," ICD code: K10.100, The cells proliferated significantly and were active. [Follow-up visit] The patient recovered well after the operation. Nothing special was found by re-examination in a half year.

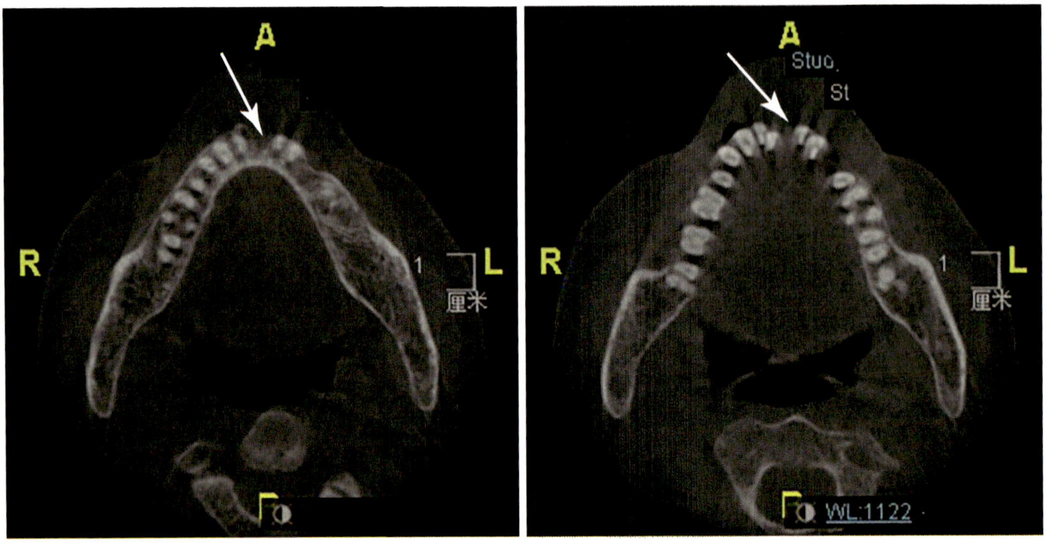

Fig. 15.9 Bone destruction of mandible chin, discontinuous bone cortex, with no obvious periosteal reaction, adjacent soft tissue swelling

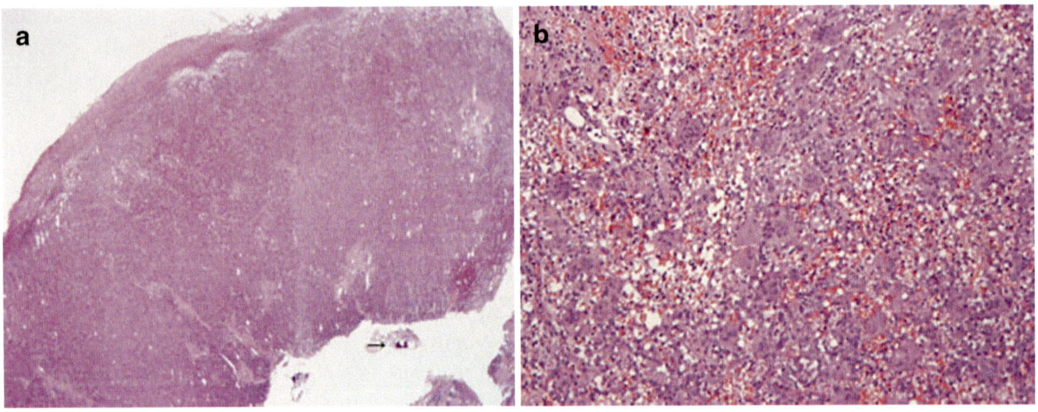

Fig. 15.10 (**a**) The lesion is located in the submucosa, and the surface epithelial ulcer is formed, being a cellulose pseudomembrane, and a small amount of dystrophic calcification (arrow) is seen below (20×). (**b**) In the background of fat spindle cells, multinucleated giant cells are infiltrated with extensive blood vessels. Giant cells are with different sizes and different nuclei number (200×)

15.4 Key Points of Diagnosis and Treatment

Imaging Characteristics The main clinical symptoms of GCG are nonspecific pain and local swelling, and the imaging shows expansive destruction, being an obvious density reduction area. Sometimes, it shows multilocular bone absorption destruction, smooth bone edge, no sclerosis, uniform density, and no bone tissue separation in the central destruction area. On a CT plain scan, it can be seen that the tumor is expanding, the density in the damaged area is even, the CT value is slightly higher than that of soft tissue, and it can be strengthened after enhancement. The damaged bone edge is thin but continuous, and no periosteal reaction is seen. Due to the expanding growth, the surrounding soft tissue is pushed, and the muscle space and normal structure are deformed with the expansion of bone.

Pathological Characteristics Pathological examination shows multinucleated osteoclastic giant cells in the stroma of highly mitotic spindle cells. Immunohistochemically, GCG is positive for macrophage and osteoclast markers, such as vascular endothelial growth factor, nuclear receptor activator factor κ(RANK) and RANKL. The increase of the RANK signal promotes the generation and differentiation of osteoclasts, leading to bone resorption [1, 5].

Treatment GCG is locally invasive and should be actively treated. At present, the following treatment methods are mainly used:

1. Scaling: GCG tends to spontaneous remission, so some scholars think that pure scaling to mandible GCG can achieve the target of cure. However, there are also reports that pure scaling has a high recurrence rate.
2. Radiotherapy: There are many debates about radiotherapy. It is reported that radiotherapy has no effect on GCG, and it may become malignant. Therefore, only when GCG involves complex structures, such as skull base, etc., and it is difficult to completely remove the lesions should postoperative radiotherapy be considered, and low dose and high voltage radiotherapy should be used.
3. Surgical resection: Thorough surgical resection is the best scheme. Aesthetic and functional reconstruction should be considered during operation.

In recent years, some scholars have studied the application of Denosumab in the treatment of GCG. Denosumab is a human monoclonal antibody binding to RANKL receptor activator. It inhibits the activation and differentiation of osteoclast-like giant cells and effectively inhibits bone resorption. Denosumab has been approved by FDA for the treatment of giant cell tumor (GCT) in adults and adolescents with mature bones. It has also been used to treat other bone diseases, such as osteogenesis imperfecta, aneurysmal bone cysts and fibrous dysplasia. It has been reported in the literature that GCG was cured by injection of Denosumab combined with oral calcium and vitamin D.

References

1. de Lange J, van den Akker HP, van den Berg H. Central giant cell granuloma of the jaw: a review of the literature with emphasis on therapy options [J]. Oral Surg Oral Med Oral Pathol Oral Radiol Endod. 2007;104(5):603–15.
2. Choe M, Smith V, Okcu MF, et al. Treatment of central giant cell granuloma in children with denosumab [J]. Pediatr Blood Cancer. 2021;68(3):e28778.
3. Lipplaa A, Dijkstra S, Gelderblom H. Challenges of denosumab in giant cell tumor of bone, and other giant cell-rich tumors of bone [J]. Curr Opin Oncol. 2019;31(4):329–35.
4. Bocchialini G, Salvagni L, Guerini A, et al. Central giant cell granuloma of the mandibular condyle: a rare case and a literature review [J]. Heliyon. 2019;6(1):e03085.
5. Itonaga I, Hussein I, Kudo O, et al. Cellular mechanisms of osteoclast formation and lacunar resorption in giant cell granuloma of the jaw [J]. J Oral Pathol Med. 2003;32(4):224–31.

Cherubism

16

Bing Liu, Hui Shan Ong, Zhen Tian, Lin Zhu, and Xiao Tang

16.1 Introduction

Cherubism is a hereditary disease characterized by symmetrical painless enlargement of bilateral jaws [1, 2]. Typical lesions begin in children aged 2–5 years, and the incidence of male and female is about 2:1 [3–5]. The lesion is characterized by painless enlargement of bilateral mandibles. The bone tissue in the lesion area is absorbed and replaced by a large number of abnormally proliferating fibrous tissues [2, 3, 6]. The lesions mainly invade the mandible and less involve the maxilla. Those with mild symptoms often need X-ray films to find out the disease, and those with serious lesions may have obvious swelling and deformity of the maxillofacial region. Most patients are accompanied by abnormal development of a dental and maxillofacial system, which can cause chewing, pronunciation and swallowing dysfunction in severe cases. Cherubism has a certain degree of self-limitation, but most patients' facial deformities can still last until adolescence.

B. Liu (✉)
Hospital of Stomatology Wuhan University, Wuhan, Hubei, China
e-mail: liubing9909@wuhan.edu.cn

H. S. Ong · Z. Tian · X. Tang
Department of Oral Maxillofacial-Head & Neck Oncology, Shanghai Ninth People's Hospital, Shanghai Jiao Tong University School of Medicine, Shanghai, China

L. Zhu
Department of Radiology, Ninth People's Hospital Affiliated to Shanghai Jiao Tong University, Shanghai, China

16.2 Case 33

The patient, female, 36 years old. The right jaw tumor recurred for more than 10 years after multiple operations.

[Present Medical History] At the age of 9, the patient underwent "scaling of right mandibular tumor" in a local hospital because of "swelling of the right mandible." After that, swelling of the right mandible recurred many times, and the maxilla also showed lesions. The patient underwent operation treatment and was diagnosed with postoperative pathology: Giant cell reparation granuloma of maxilla and mandible. Five years ago, the patient found that the right face was swollen, without obvious symptoms of pain and numbness, ignoring vague objects and dysphagia, without loosening or displacement of teeth and numbness of the lower lip. Maxillofacial CT examination in the outpatient department of our hospital showed that multiple bone structural abnormalities of the right cranial and maxillofacial bones, combined with clinical consideration, may be giant cell granuloma (may recur after the operation).

Y. He (ed.), *Inflammatory and Neoplastic Diseases of Craniofacial Bones*,
https://doi.org/10.1007/978-981-97-4155-7_16

[Specialized Examination] The maxillofacial region is asymmetrical, and the right maxilla is obviously larger than the opposite side, hard and painless. The mouth-opening degree and mouth-opening type are normal, and the vestibulum of the mouth is obviously bony, with no obvious boundary. There is no numbness in the skin of the right maxillofacial region, and the vision is normal. No obvious abnormal secretion is found in the nasal cavity, no obvious swelling in the palate, and no dysphagia. In the right mandible, the bone swelling can be palpated. However, there is no obvious ping-pong sensation, and the mucosa is intact and normal.

[Auxiliary Examination]

1. Panoramic radiographs: The bone density of the mandible is uneven and decreased, a cystic low-density area is found, the bone cortex is discontinuous, and no obvious periosteal reaction and soft tissue mass are found (Fig. 16.1).
2. Maxillofacial CT enhanced scan: Multiple bone structural abnormalities of the right cranial and maxillofacial bones: Combined with clinical consideration, maybe giant cell granuloma (may recur after operation) (Fig. 16.2).

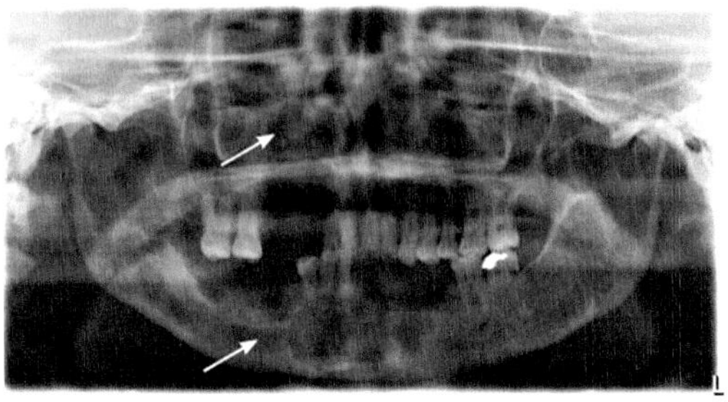

Fig. 16.1 The bone density of the mandible was uneven and decreased, a cystic low-density area was found, the bone cortex was discontinuous, and no obvious periosteal reaction and soft tissue mass were found (before the operation)

[Primary Diagnosis] Multiple space-occupying lesions of right jaw.

[Treatment] "maxilla lesion scaling" was performed under general anesthesia: A transverse incision was designed along the maxillary vestibular groove, the mucoperiosteum was cut, and the flap was turned to expose the right maxilla. Bone destruction of the maxilla was seen, local granulomatous changes were found, and the focus was scraped to the fresh bone surface. The moved parts were submitted for freezing for pathological examination. Indicating: Giant cell granuloma lesion of "right maxilla," there was no evidence of malignant tumor. The dynamic system ground off part of the bone, the wound was washed, bleeding was completely stopped, and the wound was closed by suture (Fig. 16.3).

[Pathological Examination] The part sent for pathological examination was grayish-brown broken tissues, about 2 cm*1.5 cm*0.8 cm in size. Microscopically, multinucleated giant cells were deposited in the background of proliferating fibrous tissue. The number of multinucleated giant cells was small, with different sizes and uneven distribution, and the histological morphology was similar to that of giant cell granuloma (Fig. 16.4).

[Pathological Diagnosis] Cherubism of "right maxilla," ICD code: K07.002.

[Data of Follow-Up Visit] The patient recovered well after the operation. In the follow-up visit after half a year, the appearance recovered satisfactorily, and there was no recurrence.

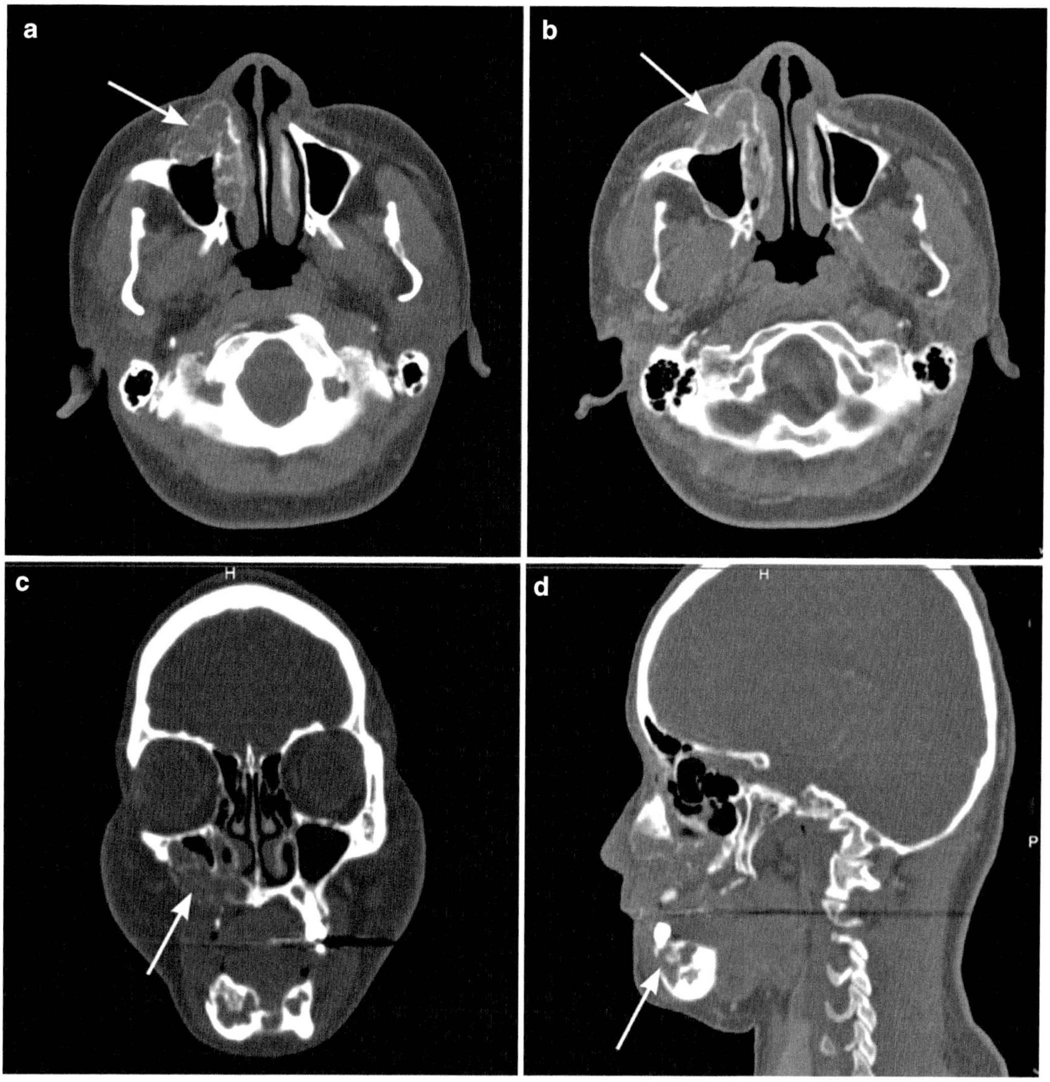

Fig. 16.2 (**a**) CT plain scan transverse view: The bone density of the right cranial and maxillofacial bone was abnormal, with bone destruction and uneven internal bone density. (**b**) Transverse view of CT enhanced scan: No significant enhancement is seen. (**c**, **d**) Coronary view and sagittal view of CT enhanced scan: Multiple abnormal bone density and bone destruction in the right cranial and maxillofacial bones

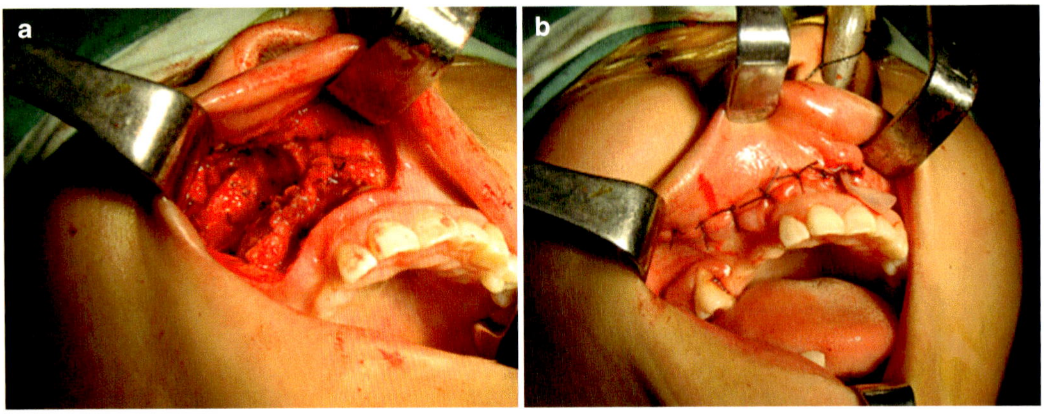

Fig. 16.3 (**a**) The diseased granulation tissue was scraped, and the dynamic system ground off part of the maxillary bone to the fresh bone surface. (**b**) Apposition suture was conducted for the mucosa, and a drainage strip of rubber was indwelled

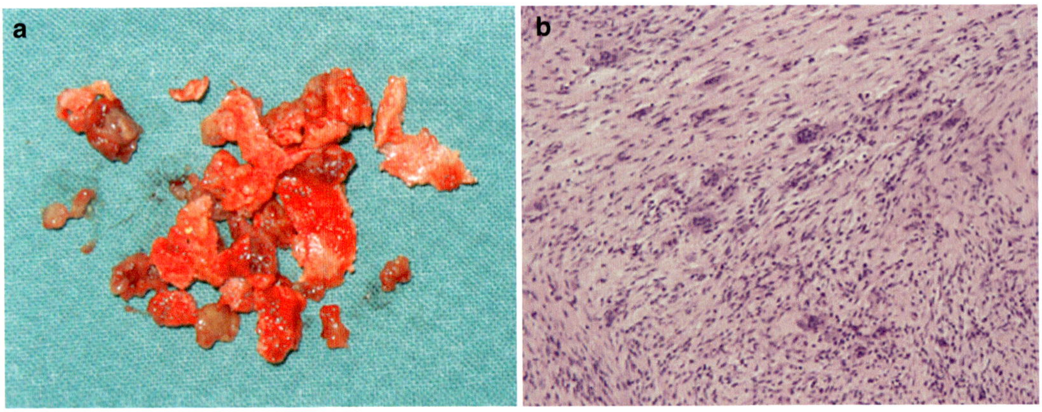

Fig. 16.4 (**a**) Right maxillary pathological tissue was scaled. (**b**) In the background of proliferating spindle cells, multinucleated giant cells were scattered, with different sizes and different numbers of nuclei (200×)

16.3 Key points of Diagnosis and Treatment

The clinical manifestations of familial cherubism vary greatly and are related to the severity of the disease. It is usually a painless enlargement of bilateral jaws, and the lesions mainly invade the mandible, mostly in the mandibular angle area, and the maxilla can also be invaded. Extensive maxillary lesions may involve the orbital floor and the orbital side wall, make the eyeballs protrude, turn upward and inward, and expose the white sclera. The infraorbital ridge can be destroyed in severe cases, and the lower eyelid will shrink after losing support. Diplopia and vision loss, etc., may be caused. The surface of the jaw is smooth or irregular, the alveolar ridge is swollen, the palpation quality is hard, and there is no tenderness. Widening of the alveolar ridge is common. When the maxilla is involved, the widening of the alveolar process can make the palate show an inverted "V" shape, and the alveolar process of the mandible expands so that the tongue is lifted, which can affect children patients' language, chewing, swallowing and breathing, and obstructive sleep apnea syndrome may also be caused. Teeth are often displaced and loose, the dentition is irregular, the gap is large, deciduous teeth fall off or stay early, and permanent teeth are not erupted or missing. Although there is no inflammation, it can often cause cervical lymph node enlargement due to reactive hyperplasia or fibrosis. In the active stage of the disease, lymph nodes are tender, active, large and discontinuous. Cherubism is usually confined to the maxilla and mandible, and no other bone is associated with it. However, there are also reports of cases invading temporal bone, ribs and some long bones. There are also reports of cases of unilateral happening in the literature. Cherubism is an autosomal dominant genetic disease; its pathogenic gene is SH3BP2 gene located in chromosome 4p16 [2].

The treatment of cherubism mainly depends on surgical operation treatment, and many scholars have different views on the selection of surgical time. It is generally believed that it should be postponed until after puberty, and premature surgery may recur. However, jaw deformity has a certain influence on children's psychological development and language function; therefore, early surgery should also be considered for children with severe jaw deformity. Scaling and osteoplasty in the rapidly progressive stage of the lesion can not only improve the tolerance but also prevent the residual lesion from growing and even stimulate the formation of new bone. In addition, calcitonin can inhibit bone resorption caused by multinucleated giant cells, which is expected to be used to treat cherubism. Because radiotherapy may inhibit the development of the jaw and lead to osteoradionecrosis of the jaws, therefore, it is a taboo for cherubism.

References

1. Jones WA. Familial multilocular cystic disease of the jaws [J]. Am J Cancer. 1933;17:946–50.
2. Reichenberger EJ, Levine MA, Olsen BR, et al. The role of SH3BP2 in the pathophysiology of cherubism [J]. Orphanet J Rare Dis. 2012;7(Suppl 1):S5.
3. Von Wowern N. Cherubism: a 36-year long-term follow-up of 2 generations in different families and review of the literature [J]. Oral Surg Oral Med Oral Pathol Oral Radiol Endod. 2000;90(6):765–72.
4. Pontes FS, Ferreira AC, Kato AM, et al. Aggressive case of cherubism: 17-year follow-up [J]. Int J Pediatr Otorhinolaryngol. 2007;71(5):831–5.
5. Chrcanovic BR, Guimarães LM, Gomes CC, et al. Cherubism: a systematic literature review of clinical and molecular aspects [J]. Int J Oral Maxillofac Surg. 2021;50(1):43–53.
6. Machado RA, Pontes H, Pires FR, et al. Clinical and genetic analysis of patients with cherubism [J]. Oral Dis. 2017;23(8):1109–15.

Part VI

Fibro-osseous Lesions

17 Fibrous Dysplasia

Yue He, Hui Shan Ong, Zhen Tian, Lin Zhu, and Yu Han

17.1 Introduction

Fibrous dysplasia, also known as fibrous dysplasia, was first reported in 1891 [1, 2]. It is characterized by progressive bone tissue defect and abnormal trabecular bone and bone marrow structure, accompanied by fibrous tissue hyperplasia, showing ground-glass changes in bone tissue in X-ray examination. Fibrous dysplasia of bone is common in femur and pelvis, and rare in the jaw [3–7]. There are three clinical types: Single type, multiple type, and cranial and maxillofacial type. The single type is usually characterized by abnormal bone structure of a single focus. It usually grows slowly and is self-limited. Multiple type can show the invasion and oppression of adjacent structures. The diagnosis of fibrous dysplasia of bone needs to combine clinical manifestations with imaging manifestations, and if necessary, gene detection (GNAS1 gene mutation) or pathological biopsy can be carried out [7, 8]. Treatment methods include observation, bisphosphonate treatment and surgical repair or resection. Bone fibrous dysplasia may recur and become malignant after operation, so it is necessary to follow up the patients for a long time.

Y. He (✉) · H. S. Ong · Z. Tian · Y. Han
Department of Oral Maxillofacial-Head & Neck Oncology, Shanghai Ninth People's Hospital, Shanghai Jiao Tong University School of Medicine, Shanghai, China

L. Zhu
Department of Radiology, Ninth People's Hospital Affiliated to Shanghai Jiao Tong University, Shanghai, China

17.2 Monostotic Fibrous Dysplasia

17.2.1 Case 34

The patient, female, 11 years old. The right maxilla tumor recurred for more than 10 years after operation.

[Present Medical History] The patient underwent resection of a "right maxillary tumor" three years ago and one year ago, respectively, due to a "right maxillary lesion." After the operation, all the patients were diagnosed with "fibrous dysplasia of the right maxilla." Ten months ago, the family members found that the tumor of the right maxilla had recurred and gradually increased. They went to the local hospital for a CT examination, considering " fibrous dysplasia of the right maxilla and sphenoid bone." In the past six months, the tumor increased rapidly and the face was asymmetric obviously.

[Specialized Examination] The face is asymmetrical, the right side of the nose and the middle part of the face are swollen, about 5.0 cm*7.0 cm in size, and the nose is pushed to the left, and the

Y. He (ed.), *Inflammatory and Neoplastic Diseases of Craniofacial Bones*,
https://doi.org/10.1007/978-981-97-4155-7_17

right nostril is larger than the left nostril. The right side of the mouth is lower than the left side; the mouth opening degree and mouth opening type are basically normal, the vestibular groove is swollen from 11 to 16, the texture is hard, the boundary is unclear, there is no fluctuation or feeling of activity, and the right side of the palate is swollen than the left side.

[Auxiliary Examination]

CT enhanced scan of maxillofacial region: After "resection of fibrous dysplasia of the right maxilla," the patient has swelling changes of the upper maxilla, sphenoid bone and hard palate, ground-glass changes of the bone marrow cavity, continuous bone cortex, obvious swelling of the upper maxilla, mass-like changes protruding to the cheek, there is no obvious enhancement after enhancement, and there is no abnormal mass in the surrounding soft tissue. The right nasal cavity is narrowed due to compression, and the right maxillary sinus changes obviously due to compression. Multiple lymph node enlargement in 1~2 regions of the neck. The adenoids are full, and the anterior nasopharyngeal cavity is slightly narrowed. The mucosa of sinus is slightly thickened (Fig. 17.1).

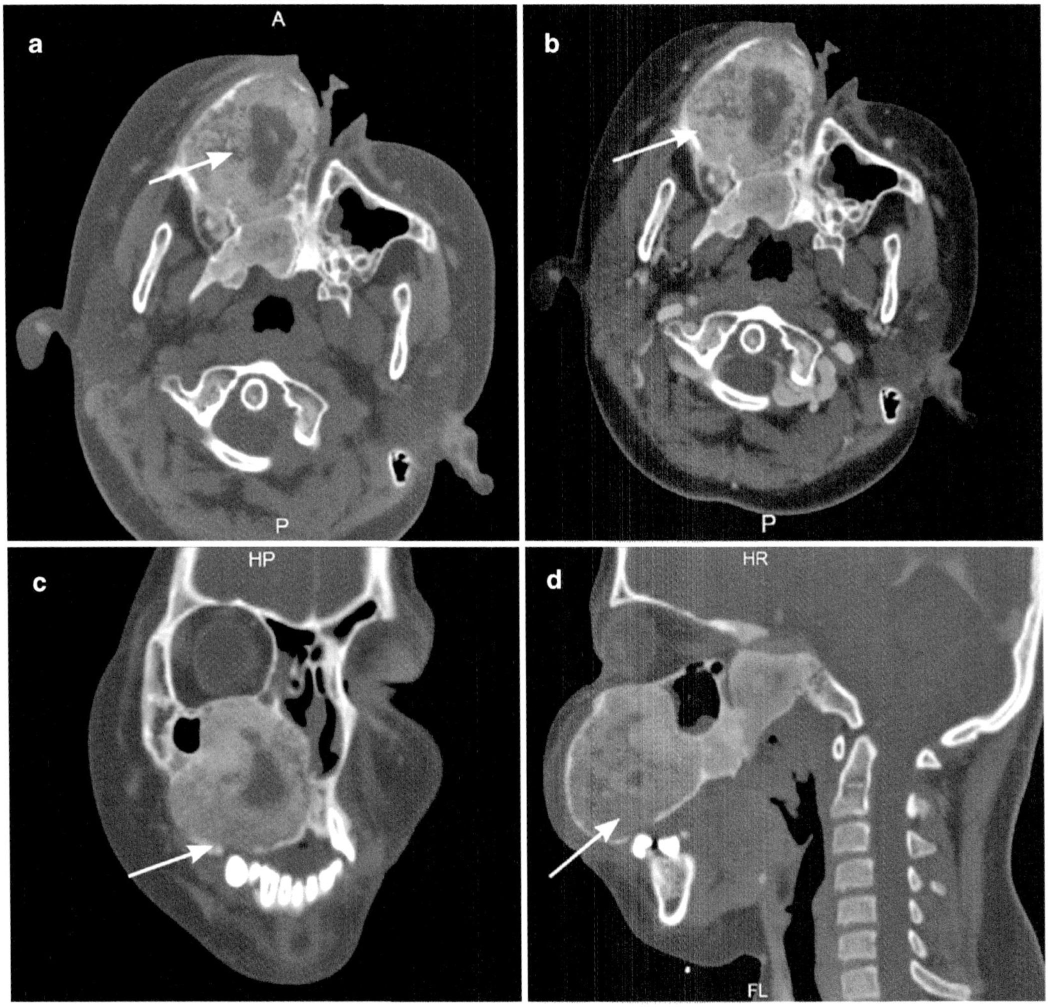

Fig. 17.1 (**a**) Transverse view of CT plain scan: Swelling changes of right maxilla, sphenoid bone and hard palate, and ground-glass changes of the bone marrow cavity. (**b**) Transverse view of CT enhanced scan: The mass has no obvious enhancement. (**c**) Coronal view of CT enhanced scan: The right nasal cavity is compressed, and the density inside the mass is uneven. (**d**) Sagittal view of CT enhanced scan: There is no obvious compression in the right maxillary sinus

[Primary Diagnosis] fibrous dysplasia of right maxilla.

[Treatment] Intra-oral approach maxilla contouring in achieving facial symmetry were performed under general anesthesia: Incision of vestibular groove, the flap was turned over to eye socket, and the lesion was exposed. The lesion was fibrous tissue, slightly softer than bone tissue, about 5.0 cm*4.5 cm in size, and there was no obvious boundary among normal maxilla, zygomatic bone and inferior orbital rim. Compared with the opposite side, the diseased tissues of the maxilla, zygomatic bone and nose were trimmed by a dynamic system, and it can be seen that the bilateral maxilla areas were symmetrical. The diseased tissue was sent for pathological examination. The operative region was rinsed, bleeding was stopped, the negative pressure drainage tube was indwelled, a full-thickness suture was conducted, and the wound was closed.

[Pathological Examination] The part sent for pathological examination was broken tissue, 7.5 cm*7 cm*5.2 cm, dark red and medium in texture. Microscopically, a braided trabecular bone was formed in the background of fibrous tissue. The trabecular bone was slender, bow-shaped and branched, and there was no connection between the trabecular bones and no osteoblasts around it. In some areas, fibroblasts were abundant and proliferated actively (Fig. 17.2).

[Pathological Diagnosis] fibrous dysplasia of "right maxilla," ICD code: K10.805.

[Follow-Up Visit] The patient recovered well after the operation, the maxillary shape was satisfactory, and the bilateral faces were basically symmetrical.

17.2.2 Case 35

The patient, female, 23 years old. The swelling and swelling of the left mandible gradually worsened for 2 weeks.

[Present Medical History] Two weeks ago, the patient found that the left mandible was swollen and gradually aggravated. There was no obvious pain, numbness of the lower lip and other sensory abnormalities, and the teeth were not loose. CT examination in the outpatient department of our hospital showed that the left mandible was proliferative, maybe ossifying fibroma.

[Specialized Examination] The face is asymmetrical from left to right, the left face is obviously swollen, and the surface skin color and temperature are normal. The mouth opening degree and mouth opening type are normal, the oral hygiene is average, the buccal side of the left mandible is obviously swollen, there is no obvious breaking or oozing of the mucosa, the teeth

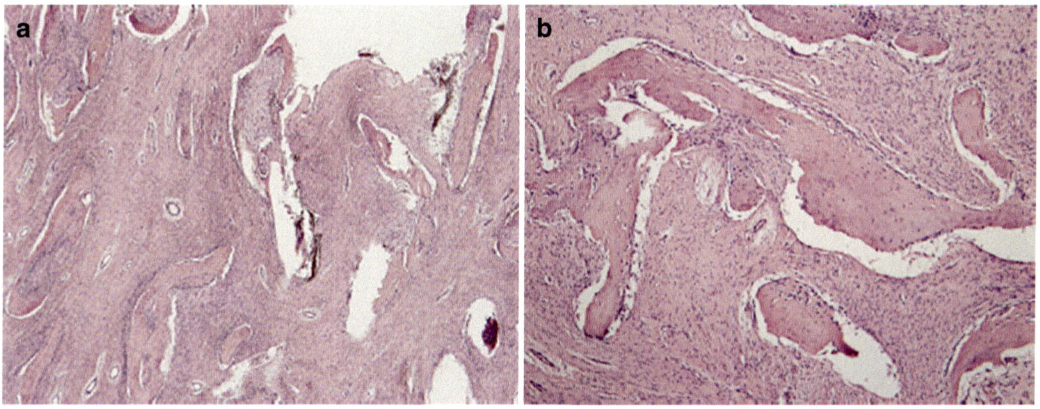

Fig. 17.2 (**a**) In the background of fibrous tissue hyperplasia, irregular trabecular bones were formed, and the trabecular bones were not connected with each other (40×). (**b**) There was no bone cell around the woven trabecular meshwork (100×)

are not loose, and no obvious lesions are found in the mucosa in the other parts of the mouth. No obvious swollen lymph nodes are seen in bilateral submandibular regions and neck.

[Auxiliary Examination]

1. Panoramic radiographs: The left mandible body has swelling changes and uneven density (Fig. 17.3a).
2. Maxillofacial CT plain scan: The left mandible bone swells with ground-glass density, about 6 cm*3 cm in size, and no abnormality is found in surrounding soft tissues (Fig. 17.3b, c).

   [Primary diagnosis] mass of left mandible (maybe ossifying fibroma).

   [Treatment] Intra-oral approach mandibular contouring in achieving facial symmetry was performed under general anesthesia: The mucoperiosteum was cut, the flap was turned over, the tumor was fully exposed, some abnormal bones were dynamically ground off, and the shapes of the two sides of the mandible were repeatedly compared. The purpose of the symmetric mandibular shape was the treatment purpose. Bleeding was completely stopped, the wound was rinsed, and apposition suture was strictly implemented.

[Pathological Examination] A pile of grayish-yellow broken bone tissue was sent for biopsy, 4 cm*3 cm*2 cm in size. Microscopically, hyperplastic trabecular bone can be seen in the background of fibrous tissue. The braided trabecular bone was slender, with different shapes, and lacked connection with each other, like an English letter.

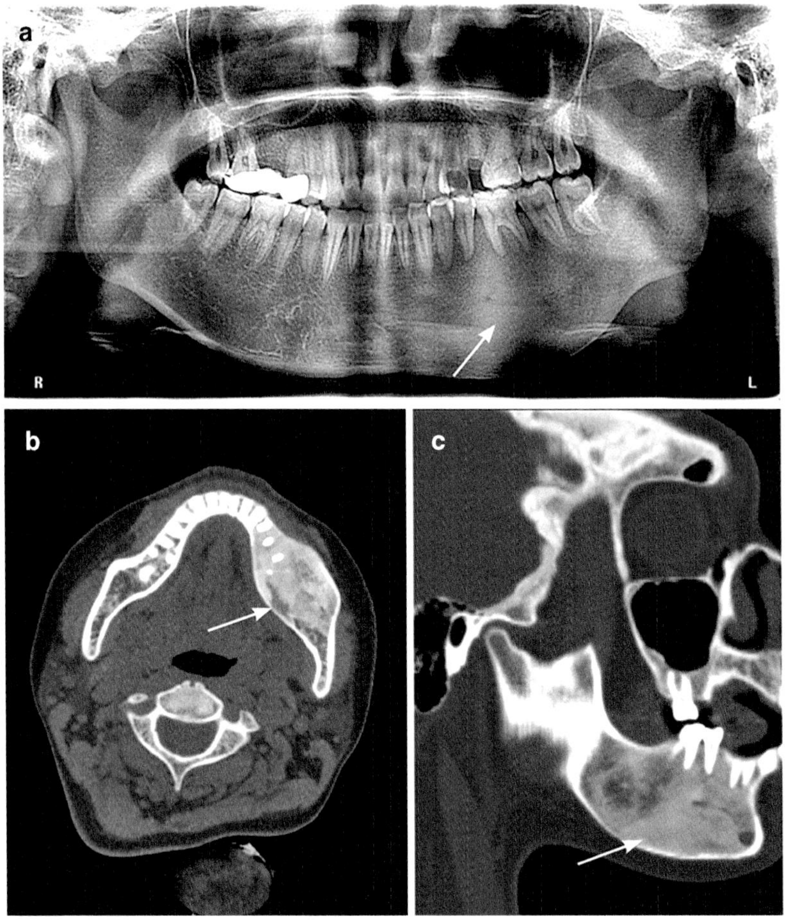

Fig. 17.3 (**a**) Panoramic radiographs: The left mandible body had swelling changes and uneven density. (**b**) Transverse view of CT plain scan: The bone of the left mandible body was swollen with ground-glass density, and the surrounding soft tissue was normal. (**c**) Reconstruction of CT plain scan thin-layer surface: There was no obvious involvement of dentition at the focus

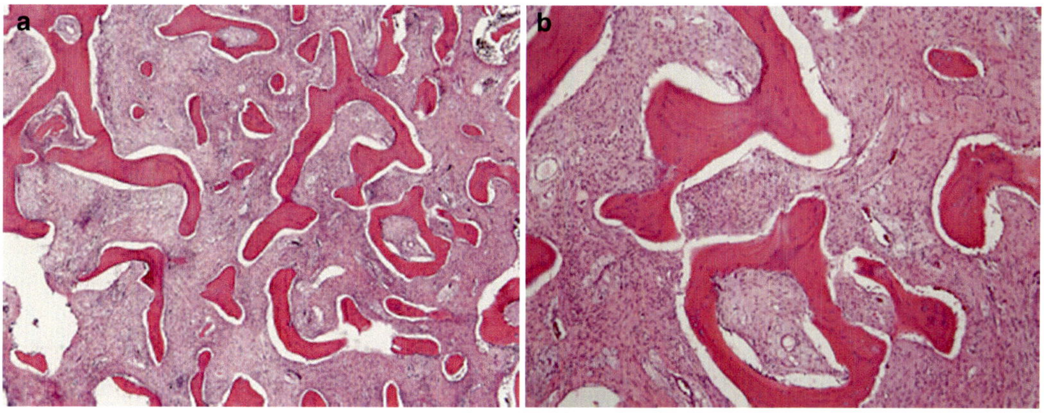

Fig. 17.4 (**a**) In the background of loose fibrous tissue, a braided trabecula was formed, and the shape of bone tissue was irregular, such as letter-like, and there was no connection between them (40×). (**b**) Osteoblasts were absent around trabecular bone, and fibrous tissue cells among trabecular bone were abundant, with vascular hyperplasia (100×)

Osteoblasts surrounded most osteoid tissues, and the diseased bone tissue was connected with the bone cortex without boundaries. Due to local secondary infection, osteoblasts and osteoclasts appeared around osteoid tissue. The fibrous stroma between trabeculae was loosely arranged, and the size of fibroblasts was consistent (Fig. 17.4).

[Pathological Diagnosis] fibrous dysplasia of "left mandible," ICD code: K10.805.

[Follow-Up Visit] The patient recovered well after the operation. The mandibular contour recovered satisfactorily, and the bilateral face was basically symmetric.

17.2.3 Case 36

The patient, male, 28 years old. Repeated swelling and pain in the mandible lasted for more than 1 year and aggravated for 4 months.

[Present Medical History] The patient underwent an "extraction of sebaceous cyst in the left submandibular region" in the local hospital more than one year ago. About one month after the operation, swelling and pain developed around the operative region. After anti-inflammatory drugs were taken orally, the symptoms were relieved, and the swelling and pain symptoms recurred. There was a history of swelling in different parts of the bilateral mandibular angle. Eleven months ago, a local hospital performed panoramic radiographs and found an abnormal density shadow of the mandible, suggesting a pathological biopsy. The patient asked for anti-inflammatory symptomatic treatment, and his symptoms worsened four months ago. He went to the other hospital for treatment and continued to be given anti-inflammatory treatment after relevant examinations, and there was no obvious improvement.

[Specialized Examination] The face is basically symmetrical. The proportion of the upper, middle and lower 1/3 face is coordinated. Slight redness, a surgical scar in the left submandibular region, unsmooth skin, no obvious ulceration, no obvious swelling and fluctuation, rough feeling on the buccal bone surface of bilateral mandible body and chin, slight swelling, unclear boundary and tenderness (−). The degree and type of mouth opening are normal, Intraoral permanent dentition, the occluding relation is normal, with no obvious tooth loosening, percussion pain (−), and there is no obvious mucosal redness, swelling or orificium fistulae. No significantly abnormally enlarged lymph nodes have been found in the bilateral submaxilla and neck.

[Auxiliary Examination]

1. Panoramic radiographs: Abnormal density of bilateral mandible body, unclear boundary and local ground glass degeneration (Fig. 17.5a).
2. Maxillofacial CT enhanced scan: Bone swelling of chin and body of bilateral mandible show ground-glass density, and local bone destruction of the buccal side of right mandible body is found, with layered periosteum reaction, swelling of surrounding soft tissues and blurred boundary, with C− of 77 Hu and C+ of 92 Hu. Bilateral submandibular and submandibular lymph nodes are slightly enlarged and strengthened, with a larger size of 14 mm-6 mm (Fig. 17.5b, c).

[Primary Diagnosis] It may be a secondary infection of mandible fibrous dysplasia.

[Treatment] Under general anesthesia, "sectional resection of mandible + fibula musculocutaneous flap transfer repair + tracheotomy" was performed. An incision of 1~2 cm was made along the inferior margin of the mandible; the flap was turned over. The mandibular marginal branch of the facial nerve was protected, and the mandible body and ascending ramus were exposed. In accordance with the design of the preoperative osteotomy guide plate, the mandible was amputated at the outer edge of bilateral mandibular angle lesions about 0.5 cm. The free fibula with vascular pedicle on the left side was prepared routinely, and the fibula with a length of about 18 cm was cut along the preoperative fibula osteotomy plate. The fibula was shaped in accordance with the design of the shaping guide plate, and the continuity of the mandible was restored. The fibula artery and vein were anastomosed with the facial artery and external jugular vein, respectively. The wound was rinsed, bleeding was stopped completely, the wound was tightly sutured, the negative pressure drainage tube was reserved, a suture was conducted in layers, and the wound was closed (Fig. 17.6).

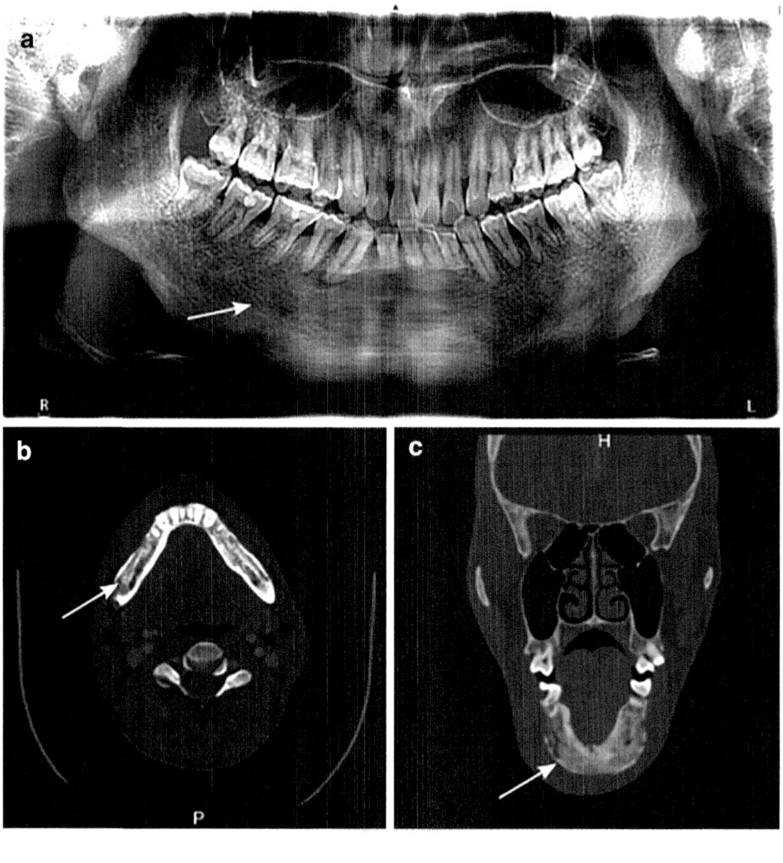

Fig. 17.5 (**a**) Panoramic radiographs: swelling changes of bilateral mandible body. (**b**) Transverse view of CT enhanced scan: bone swelling changes of bilateral mandible body, showing ground-glass density, and local bone destruction of the buccal side of the right mandible body. (**c**) Coronal view of CT enhanced scan

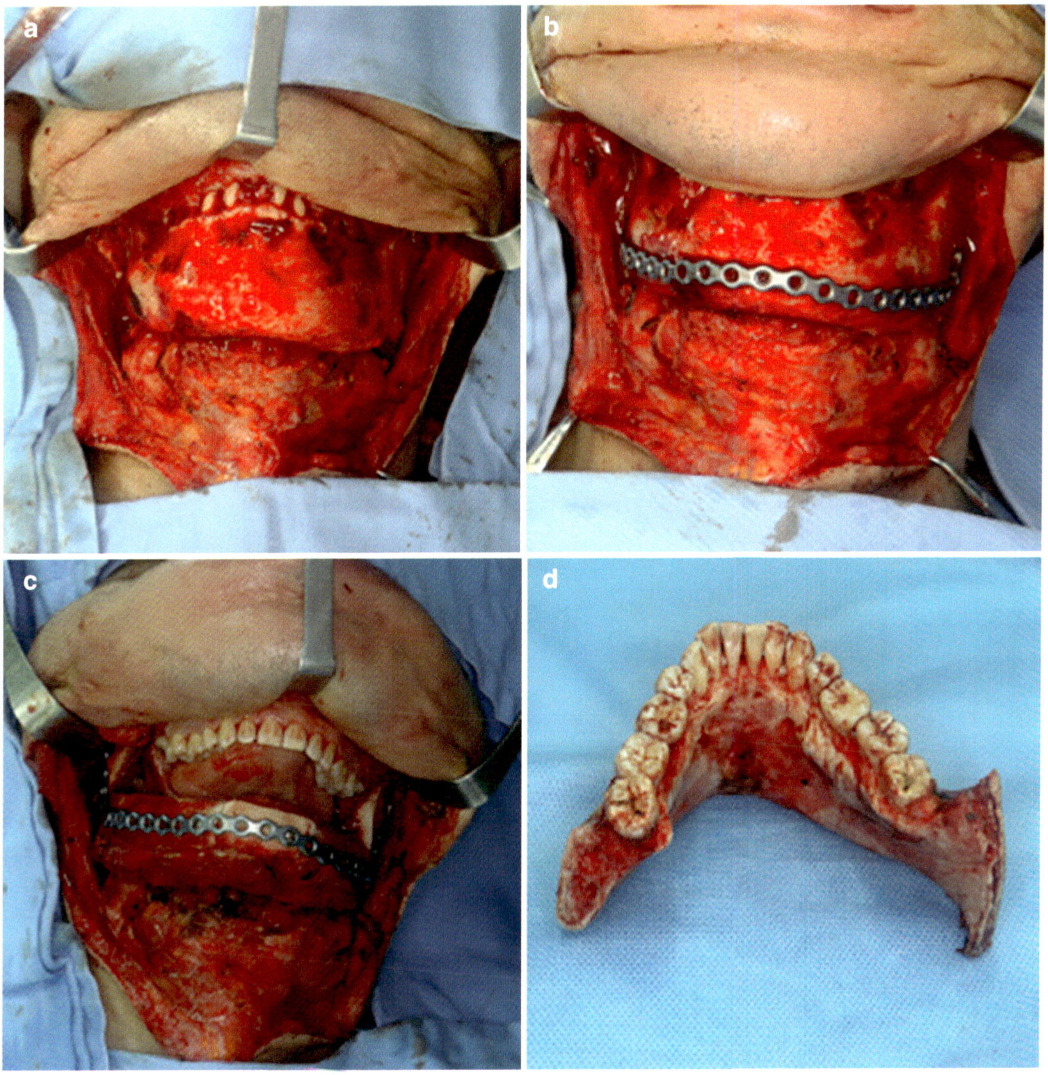

Fig. 17.6 (**a**) Bilateral mandible bodies were exposed. (**b**) Titanium plate was reconstructed by bending and forming. (**c**) Reconstructed and recovered fibula mandible continuity. (**d**) Free mandible

[Pathological Examination] The part sent for pathological examination was mandible tissue, 10 cm*7 cm*5.5 cm in size. The mandibular chin bone was slightly swollen, the section was grayish-yellow, and the texture was medium and hard. Microscopically, there were obvious hyperplasia trabeculae in the background of fibrous tissue. Some trabeculae were slender and had a lack of connection with each other, and some trabeculae were thick and connected with each other, which was related to the long course of the disease. Most of the trabecular bone lacked osteoblasts, and only a few can be seen around. Fibrous tissue between trabecular bones was loose and inflammatory cells infiltrated (Fig. 17.7).

[Pathological Diagnosis] fibrous dysplasia of "mandible," ICD code: K10.805. There was a local infection.

[Follow-Up Visit] The patient recovered well after the operation. In the follow-up visit after half a year, the reconstructed shape of the bone was satisfactory and mouth opening and closing were normal.

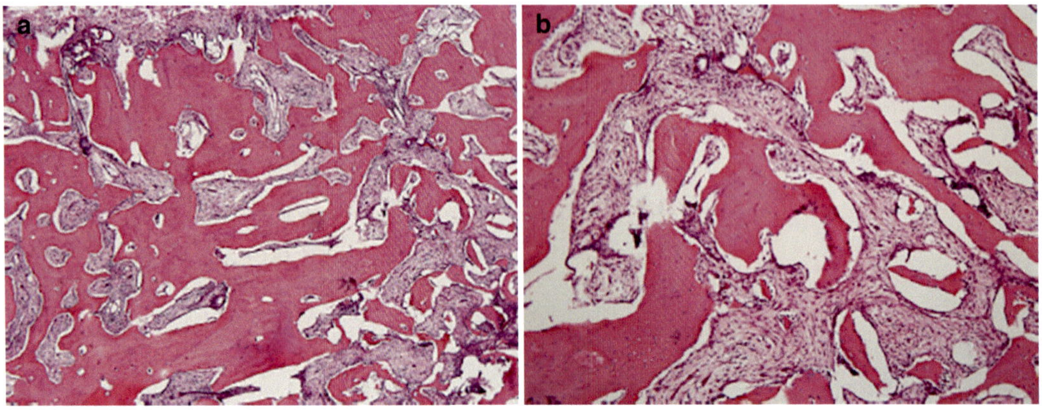

Fig. 17.7 (**a**) Irregular trabeculae were seen in the background of fibrous tissue, and some trabeculae were thick and interconnected (40×). (**b**) There were no hypertrophic osteoblasts arranged in rows around the trabecular bone, and the fibrous tissue was loose, with inflammatory cells infiltrating inside (100×)

17.3 Polyostotic Fibrous Dysplasia

17.3.1 Case 37

The patient, male, 35 years old. X-ray showed abnormal bone in the right mandible for half a year.

[Present medical history] Half a year ago, the patient planned to repair the right mandibular posterior teeth with an implant denture. Before treatment, the radiograph showed that the right mandibular bone was abnormal, and there were no obvious discomfort symptoms, such as swelling and pain, etc., and no abnormalities, such as difficulty in opening the mouth and joint snapping.

[Specialized Examination] The face is asymmetrical on the left and right. The right face is elongated, the midline of the face is left, the facial skin is complete, and the color and texture are normal. The right mandible body and buccal side of the mandibular ascending ramus can reach slight bone swelling and the mouth opening is about three horizontal fingers, and the mouth opening slightly deviates to the left. During the opening and closing of the mouth, the bilateral temporomandibular joints have no obvious abnormal movement and snapping sound. Intraoral permanent dentition, mandibular dentition is defective, root 36 is residual, 46 is missing, 45 and 47 are slightly inclined to the middle, and the occluding relation of the remaining teeth is good. The gingival mucosa is intact, and no obvious abnormal swelling and leakage and sinus fistula are found. On the buccal side of the right maxilla, bone swelling can be reached (Fig. 17.8a, b). No significantly abnormally enlarged lymph nodes have been found in the bilateral submaxilla and neck.

[Auxiliary Examination]

1. Panoramic radiographs: The density of the right maxilla and mandible decreases unevenly, and the boundary is unclear, with ground glass-like changes in some areas (Fig. 17.8c).
2. Maxillofacial CT enhanced scan: Bone swelling changes can be seen in the right mandible body—condyle, maxilla, zygomatic bone, sphenoid bone and temporal bone, with ground-glass changes in it, and low-density shadow can be seen locally. CT− is 60 Hu, CT+ is 73 Hu, and no obvious swelling is found in the surrounding soft tissues. No obvious enlarged lymph node shadows are seen in the neck (Fig. 17.9).

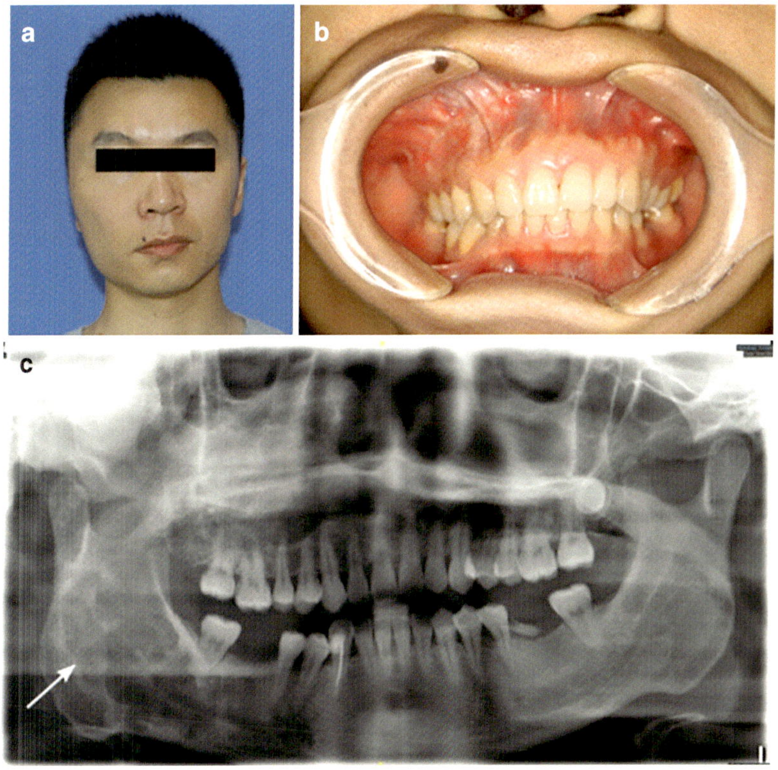

Fig. 17.8 (**a**) The face is asymmetrical in the left and right; the right face is elongated and the midline of the face is left. (**b**) The occluding relation is good, and the midline deviates. (**c**) Panoramic radiographs: The density of the right maxilla and mandible decreases unevenly, and the boundary is unclear, with ground glass-like changes in some areas

[Primary Diagnosis] polyostotic fibrous dysplasia of right cranial and maxillofacial bones.

[Treatment]

1. "Segmental resection of right mandible + vascularized fibula musculocutaneous flap transfer repair" was performed under general anesthesia: An incision was designed 1~2 cm along the lower edge of the mandible, and the mandible body and ascending ramus were exposed. The mandible was cut off in the middle of 46, and the diseased mandible body, including the condyle, was completely removed. During the operation, the condyle bone and morphology were still normal, the mandible was cut off at the condyle neck, the bone at the broken end was normal, and the condyle was replanted. The free fibula with a vascular pedicle on the left side was prepared, and the fibula with a length of about 12 cm was cut, shaped, and reconstructed, and the continuity and occluding relation of the mandible were restored. The fibula artery and vein were anastomosed with facial artery and facial vein, respectively. The operative wound was rinsed, bleeding was stopped strictly, the negative pressure drainage tube was indwelled, a suture was conducted in layers, and the wound was closed.
2. Maxillary, zygomatic, sphenoid and temporal bone lesions are temporarily considered. A close follow-up visit is required.

[Pathological Examination] The parts sent for pathological examination were the mandible body and ascending ramus, 7 cm*6.5 cm*2.5 cm in size, with local bone cortex destruction. On the sectional view, the boundary between the diseased bone and the surrounding normal tissues was unclear, involving the bone cortex, grayish yellow, tough and braided. Microscopically, in the background of fibrous tissue, there was proliferating braided trabecular bone with different shapes, the new trabecular bone was connected with cortical bone, and there was no osteoblast around the trabecular bone (Fig. 17.10).

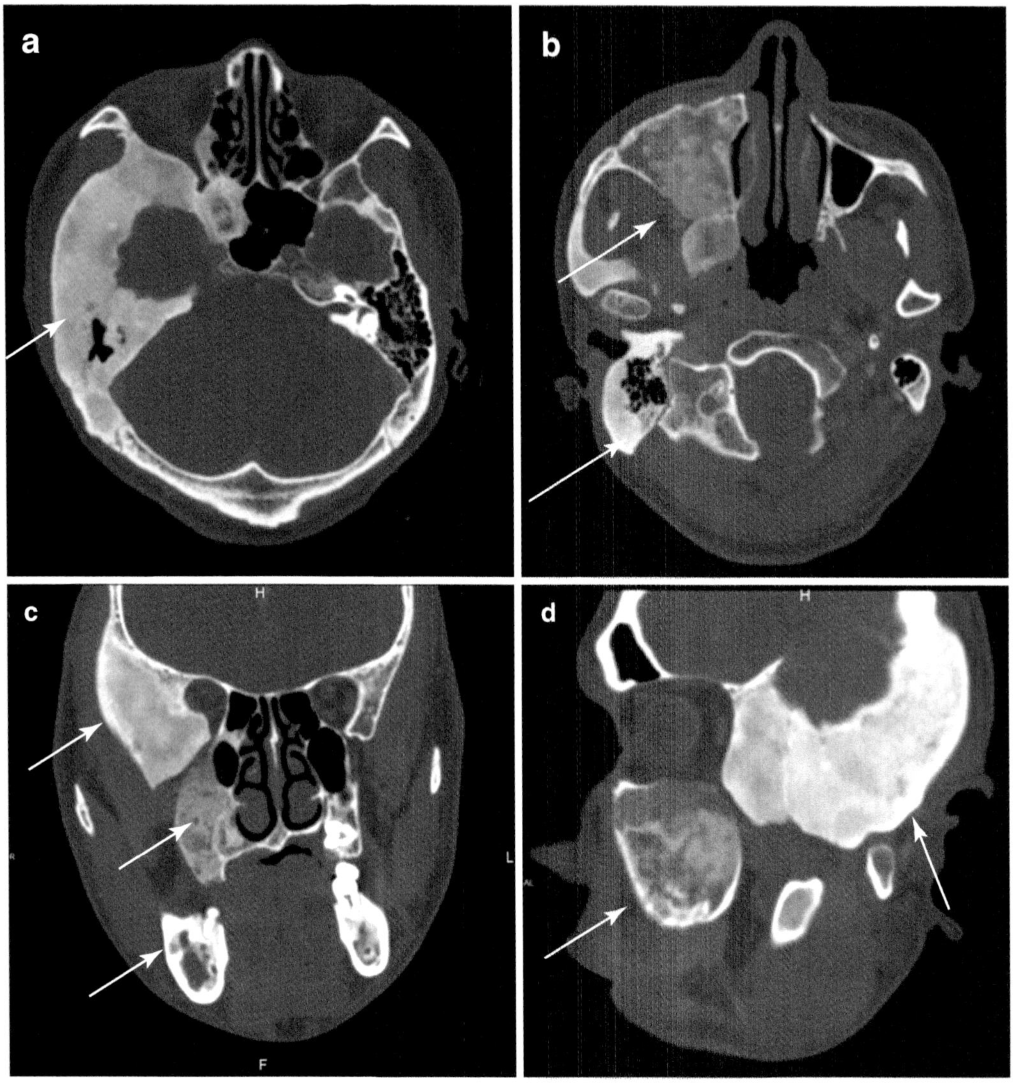

Fig. 17.9 (**a**, **b**) Transverse view. (**c**) Coronary view. (**d**) Sagittal view: Bone swelling changes can be seen in the right mandible body—condyle, maxilla, zygomatic bone, sphenoid bone and temporal bone, with ground-glass changes in it, and low-density shadow can be seen locally

[Pathological Diagnosis] fibrous dysplasia of "right mandible," some areas were rich in fibrous cells, combined with imaging findings, consistent with fibrous dysplasia of bony bones. ICD code: Q78.102.

[Follow-Up Visit] The patient recovered well after the operation. In the follow-up visit after half a year, the shape of bone reconstruction was satisfactory, and the function recovered well. There was no obvious progress in maxillary, zygomatic, sphenoid and temporal bone lesions.

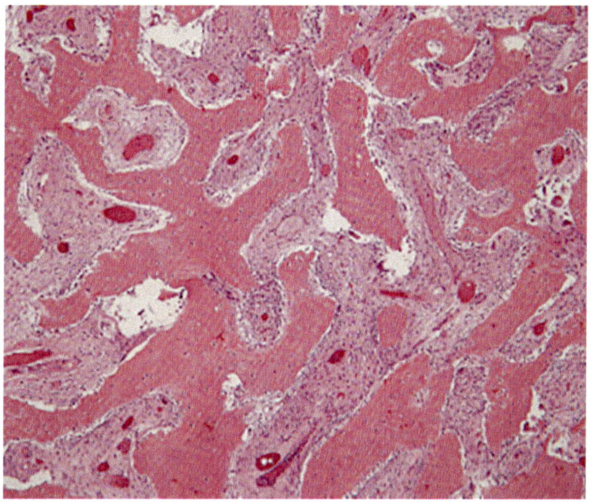

Fig. 17.10 In the background of fibrous tissue, braided trabecular bone was formed, and there were no bone cells around the trabecular bone (100×)

17.4 Key Points of Diagnosis and Treatment

Fibrous dysplasia (FD) was first proposed by Lichtenstein and Jaffe in 1942. Firstly, it was called Jaffe-Lichtenstein syndrome. The research on the pathogenesis of FD has been clear, and now, the mainstream view is that FD is a disease of bone marrow stromal cells (BMSC). During differentiation into osteoblasts, the differentiation of BMSC is blocked, proliferating and producing a fiber-like structure. Differentiation arrest of BMSC is caused by GNA gene mutation, generally occurring at 201Arg. The GNA gene encodes G protein, and the mutation of this gene prevents the activity of the endogenous GTP enzyme, leading to the accumulation of intracellular cAMP and the increase of IL-6 secretion. The secretion of IL-6 is related to the increase of osteoclasts and bone resorption observed in fibrous dysplasia of bone. Gene amplification technology such as PCR is commonly used to detect gene mutation in patients' peripheral blood samples. However, due to the interference of technical sensitivity and somatic genotype chimerism, the practicability of PCR technology in detecting mutation in blood and skin samples is limited. Alternative technologies, such as second-generation sequencing, may have higher sensitivity. It is worth noting that the level of gene mutation will change with time, and the elderly may carry fewer cells with mutations.

Clinical Manifestation The incidence of fibrous dysplasia of bone is about 0.01~0.02%, common in children or young people. There are three clinical types: Single type, multiple type, and cranial and maxillofacial type. Multiple type is common, accounting for 75~80% of FD. The commonly involved parts are ribs, long bones and cranial and maxillofacial bones; however, there are usually no obvious symptoms. The most typical single type is painless, slow growth and unilateral facial swelling. Sometimes, patients may have pain or pathological fractures with minor trauma. About 3% of the lesions are related to skin pigmentation and endocrine abnormalities, called McCone-Albright syndrome.

Diagnosis and Differential Diagnosis Because FD is often not accompanied by obvious symptoms, its diagnosis mainly depends on imaging evaluation. For example, CT and MRI are used to exclude other bone lesions and technetium radionuclide imaging is used to evaluate the severity of the disease. The diagnosis needs to be differentiated from other jaw diseases, such as ossifying fibroma, sclerosing osteomyelitis and giant cell tumor of bone. When patients have symptoms of rapid progress of lesions, severe pain and abnormal sensation, etc., other lesions should be considered, such as aneurysmal bone cyst and malignant transformation, etc.

Treatment Treatment methods include observation, medication and surgery, and the specific treatment plan should be determined in accordance with the actual situation of patients. FD of single type is usually asymptomatic, and patients of this kind can be observed and followed up regularly. Bisphosphonate drug therapy is often used to relieve osteolytic pain. Bisphosphonate can inhibit bone resorption and reduce the risk of fracture. In 2020, a retrospective study evaluated the efficacy and safety of long-term zoledronic acid in the treatment of single and multiple FD in children. The intravenous dose of zoledronic acid was 0.1 mg/kg, and the follow-up time was at least 2 years. The results indicated that the pain score was significantly improved in 6 out of 10 patients, and the alkaline phosphatase level was significantly decreased. Only one patient developed symptomatic hypocalcemia after 12 months. However, it should be noted that the follow-up time of this study is short, and it is reported that long-term and high-dose use of bisphosphonates may lead to drug-induced osteonecrosis. Therefore, whether bisphosphonates can be called first-line drugs for FD needs a randomized controlled trial with a larger sample size and longer follow-up time to determine the dose and safety of drugs.

Operation treatment is still the basic treatment of maxillofacial FD, divided into conservative dressing and osteotomy. Because of the aesthetic appearance of the maxillofacial region, cosmetic surgery is often chosen for patients with limited lesions. The biggest problem of operation is postoperative recurrence/progress. Studies have shown that the proportion of postoperative pathological changes is 68%, especially in patients with high growth hormone. This suggests that it is necessary to screen and treat endocrine diseases before operation. In addition, to avoid recurrence, many elective operations are postponed until bones mature. At this time, the lesions of FD are relatively static.

There is no uniform norm and standard for the treatment of maxillofacial FD. The newer treatment method is Denosumab treatment. Denosumab is a monoclonal antibody targeting RANKL. It has been approved to treat osteoporosis, giant cell tumors of long bone and prevent bone-related diseases caused by bone metastasis. RANKL is overexpressed in fibroblastic bone cells in FD, suggesting that it plays a role in the pathogenesis. However, in accordance with the existing clinical practice, Denosumab has some side effects, such as severe hypercalcemia, rebound bone hypermetabolic diseases after drug withdrawal, etc. Some researchers have also proposed that transplantation of bone marrow stem cells/stromal cells can treat bone fibrous dysplasia, but further transformation research is required before application.

There is less than 1% possibility that FD will become malignant, among which multiple types are more likely to become malignant. The common histological types of malignant diseases are osteosarcoma, fibrosarcoma, and chondrosarcoma, suggesting that we need to follow up closely and evaluate the invasive lesions regularly.

References

1. Schoenau E, Rauch F, et al. Fibrous dysplasia [J]. Horm Res. 2002; https://doi.org/10.1159/000058106.
2. Dicaprio MR, Enneking WF. Fibrous dysplasia. Pathophysiology, evaluation, and treatment [J]. J Bone Joint Surg Am. 2005;87(8):1848–64.
3. Chapurlat RD, Gensburger D, Jimenez-Andrade JM, et al. Pathophysiology and medical treatment of pain in fibrous dysplasia of bone [J]. Orphanet J Rare Dis. 2012;7 Suppl 1 (Suppl 1):S3.
4. Pai B, Ferdinand D. Fibrous dysplasia causing safeguarding concerns [J]. Arch Dis Child. 2013;98(12):1003.
5. Adetayo OA, Salcedo SE, Borad V, et al. Fibrous dysplasia: an overview of disease process, indications for surgical management, and a case report [J]. Eplasty. 2015;15:e6.
6. Alison M, Boyce A, et al. Surgical management of polyostotic craniofacial fibrous dysplasia: long-term outcomes and predictors for postoperative regrowth [J]. Plast Reconstr Surg. 2016; https://doi.org/10.1097/PRS.0000000000002151.
7. Okuda M, Kobayashi S, et al. Undifferentiated pleomorphic sarcoma arising in a fibrous dysplasia confirmed by GNAS mutation analysis: a case report [J]. JBJS Case Connect. 2020;10:e20.00157.
8. Tripathy SK, Swaroop S, Velagada S, et al. Response to zoledronic acid infusion in children with fibrous dysplasia [J]. Front Rediotr. 2020;8:582316.

Cemento-osseous Dysplasia 18

Yue He, Hui Shan Ong, Zhen Tian, Lin Zhu, and Qing Long Wu

18.1 Introduction

Cemento-osseous dysplasia (COD) is a non-neoplastic lesion of the jaw. In accordance with the location, quantity and imaging characteristics of the disease, COD can be divided into three categories: Focal cemento-osseous dysplasia (FCOD), periapical cemento-osseous dysplasia (PCOD?) and florid cemento-osseous dysplasia (FLCOD) [1–4]. FCOD is single, it can occur in any part of the jaw, but mostly in the back of mandible; PCOD mainly involves mandibular anterior teeth; FLCOD is multifocal involvement, not limited to mandibular anterior teeth. Generally, COD patients have no obvious symptoms and occasionally have painless jaw swelling. When the focus area is accompanied by infection, symptoms of pus overflow, swelling and pain may occur [4]. For asymptomatic patients, regular review is sufficient, and treatment is not necessary. If infection and jaw inflammation occur, surgical debridement can be performed. For patients with severe deformity or dysfunction of the maxillofacial region, surgical resection of the lesion area and reconstruction can be considered.

18.2 Periapical Cemento-osseous Dysplasia

18.2.1 Case 38

The patient, female, 58 years old. Repeated pain and discomfort of the left lower posterior teeth for 1 year.

[Present Medical History] One year ago, the patient began to suffer from repeated pain and discomfort in the left lower posterior teeth area, and the patient felt that there was a lump in the gum of the left lower back tooth area. Nine months ago, the patient was diagnosed with a "tumor in the left lower back tooth area" and suggested seeing a doctor in our hospital. A month ago, the patient went to the outpatient department of our hospital. After the panoramic film and dental CT examination, the patient was diagnosed with 28, 38 impacted teeth and 37 odontomas. Surgery was suggested.

[Specialized Examination] The face is basically symmetrical left and right, and the mouth opening degree and mouth opening type are normal. Vertical impaction of 28, there was no

Y. He (✉) · H. S. Ong · Z. Tian · Q. L. Wu
Department of Oral Maxillofacial-Head & Neck Oncology, Shanghai Ninth People's Hospital, Shanghai Jiao Tong University School of Medicine, Shanghai, China

L. Zhu
Department of Radiology, Ninth People's Hospital Affiliated to Shanghai Jiao Tong University, Shanghai, China

Y. He (ed.), *Inflammatory and Neoplastic Diseases of Craniofacial Bones*,
https://doi.org/10.1007/978-981-97-4155-7_18

knocking pain, no obvious looseness, and no redness and swelling of gums. Buccal gingival fistula of 37, no exudation was found. In the middle and lower impaction of 38, there was no knocking pain, no obvious looseness, and no redness or swelling of gums. No significantly enlarged lymph nodes have been found in the bilateral submaxilla and neck.

[Auxiliary Examination]
Panoramic Radiographs: Abnormal density shadow at root 37, adjacent to the inferior alveolar nerve canal. Impaction of 38 and 48 (Fig. 18.1).

[Primary Diagnosis] Mass of the left mandible.

[Treatment] "Radical resection of left mandible mass along with involved dental extraction" was performed under general anesthesia: An incision was conducted to buccal gingiva 37, the fistula was removed, the flap was turned over, 37 and 38 were pulled out, and buccal bone was removed, exposing space-occupying lesion of root 37. The swollen substance was hard, dense, yellow and white, and the boundary with the mandible was still clear. The swollen substance was completely removed and sent for pathological examination, hemostasis was performed, and wound closure was performed.

[Pathological Examination] The submitted specimen was a broken tissue, approximately 0.8 cm*0.5 cm*0.3 cm in size, grayish yellow, with hard nature. Microscopically, cementum-osteoid mineralization was observed in the background of fibrous connective tissue composed of fibroblasts, collagen fibers and small blood vessels (Fig. 18.2).

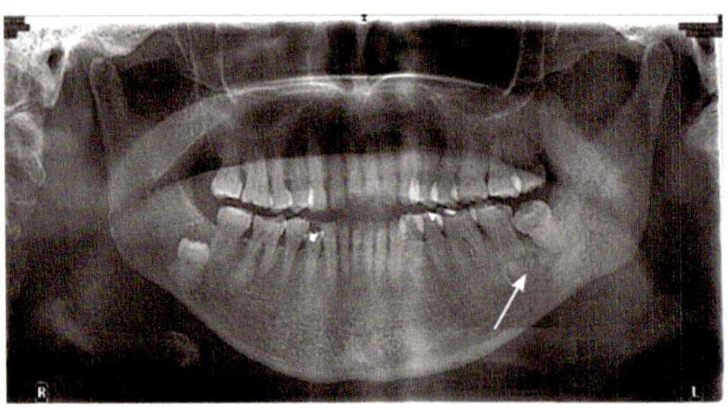

Fig. 18.1 Abnormal density shadow at root 37, adjacent to the inferior alveolar nerve canal below

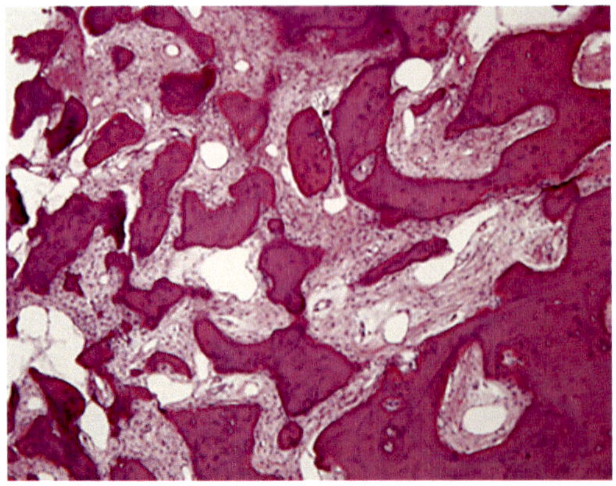

Fig. 18.2 Background of vascular fibrous connective tissue Formation of cementum-osteoid mineralization (100×)

[Pathological Diagnosis] The cementum-bone structure of periapical teeth in the "left lower posterior teeth area" was poor.

[Follow-Up Visit] The patient recovered well after the operation. Nothing special was found by re-examination in half a year after the operation.

18.3 Florid Cemento-osseous Dysplasia

18.3.1 Case 39

The patient, female, 44 years old. The mandibular posterior teeth were painful and uncomfortable for more than 2 months.

[Present Medical History] The patient suffered from pain and discomfort of mandibular posterior teeth for more than 2 months. The patient went to a local hospital for imaging examination. Multiple cysts in the jaw were considered, and the patient was recommended to go to a higher hospital.

[Specialized Examination] The bilateral maxillofacial region is basically symmetric, and the bilateral lower lip is symmetric. The mouth opening is 3.5 cm, the mouth opening type is downward, there is no elastic tenderness in bilateral condyles and the posterior disc area, and the mobility of bilateral condyles is consistent and symmetrical. Intraoral: Permanent dentition, with no percussion pain or looseness. There is a swelling on the buccal side of the right mandible, about 1.5 cm in size, without obvious ping-pong sensation, and the swelling of the right maxilla and the left maxilla and mandible is not obvious. No obvious swollen lymph nodes are seen in bilateral submandibular regions and neck.

[Auxiliary Examination]
Panoramic Radiographs: There are multiple abnormal density shadows in the bilateral maxilla and mandible, and the boundary is still clear (Fig. 18.3).

[Primary Diagnosis] c space-occupying lesion of bilateral maxilla and mandible (maybe cysts).

[Treatment] "mass resection of bilateral maxilla and mandible" was performed under general anesthesia: Incision was conducted along the gingival margin to open, the flap was turned over, grinding was conducted to remove part of the bone, the tumor was exposed, cystic and, and the tumor was peeled off along the outer wall of the cyst. Part of the bone was ground off, iodoform gauze was filled in the bone cavity, and the oral wound was tightly sutured. The right maxilla, left mandible, and left maxilla were operated as previously. There was no obvious cyst wall on the left maxillary bone cyst. The results of intraoperative frozen pathology suggested the "left lower" bone fibrotic lesion, cemento-osseous dysplasia, was to be eliminated. The "upper right" sent for pathological examination was a small amount of fibrous tissue and bone tissue. Fibrous lesions of bone cannot be completely eliminated. The "lower right" was fibrous capsule wall-like tissue. There was no obvious lining epithelium, there was bone tissue formation in the capsule wall, and an aneurysmal bone cyst was to be eliminated.

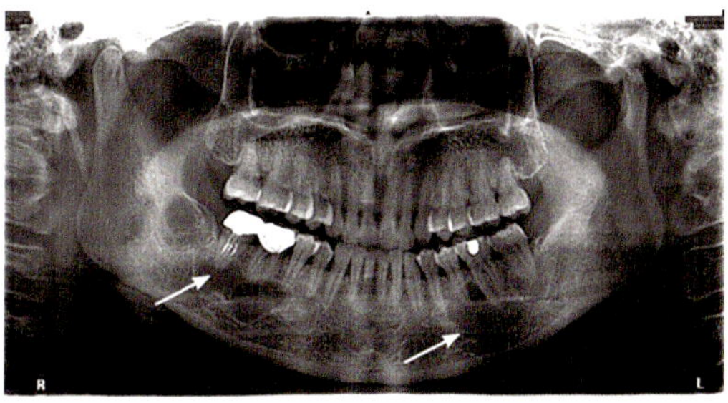

Fig. 18.3 There were multiple abnormal density shadows in bilateral maxilla and mandible, and the boundary was clear (preoperative)

[Pathological Examination] The parts sent for pathological examination were the broken tissues of the lower left, upper right and lower right parts of the jaw, 0.5 cm*0.4 cm*0.3 cm, 0.3 cm*0.2 cm*0.1 cm and 0.5 cm*0.3 cm*0.2 cm in size, respectively, grayish yellow. Microscopically, the lesion consisted of spindle-shaped mesenchymal tissue rich in cells and cementum-osteoid tissue scattered (Fig. 18.4).

[Pathological Diagnosis] Florid cemento-osseous dysplasia of "jaw," with cystic degeneration.

[Follow-Up Visit] The patient recovered well after the operation, with no obvious abnormalities in the operative area (Fig. 18.5).

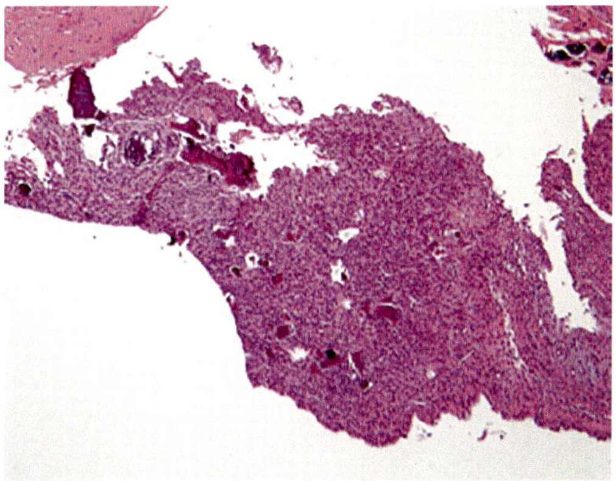

Fig. 18.4 Cementum-osteoid tissue was formed in mesenchymal tissue rich in cells (10×)

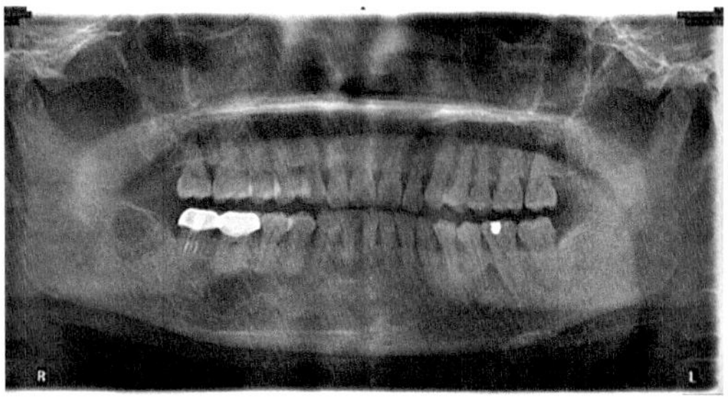

Fig. 18.5 Postoperative changes of bilateral maxilla and mandible

18.4 Key Points of Diagnosis and Treatment

COD is a non-neoplastic lesion of the jaw. The classification of head and neck tumors published by WHO in 2017 named the non-neoplastic osteofibromatosis in the dental region of the jaw as "cementum-bone dysplasia (COD)." In accordance with the location, quantity and imaging characteristics of the disease, COD can be divided into three categories: Focal cemento-osseous dysplasia (FCOD), periapical cemento-osseous dysplasia (PCOD?) and florid cemento-osseous dysplasia (FLCOD) [3]. FLCOD is multi-focus, not limited to the mandibular anterior teeth area, and often occurs bilaterally, showing a large range of high-density shadows of the jaw on imaging. Most COD patients have no obvious clinical symptoms, and lesions are often found during radiography. Some patients may show jaw swelling, while secondary infection may cause pain, pus, swelling and other symptoms. There are also cases of complications, such as lower alveolar nerve injury caused by FCOD and chronic osteomyelitis caused by FLCOD, etc.

Diagnosis The diagnosis of COD mainly depends on imaging and pathological diagnosis, and it needs to be differentiated from diseases such as radicular cysts and calcifying odontogenic cysts. Early FCOD is easily misdiagnosed as periapical abscess, granuloma or cyst, leading to unnecessary endodontic treatment. Therefore, a pulp vitality test is necessary for differential diagnosis.

Treatment If there is no serious jaw deformity or secondary infection, observation can be chosen for COD. Some scholars suggest that imaging evaluation should be carried out every 2–3 years to check whether there are related complications (such as osteomyelitis). Some scholars also believe that antibiotics can also be used preventively to prevent osteomyelitis. In addition, although histologically benign, FCOD may proliferate abnormally, thus showing jaw deformity and dysfunction. At this time, surgical resection and soft and hard tissue repair should be considered.

References

1. Amir E, Faezeh Y. CBCT findings of periapical cemento-osseous dysplasia: a case report [J]. Imaging Sci Dent. 2013;43(3):215–8.
2. Fenerty S, Shaw W, Verma R, et al. Florid cemento-osseous dysplasia: review of an uncommon fibro-osseous lesion of the jaw with important clinical implications [J]. Skeletal Radiol. 2017;46(5):581–90.
3. Wright JM, Vered M. Update from the 4th edition of the World Health Organization Classification of Head and Neck Tumours: odontogenic and maxillofacial bone tumors [J]. Head Neck Pathol. 2017;11(1):68–77.
4. Aiuto R, Gucciardino F, Rapetti R, et al. Management of symptomatic florid cemento-osseous dysplasia: literature review and a case report [J]. J Clin Exp Dent. 2018;10:e291.

19 Familial Gigantiform Cementoma

Yue He, Hui Shan Ong, Zhen Tian, Lin Zhu,
and Li Li Hou

19.1 Introduction

Familial gigantiform cementoma (FGC) is a rare autosomal dominant genetic disease and a benign proliferative lesion of cementum. The disease is easy to occur in teenagers, and the lesions progress rapidly in adolescence but tend to stagnate at the end of adolescence. Bone swelling growth above FGC and multiple quadrants of the mandible are the main manifestations, and the anterior part of the mandible is the area that occurs frequently, usually appearing with evident occlusal disorder and facial deformity, seriously affecting the maxillofacial shape and oral function [1–4]. In addition, it is often accompanied by systemic manifestations, such as long bone fractures of limbs, etc. [3–5]. Diagnosis should be combined with clinical manifestations, imaging features and pathological features. FGC recommends operation, and the operation must be thorough. Incomplete lesion resection will lead to the accelerated growth of residual lesions. For bone defects formed after resection, a fibula flap is often used for reconstruction and repair.

19.2 Case 40

The patient, female, 29 years old. Nine years after trimming the mandibular tumor outside the hospital.

[Present Medical History] The patient developed painless mandibular swelling 12 years ago, growing slowly. Nine years ago, the patient underwent "mandibular trimming" in a local stomatological hospital, and the pathology after the operation was "mandibular ossifying fibroma," the details were unknown. After that, the mandibular swelling accelerated during pregnancy five years ago, and no corresponding treatment was given. Maxillary swelling appeared after pregnancy and increased rapidly. Head CT was performed in the outpatient department of our hospital 4 months ago; Recurrence after "mandibular trimming" (maybe florid dysplasia).

[Specialized Examination] Bilateral maxillofacial regions are asymmetrical, and the left face is slightly larger than the right, the mandible is huge, involving the whole mandible, and the bilateral maxilla is larger, the left side is more obvious than the right side, the boundary is unclear and hard. The bilateral lip is numb. The

Y. He (✉) · H. S. Ong · Z. Tian · L. L. Hou
Department of Oral Maxillofacial-Head & Neck Oncology, Shanghai Ninth People's Hospital, Shanghai Jiao Tong University School of Medicine, Shanghai, China

L. Zhu
Department of Radiology, Ninth People's Hospital Affiliated to Shanghai Jiao Tong University, Shanghai, China

Y. He (ed.), *Inflammatory and Neoplastic Diseases of Craniofacial Bones*,
https://doi.org/10.1007/978-981-97-4155-7_19

degree and type of mouth opening are normal, permanent dentition of the whole mouth, 17~27, 38~48. The teeth are sparse and irregularly arranged. The maxilla and mandible are swollen to the lip, cheek, tongue, and palate, with a hard texture and no tenderness. There is no abnormality in the sensory activity of the tongue. No obvious swollen lymph nodes are seen in bilateral submandibular regions and neck.

[Auxiliary Examination]
CT enhanced scan of maxillofacial region: Bilateral maxilla and mandible are swollen with diffuse mixed density shadow, the bone cortex is still continuous, no obvious periosteal reaction and no soft tissue mass are found (Fig. 19.1).

[Primary Diagnosis] Osteogenic fibroma of maxilla and mandible after bone fiber repair.

[Treatment] "Maxillary trimming + mandibular segmental resection + fibula musculocutaneous flap transfer repair + tracheotomy" were performed: An incision of 2.0 cm was designed along the lower edge of the mandible, a cut was done, the flap was turned over, the involved range of the lesion was identified completely, the osteotomy line was adjusted by osteotomy guide and

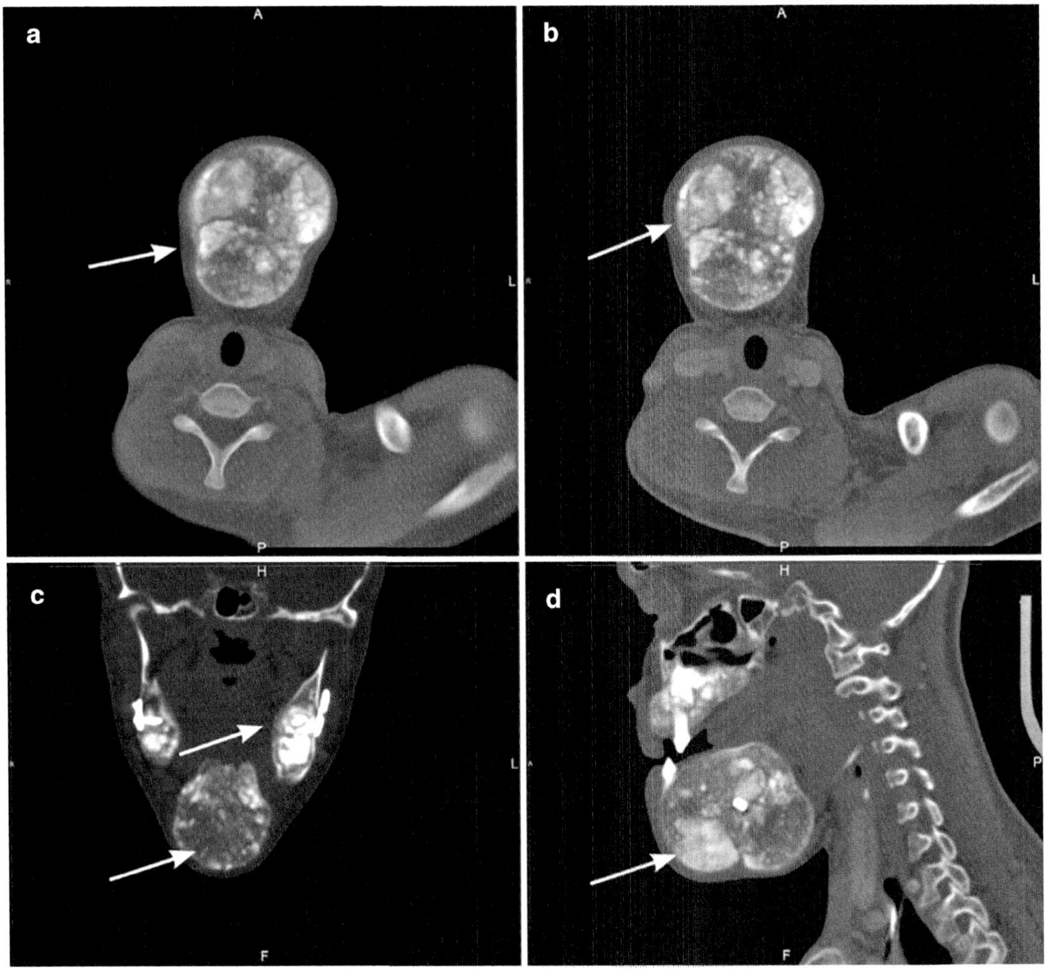

Fig. 19.1. (**a**) Transverse view of CT plain scan: Mandibular bone swelled with diffuse mixed density shadow inside. (**b**) Transverse view of CT enhanced scan: Continuous bone cortex. (**c**) Coronal view of CT enhanced scan: The maxilla and mandible were involved. (**d**) Sagittal view of CT enhanced scan: There was no obvious periosteal reaction, and there was no abnormal soft tissue mass

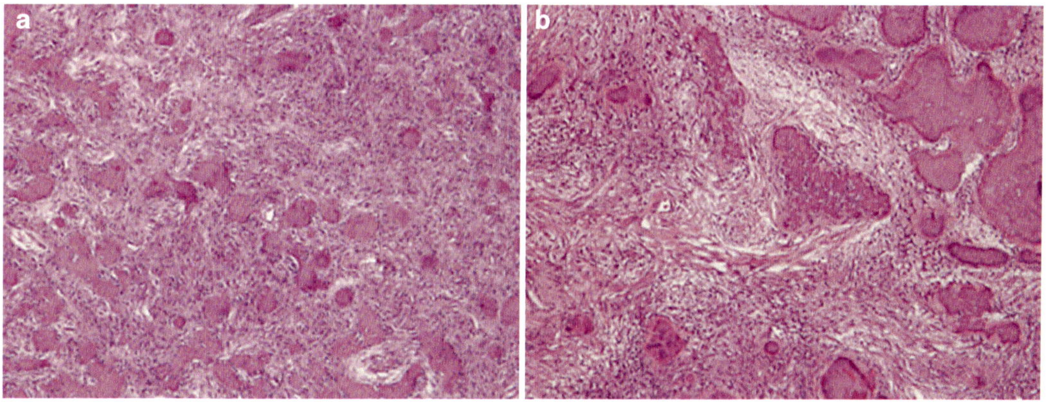

Fig. 19.2 (**a**) Bone-like (woven bone) and cementum-like mineralization with calcification were found in the fibrous tissue rich in cells (200×). (**b**) The shape of cementoid substance was irregular, and some brush-like edges can be seen (200×)

intraoperative navigation, and the mandible was cut off and sent for frozen pathological examination, indicating bone fiber disorder. There was no sufficient evidence of a malignant tumor. The fibular muscle flap was prepared routinely, and the bone flap was about 18 cm long. The continuity of the mandible was restored in accordance with the shaping and reconstruction of the osteotomy guide plate, and the peroneal artery and vein were anastomosed with the facial artery and external jugular vein, respectively. The mucoperiosteum was cut along the maxillary vestibular groove to expose the maxillary tumor, and part of the tumor was removed by osteotome to trim the appearance. The operative wound was rinsed, bleeding was stopped completely, the negative pressure drainage tube was indwelled, a suture was conducted in layers, and the wound was closed.

[Pathological Examination] The part sent for pathological examination was maxillary tissue, 9.0 cm*7.8 cm*4.7 cm in size. The jaw and gingiva were widely swollen, and the section was gray and hard. Microscopically, bone-like and cementlike substances were formed in the background of fibrous tissue, with abundant fibroblasts. There were no osteocytes around the bone-like tissue, the shape of the cementlike tissue was irregular, and there were light eosinophilic brush edges in some parts (Fig. 19.2).

[Pathological Diagnosis] familial gigantiform cementoma of "maxilla," ICD code: Partial areas of M927810 were full of cells.

19.3 Key Points of Diagnosis and Treatment

Familial gigantiform cementoma (FGC) is a rare benign fibrous bone lesion of the jaw, following the autosomal dominant genetic model.

Epidemiological Study A retrospective study on the case reports of FGC from 1966 to 2016 shows that the country with the largest number of case reports is the United States, followed by China. A study on an FGC family discovered in China in 2013 showed that all patients in the family had early onset, entered a period of rapid growth of lesions in adolescence, and the development of lesions tended to stagnate at the end of adolescence. In accordance with the clinical characteristics, the researchers divided the course of the disease into three periods of initial onset, rapid growth and growth retardation.

Clinical Characteristics FGC is characterized by widely distributed and clearly defined masses in the mandible and maxilla. It may lead to serious facial deformities. It usually occurs in the front of the mandible, leading to poor occlusion and difficulty in chewing.

Diagnosis The diagnosis mainly depends on the characteristic imaging manifestations and pathological diagnosis and should be combined with family history. The level of serum alkaline phosphatase can help to judge the development potential of the disease. In addition, it has been reported that FGC patients have a gene mutation of COLI1A2. Recently, some scholars have also found the missense mutation of the ANO5 gene in FGC patients in China's family, but there is still a lack of in-depth research on gene diagnosis of FGC. During diagnosis, FGC should also be differentiated from jaw diseases of skeletal dysplasia and cherubism.

Treatment The goal of FGC treatment is to remove lesions, preserve the mandible and restore the function of the oral and maxillofacial system. However, the lesions of FGC often progress rapidly, and the recurrence rate is high, so it is difficult to treat them. At present, the main treatment method is surgical resection of the lesion, but it has been reported that a 6-year-old child's residual lesion grew rapidly after maxilla repair, and another 20-year-old adult male underwent partial resection and reconstruction of the median mandibular joint area. Two years after the operation, the patient's maxilla and mandible showed symmetrical hyperplasia. Therefore, it is not recommended to perform incomplete resection only for aesthetic reasons or denture restoration. Only extensive resection can avoid recurrence. There are many repair and reconstruction schemes for bone defects caused by surgery, such as autogenous non-vascularized fibula and rib flap. However, these methods cannot provide enough bone for complex reconstruction, and they are only suitable for small-scale bone defects without radiotherapy. With the development of microsurgery, free vascularized bone graft has become the first choice for jaw reconstruction. The vascularized fibular flap has become the standard of mandibular reconstruction. The height of the mandible should be restored as much as possible during jaw reconstruction to facilitate the later implant repair. However, it should be noted that FGC patients may be accompanied by hypoplasia of long bones and pathological fractures at the same time as jaw disease. For this kind of patients, fibula flaps should not be used, and some scholars think that iliac bone flaps can be used for repair.

References

1. Abdelsayed RA, Eversole LR, Singh BS, et al. Gigantiform cementoma: clinicopathologic presentation of 3 cases [J]. Oral Surg Oral Med Oral Pathol Oral Radiol Endod. 2001;91(4):438–44.
2. Wang HW, Yu M, Qin XJ, et al. Familial gigantiform cementoma: analysis of a large Chinese pedigree [J]. China J Oral Maxillofac Surg. 2014;4
3. HW W, Yu M, et al. Familial gigantiform cementoma: distinctive clinical features of a large Chinese pedigree – Science Direct [J]. Br J Oarl Maxillofac Sürg. 2015;53(1):83–5.
4. Wang HW, Ma CY, Qin XJ, et al. Management strategy in patient with familial gigantiform cementoma: A case report and analysis of the literature [J]. Medicine (Baltimore). 2017;96(50):e9138.
5. Li X, Wang L, Wang HW, et al. Missense Mutation of ANO5 Affects Balance of Bone Metabolism, Leading to Occurrence of A Large Family of China Familial Giant Cementoma [A]. Chinese Stomatological Association Specialized Committee of Oral Genetic Disease and Rare Disease. Collection of Papers of Second Academic Annual Conference of Chinese Stomatological Association Specialized Committee of Oral Genetic Disease and Rare Disease [C], 2020, 1

Part VII

Benign Epithelial Odontogenic Tumor and Its Evolution

20 Ameloblastoma

Jing Song Hou, Hui Shan Ong, Zhen Tian, Lin Zhu, and Xing Zhou Qu

20.1 Introduction

Ameloblastoma is the most common benign epithelial odontogenic tumor, accounting for about 10–30% of odontogenic tumors. It is clinically classified as a "critical tumor" because of its biological characteristics of local invasion, high recurrence rate and distant metastasis [1–6]. Ameloblastoma occurs more frequently in young adults, with no significant gender difference. It is more common in the mandible than the maxilla, especially the mandibular body and mandibular angle. Among all jaw tumors, ameloblastoma has the most complex histopathological changes. The 2017 WHO classifies it into classic, unicystic, peripheral/extraosseous and metastatic ameloblastoma, with metastatic ameloblastoma as a benign tumor [1–4]. Ameloblastoma grows slowly with no obvious symptoms at the beginning but gradually expands and evolves into jaw swelling, resulting in deformity, occlusive disorder, lower lip numbness, pathological fracture and other symptoms. The typical X-ray findings show single-locular or multi-locular cystic low-density images of different sizes overlapping with clear boundaries or appearing as solid lesions [7, 8]. The lesions involving teeth may exhibit root resorption in the form of amputation. Due to the local invasive characteristics, the surgical treatment for other types of ameloblastoma, except for single cystic ameloblastoma, which can be attempted with fenestration or curettage, often requires resection of the tumor 0.5 cm outside the lesion [9, 10].

20.2 Solid or Polycystic Ameloblastoma

20.2.1 Case 41

A 41-year-old gentleman suffered from a lump in the right mandible over 8 months ago.

[History of Present Illness] When brushing teeth more than 8 months ago, the patient felt sore in the right lower gingival area and was treated in a local hospital. Panoramic radiographs showed that a honeycomb low-density shadow could be seen near the lower margin of the mandible in 46–48 root, suggesting treatment at a

J. S. Hou (✉) · X. Z. Qu
Hospital of Stomatology, Guanghua College of Stomatology, Sun Yat-sen University, Guangzhou, Guangdong, China
e-mail: houjs@mail.sysu.edu.cn

H. S. Ong · Z. Tian
Department of Oral Maxillofacial-Head & Neck Oncology, Shanghai Ninth People's Hospital, Shanghai Jiao Tong University School of Medicine, Shanghai, China

L. Zhu
Department of Radiology, Ninth People's Hospital Affiliated to Shanghai Jiao Tong University, Shanghai, China

Y. He (ed.), *Inflammatory and Neoplastic Diseases of Craniofacial Bones*,
https://doi.org/10.1007/978-981-97-4155-7_20

superior hospital. CT at a local superior hospital 1 month ago showed that the right lower mandible body presented swelling changes with internal separation. So, it was considered an odontogenic tumor.

[Specialty Examination] The oral and maxillofacial region was asymmetrical, with a slight swelling of the right mandibular body, normal skin temperature, and no redness or swelling. Subcutaneously, the mandible was palpable to bulge outward, causing tenderness (−), without a sense of a ping-pong ball. There was numbness in the lower lip (−). There was no abnormality in the mouth opening range and mouth opening pattern. The mucosa of the right mandibular lip, cheek, and lingual side was intact. No obvious swelling was seen in the vestibular sulcus, and under the mucosa, the jaw bone was palpable to bulge outward. No obvious swelling occurred on the lingual side. Intraoral examination revealed permanent dentition, with no significant abnormality in the teeth. No significant submandibular and cervical lymph node enlargement was observed.

[Auxiliary Examination]

1. Panoramic radiographs suggested a honeycomb-shaped hypodense shadow in the right mandible, involving 46–48 teeth, with no obvious absorption of the tooth root (Fig. 20.1).
2. A maxillofacial enhanced CT scan suggested a bone swelling in the right lower jaw corner, with decreased density and evolution to soft tissue protruding towards the cheek and tongue. The CT value was 40 Hu, and after enhancement, the CT+ was 90 Hu, with uneven density and visible bone septa. The bone cortex around the lesion got thinner, local continuity was interrupted, and the boundary with surrounding soft tissue was clear. No obvious enlarged lymph node shadow in the neck was observed (Fig. 20.2).

[Preliminary Diagnosis] Right mandibular odontogenic tumor (① possible mucinous tumor; ② possible ameloblastoma; ③ malignant to be ruled out).

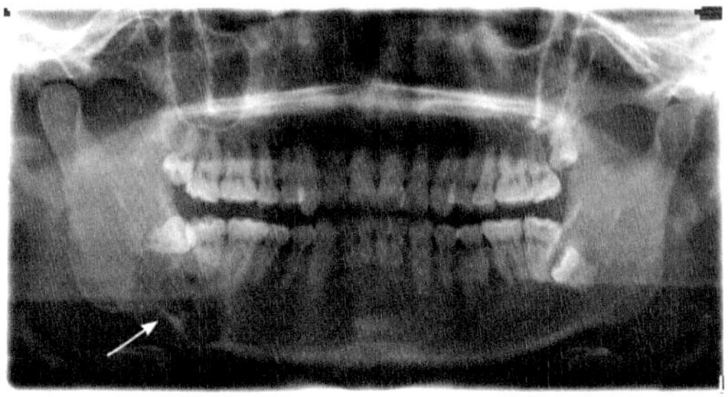

Fig. 20.1 Honeycomb shaped hypodense shadow in the right mandible, involving 46–48 teeth, with no obvious absorption of the tooth root (preoperative)

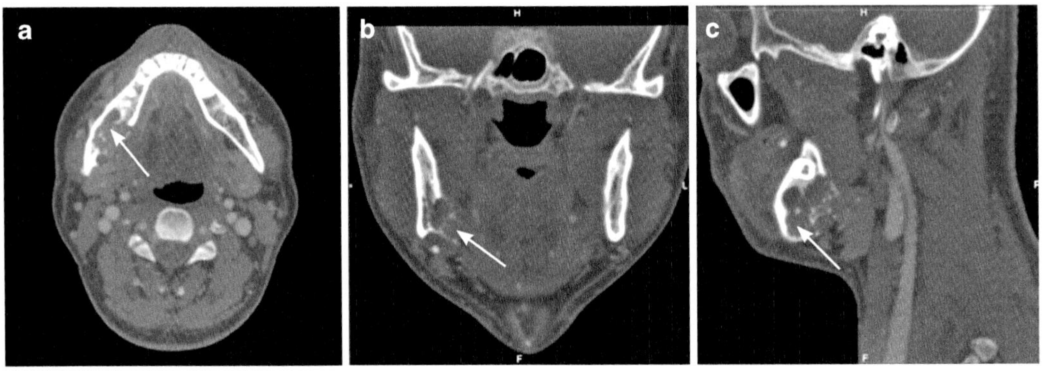

Fig. 20.2 (**a**) CT axial scan: Bone distention in the right mandibular angle, with a decrease in density and evolution to soft tissue, protruding towards the cheek and tongue, with uneven density and visible bone septa. (**b**, **c**) Coronal and sagittal images: The bone cortex around the lesion got thinner, local continuity was interrupted, and the boundary with surrounding soft tissue was clear

[Treatment] "Right segmental mandibulectomy with fibular muscle flap transfer" under general anesthesia was performed: An incision was made along the lower margin of the mandible for 1–2 cm, and the gingival flap was elevated for surgical exposure to truncate the mandible at 34 distal end to the mandibular angle, and completely remove the tumor. The peroneal muscle flap, about 14 cm in length, was shaped and double-folded to restore mandibular continuity, height and occlusal relationship. Peroneal arteriovenous anastomosis with extramaxillary artery and jugular vein was performed. The wound was rinsed, hemostasis was tight, the negative pressure drainage tube was indwelled, and a layered suture was performed to close the wound (Fig. 20.3).

[Pathological Examination] Gross pathological examination revealed a part of the mandibular tissue, which was 5.2cm × 3.9cm × 2.5cm in size, was locally swollen. The section was cyst solid, gray white, and tender. Microscopic examination showed hypercellular tumor cells interspersed between bone trabeculae and reticular connected or arranged into solid, follicular-like epithelial

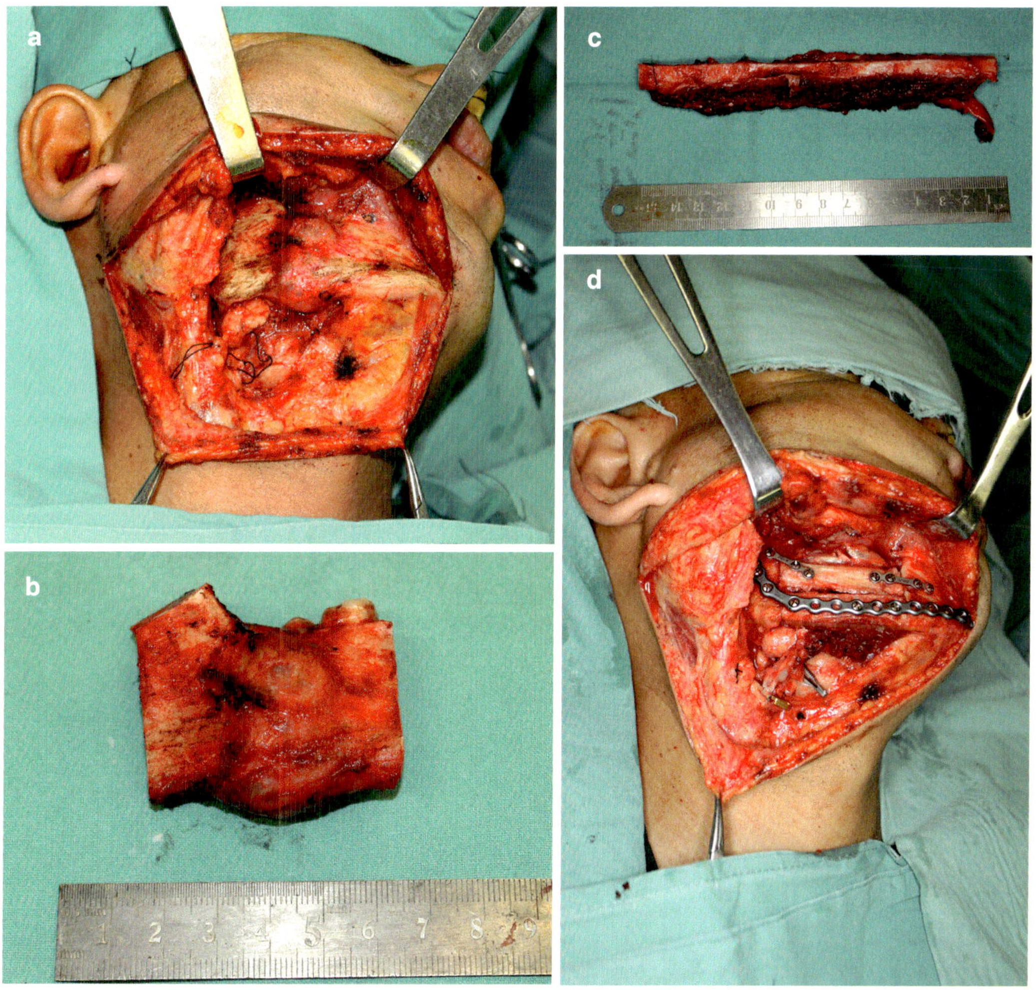

Fig. 20.3 (**a**) Expose the mandibular body and mass. (**b**) In vitro mandible. (**c**) Peroneal muscle flap, about 14 cm long. (**d**) Fibula shaped and double-fold to restore mandibular continuity and height

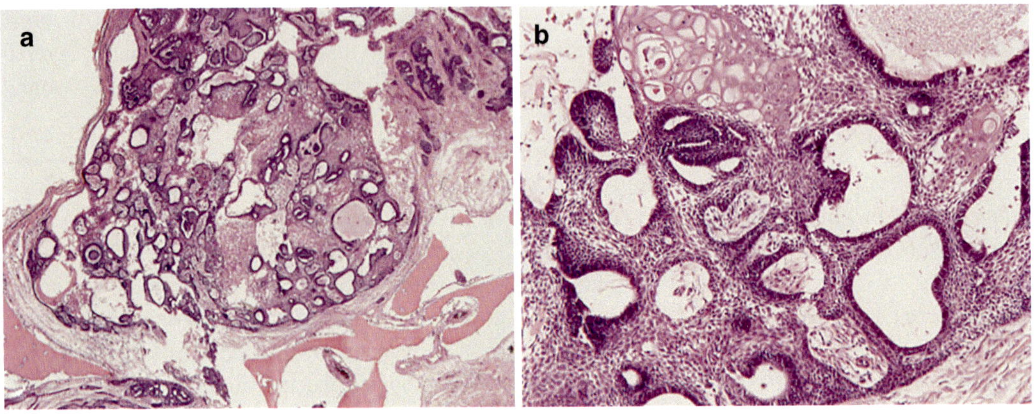

Fig. 20.4 (**a**) The tumor was interspersed between the trabeculae of the normal host bone, and the tumor cells were arranged in clumps and folliculates with local cystic changes (40×). (**b**) The cells surrounding the tumor epithelial nest were in columnar and palisade arrangement, with few intermediate cells, stellate reticulum or polygonal, loosely arranged, and some cells were accompanied by squamous metaplasia (200×)

nests. The surrounding cells were cubic or columnar cells with hyperchromatic nuclei, and they were under palisade arrangement away from the basement membrane, that is, the so-called reversed polarity, and the central cells were few and loosely arranged, similar to star reticular cells, with squamous metaplasia of some cells (Fig. 20.4).

[Pathological Diagnosis] Solid or polycystic ameloblastoma of the right mandible, with ICD-O code 9310/0, with hypercellularity and wide involvement of the trabeculae.

[Follow-Up] The patient healed uneventfully. The postoperative six-month follow-up exhibited no tumor relapse, with good recovery of the contralateral occlusal relationship and satisfactory reconstruction of the mandible.

20.2.2 Case 42

A 53-year-old woman suffered from a relapse of left mandibular ameloblastoma for 2 months after the second surgery at another hospital.

[History of Present Illness] The patient underwent "left mandibular cystic mass curettage surgery" for "left mandibular mass" at a local hospital 10 and 5 years ago, respectively. Postoperative pathology revealed ameloblastoma. About 2 months ago, the patient consciously experienced swelling and distension in the left mandibular surgical area, which gradually worsened with mild pain. Then, the patient was diagnosed at a local hospital and underwent a panoramic radiography examination to consider tumor relapse.

[Specialty Examination] The face was basically symmetrical, with a well-coordinated 1/3 proportion of the upper, middle and lower face. There was no abnormality in mouth opening range and mouth opening pattern. Intraoral examination revealed permanent dentition, anterior crossbite, anterior crossbite, postoperative changes in the left mandible, absence of 34–36 teeth, surgical scars on the mucosa, and swelling on the buccal and lingual sides from 33 to 37 teeth with a size range of approximately 3.5 cm × 2.5 cm, intact surface mucosa, no obvious rupture or fistula. It was medium hard and not movable once palpation and was well circumscribed with tenderness (±) (Fig. 20.5). The tongue had no obvious sensory or movement impairments. Bilateral submaxillary and cervical lymph nodes were not significantly enlarged.

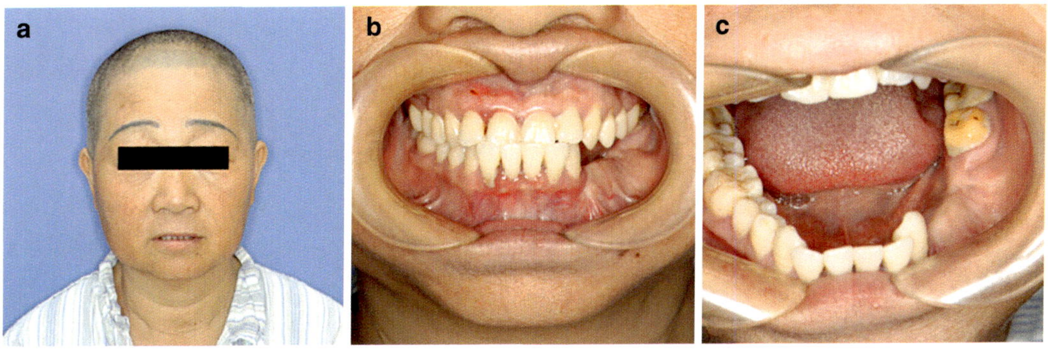

Fig. 20.5 (**a**) Basically symmetrical face. (**b**) Anterior crossbite. (**c**) Postoperative changes in the left mandible, thinning vestibular sulcus on the buccal side, and scars on the mucosa

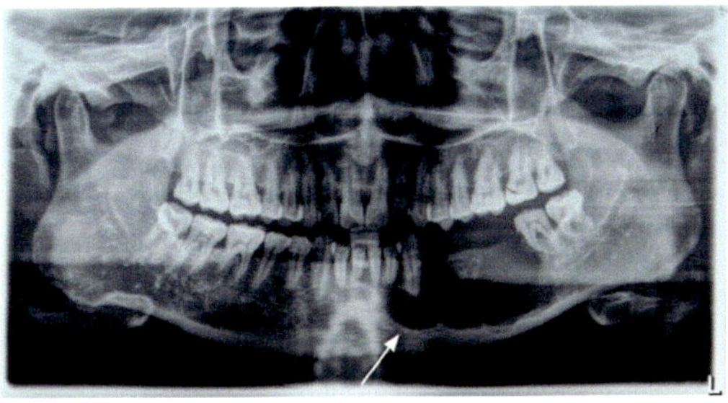

Fig. 20.6 Expansive bone destruction area in the left mandibular body, which seemed to have a little bone ridge shadow, local bone cortex was not continuous, neither obvious periosteal reaction nor abnormal soft tissue mass was observed

[Auxiliary Examination]

1. Panoramic radiographs suggested an expansive bone destruction area in the left mandibular body, which seemed to have a little bone ridge shadow; the local bone cortex was not continuous, and neither obvious periosteal reaction nor abnormal soft tissue mass was observed (Fig. 20.6).
2. Maxillofacial Enhanced CT scan suggested a swelling deformation in the bone of the left mandibular body (3–7 lower left), with a circular abnormal density shadow, a clear boundary, the size of about 36 mm × 18 mm, C− 22 Hu, C+ 29 Hu, and no obvious enhancement. The adjacent cortical bone was thinned and partially disappeared, and no obvious periosteal reaction was observed. The surrounding soft tissue density was uniform. No significant bilateral cervical lymph node enlargement was observed (Fig. 20.7).

[Preliminary Diagnosis] Relapse of left mandibular ameloblastoma after secondary surgery at another hospital.

[Treatment] "Left segmental mandibulectomy with fibular muscle flap transfer" under general anesthesia was performed: An incision was made along the lower margin of the mandible for 1–2 cm, and the gingival flap was elevated for surgical exposure of the bone distension mainly at 32–37 teeth, buccal, lingual swelling, bone cortex absorption and destruction. The mandible was truncated at the mandible midline and angle to completely remove the tumor and mandibular body. The left free fibula with vascular pedicle was prepared. The fibula, with a length of about 9 cm, was cut and shaped to reconstruct the mandibular continuity and occlusal relationship. The vascular anastomosis of the fibula and facial arteriovenous vessels was performed. The wound was rinsed and thoroughly hemostatic, a negative pressure drainage tube was indwelled, and a layered suture was performed to close the wound (Fig. 20.8).

[Pathological Examination] Gross pathological examination revealed the mandibular tissue through

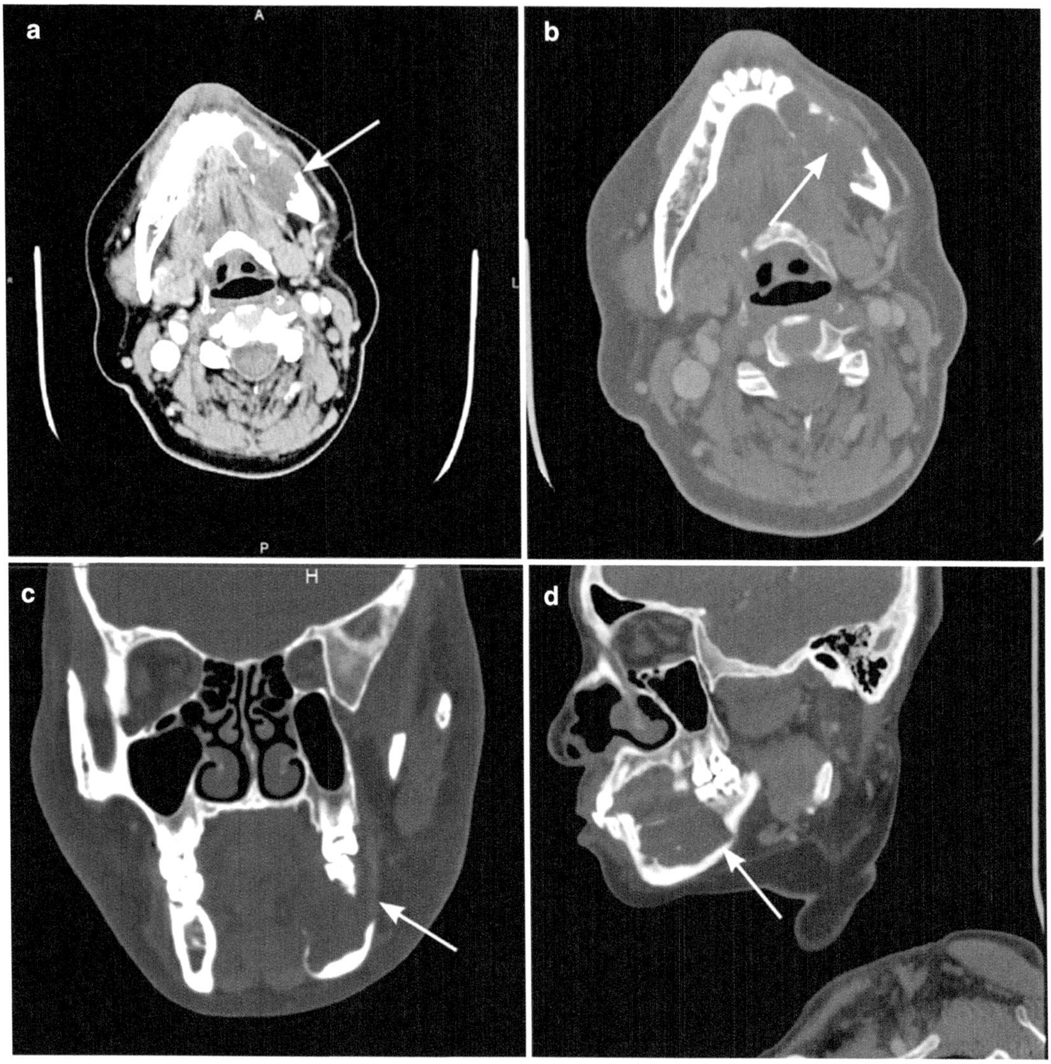

Fig. 20.7 (**a**) Enhanced CT axial scan (Soft tissue window) : Expansive bone destruction with soft tissue mass in the left mandible body, irregular shape, local mild to moderate enhancement. (**b**) Enhanced CT transversal scan (bone window) : cortical discontinuity. (**c**) Enhanced CT coronal scan (bone window): No obvious periosteal reaction was observed. (**d**) Enhanced CT sagittal scan (bone window): left inferior alveolar canal nerve involvement

segmental mandibulectomy, 7 cm × 3.8 cm × 3 cm in size. A single cystic mass was found in the mandibular body with a thin bone cortex, clear liquid content and local nodular eminences. Microscopic examination showed the tumor cells were arranged in a follicular shape, the epithelial nest was surrounded by basal-like cubic cells arranged in a palisade shape, and the central cells were arranged loosely, similar to star reticular cells, with cystic changes. In some epithelial clusters, the central cells had abundant cytoplasm and contained eosinophilic particles, indicating granulosa cell degeneration (Fig. 20.9).

[Pathological Diagnosis] Ameloblastoma of the left mandible, ICD-O code: 9310/0, with hypercellularity and local granular cell degeneration.

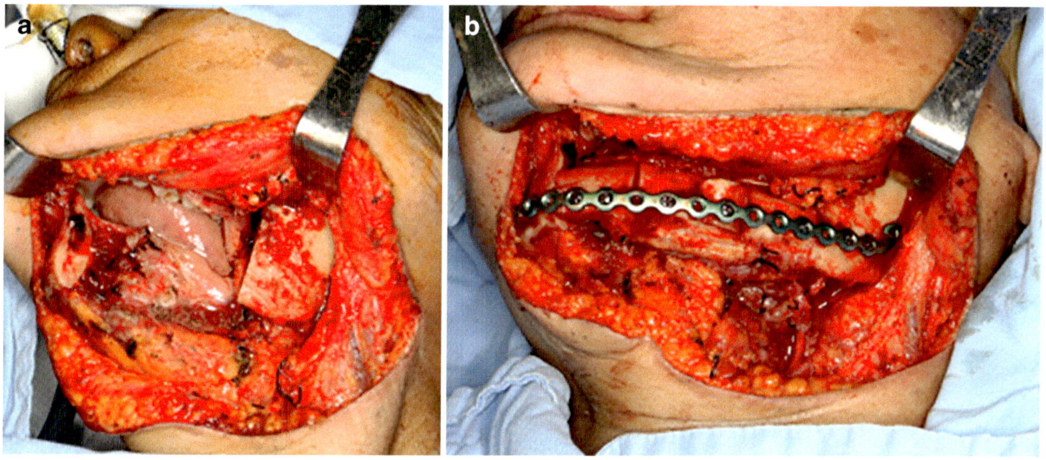

Fig. 20.8 (**a**) Wound defect after segmental resection of mandible. (**b**) Fibula reconstruction to restore mandibular continuity

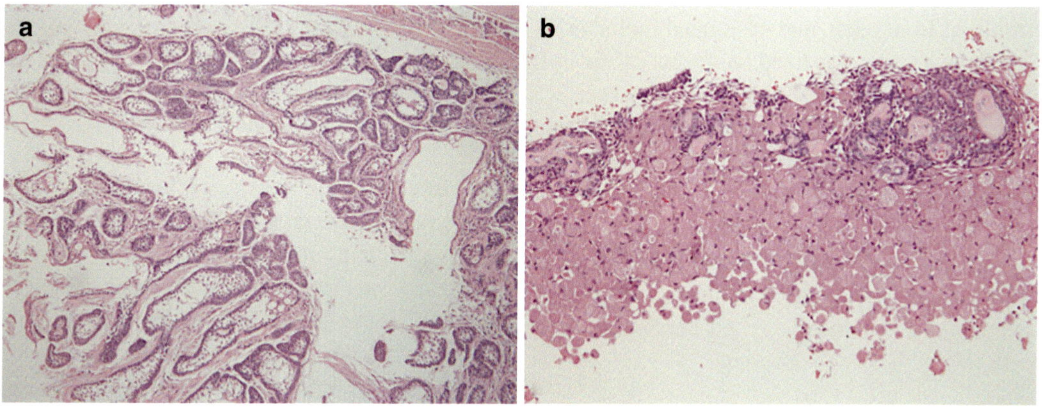

Fig. 20.9 (**a**) The cells around the odontogenic epithelial island were under palisade arrangement, with stellate reticulum cells in the middle, loosely arranged, and cystic changes in local areas (100×). (**b**) Some tumor cells had abundant cytoplasm filled with eosinophilic granules, indicating granulosa cell degeneration (200×)

[Follow-Up] The patient healed uneventfully. The postoperative six-month follow-up exhibited no tumor relapse, with good recovery of the contralateral occlusal relationship and satisfactory reconstruction of the mandible.

20.2.3 Case 43

A 16-year-old boy suffered from a right mandibular mass one and a half years after fenestration at another hospital.

[History of Present Illness] One and a half years ago, the patient accidentally found that his right cheek was slightly swollen without pain, numbness and other discomfort. Panoramic radiographs suggested a space-occupying lesion of the right mandible, and CT examination indicated "cystoid expansive bone destruction of the right mandibular angle, considering the possibility of the dental cyst." Fenestration of the right mandibular bone cyst was performed, and the postoperative pathology was unknown. After the operation, the patient washed the sac cavity with normal saline daily and received regular reexamination. Pathological section consultation at our hospital 14 months ago showed "right mandible ameloblastoma of classic type." Six months ago, the patient was found to have red new organisms in the original operation area, without abnormal sensations such as bleeding and pain. CT examination at the return visit to our hospital two months ago suggested a "benign cystic mass of the right mandible: ameloblastoma" to be considered.

[Specialty Examination] The face was symmetrical with no palpable distention in the right mandibular angle. There was no abnormality in the mouth opening range and mouth opening pattern. Intraoral examination revealed permanent dentition, poor dental hygiene, mild opening and closing of front teeth, and 46 lingual inclination. The drainage tube was fixed on the buccal side of 46 and 47 teeth, red new organisms were observed at the vestibular sulci of 46 and 47 and the distal gum of 47, which was soft without pedicles, with no pain or bleeding on the percussion, 46 and 47 teeth were loose (−) upon percussion (−). No obvious abnormalities were found in the residual mucosa. The tongue moved normally. No significant bilateral submaxillary and cervical lymph node enlargement was observed.

[Auxiliary Examination]

1. Panoramic radiographs suggested an abnormal hypodense shadow on the right mandibular body and ascending branch, including a tooth density shadow, which was well circumscribed. Maxillary margin distention was observed (Fig. 20.10).
2. Maxillofacial Enhanced CT scan suggested expansive bone destruction in the right mandibular angle and ascending branch, with a clear boundary and a size of approximately 2.8 cm × 2.1 cm, with uneven density and a mixture of cyst and solid. The solid part was significantly enhanced after enhancement, with C− 56 Hu and C+ 90 Hu. The lesion presented as unilocular, cortical bone thinning, and peripheral bone thickening, with no obvious periosteal reaction. The lower right 8 was impacted within the lesion, and the crown was oriented toward the center of the lesion. There was no significant involvement of the surrounding soft tissues. No significant bilateral cervical lymph node enlargement was observed (Fig. 20.11).

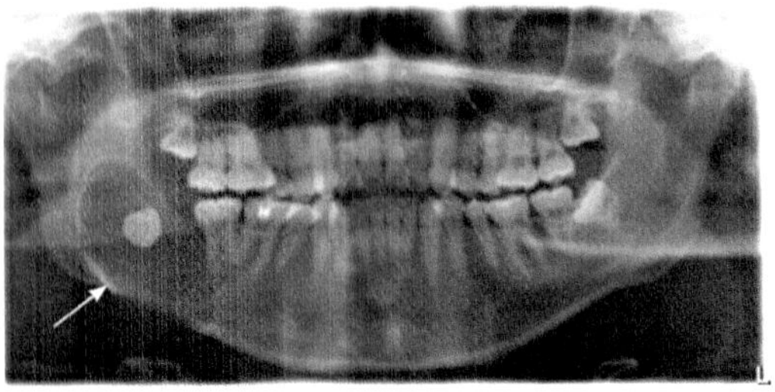

Fig. 20.10 Abnormal hypodense shadow on the right mandibular body and ascending branch, including a tooth density shadow, which was well circumscribed. Maxillary margin distention was observed

[Preliminary Diagnosis] Postoperation of fenestration of right mandibular mass.

[Treatment] "Right segmental mandibulectomy and reconstructive repair of free fibula graft with vascular pedicle" under general anesthesia was performed: An incision was made along the lower margin of the mandible for 1–2 cm, and the gingival flap was elevated for surgical exposure of the mass at the 46 and 47 teeth to the ascending mandibular rami, showing obvious buccolingual swelling. The mandibular bone was truncated using an osteotomy guide at the 46 mesial tooth, and the mandibular lesion was completely removed with the ascending ramus retaining the condyle process. Frozen pathological examination during surgery showed that lingual, buccal, internal lingual and submaxillary lymph nodes were negative. The left free fibula with vascular pedicle was prepared, and the fibula with a length of about 14 cm was cut, shaped and reconstructed to restore mandibular continuity and occlusal relationship. The vascular anastomosis of the fibula and facial arteriovenous vessels was performed. The wound was rinsed and thoroughly hemostatic, a negative pressure drainage tube was indwelled, and a layered suture was performed to close the wound (Fig. 20.12).

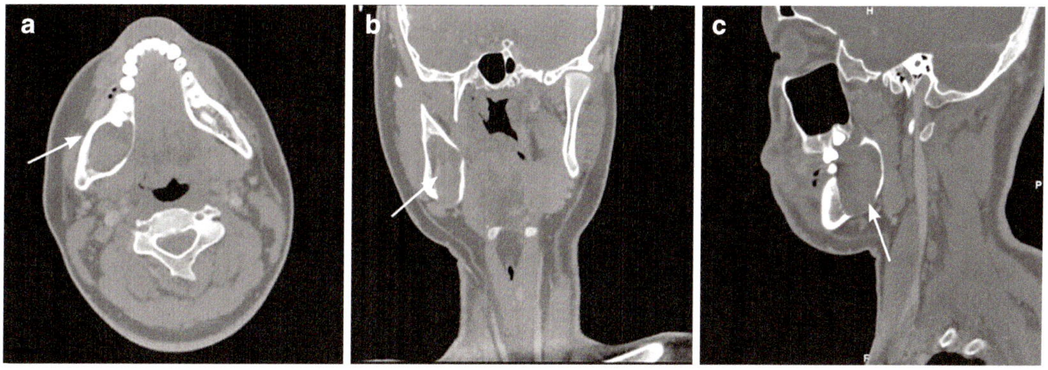

Fig. 20.11 (**a**) Expansive bone destruction in the right mandibular angle and ascending branch, with a clear boundary and a size of approximately 2.8 cm × 2.1 cm, with uneven density and a mixture of cyst and solid. The solid part was significantly enhanced after enhancement. (**b**, **c**) Coronal and sagittal scan: The lesion presented as unilocular, cortical bone thinning, peripheral bone thickening, with no obvious periosteal reaction

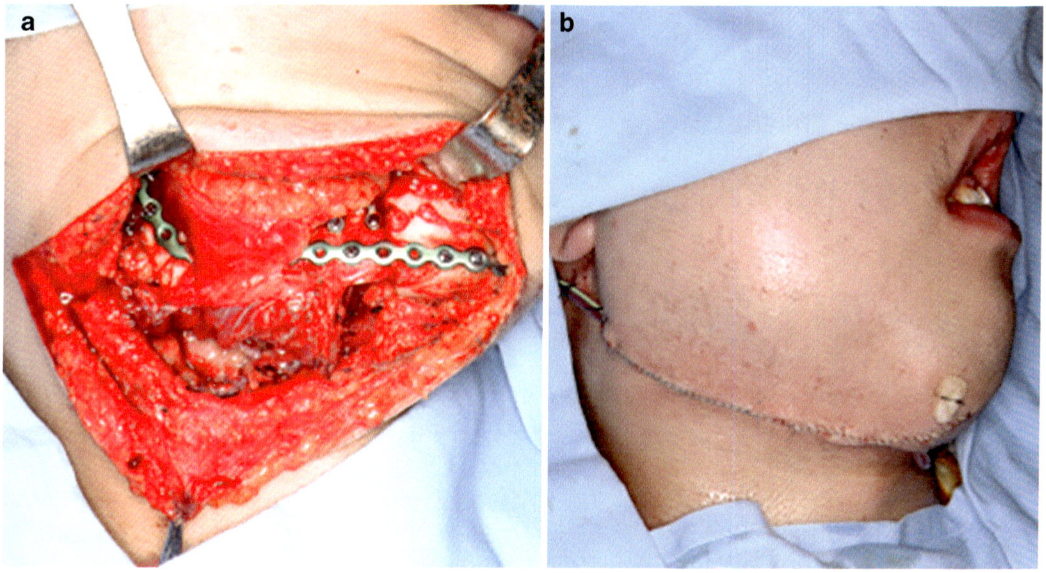

Fig. 20.12 (**a**) Fibula reconstruction to restore mandibular continuity. (**b**) Postoperative observation of fibular reconstruction

[Pathological Examination] Gross pathological examination revealed a part of the mandible through segmental mandibulectomy, 6 cm × 5 cm × 3 cm, light yellow, brittle. Microscopic examination indicated that the tumor cells were arranged in mesh-connected epithelial strips, the peripheral epithelium was a layer of cubic or columnar epithelium, and the central cells were few and loosely arranged. Local cystic lesions occurred (Fig. 20.13).

[Pathological Diagnosis] Ameloblastoma of the right mandible, ICD-O code: 9310/0, plexiform type.

[Follow-Up] The patient healed uneventfully. The postoperative six-month follow-up exhibited no tumor relapse, with good recovery of the contralateral occlusal relationship and satisfactory reconstruction of the mandible.

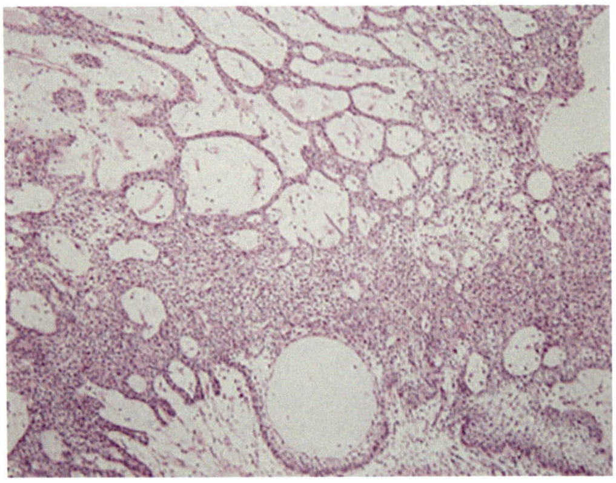

Fig. 20.13 The tumor cells anastomosed to each other into cords and clumps. The palisade arrangement and polarity inversion of peripheral cells were not as obvious as follicular cells, and the cell arrangement in the central region was more loose. Loose interstitium was seen with fewer cells and more blood vessels (100×)

20.3 Unicystic Ameloblastoma

20.3.1 Case 44

A 44-year-old gentleman suffered from a gradually growing swelling in the middle mandible accompanied by loose teeth for over 3 months.

[History of Present Illness] More than 3 months ago, the patient was found to have a "bean-sized" swelling in the middle of the mandible, which was progressively enlarged with the loosening of the lower anterior teeth. The patient had no history of dental pain in the corresponding area or trauma or swelling pain . CT examination in the outpatient department of our hospital showed that there was a cystic lesion in the middle of the mandible.

[Specialty Examination] The bilateral maxillofacial region was basically symmetrical. There was no abnormality in the mouth opening range and mouth opening pattern. The 31, 41 teeth were loose for II°, while 32, 33, 42, 43 teeth became loose on the percussion (−), and the mucosa was intact. The median 33–34 of the mandible corresponds to the labial and lingual bone swelling of about 3 cm × 3 cm, with clear boundary, smooth and continuous lingual bone cortex. The center of the lip swelling involved the cortical bone defect of about 1 cm in diameter, with no fistula inside and outside the mouth. No significant bilateral submaxillary and cervical lymph node enlargement was observed.

[Auxiliary Examination]

1. Panoramic radiographs suggested an abnormal cystic lesion in the middle of the mandible, which appeared as local swelling, thinning of bone cortex, irregular shape, and clear circumscription (Fig. 20.14).
2. A maxillofacial enhanced CT scan suggested an abnormal cystic lesion in the middle of the mandible, which appeared as local swelling, thinning of bone cortex, irregular shape, clear circumscription, and uniform density. No significant enhancement was observed after enhancement (Fig. 20.15).

[Preliminary Diagnosis] Mandible mass.

[Treatment] "Resection of mandibular mass" was performed under general anesthesia: a gingival marginal incision was made, and the gingival flap was elevated for surgical exposure of the mass after removal of cortical bone. The tumor was cystic. Brown fluid was found in the cyst cavity. The cyst wall was removed completely. Frozen pathological examination showed that the "median mandibular" lesion presented a cyst with infection and lining epitheliomatous hyperplasia. The wound was rinsed and thoroughly

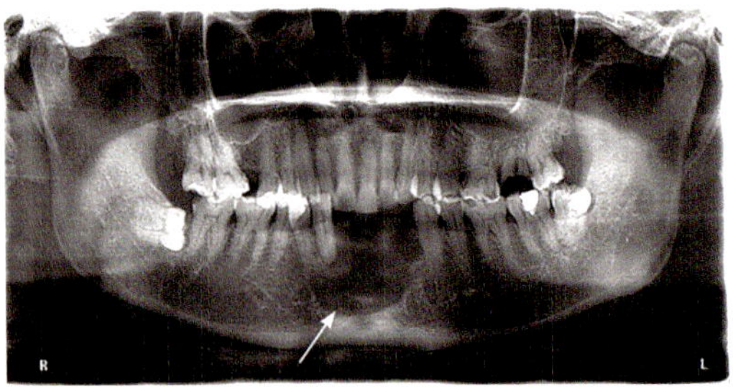

Fig. 20.14 Abnormal cystic lesion in the middle of the mandible, local swelling, thinning of bone cortex, irregular shape, and clear circumscription

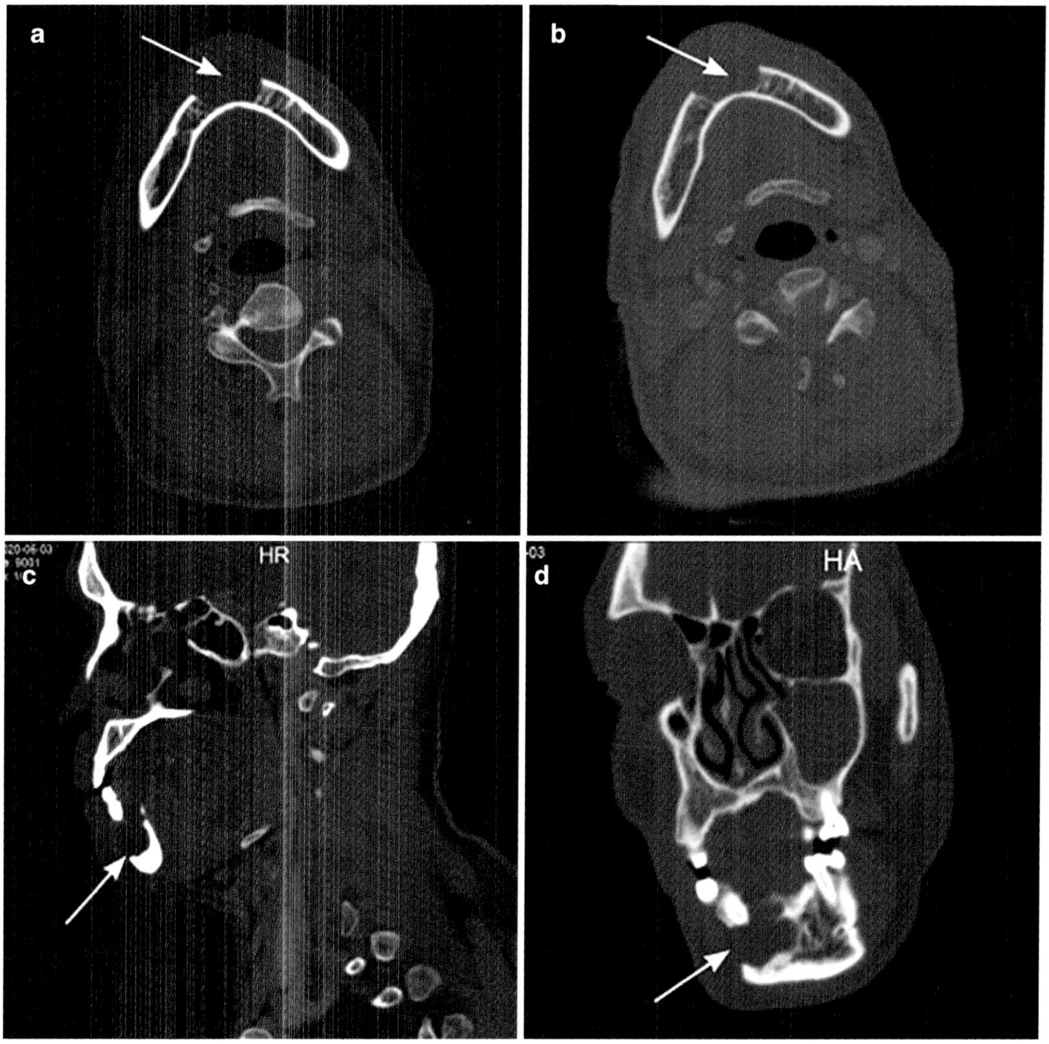

Fig. 20.15 (**a**) CT plain axial scan: Abnormal cystic lesion in the middle of the mandible, local swelling, thinning of bone cortex, irregular shape, clear circumscription, and uniform density. (**b**) Enhanced CT axial: No significant enhancement was observed. (**c**, **d**) Enhanced CT sagittal and coronal scan

hemostatic. The iodoform gauze was indwelled into the cyst cavity, and a suture was performed to close the wound.

[Pathological Examination] Gross pathological examination revealed cystoid tissue, 2.5 cm × 2 cm × 0.5 cm in size. Microscopically, the fibrous connective tissue was cystoid, lined with ameloblastomatoid epithelium. The basal layer cells were cubed and arranged in a palisade pattern, and the basal layer cells were loosely arranged, similar to the star reticular layer cells (Fig. 20.16).

[Pathological Diagnosis] Unicystic ameloblastoma "in the middle of the mandible," ICD-O code: 9310/0.

[Follow-Up] The patient healed uneventfully. The postoperative six-month follow-up exhibited no special postoperative reaction and no tumor relapse.

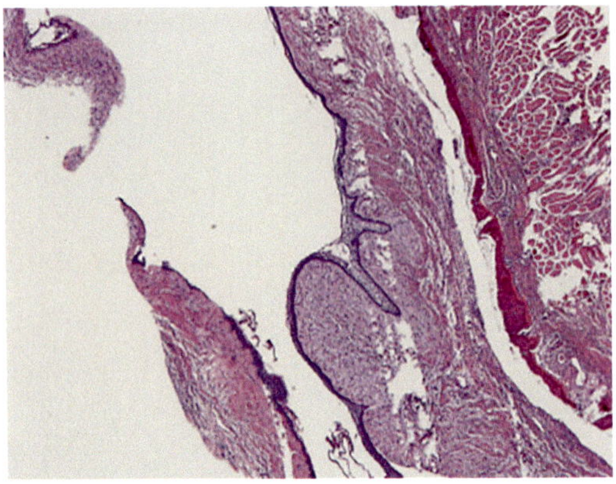

Fig. 20.16 Fibrocystic wall tissue, with normal cortical and muscle tissue laterally, lined with ameloblastoma epithelium, that is, the basal layer cells were arranged in a palisade pattern, and the basal layer cells were loosely arranged in a stellate reticulum pattern (40×)

20.4 Extraosseous or Peripheral Ameloblastoma

20.4.1 Case 45

A 46-year-old gentleman suffered from a mass in the right palate for over a year.

[History of Present Illness] More than one year ago, the patient found a mass in the right palate, which was initially about "bean" size. The patient denied a history of swelling, pain, trauma, and special drug injection. The mass gradually grew.

[Specialty Examination] The patient's bilateral maxillofacial region was basically symmetrical. There was no abnormality in the mouth opening range and mouth opening pattern. Intraoral examination revealed permanent dentition. The 18 tooth presented disuse luxatio imperfecta dentis, which was loose on the percussion (−). There was a 1.5 cm × 2.5 cm mass on the right palate near the crest of the alveolar ridge, which was medium and soft, poorly circumscribed, with no obvious tenderness and no obvious adhesion to the surrounding tissue. No significant bilateral submaxillary and cervical lymph node enlargement was observed.

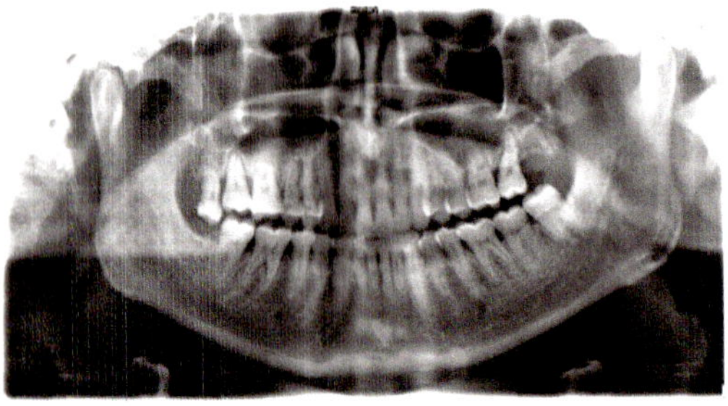

Fig. 20.17 48 loss, 18 luxatio imperfecta dentis, 16 distal, 17, 18 alveolar bone resorption, no obvious space-occupying lesion on the right maxilla (preoperative)

[Auxiliary Examination]

1. Panoramic radiographs suggested 48 loss, 18 luxatio imperfecta dentis, 16 distal, 17, 18 alveolar bone resorption, and no obvious space-occupying lesion on the right maxilla (Fig. 20.17).
2. A maxillofacial enhanced CT scan suggested a soft tissue density mass near the pterygomandibular ligament of the right palatopharyngeal arch, with a diameter of about 15 mm and a poorly defined boundary. The lesion enhanced significantly after enhancement (Fig. 20.18).

[Preliminary Diagnosis] Right palatal mass.

[Treatment] "Excision of right palatal mass with 17 and 18 exodontia" was performed under general anesthesia: The mass was completely resected at 0.5 cm outside the edge of the palatal mass. Frozen pathological examination indicated an epithelial tumor under the mucosa of the "right palate," with the nature to be determined and peripheral odontogenic tumor to be ruled out. The specific results were to be determined by paraffin and enzyme labeling. After 17 and 18 extraction, the operative area was rinsed and thoroughly hemostatic, and the wound was closed by suture. Postoperative follow-up was uneventfully, and postoperative radiographic images revealed bone formation at the surgical site (Fig. 20.20).

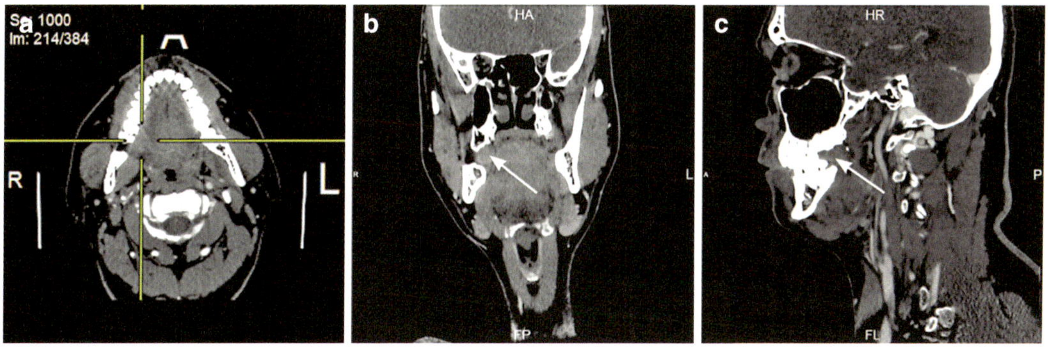

Fig. 20.18 (**a**) Enhanced CT axial scan: A soft tissue density mass was observed near the pterygomandibular ligament of the right palatopharyngeal arch, with a diameter of about 15 mm and a poorly defined boundary. The lesion enhanced significantly after enhancement. (**b**) Coronal scan. (**c**) Sagittal scan

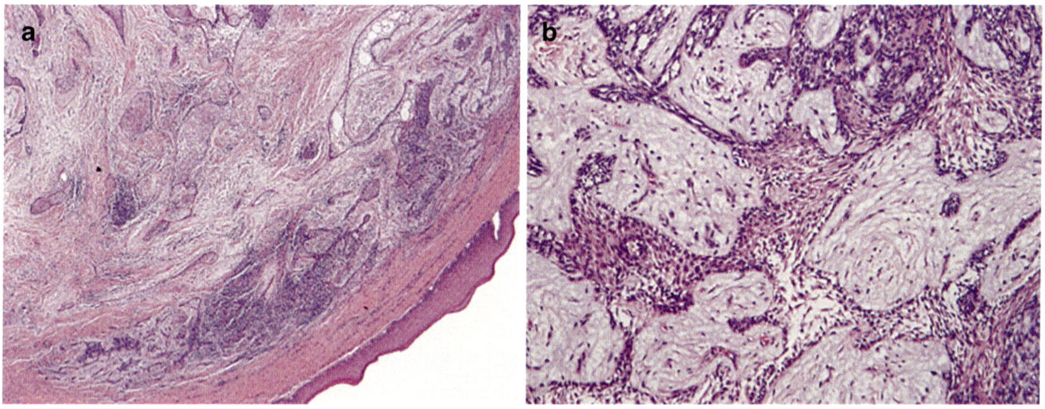

Fig. 20.19 (**a**) The lesion occurred under the mucosa and was limited to the gum. The tumor cells were arranged in follicular or clustered shapes, accompanied by secondary infection (40×). (**b**) The tumor cells were connected to each other in clumps, the peripheral cells were arranged in order, and the central cells were arranged loosely (200×)

[Pathological Examination] Gross pathological examination revealed tumor tissue, with mucosal tissue covered on one side, 1.5 cm × 1.5 cm × 1 cm, grayish white. Microscopically, tumor cells were found in the subepithelial tissue of the mucosa in the form of nest or cord. The epithelial nests were surrounded by columnar cells in a palisade arrangement, and the central cells were arranged loosely, similar to the stellate reticulum. The mucous degeneration occurred to the interfibrous interstitial epithelium, with inflammatory cell infiltration (Fig. 20.19).

[Pathological Diagnosis] Extraosseous or peripheral ameloblastoma of the right palate, ICD-O code: 9310/0, with secondary infection.

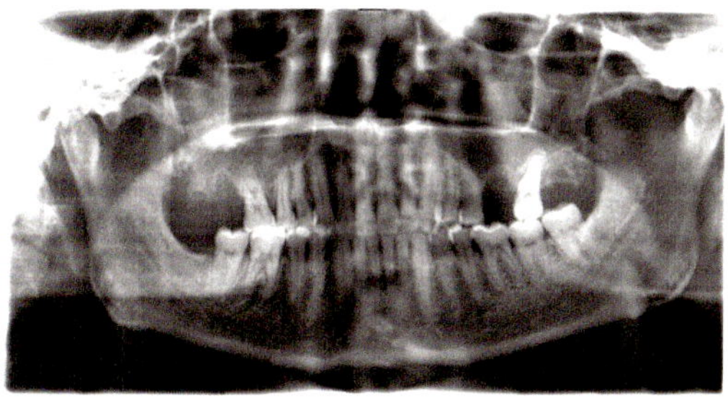

Fig. 20.20 Postoperative changes with bony healing in the right upper jaw without significant new pathological lesion

[Follow-Up] The patient healed uneventfully. The postoperative six-month follow-up exhibited no special postoperative reaction and no tumor relapse (Fig. 20.20).

20.5 Metastatic Ameloblastoma

20.5.1 Case 46

A 17-year-old girl suffered from right mandibular ameloblastoma for 3 months after multiple surgeries.

[History of Present Illness] The patient was diagnosed with "right mandibular bone cyst" at a local hospital 5 years ago due to distension of the right mandibular bone cyst and underwent "fenestration of right mandibular bone cyst." The postoperative pathology showed ameloblastoma. After surgery, the patient did not return to the clinic in time, so the right mandible appeared swollen again 2 years after surgery, and a second fenestration was performed. One year later, the right mandibular region distended again, and the patient received surgery again, with the specific operation method unknown. Now the patient once again felt the swelling of the right mandibular area. CT and MRI examinations showed that the cystic mass of the right mandibular ascending branch was accompanied by nodules in the deep lobe of the right parotid gland and neck area II: Relapse of ameloblastoma with possible metastasis.

[Specialty Examination] The face was asymmetrical. A mass was seen in the right submaxillary region, which was about 5 cm × 6 cm in size, hard, inactive, with no obvious tenderness. A postoperative scar about 6 cm long was visible on the skin surface of the tumor. There was no abnormality in the mouth opening range and mouth opening pattern. The right mandibular molar was defective, and local postoperative change was visible without obvious redness and swelling exudation. Right cervical lymph node enlargement was observed, about 3.0 cm in diameter, with moderate mobility, and no obvious adhesion to surrounding tissues. Once palpation, the mass was moderately hard and tender (−).

[Auxiliary Examination]

1. Panoramic radiographs suggested postoperative changes in the right mandible, with multiple abnormal hypodense shadows in the body and ascending branches, which presented as clear boundaries and no obvious bone white lines (Fig. 20.21).

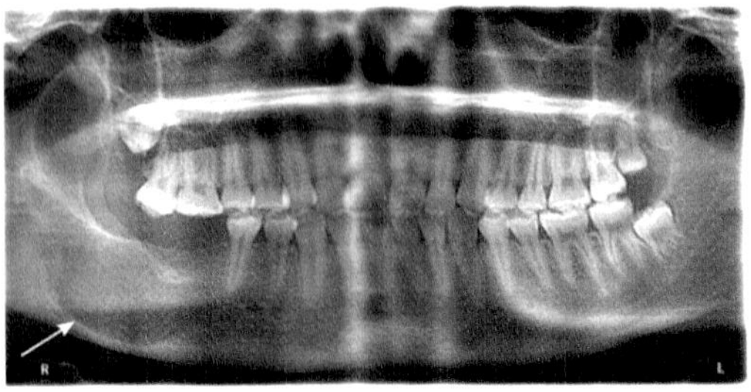

Fig. 20.21 Postoperative changes in the right mandible, with multiple abnormal hypodense shadows in the body and ascending branches, which presented as clear boundaries and no obvious bone white lines

2. Maxillofacial Enhanced CT scan suggested bone distention in the right mandible angle with bone density inside. Hypodense shadow could be seen in the swelling from the ascending branch of the right mandible to the coronal process, with a clear boundary of about 2 cm × 1.9 cm. After enhancement, uneven enhancement was observed, with C− 26,45 Hu and C+ 140,60 Hu. Local marginal cortical discontinuity was observed. There was no obvious abnormality in the structure of the skull base. The right submandibular gland was not seen. Circular enhanced nodule shadows were observed in the deep lobe of the right parotid gland and neck region II, with 32 mm in diameter (Fig. 20.22).
3. Maxillofacial Enhanced MRI scan suggested a bone distention in the right mandible angle, with uniform signal in the inner medullary cavity, high signal on T1WI and T2WI, low signal after Inhibition. A circular mass with a clear boundary and a diameter of about 2 cm can be seen in the swelling of the ascending branch of the right mandible to the coronal process, with mixed high signal on T2WI, and equisignal on T1WI, no obvious uneven enhancement after enhancement. There was no obvious abnormality in the structure of the skull base. The right submandibular gland was not seen. Circular enhanced nodules were

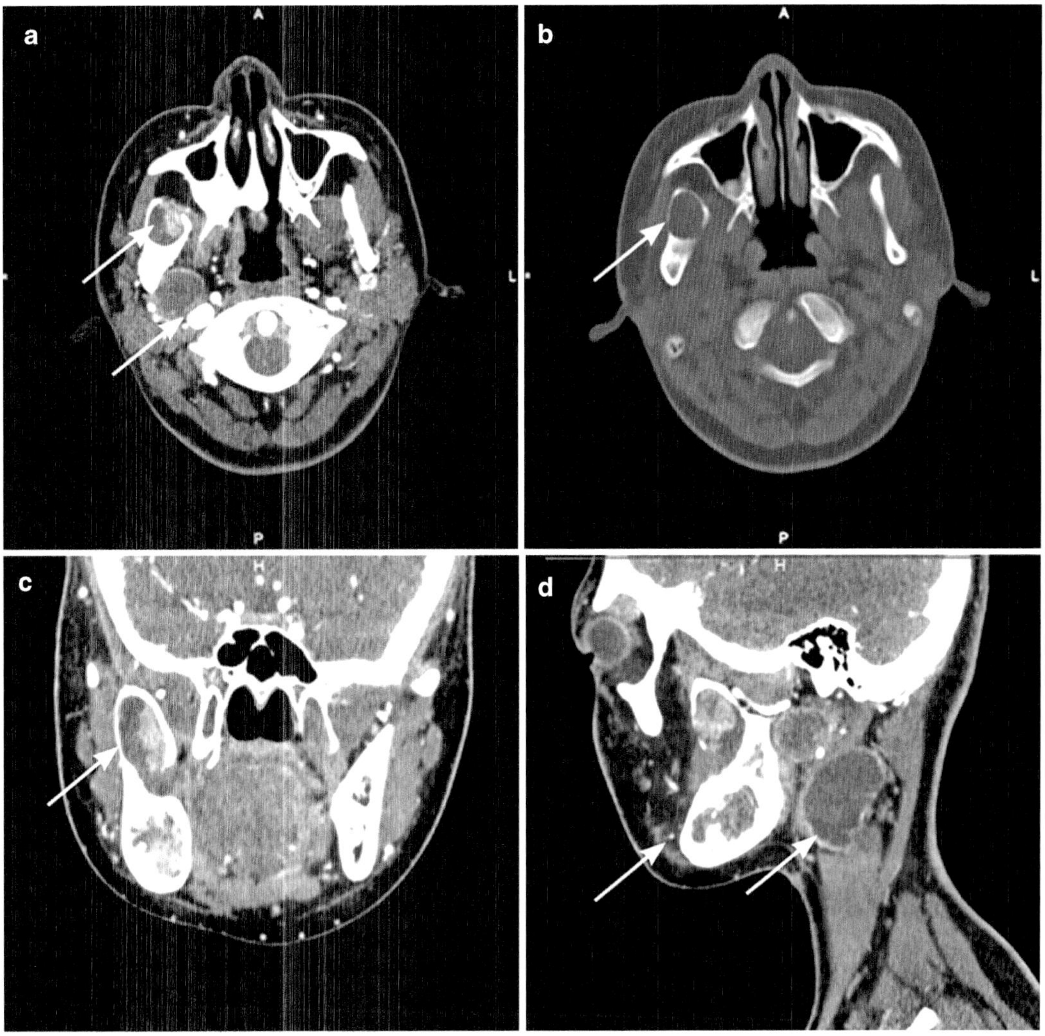

Fig. 20.22 (**a**) Enhanced CT axial scan (soft tissue window) : Abnormal soft tissue mass was observed in the mass from the right mandibular ascending ramus to the coronoid process, with clear boundary, obvious uneven enhancement, and local cortical bone discontinuity at the edge. (**b**) Enhanced CT axial scan (bone window) : bone distention in the right mandible angle with bone density inside. (**c**) Enhanced CT coronal scan (**d**) Enhanced CT sagittal scan: Circular enhanced nodules were seen in the deep lobe of the right parotid gland and neck region II

observed in the deep lobe of the right parotid gland and neck region II, with 32 mm in diameter (Fig. 20.23).

[Preliminary Diagnosis] Postoperative recurrence of ameloblastoma of the right mandible.

[Treatment] "Right mandibular marginal resection with right superior omohyoid neck lymph node dissection" was performed under general anesthesia: an incision was made along the original mandibular and parotid gland scar, and the gingival flap was elevated for surgical exposure of the mass, which extended down to the middle neck and up to the posterior part of the mandible in the deep lobe of the parotid gland. Right superior omohyoid neck lymph node dissection was performed. Intraoperative frozen pathological examination revealed that polycystic epithelial tumor in the background of lymphatic tissue of

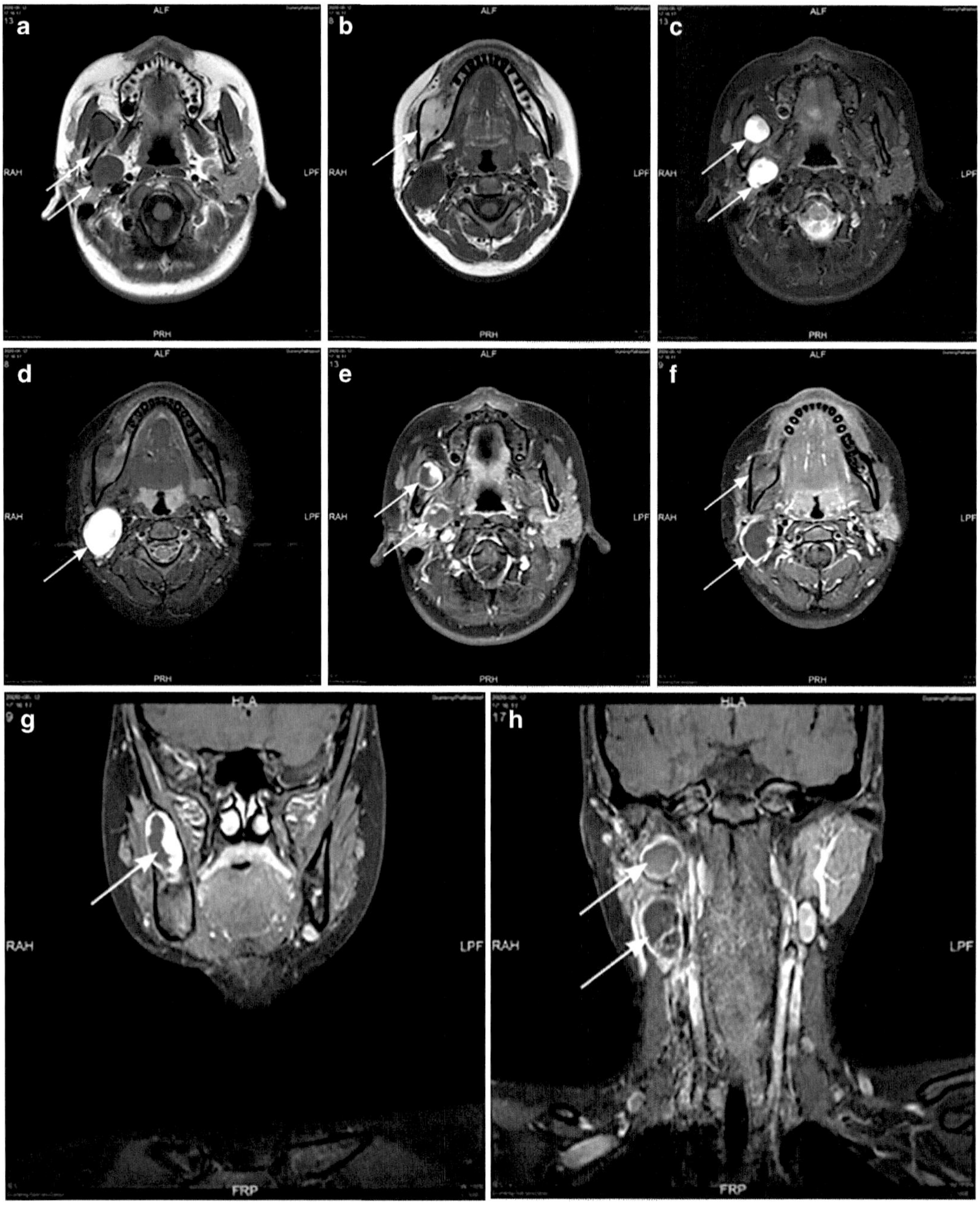

Fig. 20.23 (**a**, **b**) Axial scan T1W1: bone distention in the right mandible angle, and round mass in the ascending branch of the right mandible to the coronal process, with clear boundary and equal signal. (**c**, **d**) Axial scan T2W1: obviously high signal for the mass. (**e**, **f**) Enhanced axial scan T1W1: uneven enhancement was observed after focal enhancement. (**g**, **h**). Enhanced coronal scan T1W1: Circular enhanced nodules were seen in the deep lobe of the right parotid gland and neck

the "right neck," presenting as an ameloblastoma image containing mucinous cells; Lymph node 1 in the "deep middle neck" was negative (−). The "L" incision was sutured in the mandibular ascending branch. The coracoid process, part of the mandibular bone and the mass were removed

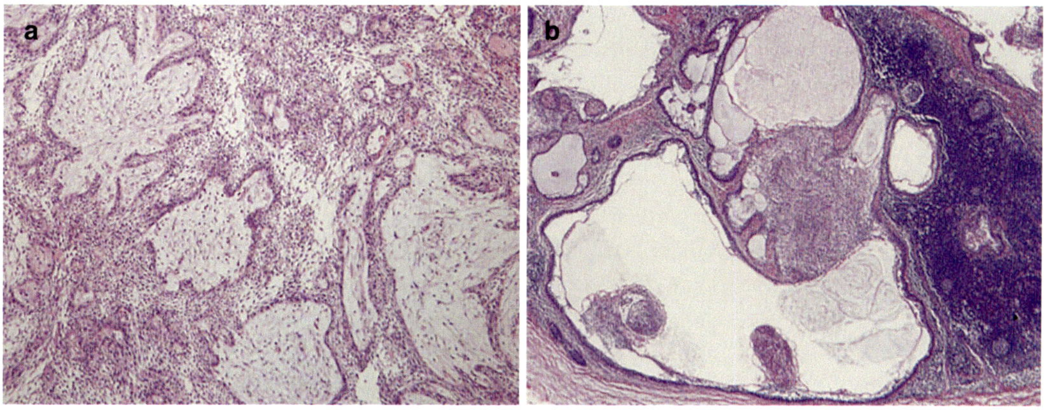

Fig. 20.24 (**a**) The proliferation of tumor cells occurred, showing flake and clumpy shape, with orderly arrangement of peripheral cells and loose arrangement of central cells. There are fewer interstitial cells and abundant blood vessels (100×). (**b**) Tumor epithelial nests can be seen in the lymph nodes, with palisade arrangement of cells around the nests, loose arrangement of central cells, accompanied by cystic transformation, unclear cell atypia, and rare mitosis (40×)

completely and sent for pathological examination. The wound was thoroughly hemostatic, a negative pressure drainage tube was indwelled into the operation area, and the layered suture was performed to close the wound.

[Pathological Examination] Gross pathological examination revealed a part of mandibular tissue and right neck mass. The mandible was locally distended, presenting as a solid cystic mass, light yellow and brittle, which was seen on the section. The mass on the right neck was about 7 cm × 5 cm × 3 cm in size, gray-red, cystic and solid in section, and contained clear, viscous liquid. Microscopc examination showed the intrajaw lesion was a cystic solid epithelial tumor. The tumor cells were arranged in clumps and sheets, the peripheral cells were arranged in order, and the central cells were fusiform and polygonal, with loose arrangement and local cystic changes. The interstitium was loose, with fewer cells and abundant blood vessels. The mass on the right neck was lymph node tissue with polycystic epithelial tumor, mild cells, no obvious atypia, and rare mitosis, appearing as an ameloblastoma view (Fig. 20.24).

[Pathological Diagnosis] "Right mandible" ameloblastoma (mainly plexiform) with local cystic change. "Right cervical lymph nodes" combined with right mandibular lesion were considered as metastatic ameloblastoma, ICD-O code: 9310/3.

[Follow-Up] The patient healed uneventfully. The postoperative six-month follow-up exhibited no tumor relapse.

20.6 Key Points of Diagnosis and Treatment

Ameloblastoma was originally known as enamel epithelioma or enamel tumor until Ivy and Churchill officially renamed it in 1930. Today, its tissue origin remains controversial. Most people believe that ameloblastoma arises from the enamel organ or dental lamella epithelium, while others believe that the epithelial remnants of the periodontal membrane or the basal cells of the oral mucosa are the tissue source of ameloblastoma. In addition, the transformation of primordial or odontogenic cysts and the ectopia of oral mucosal epithelium may also cause ameloblastoma [1–4].

Clinical Manifestations Most patients with ameloblastoma had no obvious symptoms initially until the tumor enlargement caused tooth loosening and displacement, occlusal disorder, and even maxillofacial deformity. With the gradual growth of the tumor, the normal cortex of the jaw bone is gradually destroyed and gets thinner. In severe cases, the tumor may invade the surrounding soft tissue through cortical bone. Large ameloblastoma of the maxillary bone may lead to dysfunction of the maxillary sinus, nasolacrimal duct, nasal cavity, and eye, further resulting in nasal congestion, eyeball displacement and/or protrusion, and tears. Large tumors of the mandible may cause abnormal jaw movement, affecting normal chewing, breathing and swallowing functions.

Differential Diagnosis It is difficult to distinguish small ameloblastoma without protrusion through the bone cortex from odontogenic cysts. Brown cyst fluid is extracted from ameloblastoma by puncture, while light yellow cyst fluid is extracted from a maxillary odontogenic cyst. However, cyst fluid is not a distinguishing feature between ameloblastoma and odontogenic cysts, and removing part of the tumor tissue for pathological examination is necessary. Ameloblastoma can also be distinguished from odontogenic adenoid tumors. The latter is more likely to occur in the maxillary cusp area and appears on X-ray as single-compartment shadows with calcification or dental presence, with rare recurrence after tumor resection. Other features such as cementofibroma, odontogenic calcified epithelioma, and odontogenic calcified cyst may also appear on X-ray as ameloblastoma with calcification, and their differentiation usually depends on pathological examination.

Treatment Unicystic ameloblastoma accounts for about 10% of all types of ameloblastoma. Compared with other types, unicystic ameloblastoma has low local invasivity and recurrence rate. According to a comprehensive analysis of lesion size and patient compliance, fenestration decompression or tumor curettage can be attempted at the first operation, and part of the bone wall can be removed at the same time to reduce the risk of recurrence. At present, the consensus view shows that except for unicystic ameloblastoma, the surgical resection of other types of ameloblastoma should be 0.5 cm outside the tumor, and the maxillary defect after resection can be repaired by free iliac bone, vascularized iliac bone or fibula bone. For elderly patients, patients with multiple concomitant diseases who cannot tolerate long-term surgery, or patients who cannot undergo bone graft repair at the same time due to limited conditions, reconstruction plates or other artificial replacement materials can be implanted in the defect area to maintain the gap and then bone graft repair surgery is performed later.

It is previously believed that ameloblastoma may evolve into malignant transformation, and malignant ameloblastoma is defined as metastasis of ameloblastoma. Both the primary and metastatic lesions exhibit the characteristics of benign ameloblastoma in histopathology. It is worth noting that the 2017 WHO classifies metastatic ameloblastoma as a benign tumor, which also indicates that radiotherapy and chemotherapy have no benefit for the prognosis of patients. Surgery is the effective treatment for metastatic ameloblastoma. Primary ameloblastoma, which differs from malignant ameloblastoma, is a rare epithelial malignant tumor of odontogenic origin with the histological characteristics of ameloblastoma and cellular atypia, regardless of the presence of metastasis. Primary ameloblastic carcinoma should be treated with a comprehensive treatment plan that combines surgical resection and postoperative radiotherapy [2, 8, 11, 12].

References

1. El-Naggar AK. Editor's perspective on the 4th edition of the WHO head and neck tumor classification [J]. J Egypt Natl Canc Inst. 2017;29(2):65–6.
2. Kreppel M, Zoller J. Ameloblastoma-Clinical, radiological, and therapeutic findings [J]. Oral Dis. 2018;24(1–2):63–6.
3. Loyola AM, Cardoso SV, de Faria PR, et al. Ameloblastic carcinoma: a Brazilian collaborative study of 17 cases [J]. Histopathology. 2016;69(4):687–701.

4. Almoznino G, Zadik Y, Vered M, et al. Oral and maxillofacial pathologies in young- and middle-aged adults [J]. Oral Dis. 2015;21(4):493–500.
5. Black CC, Addante RR, Mohila CA. Intraosseous ameloblastoma [J]. Oral Surg Oral Med Oral Pathol Oral Radiol Endod. 2010;110(5):585–92.
6. Laborde A, Nicot R, Wojcik T, et al. Ameloblastoma of the jaws: management and recurrence rate [J]. Eur Ann Otorhinolaryngol Head Neck Dis. 2017;134(1):7–11.
7. Weitz J, Bauer FJ, Hapfelmeier A, et al. Accuracy of mandibular reconstruction by three-dimensional guided vascularised fibular free flap after segmental mandibulectomy [J]. Br J Oral Maxillofac Surg. 2016;54(5):506–10.
8. Almeida Rde A, Andrade ES, Barbalho JC, et al. Recurrence rate following treatment for primary multicystic ameloblastoma: systematic review and meta-analysis [J]. Int J Oral Maxillofac Surg. 2016;45(3):359–67.
9. Sham E, Leong J, Maher R, et al. Mandibular ameloblastoma: clinical experience and literature review [J]. ANZ J Surg. 2009;79(10):739–44.
10. Au SW, Li KY, Choi WS, et al. Risk factors for recurrence of ameloblastoma: a long-term follow-up retrospective study [J]. Int J Oral Maxillofac Surg. 2019;48(10):1300–6.
11. Kelppe J, Hagstrom J, Sorsa T, et al. Ameloblastoma: a retrospective single institute study of 34 subjects [J]. Acta Odontol Scand. 2019;77(1):82–7.
12. Al-Rawi NH, Al-Siraj AK, Majeed AH. Comparison of osteoclastogenesis and local invasiveness of ameloblastoma and keratocystic odontogenic tumor [J]. Eur J Dent. 2018;12(1):36–42.

Calcifying Epithelial Odontogenic Tumor

21

Jing Song Hou, Hui Shan Ong, Zhen Tian, Lin Zhu, and Min Ruan

21.1 Introduction

A calcifying epithelial odontogenic tumor (CEOT), first reported by Pindborg in 1955, is a benign odontogenic epithelial tumor that may evolve into a malignant one. A calcifying epithelial odontogenic tumor is rare, accounting for about 1% of odontogenic tumors, and the mean age of onset is 36.9 years old, with no significant gender difference [1–3]. CEOT can be divided into two types, namely, intraosseous type (95%) and extraosseous type. The incidence of CEOT in the mandible is about twice that in the maxilla, and the molar area is the most commonly involved. CEOT is mainly characterized by local invasion and intratumor calcified amyloid substances. It is mostly clinically manifested as a painless mass, which gradually increases and causes later symptoms such as tooth loosening and displacement, occlusion disorder, and even maxillofacial deformity. On X-ray, CEOT usually presents as an irregular projection in the jaw bone, showing unilocular or multilocular [4–7]. The lesion may be accompanied by unerupted teeth and calcification foci of different sizes. CEOT is often misdiagnosed or relapses due to inappropriate treatment [8, 9]. Surgical resection is an effective method for the treatment of CEOT, which needs to be removed 0.5 cm outside the tumor boundary.

21.2 Case 47

A 71-year-old woman suffered from a gradually growing mandibular swelling for over 5 years.

[History of Present Illness] About 5 years ago, the patient felt a "bean-size" mandibular lingual swelling with no pain or discomfort. Due to no special diagnosis and treatment, the swelling gradually increased. A biopsy examination in our hospital a week ago showed chronic mucosal inflammation in the "premolar area and incisor area," with the formation of subepithelial inflammatory granulation tissue, surface epitheliomatous hyperplasia and mild dysplasia. Please refer to clinic examination results.

[Specialty Examination] The face is basically symmetrical. There was no abnormality in the

J. S. Hou (✉)
Hospital of Stomatology, Guanghua College of Stomatology, Sun Yat-sen University, Guangzhou, Guangdong, China
e-mail: houjs@mail.sysu.edu.cn

H. S. Ong · Z. Tian · M. Ruan
Department of Oral Maxillofacial-Head & Neck Oncology, Shanghai Ninth People's Hospital, Shanghai Jiao Tong University School of Medicine, Shanghai, China

L. Zhu
Department of Radiology, Ninth People's Hospital Affiliated to Shanghai Jiao Tong University, Shanghai, China

Y. He (ed.), *Inflammatory and Neoplastic Diseases of Craniofacial Bones*,
https://doi.org/10.1007/978-981-97-4155-7_21

mouth opening range and mouth opening pattern. Lingual swelling was seen at about 45-33 teeth in the mandible, with intact surface mucosa. The swelling was hard and palpable from the gingival margin, generating an overflow of a little yellow and white pus and causing slight pain. There was no numbness in the lower lip. No significant bilateral submaxillary and cervical lymph node enlargement was observed.

[Auxiliary Examination]

1. Panoramic radiographs suggested a bone distension with abnormal density at the upper edge of the proximal midline of the right mandible, unclear boundary, and no obvious absorption by the affected tooth root (Fig. Fig. 21.1).
2. A Maxillofacial enhanced CT scan suggested a bone distension at the upper edge of the mesial line of the mandibular bone on the right side accompanied by abnormal density, about 19 mm × 20 mm in size. It presented as local soft tissue deformation and dense shadows, swelling towards the cheek and tongue, no obvious enhancement of the lesion after enhancement, and no obvious soft tissue mass shadow around. The cortical bone of the lesion's peripheral wall was thinned and clearly separated from the surrounding soft tissue. No obvious cervical lymph node enlargement was observed. Nodular thickening of the mucosa in the left maxillary sinus was seen (Fig. Fig. 21.2).

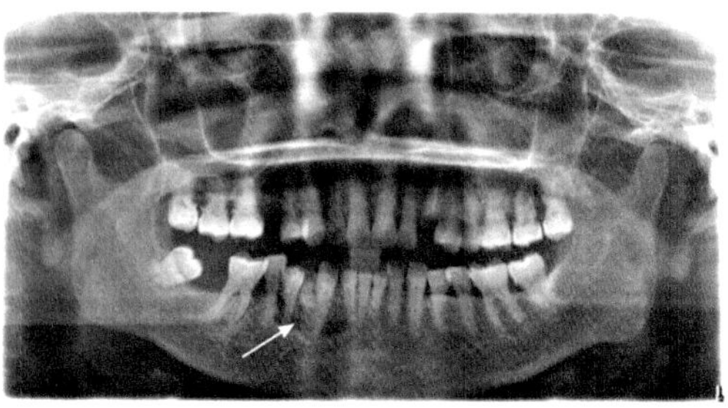

Fig. 21.1 Bone distension with abnormal density at the upper edge of the proximal midline of the right mandible, unclear boundary, and no obvious absorption by the affected tooth root (preoperative)

[Preliminary Diagnosis] Mass of the mandible.

[Treatment] "Expanded resection of mandibular mass" was performed under general anesthesia: the gum was incised at the 31st-45th teeth distal, and the lib-buccal flap was elevated for surgical exposure of the tumor. The tumor was found to be of jawbone origin and contained grayish-white soft tissue. The tumor was removed 0.5 cm outside to preserve the continuity of the mandible. Intraoperative frozen pathological examination showed a scattered epithelial mass with cells atypia. As malignant was not ruled out, please refer to clinic examination results. The wound was rinsed, thoroughly hemostatic, and closely sutured.

[Pathological Examination] Gross pathological examination revealed a part of the mandible and surrounding soft tissue, 5.5 cm × 4.5cm × 2.5 cm in size. The mandible was partially buccal-lingual swollen and the section was gray. Microscopic examination indicated that the tumor cells were arranged into small nests and cords, with clear cell boundaries, abundant eosinophilic cytoplasm, single or multiple nuclei, fine and granular chromatin, obvious nuclear polymorphism, and rare mitosis. A light eosinophilic amyloid deposit was observed between cells, often accompanied by concentric calcification (Fig. Fig. 21.3a).

[Pathological Diagnosis] Calcifying epithelial odontogenic tumor of the mandible, ICD-O code: 9340/0.

[Follow-Up] The patient healed uneventfully. The postoperative 6-month follow-up exhibited no special postoperative reaction and no tumor relapse (Fig. Fig. 21.3b).

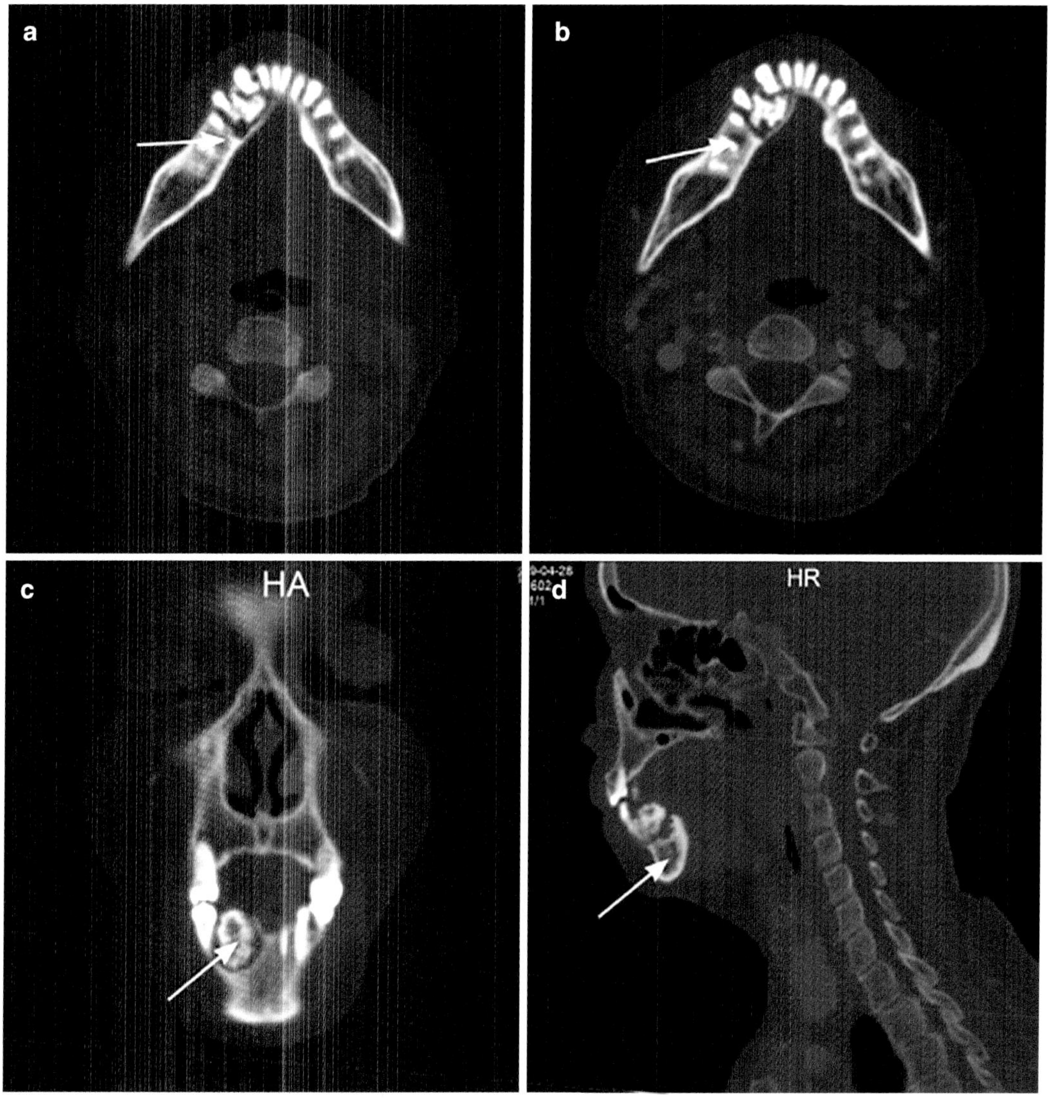

Fig. 21.2 (**a**) CT plain axial scan: bone distension at the upper edge of the mesial line of the mandibular bone on the right side accompanied with abnormal density, about 19 mm × 20 mm in size. It presented as local soft tissue deformation and dense shadow. (**b**) Enhanced CT axial scan: no obvious enhancement. (**c**, **d**). Enhanced CT coronal and sagittal scan

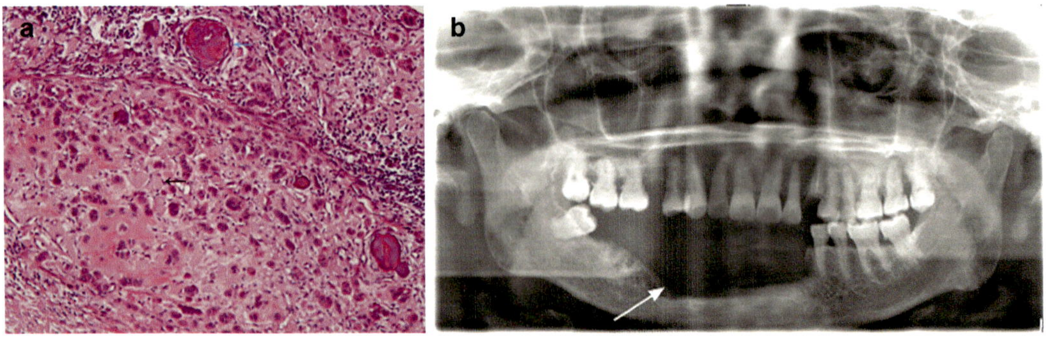

Fig. 21.3 (**a**) The tumor cells were distributed in a small nest pattern, with abundant cytoplasm and atypical nuclei but rare mitotic figures. Light eosinophilic amyloid deposit (black arrow) can be seen between the cells, and concentric circular calcification (blue arrows) occurred locally (200×). (**b**) Postoperative changes in the mandible without significant abnormalities in the surgical area (postoperative)

21.3 Key Points of Diagnosis and Treatment

A calcifying epithelial odontogenic tumor (CEOT) is formerly called "atypical ameloblastoma" or "malignant odontoma." First named by Pindborg as a separate tumor in 1955, CEOT is also known as Pindborg tumor. Although CEOT is clearly odontogenic, its histogenesis remains unclear. CEOT has a special tumor structure and cell and biological characteristics. Its pathological manifestations are large histological variation, and the tumor cells are composed of epithelial cells and fibrous stroma with variable morphology.

Clinical Manifestations Calcifying epithelial odontogenic tumors is rare clinically, accounting for less than 1% of all odontogenic tumors. CEOT usually occurs in adults aged 20–60 years, with no significant gender difference. It is more common in the lower jaw than the upper jaw, with the molar region most commonly involved. Due to no characteristic clinical symptoms, CEOT is more likely to be misdiagnosed and tends to relapse. In the early stage, CEOT is mostly painless and gradually enlarges. Initially, CEOT shows no obvious symptoms. However, in the later stage, due to the enlargement of the tumor, CEOT causes progressive destruction of the jaw, further resulting in tooth loosening and displacement and maxillofacial deformity. Maxillary lesions can also cause nasal congestion, nose bleeding, headache and other symptoms. CEOT has similar invasion characteristics to ameloblastoma, except that its local invasion is mainly manifested in the tumor envelope and surrounding connective tissue rather than the bone cancellum of the jaw bone [1–6].

Differential Diagnosis It is necessary to distinguish CEOT from ameloblastoma, odontogenic keratocyst and dentigerous cyst. CEOT can be characterized by discontinuity of the marginal bone wall, whereas ameloblastoma and other odontogenic cysts tend to cause cortical discontinuity in the case of evident buccal-lingual swelling. When there is calcification in the lesion, CEOT should be distinguished from cystic odontoma, calcifying odontogenic cystic tumor, adenoid tumor, and ossifying fibroma. The dense image of cystic odontoma usually shows a combined odontoma, with generally no scattered calcification points in other parts of the cystic cavity. The calcifying odontogenic cystic tumor usually occurs in the anterior dental region, with a clear boundary and calcification shadow mostly on one side of the lesion. Odontogenic adenoma usually occurs in the maxillary cusp region, with a clear boundary and complete and continuous envelope, mostly containing fully developed permanent cusp teeth and funnel-shaped capsular walls surrounding the tooth's root. Ossifying fibroma is a non-odontogenic tumor that usually does not involve teeth.

Treatment Surgical resection is an effective treatment method for CEOT. Extraosseous CEOT shares a treatment method similar to that of peripheral ameloblastoma. The tumor should be excised along with the surrounding oral mucosa and periosteum at 0.5 cm outside the safety boundary of the tumor, and the soft tissue boundary can be examined by freezing pathology to ensure a negative boundary. It has been reported that the recurrence rate of intraosseous CEOT ranges about from 10% to 15%, with a good prognosis. It is generally recommended to perform osteotomy in bone tissue 0.5 cm outside the tumor or osteotomy in normal bone 1.0 cm outside the tumor. Depending on the size of the defect, the bone defect area can be repaired by vascularized iliac bone graft, fibula bone graft or non-vascularized iliac bone graft [6, 7].

It is previously believed that CEOT, which has strong local invasiveness, shares similar biological characteristics with ameloblastoma. In recent years, more and more evidence has shown that the bone invasion of CEOT is relatively weak compared with ameloblastoma, and clinical views show that it is not necessary to recommend extensive jaw resection but to preserve the continuity of the jaw and reduce the scope of normal bone tissue resection. However, it should be noted that maxillary CEOT has a higher invasiveness and recurrence rate than mandibular CEOT (about three times that of mandibular CEOT) and is more likely to invade the surrounding tissue structure, so expanded resection is still recommended for the treatment of maxillary CEOT. A calcifying epithelial odontogenic tumor may evolve into malignant transformation, especially in multiple recurrences, which may transform into adenosquamous and squamous cell carcinoma, so long-term postoperative follow-up is recommended.

References

1. Philipsen HP, Reichart PA. Calcifying epithelial odontogenic tumour: biological profile based on 181 cases from the literature [J]. Oral Oncol. 2000;36(1):17–26.
2. Misra SR, Lenka S, Sahoo SR, et al. Giant pindborg tumor (calcifying epithelial odontogenic tumor): an unusual case report with radiologic-pathologic correlation [J]. J Clin Imaging Sci. 2013;3(Suppl 1):11.
3. Demian N, Harris RJ, Abramovitch K, et al. Malignant transformation of calcifying epithelial odontogenic tumor is associated with the loss of p53 transcriptional activity: a case report with review of the literature [J]. J Oral Maxillofac Surg. 2010;68(8):1964–73.
4. Venkateswarlu M, Geetha P, Lakshmi KN. CT imaging findings of a calcifying epithelial odontogenic tumour [J]. Br J Radiol. 2012;85(1009):e14–6.
5. Friedrich RE, Zustin J. Calcifying epithelial odontogenic tumour of the maxilla: a case report with respect to immunohistochemical findings [J]. In Vivo. 2011;25(2):259–64.
6. Lee SK, Kim YS. Current concepts and occurrence of epithelial odontogenic tumors: II. calcifying epithelial odontogenic tumor versus ghost cell odontogenic tumors derived from calcifying odontogenic cyst [J]. Korean. J Pathol. 2014;48(3):175–87.
7. Goode RK. Calcifying epithelial odontogenic tumor [J]. Oral Maxillofac Surg Clin North Am. 2004;16(3):323–31.
8. Cicconetti A, Tallarico M, Bartoli A, et al. Calcifying epithelial odontogenic (Pindborg) tumor. A clinical case [J]. Minerva Stomatol. 2004;53(6):379–87.
9. Angadi PV, Rekha K. Calcifying epithelial odontogenic tumor (pindborg tumor) [J]. Head Neck Pathol. 2011;5(2):137–9.

22 Adenomatoid Odontogenic Tumor

Jing Song Hou, Hui Shan Ong, Zhen Tian, Lin Zhu, and Tian Fu Wu

22.1 Introduction

An adenomatoid odontogenic tumor (AOT), also known as adenomatoid ameloblastoma, is a benign odontogenic epithelial tumor. WHO defines AOT as a slow-growing benign tumor composed of diverse odontogenic epithelium and mature connective tissue interstitium. AOT is relatively rare, accounting for about 3–7% of all types of odontogenic tumors. It occurs more often in the age of 10–30, and the incidence of women is about twice that of men. AOT can be divided into two types, namely central type (intraosseous type) and peripheral type (extraosseous type). More than 95% of AOTs occur in the bone, and the incidence in the maxillary bone is about twice that in the mandible [1–7]. Clinically, most patients with AOT are asymptomatic with slow tumor growth, and later may be accompanied by jaw swelling and pain, tooth loosening and displacement, with no tooth root absorption generally. The radiograph shows that the lesion is characterized by well-defined density-reduction shadows with punctate calcifications and unerupted teeth. It is difficult to distinguish AOT from dental cysts. The preferred treatment for AOT is complete resection or curettage. AOT has a good prognosis and a low recurrence rate.

J. S. Hou (✉)
Hospital of Stomatology, Guanghua College of Stomatology, Sun Yat-sen University, Guangzhou, Guangdong, China
e-mail: houjs@mail.sysu.edu.cn

H. S. Ong · Z. Tian
Department of Oral Maxillofacial-Head & Neck Oncology, Shanghai Ninth People's Hospital, Shanghai Jiao Tong University School of Medicine, Shanghai, China

L. Zhu
Department of Radiology, Ninth People's Hospital Affiliated to Shanghai Jiao Tong University, Shanghai, China

T. F. Wu
Hospital of Stomatology Wuhan University, Wuhan, Hubei, China

22.2 Case 48

A 65-year-old gentleman suffered from a swelling of the right mandible for six months.

[History of Present Illness] Six months ago, the patient was found swelling of the right mandible with no obvious predisposing cause. As it gradually worsened, the patient visited a local hospital but received no treatment. The patient recently felt tooth pain when eating, with no symptoms of perioral numbness or other abnormalities.

[Specialty Examination] The patient's maxillofacial region was asymmetrical, as the right mandible was swollen, with normal surface skin color and slightly higher skin temperature. There was no

Y. He (ed.), *Inflammatory and Neoplastic Diseases of Craniofacial Bones*,
https://doi.org/10.1007/978-981-97-4155-7_22

abnormality in the mouth opening range and mouth opening pattern. The vestibular sulcus in areas 34–47 teeth became thinner, extending to the swelling mass, about 3 cm × 4 cm in size. The surface mucosa was normal, and the boundary was clear. There were no obvious enlarged lymph nodes in the bilateral submaxillary region and neck.

[Auxiliary Examination]
Panoramic radiographs suggested cystic bone density reduction in the 34–47 teeth region of the mandible, with clear boundary, small incisure at the edge, obvious swelling of the jaw, truncated absorption of teeth in the lesion area, and a few punctiform calcifications in the lesion. 44 tooth was covered by the lesion (Fig. 22.1).

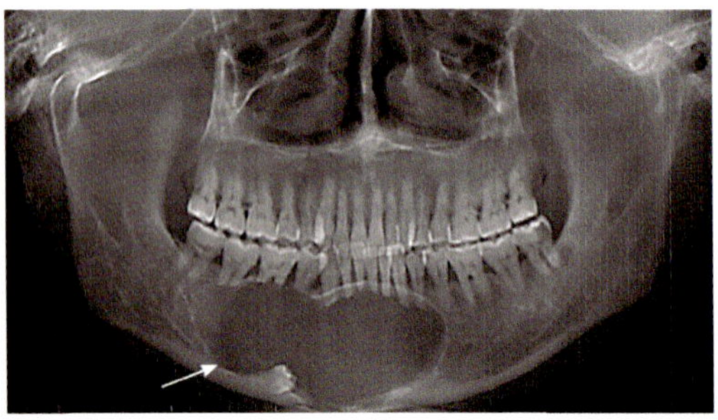

Fig. 22.1 Cystic bone density reduction in the 34–47 teeth region of, obvious swelling of the jaw the mandible, with clear boundary, small incisure at the edge, truncated absorption of teeth in the lesion area, and a few punctiform calcification in the lesion. 44 tooth was covered by the lesion

[Preliminary Diagnosis] Cystic lesion of the mandible.

[Treatment] "Segmental mandibulectomy with right iliac muscle flap transfer" was performed under general anesthesia: an incision was made along the lower margin of the mandible for 1–2 cm, and the gingival flap was elevated for surgical exposure of bone distention and local bone destruction with discontinuity observed. The mandible was truncated at the mesio-36th to the mesio-47th tooth, and the mass was completely removed. Intraoperative frozen pathological examination showed a benign odontogenic tumor of the "mandible," specifically to be determined by paraffin wax. The right vascularized iliac muscle flap was molded and reconstructed to restore mandibular continuity and occlusal relationship. The vascular anastomosis was performed. The wound was rinsed and thoroughly hemostatic, a negative pressure drainage tube was indwelled, and a layered suture was performed to close the wound.

[Pathological Examination] Gross pathological examination revealed the tissue of the mandibular lesion. Microscopic examination showed that tumor cells were arranged in solid epithelial nodules or sieve/trabecular shapes, with some areas appearing cystic (Fig. 22.2).

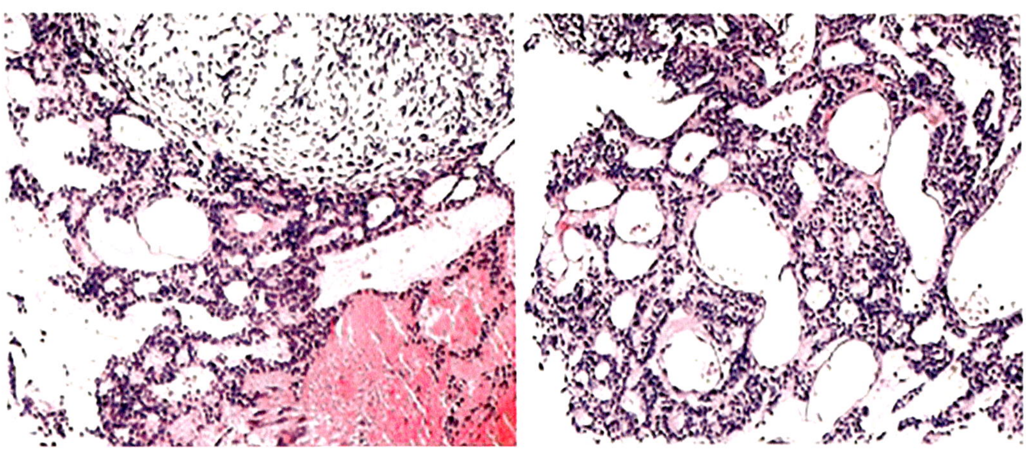

Fig. 22.2 The tumor cells were arranged in a solid epithelial nodule or sieve/trabecular shape, with some areas appearing cystic under the microscope

[Pathological Diagnosis] Adenomatoid odontogenic tumor of the mandible, ICD-O code: 9300/0.

22.3 Key Points of Diagnosis and Treatment

Adenomatoid odontogenic tumor (AOT) was originally considered a variant ameloblastoma and was therefore given the name adenomatoid ameloblastoma. Its tissue origin is still not completely clear. It may come from the ameloblast epithelium or the dental laminar epithelium residue.

AOT mainly occurs in young people between 10 and 30 years old and is quite rare for people aged at or above 30. The incidence of women is about twice that of men. It is more common in the maxilla, with the incidence twice that of the mandible, and the most common site is the anterior dental region. Most AOTs are small, with a maximum diameter generally less than 3 cm. Clinically, most patients with AOT have no obvious symptoms and are often diagnosed in routine imaging examination or special imaging examinations due to tooth failure to erupt normally. Gradual enlargement of the tumor may lead to painless enlargement of the jaw [1–5].

Differential Diagnosis On X-rays, AOT often presents as a well-circumscribed unilocular shadow, accompanied by calcified small points, and it is associated with unerupted permanent teeth (usually canines). Follicular AOT shows similar manifestations with odontogenic cysts, except that its transmittance sometimes extends along the root to the apical direction and goes beyond the enamel cementum boundary. The differential diagnosis of AOT also includes Calcifying epithelial odontogenic tumor, ameloblastoma, etc. The calcifying epithelial odontogenic tumor has no capsule with multinucleated tumor giant cells, while AOT has a clear and thick capsule. Ameloblastoma has neither a glandular tubular structure nor an eosinophilic homogenous substance, which is locally invasive. The cells around the solid epithelial mass of AOT can be columnar with a petal structure, but it has no stellate reticular cell, which is not locally invasive [6–9].

Pathological Characteristics AOT presents as well circumscribed and tumors often have a thick fibrous envelope. The tumor composed of fusiform epithelial cells and fibrous stromal cells. Epithelial components express epithelial markers, and stromal components interstitial markers. The epithelial cells are arranged in flake, ribbon or vortex mass, forming a variety of different morphological structures: (1) Nodular solid cell nest: the cells are fusiform or cube, rose-shaped, with eosinophilic amorphous substances in the middle of the cell nests; (2) Glandular tubular structure: cubic or columnar cells, with polar arrangement of nuclei, eosinophilic substances in cavity; (3) Small nodules: polygonal eosinophilic squamous cells with intercellular bridges and calcified clumps and amyloid substances; (4) Beam or sieve structure: found around the tumor or between solid cell nests, round or fusiform cells, deep nuclear staining; (5) Dysplastic dentin, enamel matrix and cementoid [10, 11].

AOT is a rare benign odontogenic tumor, and its diagnosis often requires a combination of pathological examination and immunohistochemical examination. AOT is easy for complete removal or curettage because of its thicker envelope, less recurrence, and good prognosis [12].

References

1. Chrcanovic BR, Gomez RS. Adenomatoid odontogenic tumor: an updated analysis of the cases reported in the literature [J]. J Oral Pathol Med. 2019;48(1):10–6.
2. Karam Genno N, Aoun N, El Toum S. Adenomatoid odontogenic tumor associated with an impacted maxillary lateral incisor: a case report with five-year follow-up [J]. Case Rep Dent. 2017;2017:1709492.
3. Shukla P, Prabhu S, Jose M, et al. Comparative immunohistochemical study of Bcl-X in ameloblastoma, keratocystic odontogenic tumor and adenomatoid odontogenic tumor [J]. J Oral Maxillofac Pathol. 2017;21(1):51–7.
4. Sethi S, Kumar M, Aggarwal P, et al. A case report and short review on changing trends in the site of occurrence of adenomatoid odontogenic tumor:

unravelling the past 15 years [J]. Dent Res J (Isfahan). 2016;13(5):462–71.
5. Jiang M, You M, Wang H, et al. Characteristic features of the adenomatoid odontogenic tumour on cone beam CT [J]. Dentomaxillofac Radiol. 2014;43(6):20140016.
6. Reichart PA, Philipsen HP, Khongkhunthian P, et al. Immunoprofile of the adenomatoid odontogenic tumor [J]. Oral Dis. 2017;23(6):731–6.
7. Bilodeau EA, Collins BM. Odontogenic cysts and neoplasms [J]. Surg Pathol Clin. 2017;10(1):177–222.
8. Bhatt R, Dave J, Nalawade TM, et al. Adenomatoid odontogenic tumour in mandible in a 14-year-old boy [J]. BMJ Case Rep. 2013;2013:bcr 2013010287.
9. Kalia V, Kalra G, Kaushal N, et al. Maxillary adenomatoid odontogenic tumor associated with a premolar [J]. Ann Maxillofac Surg. 2015;5(1):119–22.
10. de Matos FR, Nonaka CF, Pinto LP, et al. Adenomatoid odontogenic tumor: retrospective study of 15 cases with emphasis on histopathologic features [J]. Head Neck Pathol. 2012;6(4):430–7.
11. Philipsen HP, Reichart PA, Siar CH, et al. An updated clinical and epidemiological profile of the adenomatoid odontogenic tumour: a collaborative retrospective study [J]. J Oral Pathol Med. 2007;36(7):383–93.
12. Leon JE, Mata GM, Fregnani ER, et al. Clinicopathological and immunohistochemical study of 39 cases of adenomatoid odontogenic tumour: a multicentric study [J]. Oral Oncol. 2005;41(8):835–42.

Part VIII

Benign Epithelial Mesenchymal Complex Odontogenic Tumor

Ameloblastic Fibroma

23

Jing Song Hou, Hui Shan Ong, Zhen Tian, Lin Zhu, and Yang Wang

23.1 Introduction

Ameloblastic fibroma (AF) is a rare mixed epithelial and ectodermal mesenchymal tissue tumor, defined by the World Health Organization (WHO) as "a tumor that consists of proliferating odontogenic epithelial cells and extracellular interstitial tissue, similar to dental papillae, and has varying degrees of induced changes and hard tissue formation of teeth" [1–4]. AF accounts for about 2.5% of odontogenic tumors, and tends to occur in the posterior dental region of the mandible [1–5]. It is common in children and young adults with an average age of 15 years old and no obvious gender orientation. Its main manifestations are painless and progressive swelling of the jaw, occasionally ulcer, pain and swelling. The X-ray examination mainly shows unilocular or multilocular projection shadow, which may contain unerupted teeth, with sclerotic edges visible at the border. It does not invade trabeculae, but displacement of adjacent teeth may happen. The main treatment methods for AF are extirpation or curettage [5–9]. For a large range of multiple recurrent AF, segmental resection of the jaw and simultaneous reconstruction of the jaw are considered. It should be noted that AF has the possibility of recurrence and malignant transformation, so long-term follow-up is required after surgery. Study shows that the age of AF patients is greatly associated with malignant degeneration, and patients younger than 22 years of age were less likely to develop AF malignant degeneration than patients older than 22 years of age.

23.2 Case 49

A 12-year-old boy received fenestration for right maxillary ameloblastoma more than two months ago.

[History of Present Illness] Six months ago, the patient's parent found a swelling in the right middle face of the patient, without pain, numbness, or loose teeth. More than two months ago, the patient received "partial resection of benign lesion in the right maxilla with fenestration decompression and dental extraction" under general anesthesia. The postoperative pathology showed that (the right maxilla) ameloblastoma

J. S. Hou (✉)
Hospital of Stomatology, Guanghua College of Stomatology, Sun Yat-sen University, Guangzhou, Guangdong, China
e-mail: houjs@mail.sysu.edu.cn

H. S. Ong · Z. Tian · Y. Wang
Department of Oral Maxillofacial-Head & Neck Oncology, Shanghai Ninth People's Hospital, Shanghai Jiao Tong University School of Medicine, Shanghai, China

L. Zhu
Department of Radiology, Ninth People's Hospital Affiliated to Shanghai Jiao Tong University, Shanghai, China

Y. He (ed.), *Inflammatory and Neoplastic Diseases of Craniofacial Bones*,
https://doi.org/10.1007/978-981-97-4155-7_23

fibroma. The doctor suggested further treatment. The consultation of the Oral Pathology Department concluded that ameloblastoma fibroma of the "right maxilla" was combined with imaging findings.

[Specialty Examination] The face was asymmetrical, and the right face was swollen, with a well-coordinated 1/3 proportion of the upper, middle and lower face. There was no abnormality in the mouth opening range and mouth opening pattern. Intraoral examination revealed permanent dentition, postoperative changes of right maxillary fenestration, and absence of 14 and 15 teeth. The fenestration wound narrowed. The mucosa showed no obvious redness. The swelling in the buccal side of the right maxilla was about 4.0 cm × 2.0cm. The buccal cortex was damaged, and a solid mass was palpated, with unclear boundaries, poor mobility and tenderness (−). No obvious abnormality was found in the palatal mucosa. The left posterior crowed dentition was seen with 25 was palatally erupted and 35 was not erupted. Eye movement was normal without double vision. Right rhinostegnosis happened occasionally (Fig. 23.1a, b). Submaxillary and cervical lymph nodes were not significantly enlarged.

[Auxiliary Examination]

1. Panoramic radiographs suggested a postoperative change of the right maxilla, with abnormal maxillary density space-occupying shadow, which appeared as poorly circumscribed (Fig. 23.1c).
2. A Maxillofacial enhanced CT scan suggested expansive bone destruction in the "right maxillary bone" after fenestration of the right maxillary enamel fibroma. The range was about 4.5 cm × 2.6 cm, with inhomogeneous density. After enhancement, segmental enhancement was observed, with C− 32 Hu and C+ between 40 and 68 Hu. Multiple spot-like and linear high-density shadows were

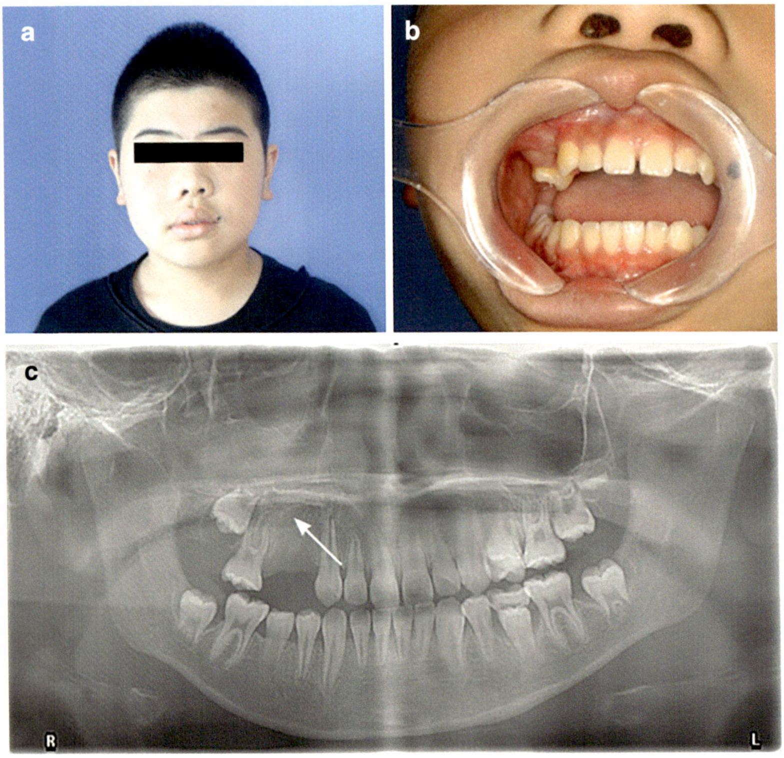

Fig. 23.1 (**a**) Asymmetrical face, with a slight swelling in the middle of the right face. (**b**) Postoperative changes in the right upper jaw, with visible buccal vestibular sulcus swelling. (**c**) Panoramic radiograph: postoperative change of the right maxilla, abnormal maxillary density space-occupying shadow, poorly circumscribed (preoperative)

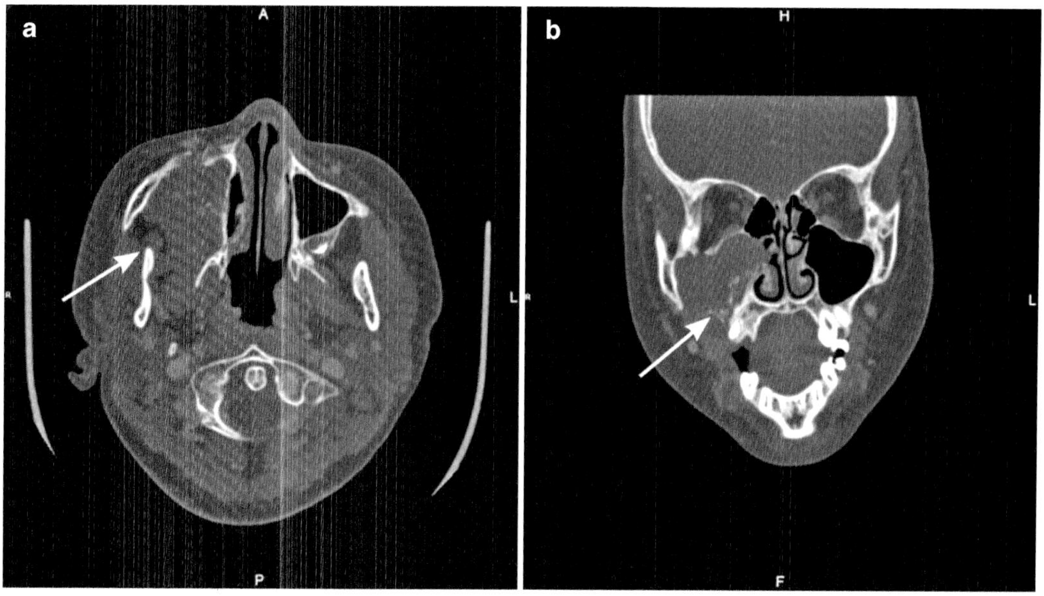

Fig. 23.2 (**a**) Expansive bone destruction was observed in the right maxilla, about 5.0 cm × 2.8 cm, and low-density shadow was seen in the lesion, with CT value of about 26 Hu. Multiple spot-like and linear high-density shadow was observed in the lesion, with noncontinuous local cortical bone, and no obvious periosteum reaction. (**b**) The lesion expanded into the maxillary sinus cavity, and the maxillary sinus cavity shrank

observed in the lesion, with noncontinuous local cortical bone and no obvious periosteum reaction. The lesion expanded into the maxillary sinus cavity, and the maxillary sinus cavity shrank. No obvious mass was found in the surrounding soft tissue (Fig. 23.2).

[Preliminary Diagnosis] After fenestration for right maxillary ameloblastoma at another hospital.

[Treatment] "Right maxilla subtotal resection with skull base tumor resection and partial zygomatic bone resection" was performed under general anesthesia: extraoral Weber incision was made to perform subtotal maxilla resection. During the operation, the tumor involved the sphenoid sinus, so it was carefully exfoliated from the cavitary sinus. The incision margin was removed and sent for intraoperative frozen pathological examination, showing epithelial odontogenic mass and fiber components were found in the tissue of the "right maxillary bone," considered as ameloblastoma combined with medical history. No tumor cells (−) were found in frozen sections of the incisal margin. The sharp bone tip and bone margin were trimmed, the surgical wound was rinsed and thoroughly hemostatic, the soft tissue wound was covered with artificial repair film and iodoform oil gauze, the extraoral wound was sutured in layers, and the right nasal indentation catheter was indwelled (Fig. 23.3).

[Pathological Examination] Gross pathological examination revealed a part of the maxilla and the surrounding soft tissues, 6.5 cm × 6 cm × 5 cm. The maxilla was swollen to the buccal and lingual side, and a mass was found on the section, which was 4.5 cm × 4 cm × 4 cm, grayish-white and tender. Microscopic examination showed that the tumor was composed of epithelial and mesenchymal components, and the embryonic mucous fibers similar to dental papillae showed long, narrow cords or island-like odontogenic epithelium. These cords usually consisted of two thick layers

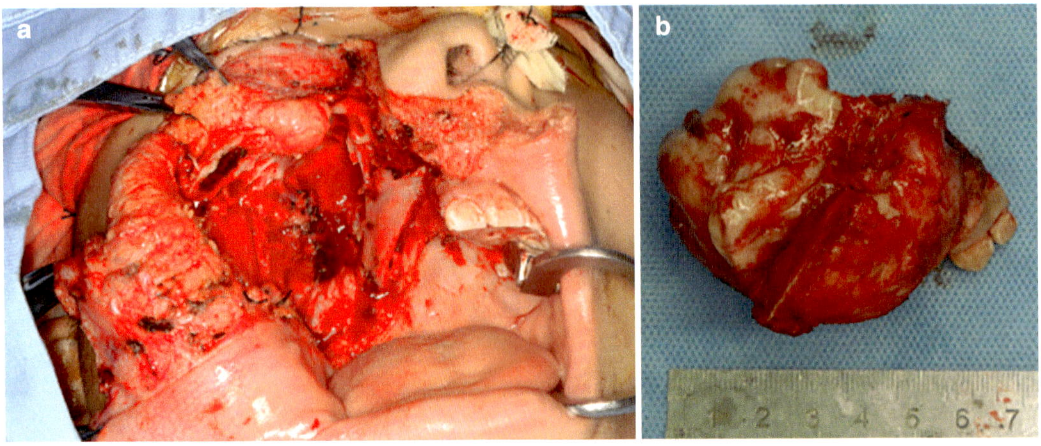

Fig. 23.3 (**a**) The tumor was completely resected and the sinus mucosa was cleared. The intraoperative margin was negative. (**b**) View of the right maxillary mass resected

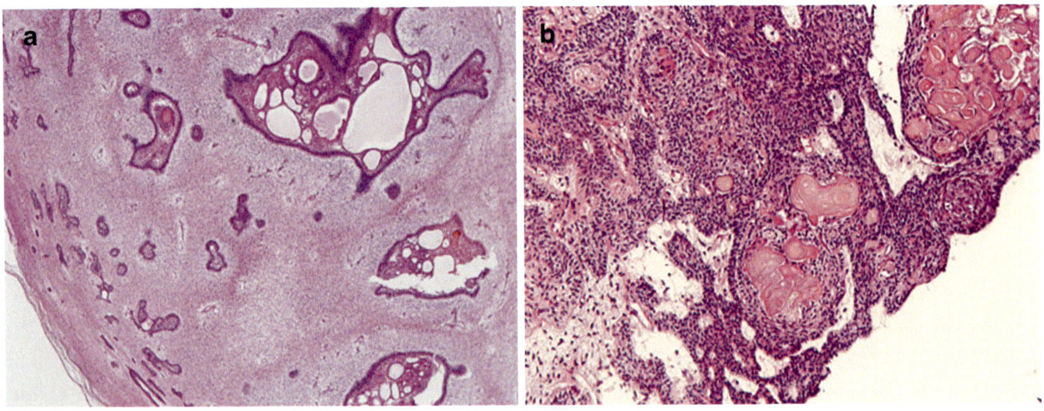

Fig. 23.4 (**a**) Odontogenic epithelial cords and upper skin islands were seen in the embryonal mucinous mesenchyme tissue, with island-like arrangement of cells and ameloblastoma-like image (40×). B. Shadow cell mass in the epithelium (200×)

of cubic or columnar cells, with palisade arrangement around the upper insula and fewer central cells, loosely arranged, similar to stellate reticulum cells. Scattered, clumpy eosinophil homogeneous mineralides were seen locally, the nucleus disappeared, and the surrounding region was hypercellular and prolifically active (Fig. 23.4).

[Pathological Diagnosis] Ameloblastoma of the "right maxillary," ICD-O code: 9330/0, with active mesenchymal cell proliferation.

[Follow-Up] The patient healed uneventfully. The postoperative six-month follow-up exhibited no tumor relapse (Fig. 23.5).

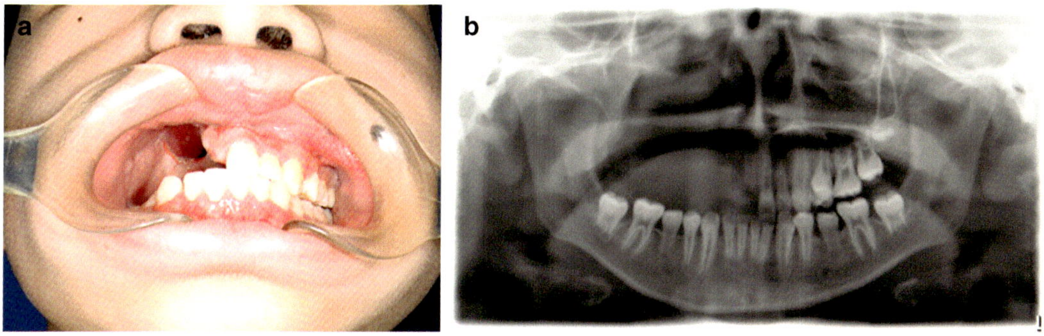

Fig. 23.5 (**a**) After subtotal resection of the right maxilla, oral and nasal communication was observed, with no obvious new organisms. (**b**) Postoperative changes of the right maxilla, bone defect in the operative area, no obvious space-occupying change

23.3 Key Points of Diagnosis and Treatment

Ameloblastic fibroma (AF) is a rare benign odontogenic tumor that mainly presents as a slow-growing painless mass with occasional pain. 88% of AF occurs in the posterior dental region of the mandible and is most common in children and young adults. AF has no specific radiological manifestations and usually shows a scalloped outline of unilocular ameloblastoma or soap bubble appearance of multilocular ameloblastoma. It is well circumscribed, usually with hardened edges, and may contain unerupted teeth. The buccolingual cortical bone of the jaw may show expansion, which is easily overlooked in 2D images, so CT scan is recommended to evaluate the extent and invasion of the tumor. MRI should be considered when soft tissue invasion is suspected. The diagnosis of AF mainly depends on histopathological examination. Microscopic examination suggests that the tumor is composed of epithelial and mesenchymal tissues, and the mesenchymal component is similar to the dental papillary mesenchymal component, with stellate reticular cells and oval cells embedded in the porous matrix. The epithelial component comprises cubic or columnar cells arranged into strips or islands, with no obvious mitosis or tooth-hard tissue in the tumor cells.

Differential Diagnosis AF generally presents as an asymptomatic, slow-growing distensible jaw mass, so it should be distinguished from other asymptomatic jaw masses in clinical diagnosis. The differential diagnosis mainly includes but is not limited to ameloblastoma, odontogenic calcified epithelioma, odontogenic adenoma, odontoma (in the old classification of ameloblastic fibroodontoma), etc. The differential diagnosis mainly relies on histopathology to confirm the diagnosis, and the diagnostic effect of immunohistochemistry is limited. Ki-67, p53 and PCNA can be used as biomarkers to distinguish whether AF has malignant transformation, and these markers have a high positive rate in AF malignant transformation cases [2, 4, 7, 8].

Treatment AF tends to grow slowly. Small tumors are generally unilocular lesions with clear boundaries, while large tumors are mostly multilocular lesions. The local recurrence rate after treatment is about 16.3–33.3%. No unified consensus has been reached on the treatment of AF, so a surgical plan is recommended according to the specific situation. In principle, while removing the tumor, attention should be paid to preserving adjacent important structures. The treatment plan needs to consider the patient's age, lesion range, and involvement of the tissue. AF is less aggressive than ameloblastoma, but recurrence and malignant transformation may happen according to the report. The surgical methods are mainly local curettage or extraction. Most literature supports the initial conservative surgical protocol, and more aggressive resection may be performed for recurrent lesions, very large tumors or tumors involving the maxillary bone. For child patient, local exfoliation and curettage are more appropriate to reduce the appearance changes caused by local tissue defects and the impact of surgery on children's growth and development. Long-term postoperative follow-up should be conducted, and further treatment should be done in case of recurrence during the follow-up. Attention should be paid to the possibility of local malignancy in cases of multiple recurrence.

In this case, AF occurs in the maxilla of a 15-year-old patient with a large lesion range (4.5 cm × 2.6 cm). CT findings show multilocular lesions with unclear local boundaries and ethmoid sinus and zygomatic bone involved. Considering the patient's age, lesion scope, and location, subtotal maxillary resection is more appropriate, with extended resection of the tumor and later restoration of maxillary defect with pseudocomplex or adult autogenous bone transplantation.

References

1. Kumar RM, Bavle R, Srinath N, et al. Ameloblastic fibroma in a young adult [J]. J Oral Maxillofac Pathol. 2019;23(Suppl 1):63–5.
2. Kramer IRH, Pindborg JJ, Shear M. Histological typing of odontogenic tumors. In: WHO international histological classification of tumors. 2nd ed. Berlin: Springer Verlag; 1992. p. 16–8.
3. DeLair D, Bejarano PA, Peleg M, et al. Ameloblastic carcinosarcoma of the mandible arising in ameloblastic fibroma: a case report and review of the literature [J]. Oral Surg Oral Med Oral Pathol Oral Radiol Endod. 2007;103(4):516–20.
4. Bertoni F, Del Corso G, Bacchini P, et al. Ameloblastic Fibrosarcoma of the mandible evolving from a prior Ameloblastic Fibroma after two years: an unusual finding [J]. Int J Surg Pathol. 2016;24(7):656–9.
5. Chen Y, Wang J, Li T. Ameloblastic fibroma: a review of published studies with special reference to its nature and biological behavior [J]. Oral Oncology. 2007;43(10):960–9.
6. Darling MR, Daley TD. Peripheral ameloblastic fibroma [J]. J Oral Pathol Med. 2006;35(3):190–2.
7. Buchner A, Vered M. Ameloblastic fibroma: a stage in the development of a hamartomatous odontoma or a true neoplasm? Critical analysis of 162 previously reported cases plus 10 new cases [J]. Oral Surg Oral Med Oral Pathol Oral Radiol. 2013;116(5):598–606.
8. Muller S, Parker DC, Kapadia SB, et al. Ameloblastic fibrosarcoma of the jaws. A clinicopathologic and DNA analysis of five cases and review of the literature with discussion of its relationship to ameloblastic fibroma [J]. Oral Surg Oral Med Oral Pathol Oral Radiol Endod. 1995;79(4):469–77.
9. Carroll C, Gill M, Bowden E, et al. Ameloblastic fibroma of the mandible reconstructed with autogenous parietal bone: report of a case and literature review [J]. Case Rep Dent. 2019;2019:5149219.

24 Odontoma

Jing Song Hou, Hui Shan Ong, Zhen Tian, Lin Zhu, and Xing Zhou Qu

24.1 Introduction

Odontoma is the most common type of odontogenic tumor in the mouth, accounting for more than 50% of odontogenic tumors [1, 2]. It is often considered a developmental abnormality (hamartoma) rather than a true tumor [3–6]. The 2017 WHO classifies odontoma as a mixed epithelial and ectodermal mesenchymal tumor. The etiology of odontoma remains unknown and may be related to trauma, inflammation, infection, genetic abnormalities, and genetic mutations in the deciduous teeth. It is common in young people before the age of 20, without large gender differences. The fangs, maxillary central incisor and third molar teeth are the most commonly affected teeth. Most patients with odontoma present no conscious symptoms and are often diagnosed by X-ray due to abnormal tooth eruption. The main treatment protocol is surgical curettage, which leads to a good prognosis and rare recurrence [5, 6] The earlier the diagnosis and treatment, the less the impact on affected teeth.

24.2 Compound Odontoma

24.2.1 Case 50

A 6-year-old boy suffered from a left mandibular lesion for two months.

[History of Present Illness] Two weeks ago, the patient received a panoramic radiography examination at another hospital for dental treatment, which suggested possible space-occupying of the left mandible, with no special discomfort.

[Specialty Examination] The face was symmetrical, with a well-coordinated 1/3 proportion of the upper, middle, and lower face. There was no abnormality in the mouth opening range and mouth opening pattern. Intraoral examination revealed mixed dentition, with odontosis of 16, 26, 36, 46 teeth, 71, 72 buccal bone swelling, thin mucosa, the range of about 1.5 cm × 1 cm; 7A, 7B loose (-) on the percussion (-). The gingival margin showed no redness, swelling, and exudation.

J. S. Hou (✉) · X. Z. Qu
Hospital of Stomatology, Guanghua College of Stomatology, Sun Yat-sen University, Guangzhou, Guangdong, China
e-mail: houjs@mail.sysu.edu.cn

H. S. Ong · Z. Tian
Department of Oral Maxillofacial-Head & Neck Oncology, Shanghai Ninth People's Hospital, Shanghai Jiao Tong University School of Medicine, Shanghai, China

L. Zhu
Department of Radiology, Ninth People's Hospital Affiliated to Shanghai Jiao Tong University, Shanghai, China

Y. He (ed.), *Inflammatory and Neoplastic Diseases of Craniofacial Bones*,
https://doi.org/10.1007/978-981-97-4155-7_24

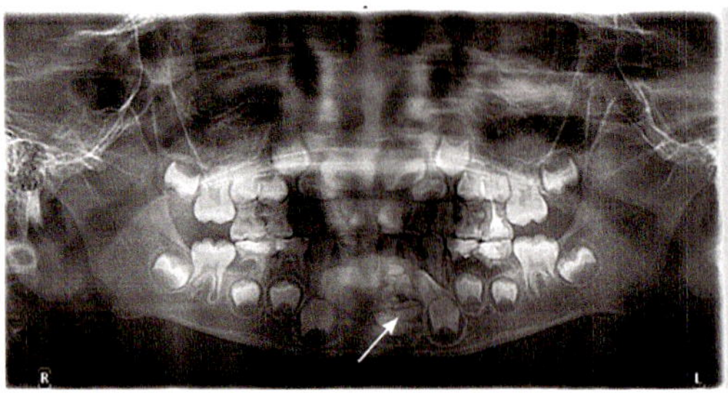

Fig. 24.1 Hard tissue density shadow with clear boundary and nodular calcification in the left inferior deciduous tooth 1 to left inferior deciduous tooth 3 (preoperative)

[Auxiliary Examination]

1. Panoramic radiographs suggested high-density shadows in the apical areas of 71, 72 and 73 roots, chaotic intraoral teeth structure, with relatively clear boundary, and no permanent tooth embryo below (Fig. 24.1).

[Preliminary Diagnosis] Left mandibular mass (odontoma possible).

[Treatment] "Resection of left mandibular mass" was performed under general anesthesia: the gingiva was incised on the 71 and 72 buccal sides, and the gingival flap was elevated for surgical exposure of the bone surface to remove part of the bone, and the tumor completely. The tumor was found to contain dental tissue of different development degrees. The wound was rinsed, thoroughly hemostatic and sutured.

[Pathological Examination] Gross pathological examination revealed a pile of deformed dental tissue, 1.8 cm × 1.5 cm × 0.8 cm, gray-white and hard. Microscopic examination showed that multiple dentin structures were observed, and the dentin, enamel, cementum and pulp tissues were arranged like normal teeth. Still, they were different in shape and size, and dysplasia was observed (Fig. 24.2).

[Pathological Diagnosis] Compound odontoma, ICD-O code: 9281/0.

[Follow-Up] The patient healed uneventfully. The postoperative six-month follow-up exhibited no tumor relapse (Fig. 24.3).

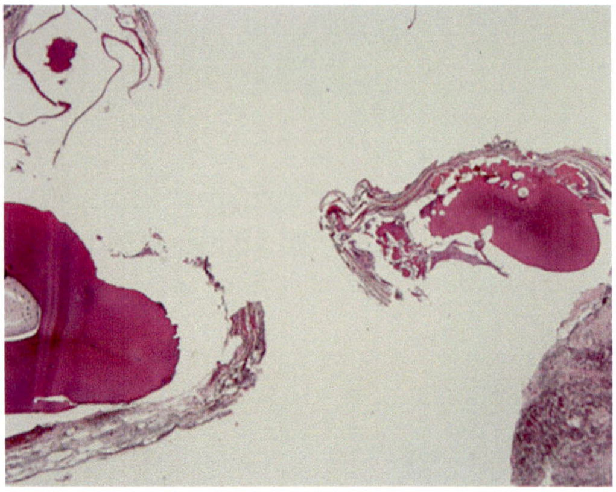

Fig. 24.2 Multiple malformed odontoid corpuscles with teeth arranged like normal teeth (20×)

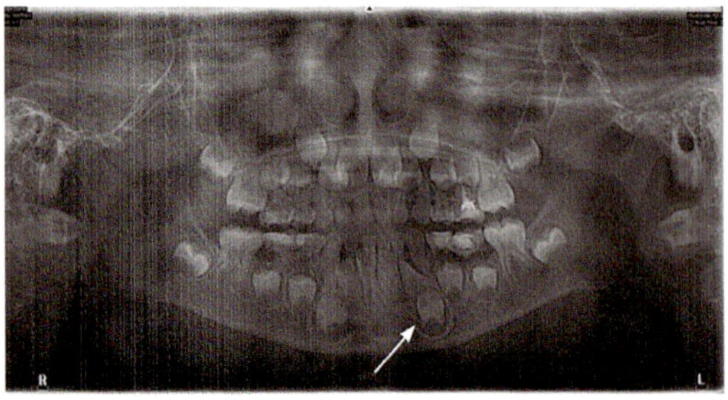

Fig. 24.3 Postoperative changes in the left mandible without abnormal shadow that has significant increase in density (postoperative)

24.3 Mixed Odontoma

24.3.1 Case 51

A 11-year-old boy suffered from a painless mass in the left mandible for over a month.

[History of Present Illness] The patient received a panoramic radiograph examination due to the delayed emergence of the left first molar 1 month ago. Panoramic radiographs showed that the left mandible was occupied by high-density shadow, accompanied by no eruption of permanent teeth, mandibular swelling, and previous symptoms such as pain, lower lip numbness, ulcers and bleeding.

[Specialty Examination] The face was basically symmetrical, with a well-coordinated 1/3 proportion of the upper, middle, and lower face. No swelling was observed in the soft tissue of the left mandibular body, with no tenderness and no ping-pong or mobility sensation. Bilateral lower lip tactile pain was symmetrical. There was no abnormality in the mouth opening range and mouth opening pattern. Intraoral examination revealed mixed dentition, with the absence of 36 and no percussion pain of 75. There was no redness or swelling of the gingiva in the posterior area of the molars and no rupture or bleeding. Slight swelling was seen in the buccal and lingual mandible without tenderness. No significant bilateral submandibular and cervical lymph node enlargement was observed.

[Auxiliary Examination]
Panoramic radiographs suggested 36 tooth impacted, distally mixed heterogeneous high-density shadows, 37 permanent tooth embryo not seen (Fig. 24.4).

[Preliminary Diagnosis] Mixed odontoma of the left mandible.

[Treatment] "Resection of left mandibular mass" was performed under general anesthesia: the gingival flap was incised and elevated along the left mandibular buccal gingiva for surgical exposure of bone surface. The bone was removed to expose the tumor for thorough curettage. There was no nerve exposure and no damage to the permanent tooth embryo during the operation. The marginal bone was trimmed to stop bleeding. The wound was rinsed and closed tightly.

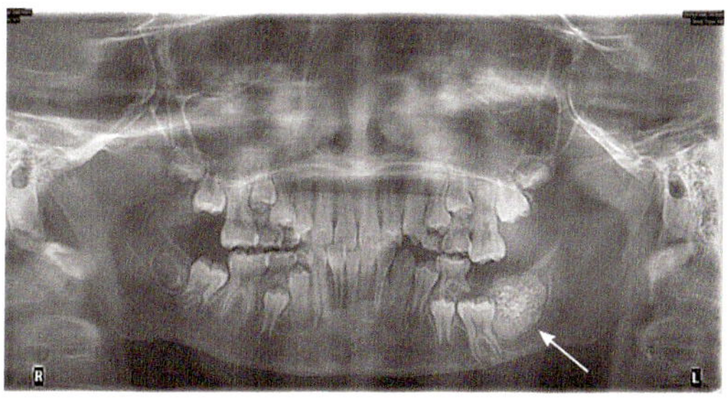

Fig. 24.4 36 tooth impacted, distally mixed heterogeneous high-density shadows, 37 permanent tooth germ was not seen

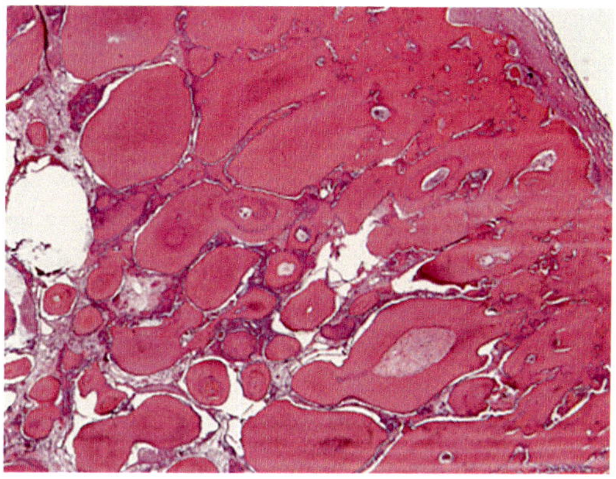

Fig. 24.5 Dental tissues of various components are mixed and fused into clumps (40×)

[Pathological Examination] Gross pathological examination revealed the hard issue, about 3 cm × 2 cm × 1 cm in size, gray-white. Microscopic examination showed that red-stained dentin substances were mixed and interconnected, and dentin tubules were seen inside. Irregular cavities were found between dentin lumps, containing weakly basophilic vesicular substances in the form of a grid or fish scale, i.e., residual enamel after decalcification. Cementoid substances with alkaline reflexes were also observed. Part of the tooth tissue was arranged as normal teeth (Fig. 24.5).

[Pathological Diagnosis] Mixed odontoma of the left mandible, ICD-O code: 9282/0.

[Follow-Up] The patient healed uneventfully. The postoperative six-month follow-up exhibited no tumor relapse.

24.4 Key Points of Diagnosis and Treatment

Diagnosis Odontoma, consisting of various dental tissue components, is an abnormality that occurs during the growth of fully differentiated epithelial and mesenchymal cells into ameloblasts and odontoblasts. According to the arrangement of dental tissue components, it can be divided into two categories, namely, compound odontoma and mixed odontoma. Compound odontoma consists of deformed teeth that are arranged in order similar to normal dental tissue components, while mixed odontoma consists of disordered tissue components. In addition, some lesions may be composed of compound odontoma and mixed odontoma occasionally. Epidemiological analysis suggests that compound odontoma is more common and usually occurs in the maxillary incisor and cusp region, followed by the anterior and posterior mandibular regions, and mixed odontoma is more common in the mandibular second molar and third molar region. Clinically, odontoma is usually a slow, painless growing jaw lesion. Routine X-ray examination shows that odontoma usually appears as a unilocular mass, which may contain blocked projections of multiple tiny tooth structures or non-transmitted dense masses surrounded by thin transmitted edges. The lesions tend to happen between the roots of unerupted teeth or between deciduous permanent denticles. Compound odontoma is rarely confused with other diseases, while mixed odontoma may be confused on imaging examination with osteomas or other calcifying diseases of the jaw, such as fibrodysplasia and ossifying fibroma [5, 6].

Treatment Odontoma has benign characteristics and limited growth potential, and surgical resection is an effective clinical treatment method. No treatment for odontoma often results in tissue degradation, cyst formation, tooth eruption disorder, mandibular fracture, odontoma exposure in the mouth or infection. Small odontomas can be removed surgically. Whether to retain impacted teeth depends on the specific clinic results. The affected permanent teeth should be protected as much as possible during the operation, and auxiliary orthodontic treatment can be performed if necessary. Studies have found that 75% of associated impacted teeth erupt gradually after odontoma removal, so it is necessary to carefully evaluate the removal of affected impacted teeth. In rare cases, giant odontoma can cause significant cortical swelling, resulting in local swelling and facial asymmetry, restricted mouth opening, pain, and tooth displacement. The operative approach should be selected carefully, taking into account the possibility of fracture of the remaining mandible. Therefore, early diagnosis and early treatment are conducive to minimizing potential complications.

References

1. Soluk Tekkesin M, Pehlivan S, Olgac V, et al. Clinical and histopathological investigation of odontomas: review of the literature and presentation of 160 cases [J]. J Oral Maxillofac Surg. 2012;70(6):1358–61.
2. Isola G, Cicciu M, Fiorillo L, et al. Association between odontoma and impacted teeth [J]. J Craniofac Surg. 2017;28(3):755–8.
3. Yassin OM. Delayed eruption of maxillary primary cuspid associated with compound odontoma [J]. J Clin Pediatr Dent. 1999;23(2):147–9.
4. Morning P. Impacted teeth in relation to odontomas [J]. Int J Oral Surg. 1980;9(2):81–91.
5. Park JC, Yang JH, Jo SY, et al. Giant complex odontoma in the posterior mandible: a case report and literature review [J]. Imaging Sci Dent. 2018;48(4):289–93.
6. Bueno NP, Bergamini ML, Elias FM, et al. Unusual giant complex odontoma: a case report [J]. J Stomatol Oral Maxillofac Surg. 2020;121(5):604–7.

Ameloblastic Fibro-Odontoma

25

Jing Song Hou, Hui Shan Ong, Zhen Tian, Lin Zhu, and Xiao Mei Zhao

25.1 Introduction

Ameloblastic fibro-odontoma (AFO) is an expansive, slow-progressing odontogenic tumor that accounts for 0.3–1.7% of jaw tumors. The 2005 WHO Classification of Tumors (3rd Edition) defines it as "a tumor composed of proliferating epithelial odontogenic cells in extracellular stromal tissue, with varying degrees of induced deformation and hard tissue formation of teeth" [1, 2]. Ameloblastic fibro-odontoma is a lesion that combines soft and hard tissue components, accompanied with dentin and enamel. In very few cases, AFO is called ameloblastic fibrodentinoma as long as dentin is present. The 2017 WHO Classification of Odontogenic Tumors considered that the hard tissue of dysplastic teeth in the lesions of ameloblastic fibro-odontoma and ameloblastic fibrodentinoma eventually developed into mature dentin or enamel, which means ameloblastic fibro-odontoma and ameloblastic fibrodentinoma are only a stage in the development of odontoma, with no enough evidence to support the classification of the two as independent disease types [1–4]. So, in 2017, WHO classified them as odontomas of different degrees of development [1, 4, 5]. AFO occurs primarily in children and young adults (before the age of 20 years) with no significant gender orientation. AFO tends to occur in the posterior dental region of the mandible and usually presents as a painless, slow-growing lesion of the jaw that prevents normal tooth eruption. Surgical excision is the main treatment method for AFO. The removal of the affected unerupted teeth depends on the circumstances. AFO has a low recurrence [3, 4].

25.2 Case 52

A 8-year-old girl suffered from left mandibular distention for three weeks.

[History of Present Illness] The patient happened to find left mandibular distention 3 weeks ago, with no obvious pain. Panoramic radiographs at a local hospital suggested a "bone tumor" possibly. The enhanced CT at our outpatient department showed "the possibility of benign odontogenic tumor in the mandible: odontoma."

J. S. Hou (✉)
Hospital of Stomatology, Guanghua College of Stomatology, Sun Yat-sen University, Guangzhou, Guangdong, China
e-mail: houjs@mail.sysu.edu.cn

H. S. Ong · Z. Tian · X. M. Zhao
Department of Oral Maxillofacial-Head & Neck Oncology, Shanghai Ninth People's Hospital, Shanghai Jiao Tong University School of Medicine, Shanghai, China

L. Zhu
Department of Radiology, Ninth People's Hospital Affiliated to Shanghai Jiao Tong University, Shanghai, China

Y. He (ed.), *Inflammatory and Neoplastic Diseases of Craniofacial Bones*,
https://doi.org/10.1007/978-981-97-4155-7_25

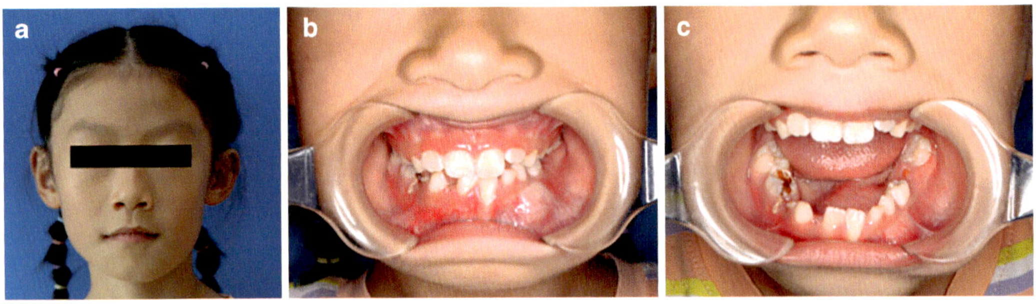

Fig. 25.1 (**a**) Facial asymmetry, left mandible bulge. (**b**) Mixed dentition, none distention of the left mandibular buccal side, intact mucosa. (**c**) Obvious lingual distention in the anterior part of mandible

[Specialty Examination] The face was asymmetrical, and the left mandible body was more swollen than the right mandible, with normal surface skin color and temperature. There was no abnormality in the mouth opening range and mouth opening pattern. 72-36 buccal vestibular sulcus swelling and 74-83 lingual sulcus swelling were seen with hard texture, normal surface mucosal color, no ulceration, clear boundary, no mobility, no tenderness (Fig. 25.1). No obvious bilateral submandibular and cervical lymph node enlargement was observed.

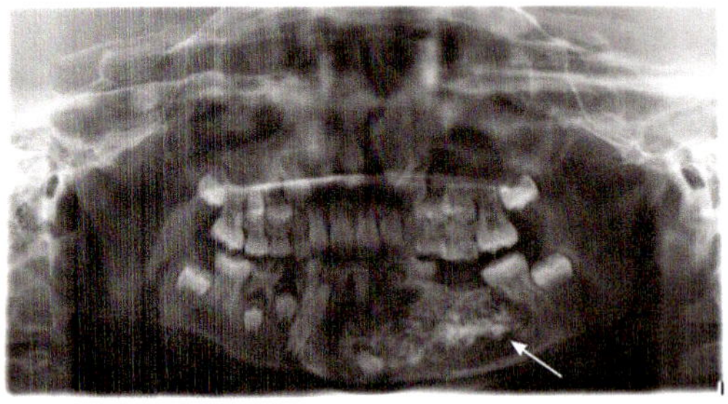

Fig. 25.2 Apace-occupying shadow with abnormal density in the anterior of the mandible and the left of the mandible, with uneven increase in density inside the lesion and unclear boundary

[Auxiliary Examination]

1. Panoramic radiographs suggested a space-occupying shadow with abnormal density in the anterior of the mandible and the left of the mandible, with an uneven increase in density inside the lesion and unclear boundary (Fig. 25.2).
2. Maxillofacial Enhanced CT scan suggested a bone distention of the mandible (lower right 3- lower left 6). A circular abnormal density shadow with a clear boundary was observed, about 5.3 cm × 2.8 cm in size, 64 Hu for C× and 75 Hu for C+. Multiple dense shadows were seen in the lesion, some of which were enamel dense. The adjacent cortical bone was thinned and partially disappeared, with no obvious periosteal reaction. No abnormal swelling was seen in the surrounding soft tissue. No obvious bilateral cervical lymph node enlargement was observed (Fig. 25.3).

[Preliminary Diagnosis] Mass of the mandible.

[Treatment] "Expanded resection of mandibular masses" was performed under general anesthesia: a gingival incision was made along the crest of the mesial alveolar ridge from 82 to 36, and the gingival flap was elevated for surgical exposure of the thin buccal bone wall. After the in thin buccal bone wall was removed, a large number of white nodular contents were visible in the bone cavity, along with dentin substances. Frozen pathological examination suggested the tumor was composed of odontogenic epithelium, odontogenic mesenchymal tissue and dental tissue in the mandible, considered to be mixed odontoma or ameloblastic fibro-odontoma, and to be determined after paraffin decalcification. The wound was rinsed and thoroughly hemostatic, the iodo-

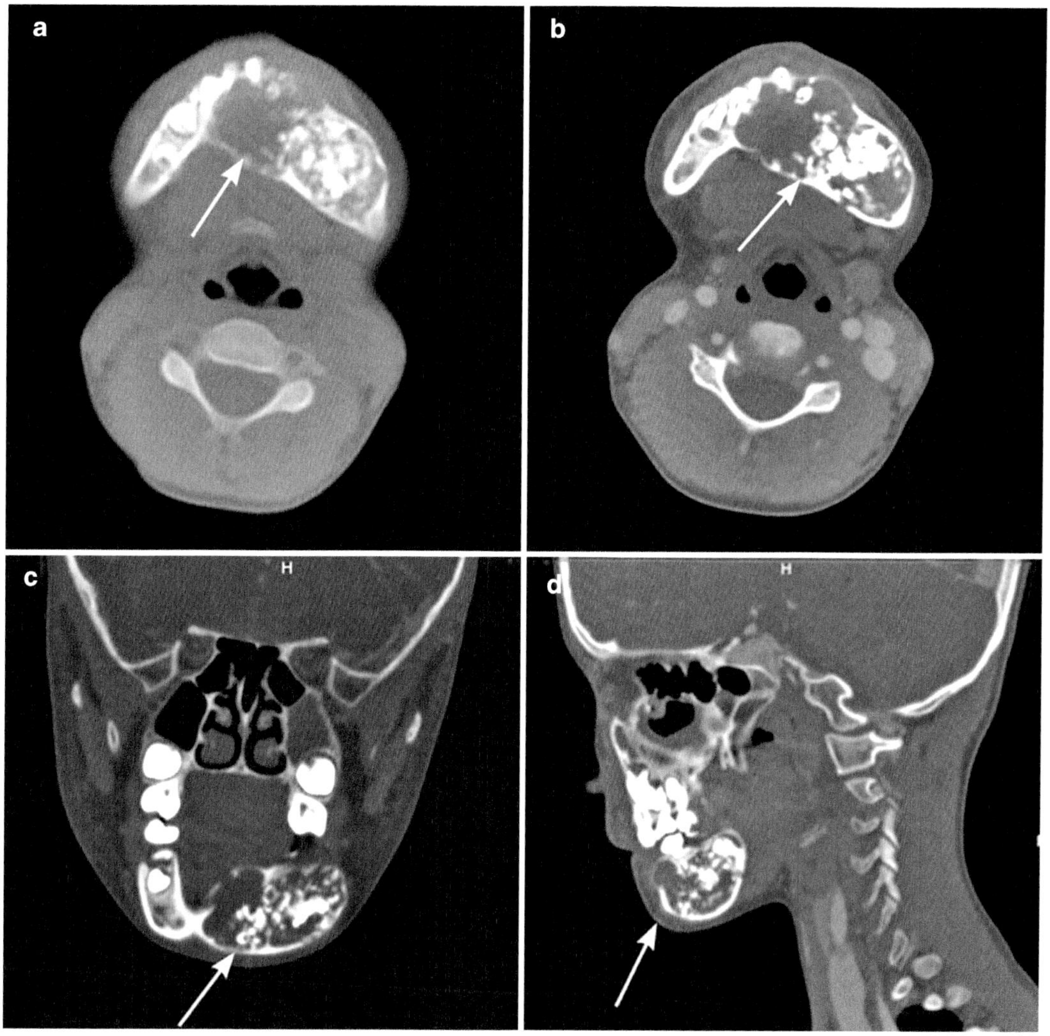

Fig. 25.3 (**a**) CT plain axial scan: bone distention of the mandible (lower right 3- lower left 6). A circular abnormal density shadow with a clear boundary was observed, about 5.3 cm × 2.8 cm in size. Multiple dense shadows were seen in the lesion, some of which were enamel dense. The adjacent cortical bone was thinned and partially disappeared, with no obvious periosteal reaction. (**b**) Enhanced CT axial scan: No abnormal swelling or enhancement of the surrounding soft tissue. (**c**, **d**) Enhanced CT of coronal and sagittal views show the similar well demarcated expansile bony lesion

form gauze strip was indwelled into the bone cavity, and layered suture was performed to close the wound (Fig. 25.4).

[Pathological Examination] Gross pathological examination revealed a heap of issues, 8 cm × 7 cm × 2 cm, and partially phymatoid, 2.5 cm × 3.5 cm × 2 cm, gray yellow, gray-white, partly hard. Microscopic examination suggested the tumor was composed of odontogenic epithelium, odontogenic mesenchymal tissue and dental tissue in a mixed arrangement. Locally, odontogenic epithelial cords and epithelial masses were seen. The surrounding epithelium was columnar and palisade, and the central cells were few and loosely arranged like stellate reticular cells (Fig. 25.5).

[Pathological Diagnosis] Ameloblastic fibro-odontoma.

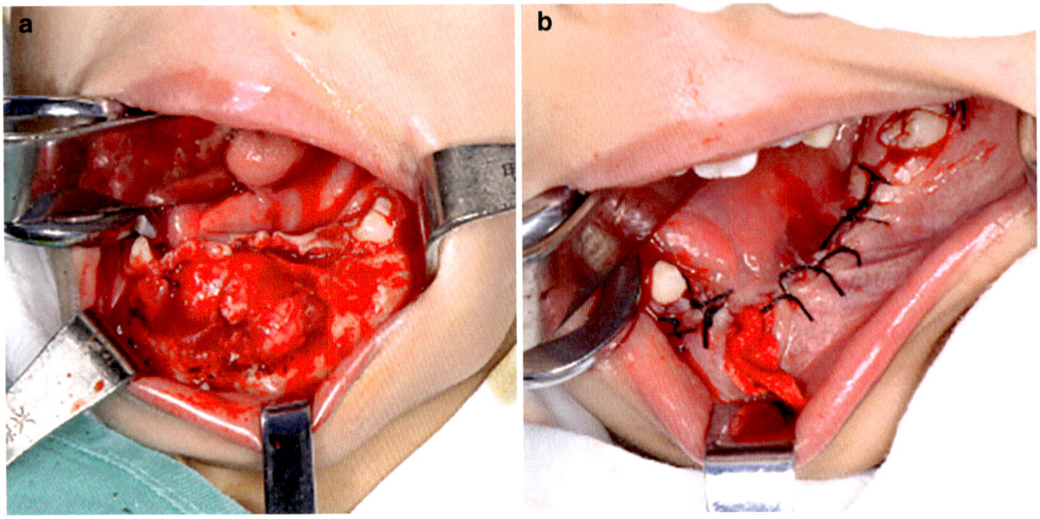

Fig. 25.4 (**a**) Curettage of mandibular mass, with fresh bleeding exudated on the bone surface. (**b**) Iodoform gauze strip indwelled in bone cavity, and mucosal transposition suture

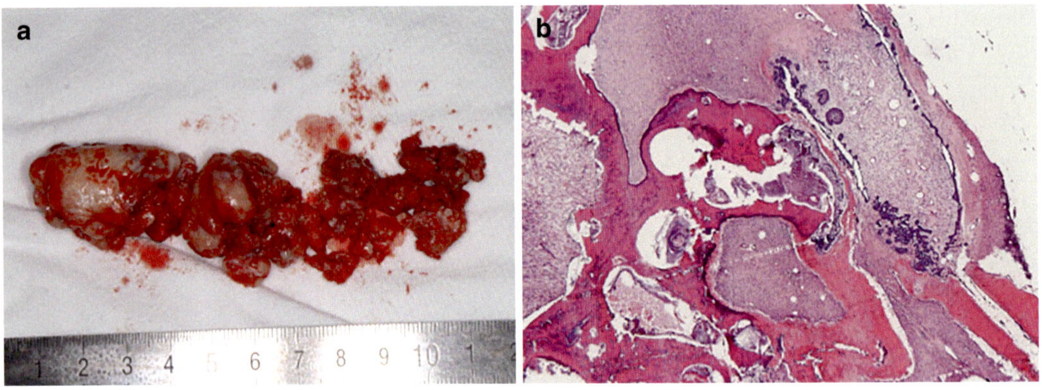

Fig. 25.5 (**a**) Partially phymatoid, grayish yellow, grayish white, partly hard, denti-like substance. (**b**) Dental tissues such as dentin, enamel and cementum under mixed arrangement, and ameloblastoma odontogenic epithelial mass in embryonic mucinous interlobar tissue (40×)

[Follow-Up] The patient healed uneventfully. The postoperative six-month follow-up exhibited no obvious postoperative reaction and no tumor relapse.

25.3 Key Points of Diagnosis and Treatment

Imaging Characteristics and Imaging Characteristics Most AFOs are detected in routine X-ray examination for jaw swelling or tooth eruption abnormalities. On X-ray, the lesion appears as a well-circumscribed and unicystic shadow and occasionally as a polycystic shadow, containing varying amounts of dental-dense calcifications. The unerupting teeth are usually located at the lesion edge, or the tooth crown is included in the shadow. In some cases, only a small amount of calcified enamel and dentin are present, similar to unicystic lesion in imaging examination. In some cases, a large number of calcified masses are visible in imaging examination, and only narrow rays appear at the edge.

According to clinical manifestations and imaging examinations, AFO is easily considered as a dental tumor. In addition, atypical AFO should be distinguished from calcifying epithelial odontogenic tumor, an intraosseous lesion that often occurs in the posterior part of the mandible and is often associated with impacted molars. Complex or immature odontoma, calcifying epithelial odontogenic tumor and AFO appear similar on X-ray and are easily confused, so pathological examination is crucial [1, 2].

Pathological Characteristics AFO is pathologically similar to ameloblastoma, with long, narrow odontogenic epithelium visible in loose connective tissue. Calcifying components consist of enamel and dentin matrix. Dentin is deposited as an eosinophilic mineralization with tubules, similar to normal teeth, but dentin may also appear as a uniform eosinophilic mass containing few cells. Similar to the normal tooth development process, the formation of dentin matrix is closely associated with epithelial cell nests. With the increase of matrix deposition, a large area of dentin surrounding the epithelial island can be formed, and eventually, the epithelial island degenerates and may disappear completely, leaving a cavity where some residual epithelial or enamel deposits may still be found. If the amount of soft tissue is limited, the majority of the lesion consists of mature hard tooth tissue.

Treatment Conservative surgical curettage is usually adopted for the treatment of AFO, because of clear boundary for the convenience of complete curettage. AFO has a good prognosis, rare recurrence and malignant transformation. AFO recurrence is often associated with inadequate resection of the tumor, especially for large ones. Residual tumor edges or affected teeth may cause AFO recurrence. Therefore, for large AFO, a special complete resection of the tumor should be noted to reduce the risk of tumor residue and recurrence.

References

1. Barnes L, Eveson JW, Reichart PA, et al. World Health Organization classification of tumours. Pathology and genetics of head and neck tumours [M]. Lyon: IARC Press; 2005.
2. El-Naggar A, Chan J, Grandis J, et al. WHO classification of head and neck tumours [M]. International Agency for Research on Cancer; 2017.
3. Philipsen HP, Reichart PA, Praetorius F. Mixed odontogenic tumours and odontomas. Considerations on interrelationship. Review of the literature and presentation of 134 new cases of odontomas [J]. Oral Oncol. 1997;33(2):86–99.
4. Ribeiro CM, Santos TT, de Castro SR, et al. Extensive mandibular ameloblastic fibro-odontoma [J]. J Craniofac Surg. 2016;27(6):e563–5.
5. Pontes HA, Pontes FS, Lameira AG, et al. Report of four cases of ameloblastic fibro-odontoma in mandible and discussion of the literature about the treatment [J]. J Craniomaxillofac Surg. 2012;40(2):e59–63.

26 Dentinogenic Ghost Cell Tumor

Jing Song Hou, Hui Shan Ong, Zhen Tian, Lin Zhu, and Min Ruan

26.1 Introduction

Dentinogenic ghost cell tumor (DGCT) is a rare odontogenic tumor considered as a solid variant of calcifying odontogenic cyst, accounting for about 1% of odontogenic tumors. With unknown etiology, it is locally invasive and characterized by ameloblastomatoid epithelial island, ghost cells, and dentin components. DGCT is common in middle-aged and elderly people (average age 50 years), with slightly more males than females. It is mainly an intraosseous lesion, and a few cases occur in gingiva or alveolar mucosa and other peripheral soft tissues [1–5]. The intraosseous lesion mainly occurs in the region from the first molar to the cusp, with varying size [5–7]. Patients often have no obvious symptoms, with the main symptoms as maxillary swelling, tooth displacement or loosening, possibly accompanied by pain and occasionally pus discharge. Peripheral DGCT mainly occurs in the anterior part of the mandible and is characterized by pedicled or non-pedicled external nodules confined to the gingivitis mucosa, which can be easily confused with gingivitis [8–10]. In some cases, mild invasion or acetabuliform of the deep cortical bone can take place. In 2005, the World Health Organization (WHO) defined DGCT as "a locally aggressive tumor characterized by ameloblastomato epithelial cell island in the interstitium of mature connective tissue, with abnormal keratosis in the form of ghost cells, accompanied by varying amounts of dysplastic dentin." In the 2017 WHO Classification of Odontogenic Tumors, DGCT was classified as mixed epithelial and mesenchymal tumor. Surgical resection is the main treatment method for DGCT [5]. Intraosseous DGCT is an aggressive tumor with local invasion feature and a recurrence rate of up to 71%. Peripheral DGCT is less aggressive than central type and has rare recurrence. DGCT is prone to malignant transformation into odontogenic ghost cell carcinoma [7].

J. S. Hou (✉)
Hospital of Stomatology, Guanghua College of Stomatology, Sun Yat-sen University, Guangzhou, Guangdong, China
e-mail: houjs@mail.sysu.edu.cn

H. S. Ong · Z. Tian · M. Ruan
Department of Oral Maxillofacial-Head & Neck Oncology, Shanghai Ninth People's Hospital, Shanghai Jiao Tong University School of Medicine, Shanghai, China

L. Zhu
Department of Radiology, Ninth People's Hospital Affiliated to Shanghai Jiao Tong University, Shanghai, China

26.2 Case 53

An 18-year-old gentleman suffered from a relapse of right mandibular mass for half a year after multiple operations at other hospital.

Y. He (ed.), *Inflammatory and Neoplastic Diseases of Craniofacial Bones*, https://doi.org/10.1007/978-981-97-4155-7_26

[History of Present Illness] The patient found a hard bean-size mass on the right mandible 4 years ago, without spontaneous pain. Diagnosed as "right mandibular bone cyst" at a local hospital, the patient received "curettage of right mandible bone cyst with impacted tooth extraction." The tumor was found to appear again on the right mandible 2 years ago, and "fenestration of right mandible cystic mass" was performed. Postoperative pathology suggested ameloblastoma, and the patient was recommended to receive surgical treatment until he grows to an adult. Six months ago, the right mandibular mass was found to gradually enlarge. The pathological section was taken one week ago, and the consultation at our oral pathology department came into conclusion of dentinogenic ghost cell tumor.

[Specialty Examination] No obvious deformity was seen in the oral and maxillofacial region, and the right mandibular swelling was about 2 cm × 1 cm in size, painless on palpation, medium hard, with no numbness around the mouth and face. There was no abnormality in mouth opening range and mouth opening pattern. Intraoral examination revealed permanent dentition. Postoperative change was observed in the right mandibular posterior dental area. A submucosal mass was found in the posterior molar area, about 1.5 cm × 1.0 cm in size, with clear boundary and not tender to palpation (−). There was a small amount of yellow and white exudation at the fenestration site (Fig. 26.1a). No obvious submandibular and cervical lymph node enlargement was observed.

[Auxiliary Examination]
1. Panoramic radiographs suggested a hypodense space-occupying shadow on the right mandibular body and angle, with local swelling, and high density strip shadow inside (Fig. 26.1b).
2. Maxillofacial enhanced CT scan suggested a distention of the right mandible, with an oblong mass shadow, ranging from 2.6 cm × 1.6 cm × 3.3 cm, bone hardening at the edge, with about 10 Hu and 36 Hu for plain scan CT, and 57 Hu, 86 Hu for enhanced CT. High density strip shadow, discontinuous buccal bone, and displacement of the right mandibular neural tube were seen. No cervical lymph node enlargement was observed (Fig. 26.2).

[Preliminary Diagnosis] Relapse of right mandibular dentinogenic ghost cell tumor after surgery.

[Treatment] "Right segmental mandibulectomy with fibular flap transfer" was performed under general anesthesia: an incision was made along the lower margin of the mandible for 1–2 cm, and the gingival flap was elevated for surgical exposure of the tumor mainly located at the right mandible body. The buccal side was obviously swollen. According to the preoperative osteot-

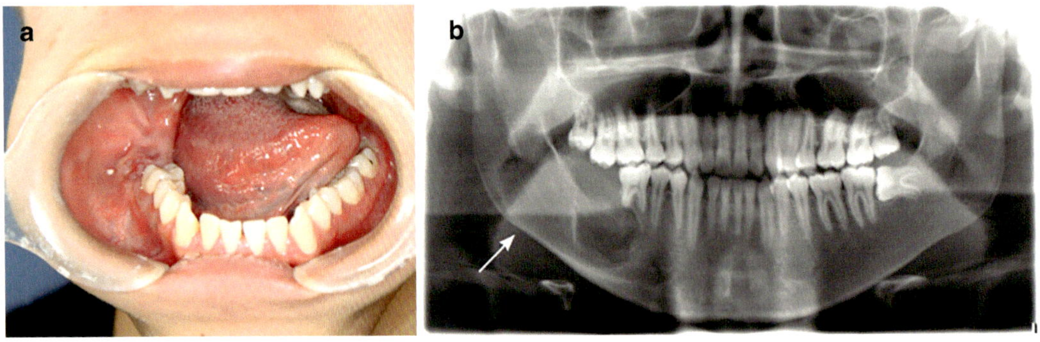

Fig. 26.1 No abnormality in mouth opening range and mouth opening pattern. (**a**) mass was found in the posterior molar area, protruding the mucosal surface, there was a small amount of yellow and white exudation at the fenestration site. (**b**) hypodense space-occupying shadow on the right mandibular body and angle, with local swelling, and high density strip shadow inside (preoperative)

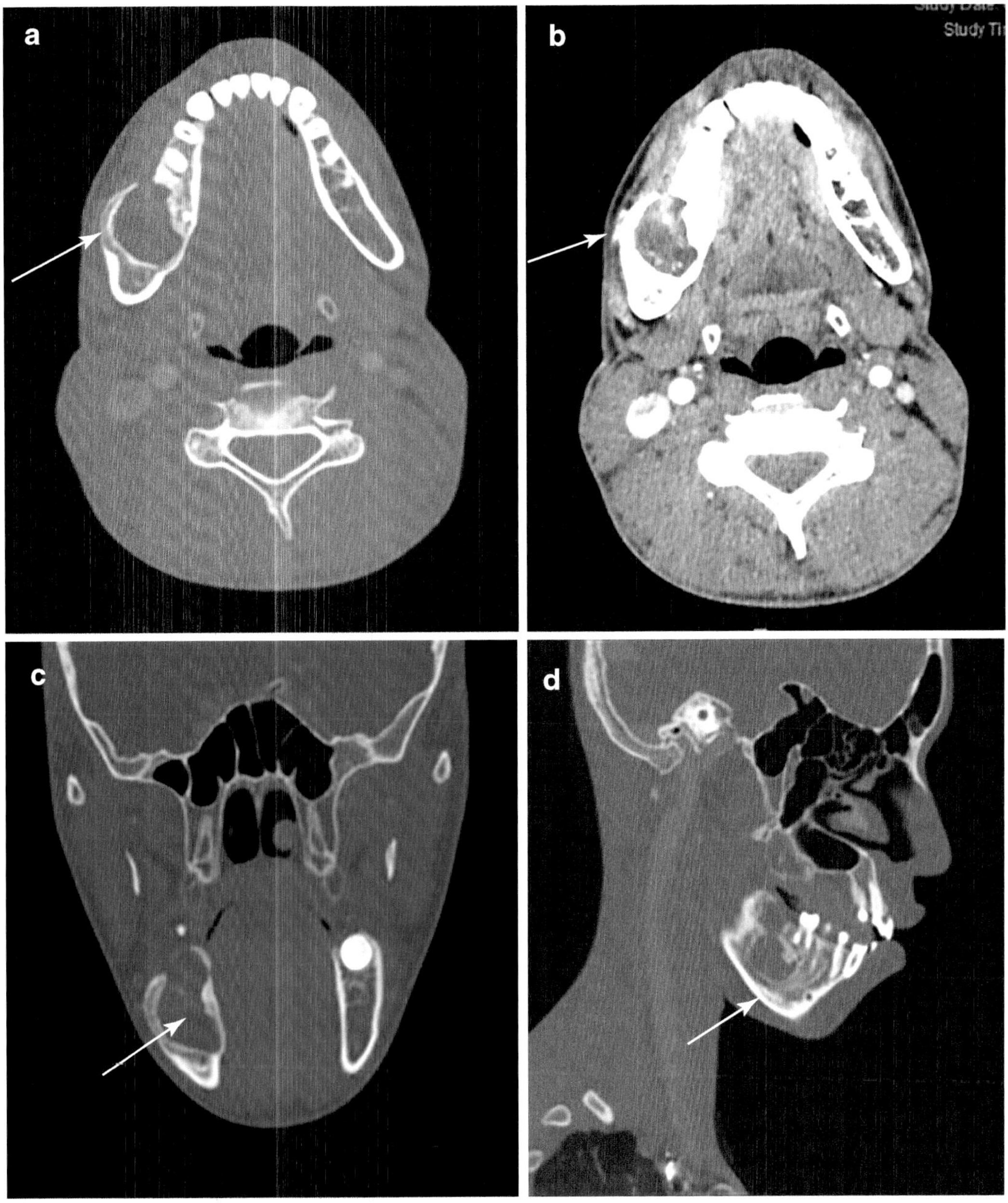

Fig. 26.2 (**a**) Enhanced CT axial scan (bone window): Right mandibular distension, with ellipsoidal mass shadow and marginal bone hardening. (**b**) Enhanced CT enhanced axial scan (soft tissue window): No significant swelling or abnormal enhancement of soft tissue was observed. (**c**, **d**) coronal and sagittal scan.

omy guide design, the mandible was cut off distal at 44 and 48 respectively, and the tumor and mandible were completely removed. The left free fibula with vascular pedicle was prepared, and the fibula with a length of about 7 cm was cut along the preoperative osteotomy guide and shaped to reconstruct the continuous occlusal relationship of the mandible. The vascular anastomosis of the fibula and right facial arteriovenous vessels was performed. The epithelial island was trimmed and shaped to repair the defects of mucous tissue in the mouth, mouth floor and lip and buccal. The wound was rinsed and thoroughly hemostatic, negative pressure drainage tube was indwelled, and layered suture was performed to close the wound (Fig. 26.3).

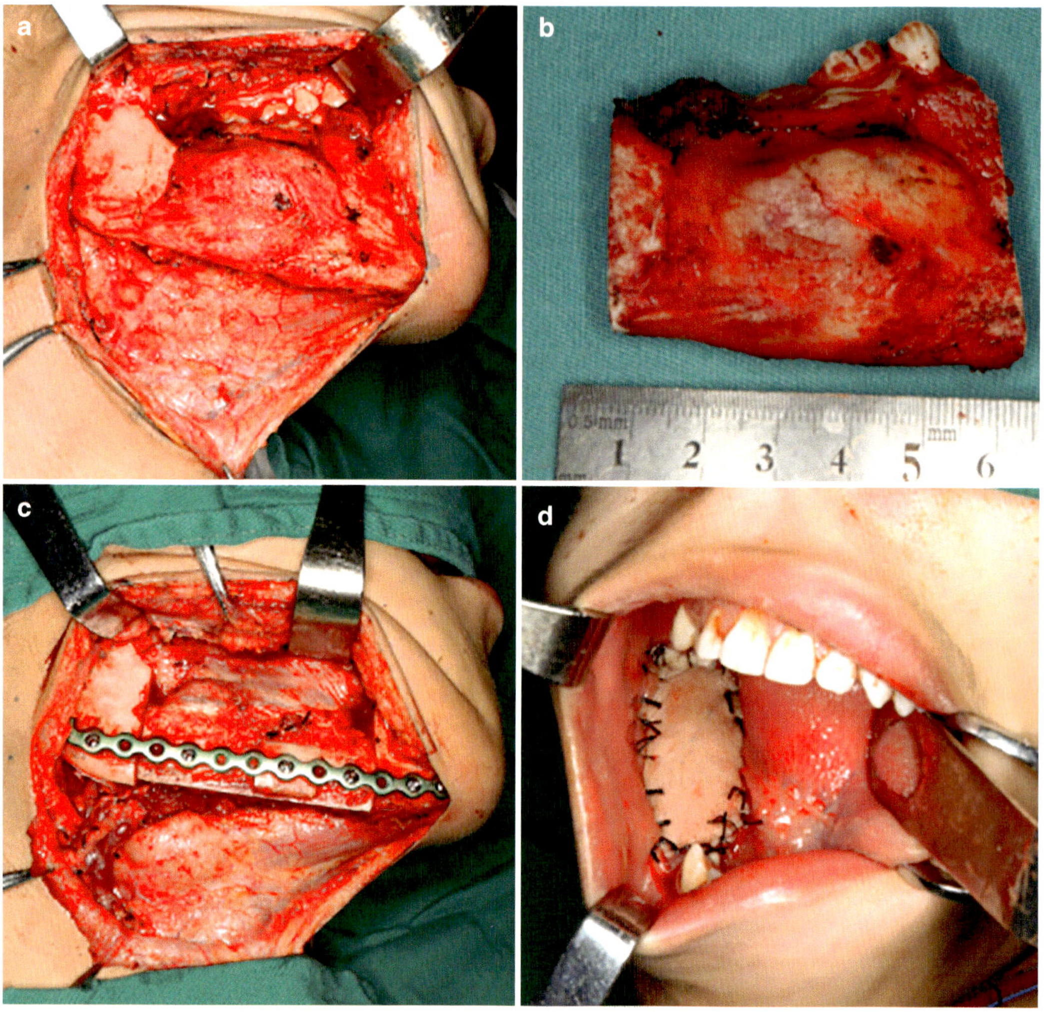

Fig. 26.3 (**a**) Exposed mandible, with bone distention visible. (**b**) Excised mandible. (**c**) Fibula reconstruction to restore mandibular continuity. (**d**) Repair of oral mucosal defect by epithelial island

[Pathological Examination] Gross pathological examination revealed a part of the mandible tissues, 5.8 cm × 4.6 cm × 3.2 cm in size. The buccal-lingual bone was swollen, the section was cystic, grayish yellow, grayish red. The lesion involved the surface gingival mucosa. Microscopic examination showed that the ameloblastomatoid epithelial nests were arranged in clumpy and cord shape, with hypercellular, occasional mitotic views, cystic deformation, local ghost cell clusters, accompanied by calcification, clear ghost cell boundary, abundant cytoplasm, eosinophilic, and absence of nuclei. Dysplastic dentin formation was observed in the tumor stroma (Fig. 26.4).

[Pathological Diagnosis] Dentinogenic ghost cell tumor of the "right mandible," ICD-O code: 9302/0, with hypercellularity, active growth, and lesion that destroys cortical bone.

[Follow-Up] The patient healed uneventfully. The postoperative 6-month follow-up exhibited no tumor relapse, with satisfactory mandibular reconstruction and good recovery of occlusal relationship (Fig. 26.5).

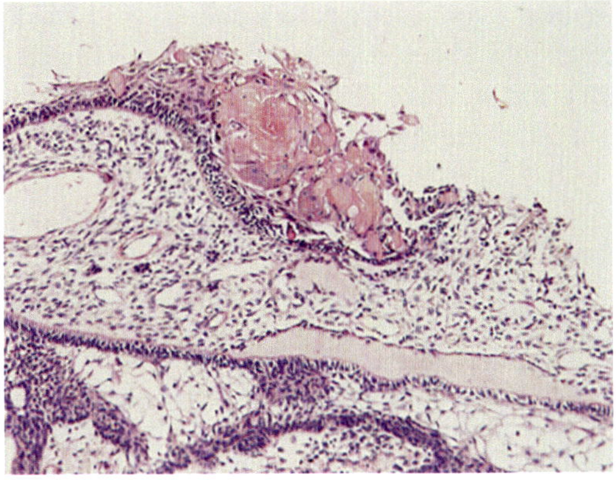

Fig. 26.4 The tumor epithelium presented an ameloblastoma image, ghost cells with lost nuclei were observed (200×)

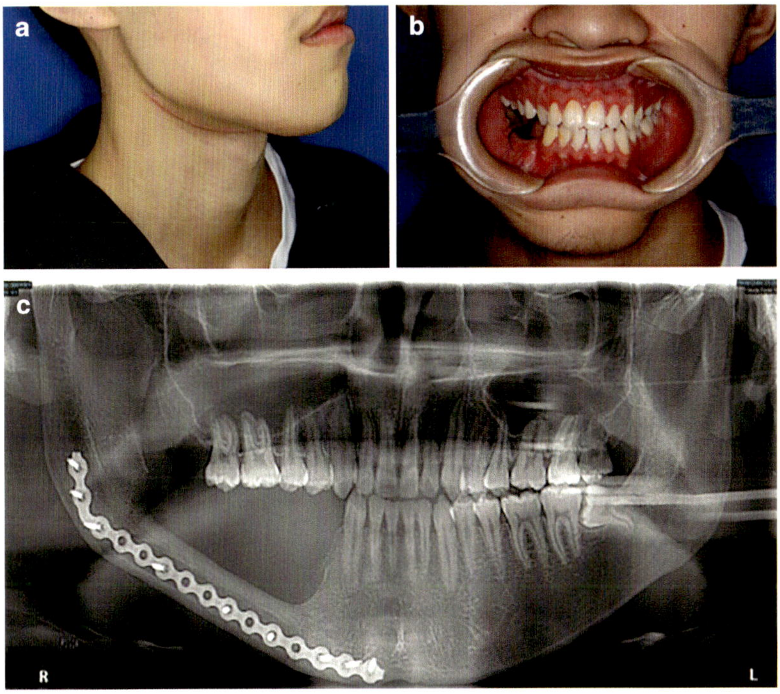

Fig. 26.5 (**a**) Postoperative changes of the right mandible, good recovery of mandible outline. (**b**) The occlusal relationship between the anterior teeth and the left posterior teeth was similar to that before surgery. Oral epithelial island survived. (**c**) Postoperative changes of the mandible, internal fixation, bone fracture healing well

26.3 Key Points of Diagnosis and Treatment

Diagnosis and Differential Diagnosis DGCT usually has no obvious symptoms in the early clinical stage, but with the development of the disease, swelling and facial asymmetry gradually appear. According to the presence and degree of calcification, it is classified into radiotransparent, opaque, or mixed lesion on the X-ray manifestations, which can be unilocular or multilocular lesion with clear or unclear marginal boundaries, root absorption of the affected tooth, displacement of adjacent teeth, and the presence of impacted teeth. It is often difficult to diagnose DGCT solely based on clinical symptoms and imaging. It should be noted to distinguish benign non-odontogenic tumors with local aggressiveness and odontogenic tumors containing hard tissue, such as calcifying epithelial odontogenic tumor, calcifying odontogenic cystic tumor, and odontogenic adenoid. Histopathology is the main diagnostic basis of DGCT.

Pathological Characteristics Either central or peripheral DGCT is histopathologically characterized by the presence of lamellate and round odontogenic epithelial island cells in mature connective tissue, and the epithelium resembles ameloblastoma without mitosis. A typical pathological feature of DGCT is the transformation of epithelial cells into ghost cells, and another is the formation of dentin or osteoid substance. Ghost cells are essentially swollen ellipsoid keratinized epithelial cells characterized by loss of nucleus, retention of basic cell contour, induction of foreign body granuloma, and potential calcification. Ghost cells may originate from epithelial transformation, odontogenic metaplasia, ischemia-induced squamous metaplasia secondary calcification, epithelial degeneration, or apoptosis. Although ghost cells are the basis of DGCT diagnosis, it must be noted that ghost cells are not only found not only in DGCT but also in other tumors such as odontoma, ameloblastoma, and ameloblasto fibro-odontoma, which can be identified histopathologically by protocellular exostroma similar to dental papillae.

Treatment Compared with peripheral DGCT, central DGCT is more invasive with a higher recurrence rate and the possibility of malignant transformation. Expanded radical resection is recommended in clinical practice. Segmental mandibulectomy or maxillectomy may be adopted to ensure sufficient resection range of tumor, and jaw reconstruction should be performed simultaneously according to clinical conditions to better restore the patient's appearance and occlusal function. Regular postoperative follow-up should be carried out.

References

1. de Arruda JAA, Monteiro J, Abreu LG, et al. Calcifying odontogenic cyst, dentinogenic ghost cell tumor, and ghost cell odontogenic carcinoma: a systematic review [J]. J Oral Pathol Med. 2018;47(8):721–30.
2. Bafna SS, Joy T, Tupkari JV, et al. Dentinogenic ghost cell tumor [J]. J Oral Maxillofac Pathol. 2016;20(1):163.
3. Buchner A. The central (intraosseous) calcifying odontogenic cyst: an analysis of 215 cases [J]. J Oral Maxillofac Surg. 1991;49(4):330–9.
4. Praetorius F, Ledesma-Montes C. Dentinogenic ghost cell tumour [M]. In: Barnes L, Eveson JW, Reichart P, Sidransky D, editors. World Health Organization classification of tumours. Pathology and genetics of head and neck tumours. Lyon: IARC Press; 2005. p. 314.
5. El-Naggar A, Chan J, Grandis J, et al. WHO classification of head and neck tumours [M]. International Agency for Research on Cancer; 2017.
6. Fejerskov O, Krogh J. The calcifying ghost cell odontogenic tumor—or the calcifying odontogenic cyst [J]. J Oral Pathol. 1972;1(6):273–87.
7. Sun G, Huang X, Hu Q, et al. The diagnosis and treatment of dentinogenic ghost cell tumor [J]. Int J Oral Maxillofac Surg. 2009;38(11):1179–83.
8. Gupta S, Singh S, Anjum R, et al. Dentinogenic ghost-cell tumor of the maxilla: a case report and review of literature [J]. J Oral Maxillofoc Pathol. 2019;23(3):478.
9. Gagari E, DeVilliers P, Antoniou C. Clinicopathologic conference: case 5 [J]. Head Neck Pathol. 2009;3(4):295–8.
10. Ravi B, Kamath G, Srivathsa S, et al. Dentinogenic ghost cell tumor—a rare case report [J]. J Stomatol Oral Maxillofac Surg. 2020;121(2):186–8.

Part IX

Benign Mesenchymal Odontogenic Tumor and Its Evolution

Odontogenic Myxoma/ Myxofibroma 27

Jing Song Hou, Hui Shan Ong, Zhen Tian, Lin Zhu, and Wen Yu Yang

27.1 Introduction

Odontogenic myxoma (OM) is a rare benign tumor of the jaw derived from ectodermal mesenchymal cells. It is called odontogenic myxofibroma (OMF) when the tumor is dominated by collagen fibers. Odontogenic myxoma mostly presents as painless, slow-growing mass in the jaw, and is usually diagnosed for maxillofacial malformation caused by bone distention. Odontogenic myxoma has a low incidence, accounting for 3–20% of all odontogenic tumors [1–5]. The range of onset age is wide, from 5 to 56 years old, but it mainly occurs in young people, especially in adults between 20 and 40 years old, with no significant gender difference [5–8]. Tumors may occur in almost any part of the jaw, and is more common in the mandible than the maxilla, accounting for about two-thirds. Despite a benign tumor, OM is locally aggressive with a high recurrence rate after surgical treatment [3, 5, 8, 9].

27.2 Odontogenic Myxoma

27.2.1 Case 54

A 57-year-old woman suffered from right maxillary odontogenic myxoma 3 months after incomplete surgery.

[History of Present Illness] The patient received "resection of the right maxillary mass" at another hospital 3 months ago. Postoperative pathology suggested odontogenic myxoma. There was no obvious postoperative discomfort. CT during follow-up visit showed possible postoperative recurrence of right maxillary odontogenic myxoma. Pathological reprints supported the original diagnosis.

[Specialty Examination] The bilateral submandibular region is symmetrical, with no tenderness and snapping of temporomandibular joint.There was no abnormality in mouth opening range and mouth opening pattern. Intraoral examination revealed permanent dentition, general oral hygiene, postoperative change of the right maxilla, absence of 15–17 teeth, no significant maxillary swelling, no obvious rupture, and exudation of mucosa. The tongue moved freely, and the taste was normal. No

J. S. Hou (✉)
Hospital of Stomatology, Guanghua College of Stomatology, Sun Yat-sen University, Guangzhou, Guangdong, China
e-mail: houjs@mail.sysu.edu.cn

H. S. Ong · Z. Tian · W. Y. Yang
Department of Oral Maxillofacial-Head & Neck Oncology, Shanghai Ninth People's Hospital, Shanghai Jiao Tong University School of Medicine, Shanghai, China

L. Zhu
Department of Radiology, Ninth People's Hospital Affiliated to Shanghai Jiao Tong University, Shanghai, China

Y. He (ed.), *Inflammatory and Neoplastic Diseases of Craniofacial Bones*,
https://doi.org/10.1007/978-981-97-4155-7_27

significant bilateral submaxillary and cervical lymph node enlargement was observed.

[Auxiliary Examination]

1. Panoramic radiographs suggested distensible bone destruction of the right maxilla with irregular morphology after surgery for the right maxillary odontogenic myxoma (Fig. 27.1).
2. Maxillofacial enhanced CT scan suggested distensible bone destruction of the right maxilla with irregular morphology. A cordlike bony prominence was seen on the medial side, the local cortical bone was not continuous. A maximum cross-section was 2.8 cm × 2.1 cm × 3.8 cm, with C- of 32 Hu and C+ 34 Hu. There was no obvious absorption in the adjacent root, and some dentition was missing. There were no abnormalities in the structure of the skull base. No obvious bilateral cervical lymph node enlargement was observed (Fig. 27.2).

[Preliminary Diagnosis] Relapse of the right maxillary odontogenic myxoma after surgery at other hospital.

[Treatment] "Right subtotal maxillectomy with fibular flap transfer" was performed under general anesthesia: a Weber incision was made along the right maxilla, and the gingival flap was elevated to disconnect the palate and the base of the orbit, internally to the turbinate, upper to the lower margin of the base of the orbit. The maxilla was severed, and the tumor was removed together, and the incisal margin was negative (-). Fibular myocutaneous flap was prepared and shaped. The vascular anastomosis of the fibula and facial arteriovenous vessels was performed. The epithelial island repaired palate and nasal side defects. The wound was rinsed and thoroughly hemostatic, negative pressure drainage tube was indwelled, and layered suture was performed to close the wound (Fig. 27.3).

[Pathological Examination] Gross pathological examination revealed a part of the right maxillary tissues, 5.5 cm × 3.5 cm × 3 cm, with 2 teeth attached. A grayish white and translucent mass of 2 cm × 1.5 cm × 1 cm was found on the soft tissue section beside the maxillary sinus. Microscopic examination showed that the tumor was poorly circumscribed, appearing as mucofibriform connective tissue with few tumor cells in stellate or spindle shape, loose arrangement, no odontogenic epithelium. Many collagen fibers were seen in the tumor, and the lesion involved bone trabeculae (Fig. 27.4).

[Pathological Diagnosis] Odontogenic myxoma of the "right maxilla," ICD-O code: 9320/0.

[Follow-Up] The patient healed uneventfully. The postoperative 6-month follow-up exhibited no obvious postoperative reaction and no tumor relapse, with satisfactory reconstruction of the maxilla and good recovery of occlusal relationship.

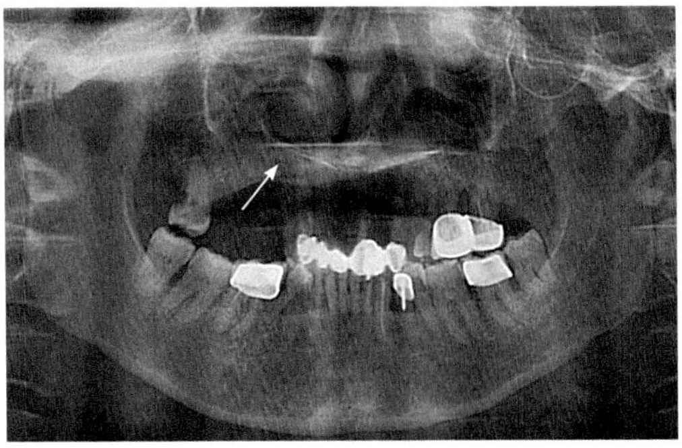

Fig. 27.1 Distensible bone destruction of the right maxilla with irregular morphology after surgery for the right maxillary odontogenic myxoma (preoperative)

27.2.2 Case 55

A 40-year-old gentleman suffered from a gradually growing mass in his left mandible for 1 year.

[History of Present Illness] The patient was found to have a swollen mass in the posterior dental area of the left mandible for unknown predisposing factors 1 year ago. The mass gradually grew as the patient didn't receive examination and treatment. The panoramic radiographs at other hospital 1 month ago suggested abnormal density shadow of the left mandible.

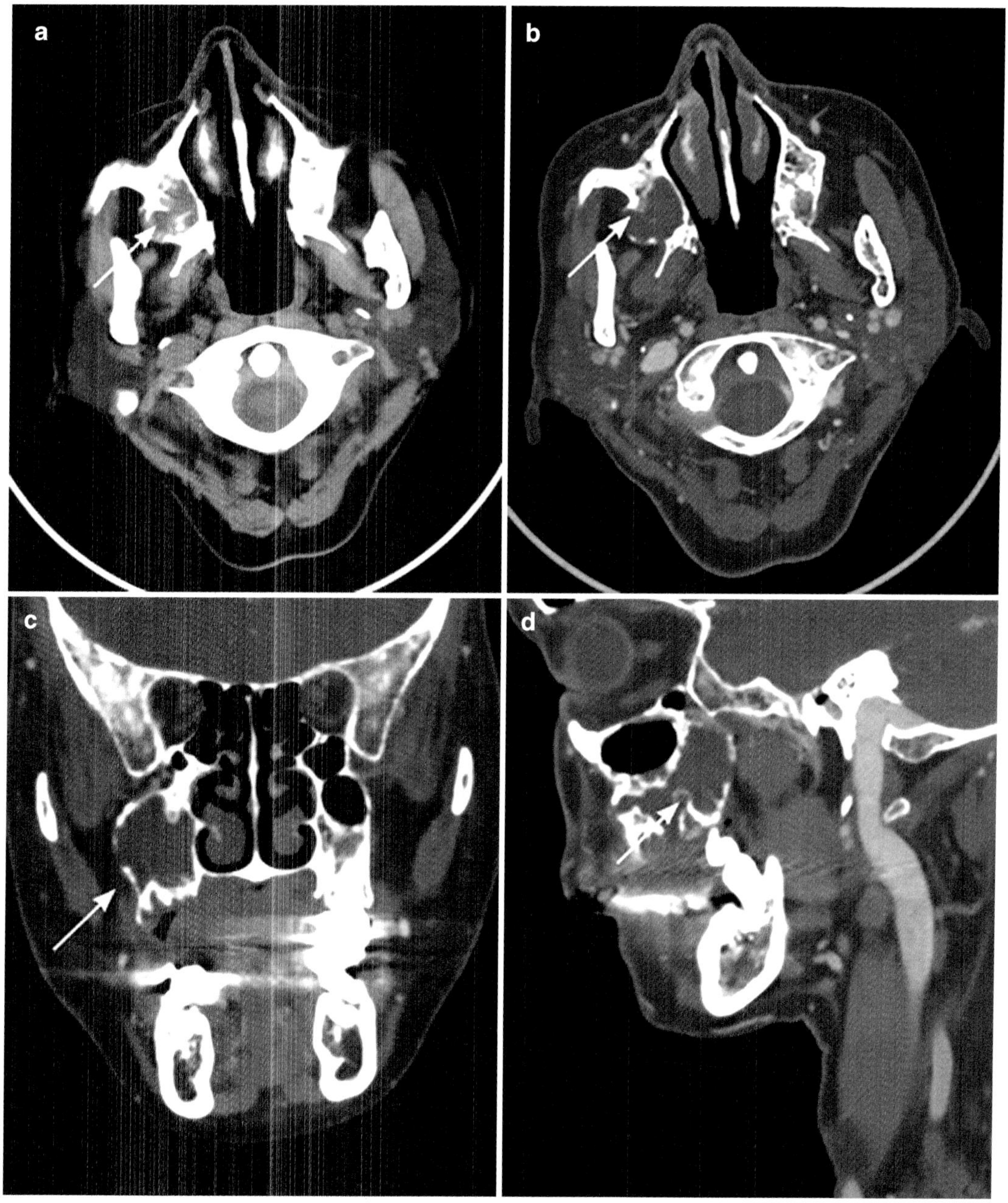

Fig. 27.2 (**a**) CT plain axial scan: distensible bone destruction of the right maxilla with irregular morphology. A cordlike bony prominence was seen on the medial side, the local cortical bone was not continuous. A maximum cross-section was 2.8 cm × 2.1 cm × 3.8 cm, with C− of 32 Hu. (**b**) Enhanced CT axial scan: Local slight reinforcement. (**c**, **d**) Enhanced CT coronal and sagittal scan: distensible bone destruction of the right maxilla, no obvious absorption of adjacent roots within the lesion, partial dentition defect

[Specialty Examination] The patient's bilateral maxillofacial region was basically symmetrical, but the left mandible was slightly swollen, with no obvious pain on palpation, the skin color and skin temperature around the left mandible were normal, and no obvious numbness symptoms were observed. The mouth opening pattern was normal, but the mouth opening range was about two transverse fingers. Intraoral examination revealed poor oral hygiene. The left mandibular

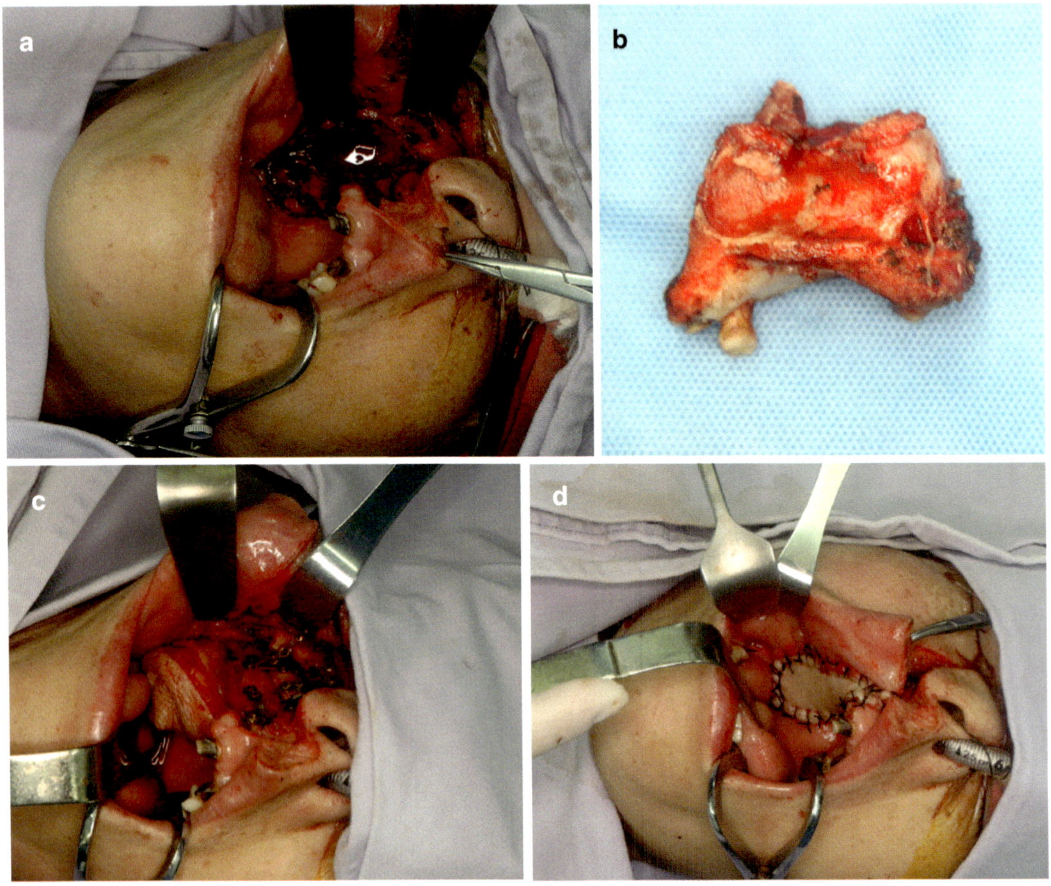

Fig. 27.3 (**a**) Postoperative of right subtotal maxillectomy. (**b**) Isolated right maxilla and mass. (**c**) Reconstruction of maxillary defect by free fibula. (**d**) Repair of palate defect by epithelial island

posterior dental area was swollen, which was more obvious at the lingual side of 36–38, involving mandibular angle and ascending branch. It was about 6.3 cm × 3 cm × 6 cm in size, hard, with no obvious pain on palpation. The surrounding mucosa was intact with no exudation, no numbness. 37, 38 buccal side was tilted, with no obvious loosening on the percussion (−) (Fig. 27.5). No significant submaxillary and cervical lymph node enlargement was observed.

[Auxiliary Examination]
Maxillofacial enhanced CT scan suggested bond distention of the left mandible body, angle and ascending branch. An elliptic mass shadow was seen, ranging from 6.3 cm × 2.2 cm × 6.2 cm, with clear boundary and local bone cortical absorption. The plain CT value was about 23 Hu, and no obvious enhancement was observed after enhancement. Enhanced coronal and sagittal scan showed multiple small bony compartments, some of which appeared to be "flame-like" (Fig. 27.6).

[Preliminary Diagnosis] Mass of the left mandible (odontogenic myxoma possible).

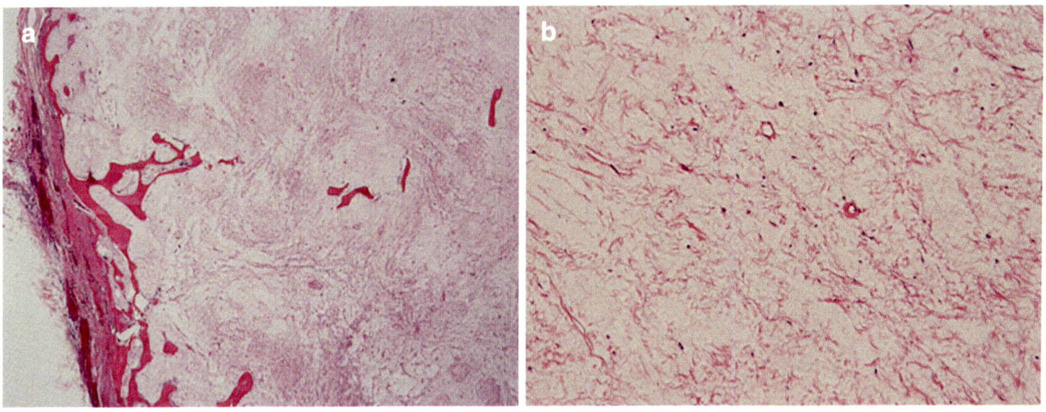

Fig. 27.4 (**a**) The tumor presented as no clear boundary and infiltrated between bone trabeculae, with the residual bone trabeculae indicated by the arrow (20×). (**b**) The lesion is mainly composed of loose mucous fiber tissue, with small and few tumor cells, no obvious atypia, and loose arrangement (200×)

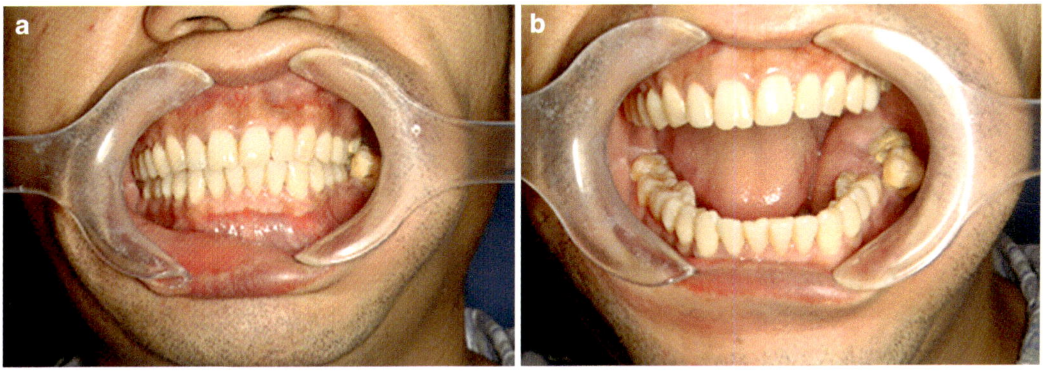

Fig. 27.5 (**a**) Permanent dentition, normal occlusal relationship of right and anterior teeth. (**b**) Mouth opening range was about two transverse fingers, with obvious lingual bone swelling, intact mucosa and buccal displacement in the left lower posterior dental region

Treatment] "Left segmental mandibulectomy with fibular flap transfer and tracheotomy" was performed under general anesthesia: an incision was made along the lower margin of the mandible for 1 to 2 cm, and the gingival flap was elevated for surgical exposure of the mass which was located from 33 to the ascending mandibular branch and involved the lingual mucosa. Using the osteotomy guide, the mandible was truncated along 31 tooth extraction wound, the condyle was retained, and the tumor and the affected mandible were completely removed. Intraoperative frozen pathological examination showed that scattered fusiform and stellate cells were found in the mucoid matrix of the left mandible, which was considered to be odontogenic myxoma. The left fibular myocutaneous flap with fibular length of about 10 cm was made and reconstructed to restore mandibular continuity and occlusal relationship. The fibular arteriovenous anastomosis with the superior thyroid artery and the facial vein was performed. The defect of oral mucosa was repaired by epithelial island. The wound was rinsed and thoroughly hemostatic, negative pres-

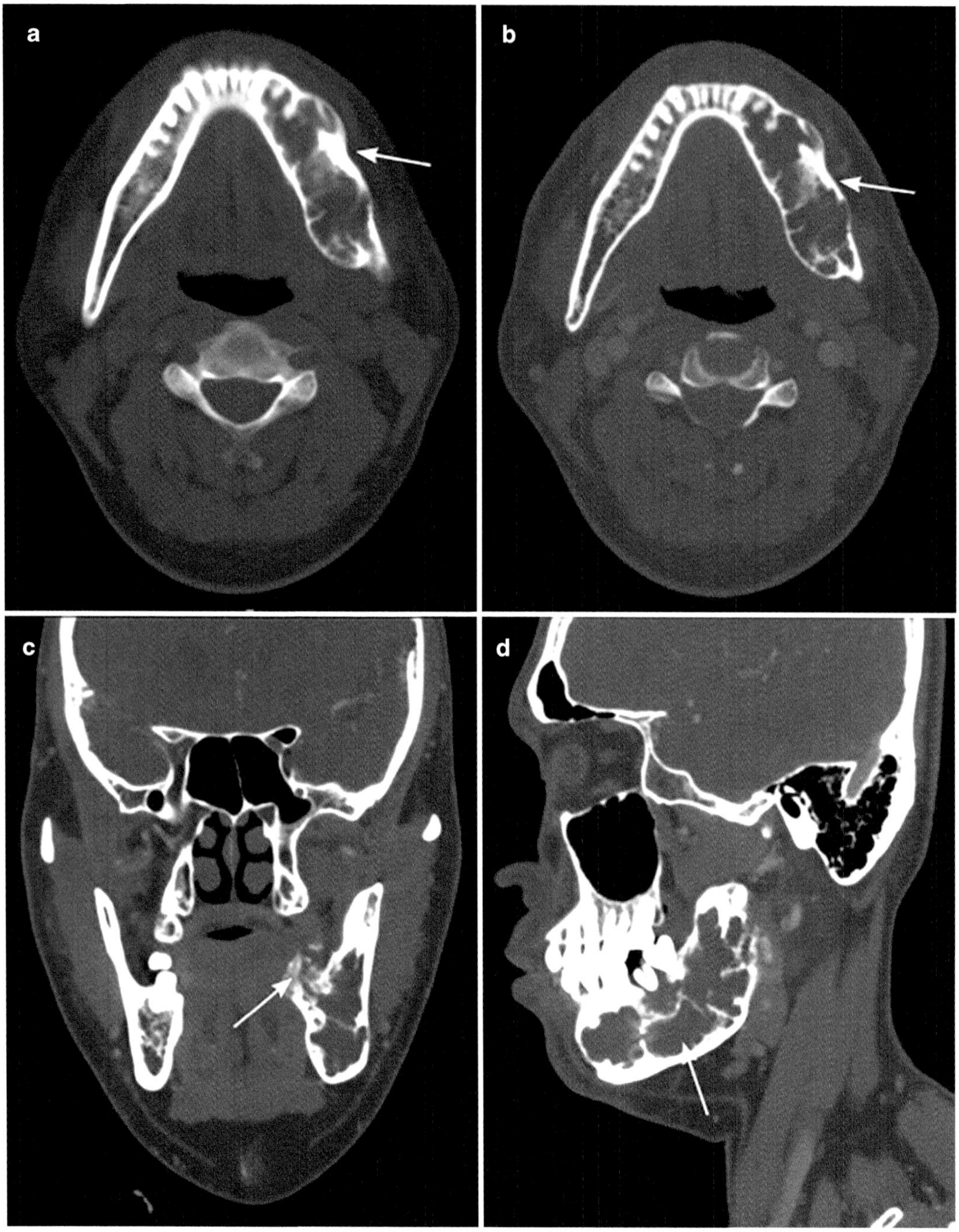

Fig. 27.6 (**a**) CT plain axial scan: bond distention of the left mandible body, angle and ascending branch. An elliptic mass shadow was seen, with clear boundary and local bone cortical absorption. The plain CT value was about 23 Hu. (**b**) Enhanced CT axial scan: No obvious enhancement was observed for the lesion. (**c**, **d**) Enhanced CT coronal and sagittal scan: multiple small bony compartments, some of which appeared to be "flame-like"

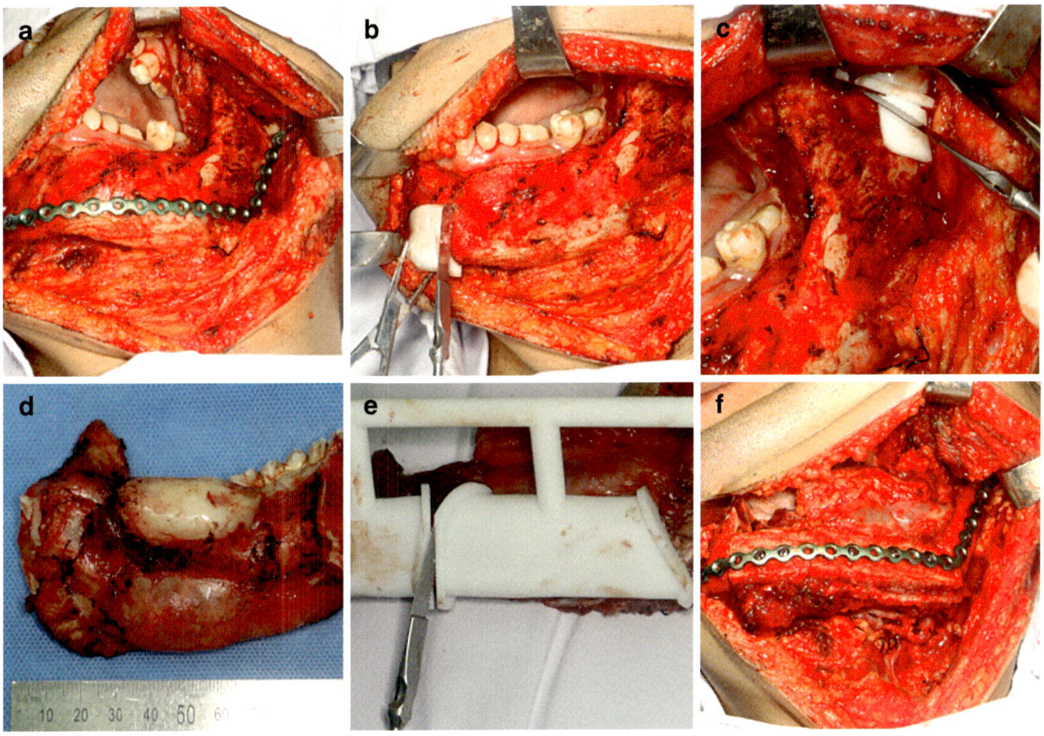

Fig. 27.7 (**a**) Pre-bending reconstruction of titanium plate. (**b**, **c**) Design the osteotomy line according to the osteotomy guide plate and truncate the mandible. (**d**) Isolated mandible and mass (lateral tongue). (**e**) Fibula is shaped according to the shaping guide. (**f**) Fibula reconstruction to restore mandibular continuity

sure drainage tube was indwelled, and layered suture was performed to close the wound (Fig. 27.7).

[Pathological Examination] Gross pathological examination revealed a part of the mandibular body and ascending branch, 10 cm × 3.5 cm × 3 cm, with 7 teeth attached to the upper part. Mass was found in mandibular body, and the palate was distended, about 4 cm × 2.5 cm. The section was solid, translucent, and gelled. Microscopic examination showed that mucous fibrous connective tissue with neoplastic hyperplasia was locally infiltrated between the residual bone trabecular tissues. The tumor cells were spindle and stellate shaped, with long cytoplasm protrusions and loose arrangement, and the lesion protruded from the bone cortex to the submucosa (Fig. 27.8).

[Pathological Diagnosis] Odontogenic myxoma of "left mandible," ICD- O code: 9320/0.

[Follow-Up] The patient healed uneventfully. The postoperative 6-month follow-up exhibited no tumor relapse, with satisfactory mandibular reconstruction and good recovery of occlusal relationship.

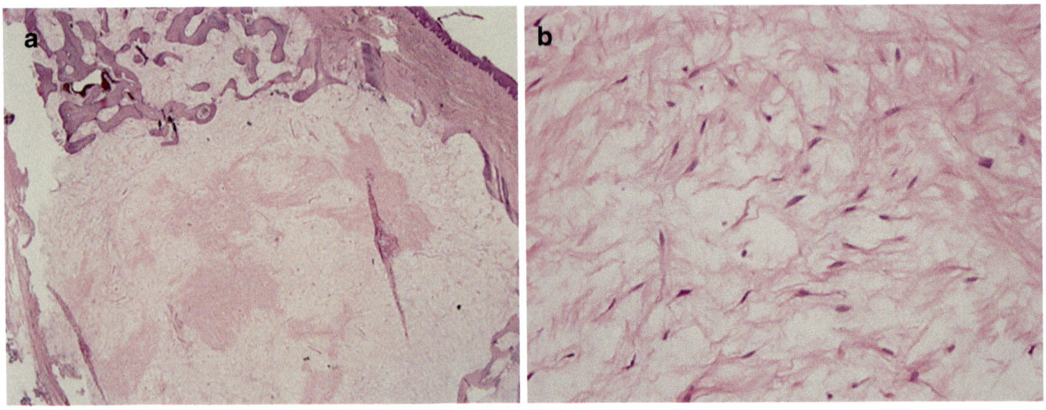

Fig. 27.8 (**a**) The lesions were interspersed between bone trabeculae and locally penetrated the bone cortex to submucosa (20×). (**b**) Tumor cells were fusiform and stellate, dispersed in mucous fibrous tissues (400×)

27.3 Odontogenic Myxofibroma

27.3.1 Case 56

A 64-year-old woman suffered from a right upper posterior dental mass for more than 7 months.

[History of Present Illness] More than 7 months ago, the patient was found to have a mass in the right maxillary molar area, about fingernail size, with no obvious bleeding, pain, nasal congestion and other symptoms, no swallowing restriction, no influence on eating, no numbness in the infraorbital area and no blurred vision. The mass was gradually enlarged with progressive swelling of the right face.

[Specialty Examination] The bilateral maxillofacial region is asymmetrical, with the right slightly higher than the left. No redness, numbness, and tenderness were observed. There was no abnormality in mouth opening range and mouth opening pattern. A mass about 4 cm × 2.5 cm in size was found in the right maxillary molar area, with medium hard, solid base, surface bulge, no obvious tenderness, no bleeding, and unclear boundary. Bilateral submaxillary and cervical lymph nodes were not significantly enlarged.

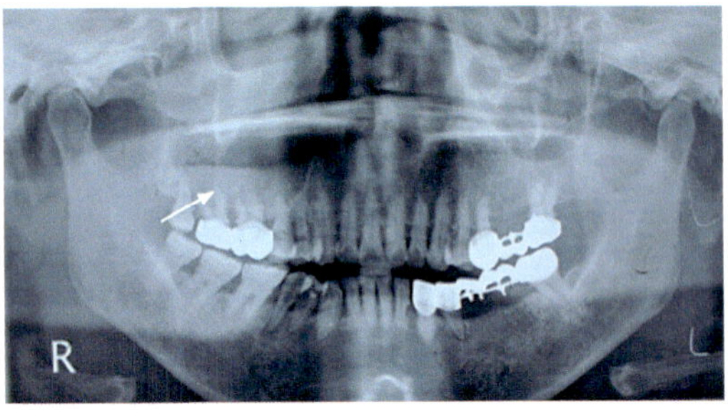

Fig. 27.9 Hypodense space-occupying shadow of the right maxilla, with local bone destruction, not well circumscribed

[Auxiliary Examination]

1. Panoramic radiographs suggested a hypodense space-occupying shadow of the right maxilla, with local bone destruction, which appeared as not well circumscribed (Fig. 27.9).
2. Maxillofacial enhanced CT scan suggested expansive bone destruction of the right maxilla, with abnormal soft tissue mass, uneven enhancement after enhancement, scattered patchy enhancement (Fig. 27.10).

[Preliminary Diagnosis] Mass of the right maxilla.

[Treatment] "Right subtotal maxillectomy" was performed under general anesthesia: a Weber incision was made, and the gingival flap was ele-

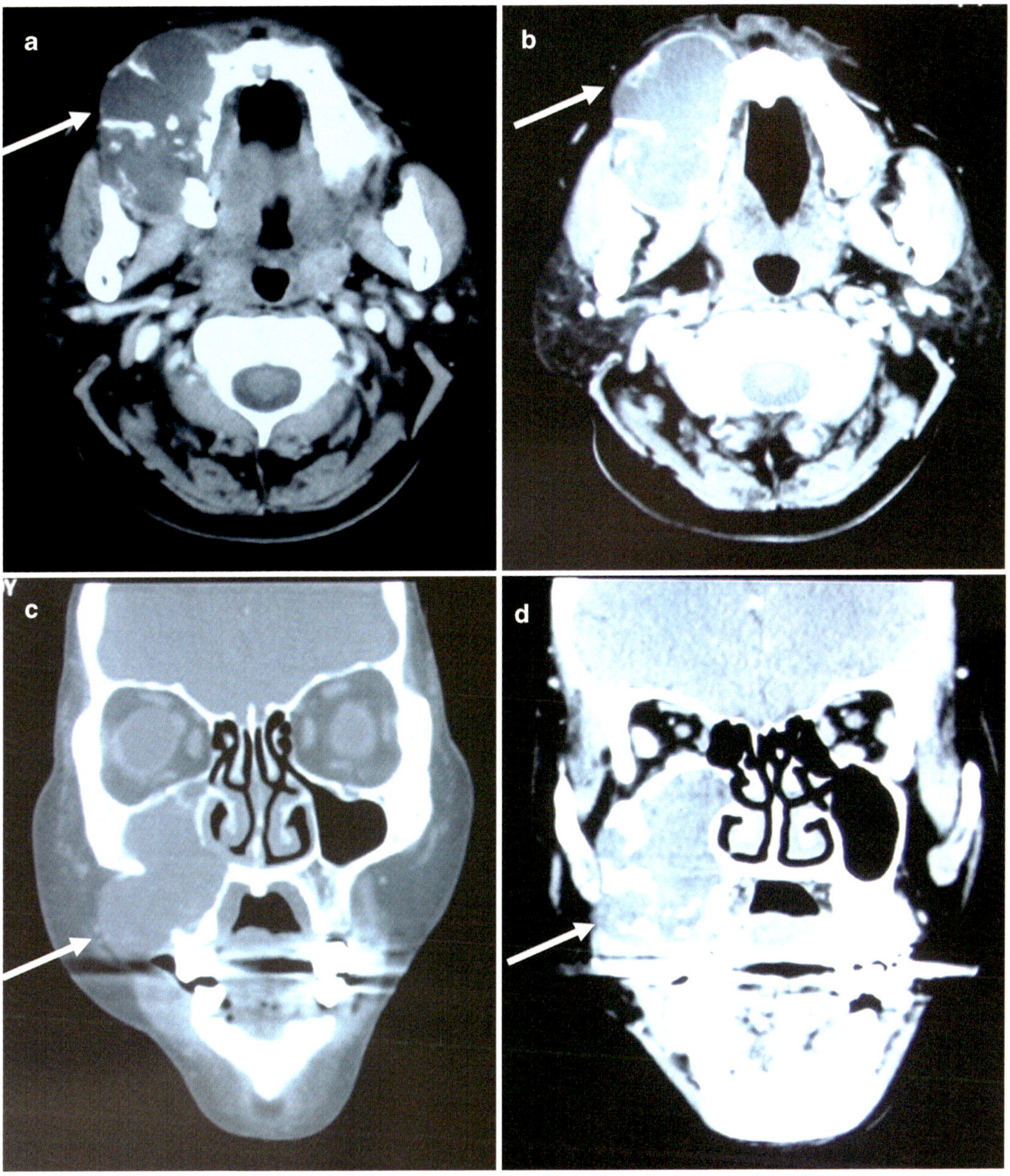

Fig. 27.10 (**a**, **b**) Enhanced CT axial scan: Expansive bone destruction of the right maxilla accompanied by abnormal soft tissue mass, uneven enhancement after enhancement, and scattered patchy enhancement. (**c**, **d**) Enhanced CT coronal scan

vated for surgical exposure of the right maxilla for truncation from the midline, maxillary process of zygomatic bone and pterygoid process of sphenoid bone. The internal maxillary artery was ligated and the orbital contents were preserved. Intraoperative frozen pathological examination showed that the tumor was mainly composed of the myxoid tissue of the "right maxilla," with cell atypia, tending to be myxoma, fibromyxoma, progressive or low-grade malignancy to be ruled out. The incisal margin was negative. The wound was rinsed and thoroughly hemostatic. The base of the orbit and the anterior part were fixed with titanium mesh. The wound was covered with buccal fat pad flap. Layered suture was performed to close the wound.

[Pathological Examination] Gross pathological examination revealed a part of the maxilla and its surrounding soft tissues, 8 cm × 6.5 cm × 6 cm in size, with five attached teeth. A mass of 6 cm × 6 cm × 5 cm was found in the section of the posterior molar region and maxillary sinus, with local envelope, and it was pale and translucent on the section. Microscopic examination indicated that the tumor cells were stellate and fusiform, with oval nuclei and loose arrangement. The intercellular interstitium was rich in mucus and contained more collagen fibers. No odontogenic epithelial island was observed (Fig. 27.11).

[Pathological Diagnosis] Odontogenic myxoma of "left mandible," ICD- O code: 9320/0.

[Follow-Up] The patient healed uneventfully. The postoperative 6-month follow-up exhibited no obvious postoperative reaction and no tumor relapse.

27.3.2 Case 57

A 52-year-old gentleman suffered from a gradually increasing mandibular distention for 4 years.

[History of Present Illness] The patient found swelling and distention in the left mandibular region 4 years ago, with no obvious pain or numbness, obvious gingival bleeding or tooth loosening, no restriction on opening of the mouth, and no influence on eating and breathing. The patient received no treatment. CT examination at other hospital 3 months ago suggested low density lesion in the left mandible with bone destruction.

[Specialty Examination] The face was asymmetrical, and the left mandibular body region was slightly swollen, with normal surface skin color and temperature. There was no abnormality in mouth opening range and mouth opening pattern. The left mandible 35-27 teeth region was swollen significantly to the lingual side and slightly to the buccal side, with intact surface mucosa. The swelling was about 5 cm × 3 cm in size, hard, with no obvious tenderness, ping-pong sensation, and loose teeth.

[Auxiliary Examination]

1. Panoramic radiographs suggested expansive bone destruction of the left mandible, thin bone cortex, and multiple bone partitions (Fig. 27.12).
2. Maxillofacial enhanced CT scan suggested expansive bone destruction of the left mandible accompanied by abnormal soft tissue mass, with residual bone seen at the margin. The mass in the rami region protruded from the bone cortex and involved the left pterygopalatine fossa (Fig. 27.13).

[Preliminary Diagnosis] Mass of the left mandible.

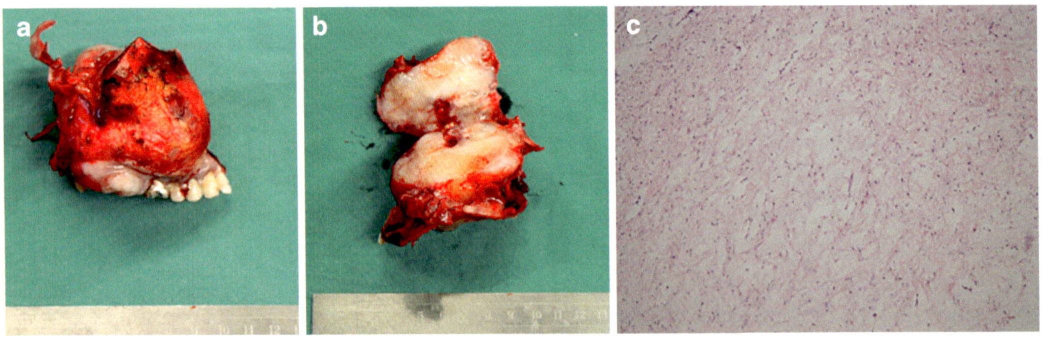

Fig. 27.11 (**a**) A mass of 6 cm × 6 cm × 5 cm was found in the posterior molar region and maxillary sinus section. (**b**) Local envelope, gray and translucent on the section. (**c**) Loose arrangement of tumor cells was observed in the collagen-rich mucous fiber tissue, and no obvious odontogenic epithelium was observed (100×)

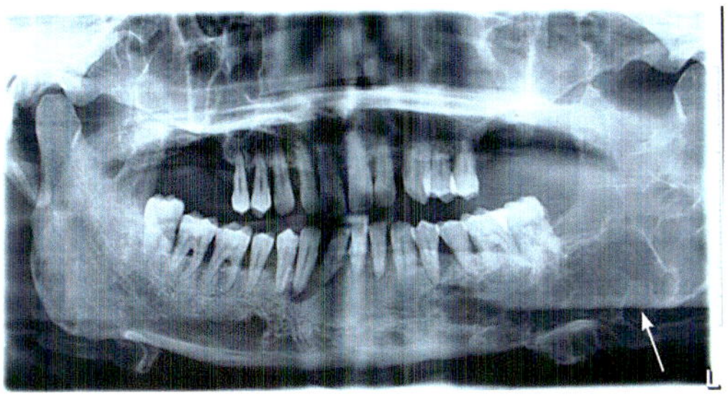

Fig. 27.12 Expansive bone destruction of the left mandible, thin bone cortex, and multiple bone partitions

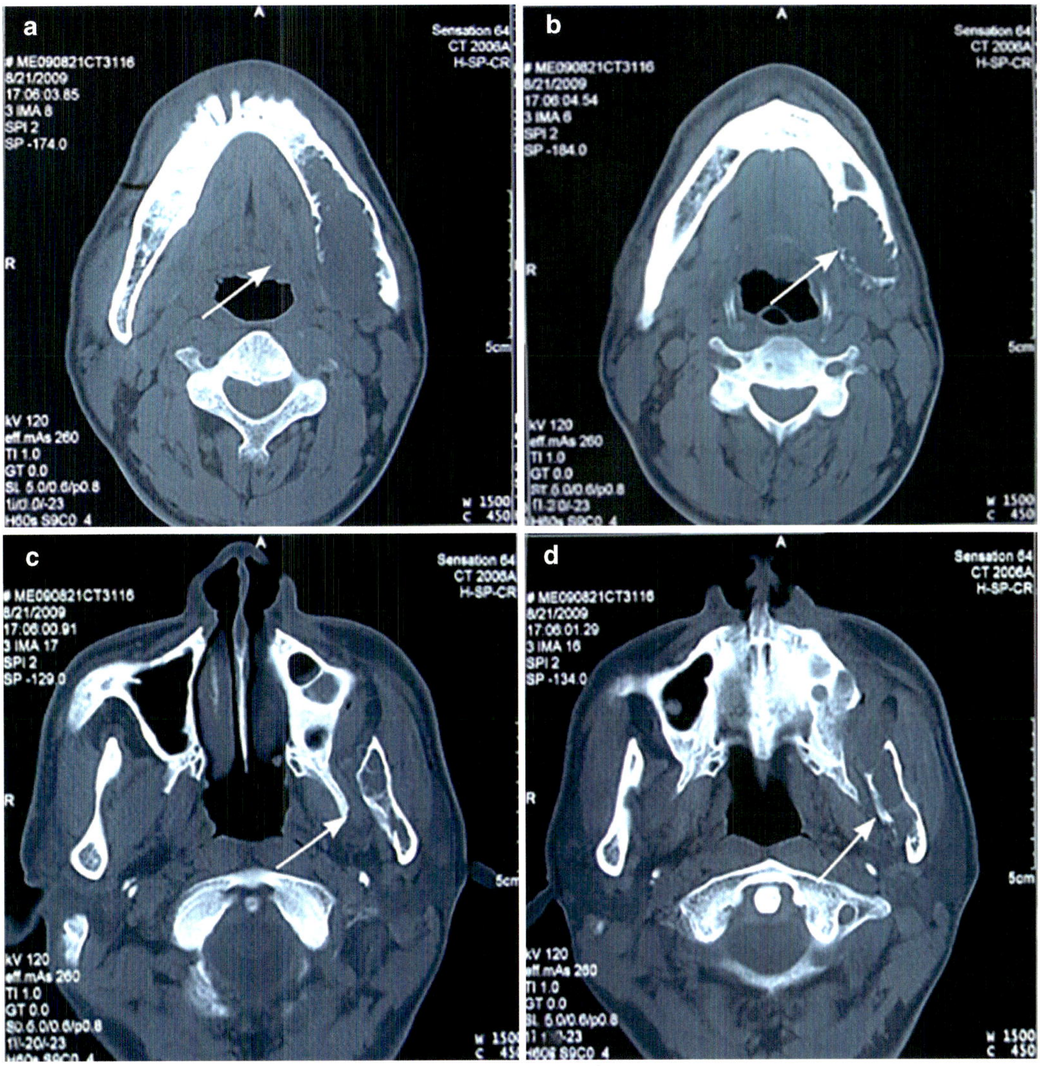

Fig. 27.13 (**a**, **b**) Expansive bone destruction of the left mandible accompanied by abnormal soft tissue mass, with residual bone seen at the margin. (**c**, **d**) Distention in the mandibular branch of the zygomatic arch of the maxilla, involving the left pterygopalatine fossa

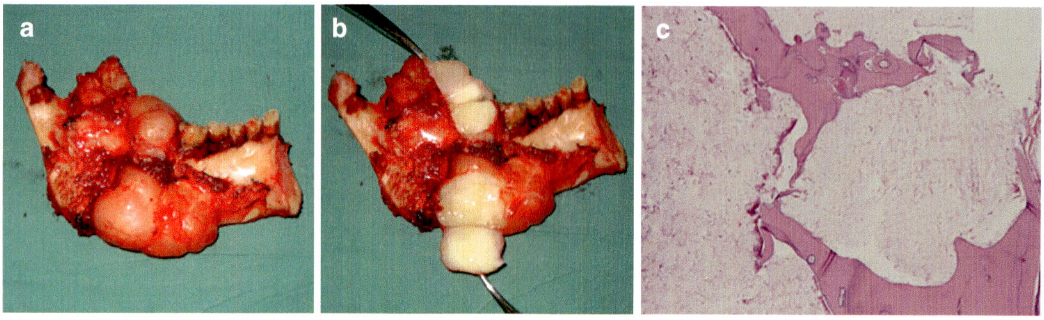

Fig. 27.14 (**a**) Mandible, ascending branch and covering gingival tissue. A mass was found inside the mandible, 5 cm × 3 cm × 2.3 cm. (**b**) The section was gray and translucent. (**c**) Mucous fibrous tissue hyperplasia, deficient cells, interspersed between bone tissues (40×)

[Treatment] "Left segmental mandibulectomy with fibular flap transfer and tracheotomy" was performed under general anesthesia: an incision was made along the lower margin of the mandible for 1–2 cm, and the gingival flap was elevated. The mandible was amputated at 31 distally to completely remove the mandible, including condyle, and the mass. Fibular myocutaneous flap, about 14 cm long, was shaped and reconstructed to restore mandibular continuity and occlusal relationship. Fibular arteriovenous anastomosis with external maxillary artery and internal jugular vein branch was performed. The wound was rinsed and thoroughly hemostatic, negative pressure drainage tube was indwelled, and layered suture was performed to close the wound.

[Pathological Examination] Gross pathological examination revealed a part of the mandible, ascending branch and covering gingival tissue, 12 cm × 8 cm × 3.7 cm. A mass was found inside the mandible, 5 cm × 3 cm × 2.3 cm, gray and translucent. The mass was covered with thin cortical bone. Microscopically, myxoid connective tissue tumor hyperplasia was observed, interspersed between residual host bone, with few and small tumor cells, loose arrangement, collagen fiber components. No odontogenic epithelial mass was seen (Fig. 27.14).

[Pathological Diagnosis] Odontogenic myxofibroma of the "left mandible," ICD-O code: 9320/0, with damage to bone tissue.

[Follow-Up] The patient healed uneventfully. The postoperative 6-month follow-up exhibited no obvious postoperative reaction and no tumor relapse, with good recovery of contralateral occlusal relationship.

27.4 Key Points of Diagnosis and Treatment

Myxoma is a rare benign mesenchymal tumor which is locally invasive and may occur in various organs and tissues such as heart, skin, subcutaneous tissue, aponeurosis, urogenital tract, bone, and skeletal muscle. Head and neck tumors occur mostly in the jaw, and rarely in the larynx, pharynx, paranasal sinuses, and other soft tissues. In 1947, Thomas and Goldman first reported the occurrence of odontogenic myxoma in the jaw.

Clinical Manifestations Odontogenic myxoma usually presents as a slow-growing mass that is usually asymptomatic. As the tumor grows, clinical symptoms occur, including pain, paresthesia, ulcers, and tooth displacement will appear. Odontogenic myxoma rarely crosses the midline, which may be related to early medical attention.

Imaging Characteristics According to imaging manifestations, odontogenic myxoma can be classified into four types, namely, unicystic, multilocular, pericoronal (few), and mixed radioparent–radioopaque (rare). More than 50% of

OM cases are multilocular. Unicystic lesions were small in scope and mostly located in the anterior dental region. Larger lesions are often multilocular and located in the posterior dental region. Thin, sparse bone trabeculae can be seen in radioparent region of most multilocular and some unicystic lesions, which can be manifested as soap bubble, honeycomb, or tennis racquet reflections. The radioparent projection edge is irregular and may fan out between the roots of the teeth, sometimes accompanied by hardening of the edges. It should be differentiated from odontogenic keratocyst, ameloblastoma, ameloblastic fibroma, calcifying epithelial odontogenic tumor and calcifying odontogenic cyst on imaging examination.

Pathological Characteristics Odontogenic myxoma was generally soft, transparent, gelatinous, unenveloped, and poorly circumscribed with the surrounding tissue. Microscopically, the tumor is low in cell content and consists mainly of a large number of loose mucoid matrix with irregular arrangement of stellate, fusiform, and round cells and a small number of collagen fibers. Odontogenic epithelial nests may occasionally be seen, but it is not necessary for pathological diagnosis. Some tumors contain more collagen fibers, which is often referred to as fibromyxoma or myxofibroma [4].

Histopathologically, myxoma should be distinguished from chondromyxoid fibroma and myxoid neurofibroma. Chondromyxoid fibroma is a well circumscribed tumor consisting of nodular myxoid tissue, scattered giant cells, and cartilage differentiation areas. It is most common in the metaphyseal of long bone and rarely involves the jaw bone. However, myxoid neurofibroma tends to have pathological cells that are positive for S-100 protein antibody. Developing teeth with myxoid change may also have enlarged dental sacs or papillae that resemble myxoma [4].

Treatment Myxoma is mainly treated with surgery, and the treatment protocol depends on the site and size of the tumor. Small myxoma is usually treated with curettage, but must be followed closely for at least 5 years. If large myxoma cannot be completely removed by curettage, an extended resection is required. As myxoma lacks a distinct envelope, it is easy to invade the surrounding bone, especially the posterior lesions of the maxilla, and should be treated with radical surgery. Allphin et al proposed that OM could be treated relatively conservatively for the first time, followed by radical surgery if necessary. When radical surgery is performed, secondary reconstruction is recommended due to the high recurrence rate of about 25%, which usually occurs within the first 2 years after resection, depending on surgical resection. Odontogenic myxoma is radio-resistant. Despite radiotherapy recommended before or after surgery according to few studies, the current consensus is that radiotherapy has no significant role in the treatment of odontogenic myxoma. In addition, better clinical efficacy could be achieved on the basis of radical surgery, combined with cryotherapy.

References

1. Abrahams JM, McClure SA. Pediatric odontogenic tumors [J]. Oral Maxillofac Surg Clin North Am. 2016;28(1):45–58.
2. Leiser Y, Abu-El-Naaj I, Peled M. Odontogenic myxoma—a case series and review of the surgical management [J]. J Craniomaxillofac Surg. 2009;37(4):206–9.
3. Francisco AL, Chulam TC, Silva FO, et al. Clinicopathologic analysis of 14 cases of odontogenic myxoma and review of the literature [J]. J Clin Exp Dent. 2017;9(4):e560–3.
4. Gomes CC, Diniz MG, Duarte AP, et al. Molecular review of odontogenic myxoma [J]. Oral Oncol. 2011;47(5):325–8.
5. Lo Muzio L, Nocini P, Favia G, et al. Odontogenic myxoma of the jaws: a clinical, radiologic, immunohistochemical, and ultrastructural study [J]. Oral Surg Oral Med Oral Pathol Oral Radiol Endod. 1996;82(4):426–33.
6. Shivashankara C, Nidoni M, Patil S, et al. Odontogenic myxoma: a review with report of an uncommon case with recurrence in the mandible of a teenage male [J]. Saudi Dent J. 2017;29(3):93–101.
7. Dotta JH, Miotto LN, Spin-Neto R, et al. Odontogenic myxoma: systematic review and bias analysis [J]. Eur J Clin Invest. 2020;50(4):e13214.
8. Kumar N, Kohli M, Pandey S, et al. Odontogenic myxoma [J]. J Maxillofac Oral Surg. 2014;13(2):222–6.
9. Rocha AC, Gaujac C, Ceccheti MM, et al. Treatment of recurrent mandibular myxoma by curettage and cryotherapy after thirty years [J]. Clinics (Sao Paulo). 2009;64(2):149–52.

28 Cementoblastoma

Jing Song Hou, Hui Shan Ong, Zhen Tian, Lin Zhu, and Ze Hang Zhuang

28.1 Introduction

Cementoblastoma is a slow-growing benign odontogenic tumor which is derived from the ectodermal mesenchymal cells of periodontal tissue and contains cementoblasts [1–4]. Cementoblastoma is a rare jaw tumor, accounting for about 1% of all odontogenic tumors [5, 6]. It mainly occurs in children and young adults, with about 50% of cases in the age of 20 years old, 75% in the age of 30 years old, without significant gender difference. It is more common in the mandible than maxilla, and is prone to involve the mandibular first permanent molar teeth, and rarely invade the deciduous teeth. At present, the main treatment is surgery, which includes extensive resection of the lesion and extraction of the affected tooth. After surgery, it has an overall recurrence rate of 21.7–37.1% [5–7]. It is important to carefully select the surgical method for better clinical prognosis.

J. S. Hou (✉) · Z. H. Zhuang
Hospital of Stomatology, Guanghua College of Stomatology, Sun Yat-sen University, Guangdong, China
e-mail: houjs@mail.sysu.edu.cn

H. S. Ong · Z. Tian
Department of Oral Maxillofacial-Head & Neck Oncology, Shanghai Ninth People's Hospital, Shanghai Jiao Tong University School of Medicine, Shanghai, China

L. Zhu
Department of Radiology, Ninth People's Hospital Affiliated to Shanghai Jiao Tong University, Shanghai, China

28.2 Case 58

A 21-year-old woman suffered from swollen pain in the posterior region of the right mandibular molar for 1 week.

[History of Present Illness] The patient felt pain in the right mandibular posterior tooth 1 week ago. Panoramic radiographs suggested space-occupying of the right mandible.

[Specialty Examination] The face was basically symmetrical. There was no abnormality in mouth opening range and mouth opening pattern. Intraoral examination revealed 48 mesio-impacted, 46, 47 gingival buccal and lingual swelling, bleeding upon percussion, 46, 47 loosening for I, no fistula formation. The tongue moved freely, without abnormal oral mucosa and lip skin. No bilateral submandibular and cervical lymph node enlargement was observed.

[Auxiliary Examination]

1. Panoramic radiographs suggested 48 mesio-impacted, 46 and 47 increased bone density shadow in root tip, and decreased in peripheral ring bone mineral density (Fig. 28.1).

Y. He (ed.), *Inflammatory and Neoplastic Diseases of Craniofacial Bones*,
https://doi.org/10.1007/978-981-97-4155-7_28

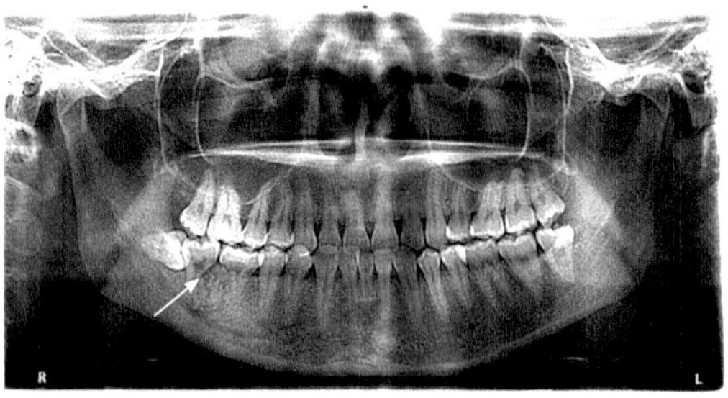

Fig. 28.1 46 and 47 bone high-density shadow, with heterogeneous density (preoperative)

2. Maxillofacial enhanced CT scan suggested 46 and 47 bone high-density shadow, ranging from 16 mm × 11 mm × 14 mm, with heterogeneous density. Low density shadow was seen around the edges, with bone absorption in adjacent roots. No obvious abnormal density shadow was seen in the surrounding soft tissues. There was no abnormal enhancement after enhancement. No obvious cervical lymph node enlargement was observed (Fig. 28.2).

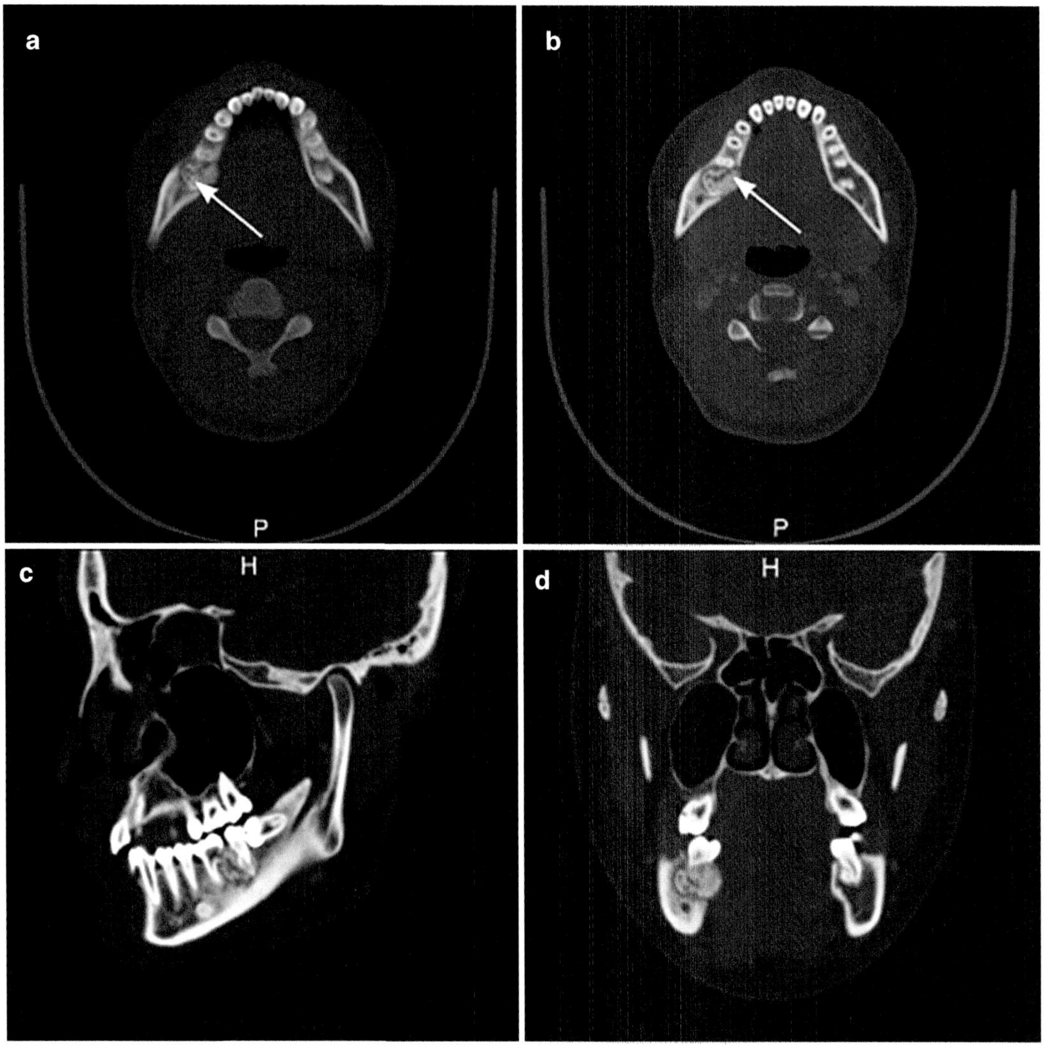

Fig. 28.2 CT plain axial scan: 46 and 47 bone high-density shadow, with heterogeneous density. (**a**) Radioopqaue lesion over the molar region of Right mandible. (**b**) Enhanced CT axial scan: no obvious enhancement in the lesion. (**c**) Enhanced CT sagittal scan: bone resorption of adjacent roots. (**d**) Enhanced CT coronal scan

[Preliminary Diagnosis] Mass of the right mandible.

[Treatment] "Resection of right mandibular mass" was performed under general anesthesia: a gingival marginal incision was made, and the gingival flap was elevated for 46 and 47 tooth extraction. It was found that 46 distal root was damaged by absorption and 47 root had osteoid mass of about 1.5 cm × 1.0 cm. The mass was completely removed, and alveolar bone was trimmed. The wound was rinsed, thoroughly hemostatic, and closed properly. Intraoperative frozen pathological examination suggested "right mandibular" mucosa chronic inflammation, fibrous tissue hyperplasia, tissue edema. The hard tissue was sent for gross pathological examination. The specific result was to be determined by paraffin wax examination.

[Pathological Examination] Gross pathological examination revealed one molar with bony tissue covering the root tip, 2.5 cm × 1.8 cm × 1.5 cm, grayish yellow. Microscopically, hyperplasia of cementoid hard tissue at the root of the tooth was observed, which was fused into a mass containing basophilic reverse line. Hypertrophic cementoblast and osteoclast multinucleate giant cells were observed around the hard tissue (Fig. 28.3).

[Pathological Diagnosis] "Right mandibular" cementoblast, ICD-O code: 9273/0.

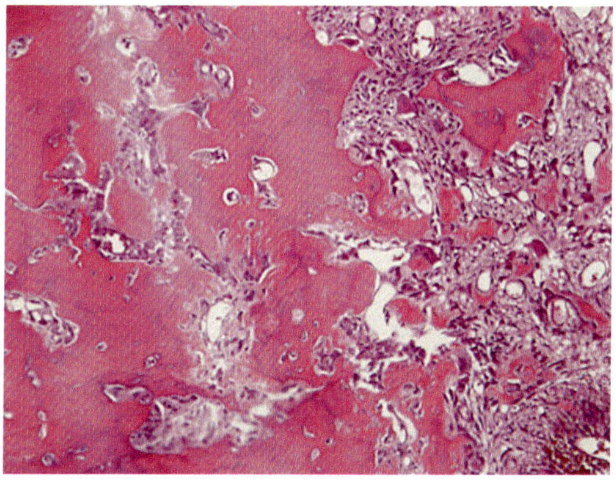

Fig. 28.3 Cementoid hyperplasia, cementoblast and a few osteoclast-like multinucleated giant cells (200×)

[Follow-Up] The patient healed uneventfully. The postoperative 6-month follow-up exhibited no obvious postoperative reaction and no tumor relapse.

28.3 Key Points of Diagnosis and Treatment

Cementoblastoma was first reported by Dewey in 1927 and was defined as a benign tumor in the 2017 WHO classification of Odontogenic Tumors. Cementoblastoma is characterized by cementoid tissue that forms and attaches to the root of the tooth. Cementoblasts usually involve the mandible, especially the molar and premolar regions of the mandible, with less than 25% of cases occurring in the maxilla.

Clinical Manifestations Cementoblastoma usually presents in clinical examination as local swelling and pain caused by swelling of the bone on the buccal or lingual side of the alveolar crest. It has been reported that the lesion is locally invasive, causing maxillary enlargement, displacement of adjacent teeth, and involvement of maxillary sinuses.

Imaging and Pathological Characteristics Cementoblastoma originates from odontogenic external mesenchymal functional cementoblasts. The lesion is connected to 1/3 of the cementum layer of the root tip and separated from the surrounding bone through the periodontal membrane, supporting the odontogenic origin to a certain extent. Radiographically, it is a well-circumscribed dense mass within the jaw, fused with 1/3 of the apex of the root, surrounded by a clear margin. Histopathologically, it presents as a lamellar cementoid structure that is continuous with the root of the tooth. Cementoblastoma mostly contains sheets of thick mineralized tissue with many plump cementoblastoid cells and notable basophilic reflexes, as well as abundant fibrous vascular tissue, in addition to multinucleated giant cells. The surrounding is often composed of noncalcified stroma arranged in radiating columns perpendicular to the fiber wall, which is consistent with the area of increased radiographic opacity.

Differential Diagnosis Cementoblastoma should be distinguished from osteoblastoma and osteosarcoma. Osteoblastoma and cementoblastoma are basically the same histopathologically, the only difference is that cementoblastoma is attached to the tooth root and fused with it. In addition, it is important to distinguish cementoblastoma from osteosarcoma. Histopathologically, cementoblastoma cells may be plump, with polymorphic and deeply stained nuclei, but without mitosis unlike osteosarcoma. In addition to the pathological findings, the differentiation of these lesions and cementoblastoma requires a comprehensive judgment combined with clinical symptoms and imaging findings.

Treatment Cementoblastoma is treated by complete removal of the tumor along with extraction of the affected tooth. Incomplete resection tends to cause tumor recurrence, with a recurrence rate of 37.1%. Therefore, some people advocate that the tumor should be removed after tooth extraction to reduce the recurrence rate. No reports about the malignant transformation of cementoblastoma have been published.

References

1. Pynn BR, Sands TD, Bradley G. Benign cementoblastoma: a case report [J]. J Can Dent Assoc. 2001;67(5):260–2.
2. Subramani V, Narasimhan M, Ramalingam S, et al. Revisiting Cementoblastoma with a rare case presentation [J]. Case Rep Pathol. 2017;2017:8248691.
3. Brannon RB, Fowler CB, Carpenter WM, et al. Cementoblastoma: an innocuous neoplasm? A clinicopathologic study of 44 cases and review of the literature with special emphasis on recurrence [J]. Oral Surg Oral Med Oral Pathol Oral Radiol Endod. 2002;93(3):311–20.
4. Chrcanovic BR, Gomez RS. Cementoblastoma: an updated analysis of 258 cases reported in the literature [J]. J Craniomaxillofac Surg. 2017;45(10):1759–66.
5. Ackermann GL, Altini M. The cementomas — a clinicopathological re-appraisal [J]. J Dent Assoc S Afr. 1992;47(5):187–94.
6. Slootweg PJ. Cementoblastoma and osteoblastoma: a comparison of histologic features [J]. J Oral Pathol Med. 1992;21(9):385–9.
7. Pathak J, Hosalkar RM, Sidana S, et al. Benign cementoblastoma involving left deciduous first molar: a case report and review of literature [J]. J Oral Maxillofac Pathol. 2019;23(3):422–8.

Odontogenic Fibroma

29

Jing Song Hou, Hui Shan Ong, Zhen Tian, Lin Zhu, and Bing Bing Sun

29.1 Introduction

Odontogenic fibroma is a benign mesenchymal odontogenic tumor typically characterized by a varying number of odontogenic epithelium in a mature fibrous matrix. It is divided into two types, namely, intraosseous /central odontogenic fibroma (COF) and extraosseous /peripheral odontogenic fibroma (POF) [1–6]. Histologically, COF has two main subtypes, namely simple COF (epithelial-poor) and complex COF (epithelial-rich) [7–10]. In the 2017 WHO classification, the panel excluded the subtype pf "epithelial-poor or simple" of odontogenic fibroma for poor definition [8–13]. COF typically includes granular cell odontogenic fibroma, odontogenic fibroma consisting of pleomorphic fibroblasts, and odontogenic fibroma exhibiting giant cell response [9, 14–17]. COF is a rare odontogenic tumor, which occurs mostly in females, with a male to female ratio of about 1:2.2. The age of onset is 4–80 years old (average 40 years old). It can occur in both maxilla and mandible, usually before the maxillary first molar and behind the mandibular first molar [9]. About 1/3 of COF may be associated with unerupted third molar. Peripheral odontogenic fibroma is more common than COF, with a wide age range of onset. It has been reported in literature that odontogenic fibroma may strike to people at the age between 11 and 90, with a peak at the age between 20 and 40 years. It is more common in females, and can occur in both maxilla and mandible, usually in mandibular buccal gums. The main treatment of odontogenic fibroma is surgical curettage or excision. Odontogenic fibroma has a prognosis with no tendency of recurrence.

J. S. Hou (✉)
Hospital of Stomatology, Guanghua College of Stomatology, Sun Yat-sen University, Guangdong, China
e-mail: houjs@mail.sysu.edu.cn

H. S. Ong · Z. Tian · B. B. Sun
Department of Oral Maxillofacial-Head & Neck Oncology, Shanghai Ninth People's Hospital, Shanghai Jiao Tong University School of Medicine, Shanghai, China

L. Zhu
Department of Radiology, Ninth People's Hospital Affiliated to Shanghai Jiao Tong University, Shanghai, China

29.2 Central Odontogenic Fibroma

29.2.1 Case 59

A 6-year-old boy suffered from a space-occupying of the right mandible for 3 months.

[History of Present Illness] Three months ago, the patient received root canal treatment at other hospital for pain in the left lower posterior tooth. Panoramic radiographs suggested the possibility of cystic space-occupying in the

Y. He (ed.), *Inflammatory and Neoplastic Diseases of Craniofacial Bones*,
https://doi.org/10.1007/978-981-97-4155-7_29

right mandible, without obvious pain and discomfort. The patient was advised to seek medical treatment at our hospital.

[Specialty Examination] The face was basically symmetrical, with a coordinated proportion between the upper, middle, and lower face. No deformity or numbness was observed in the lip. There was no abnormality in the mouth opening range and the mouth opening pattern. Intraoral examination revealed absence of 84 tooth, no obvious swelling of buccal-lingual gingiva, no ulcer in the palate, and no deviation in the palate sag. The soft palate moved normally. No significant bilateral submental, submaxillary, and cervical lymph node enlargement was observed.

[Auxiliary Examination] Panoramic radiographs suggested a low-density shadow of about 1.5 cm in diameter in the alveolar bone in tooth 84 region, adjacent to the lower margin of the mandible. Two high-density images, resembling teeth, were seen in the low-density shadow (Fig. 29.1).

[Preliminary Diagnosis] Mass of the right mandible (nature to be determined).

[Treatment] "Resection of right mandibular mass" was performed under general anesthesia: a trapezoidal incision was made on the lateral vestibular groove, and the gingival flap was elevated for surgical exposure of the bone cortex for removal. Solid space-occupying was found in the right mandible. The tumor, which was downward near the lower margin of the mandible, was completely removed, while the tooth tissue in the tumor was retained. Frozen pathology examination suggested odontogenic fibroma /odontogenic fibromyxoma of the "right mandible," with hypercellularity and mild atypia. The wound was rinsed, covered with iodoform strip, and sutured.

[Pathological Examination] Gross pathological examination revealed tumor tissue, 0.4 cm × 0.3 cm × 0.3 cm, grayish white. Microscopically, fusiform and short-fusiform cells were proliferated in the fibrous tissue, with hypercellularity and mild atypia. Odontogenic epithelial clusters were seen inside (Fig. 29.2a).

[Pathological Diagnosis] Central odontogenic fibroma of the "right mandible," ICD-O code: 9330/0.

[Follow-Up] The patient healed uneventfully. The postoperative 3-month follow-up exhibited no obvious postoperative reaction and no tumor relapse (Fig. 29.2b).

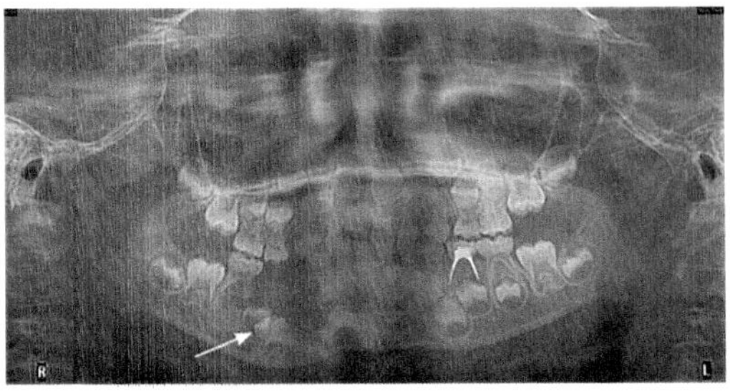

Fig. 29.1 Low-density shadow of about 1.5 cm in diameter in the alveolar bone in tooth 84 region, adjacent to the lower margin of the mandible. Two high-density images, resembling teeth, were seen in the low-density shadow

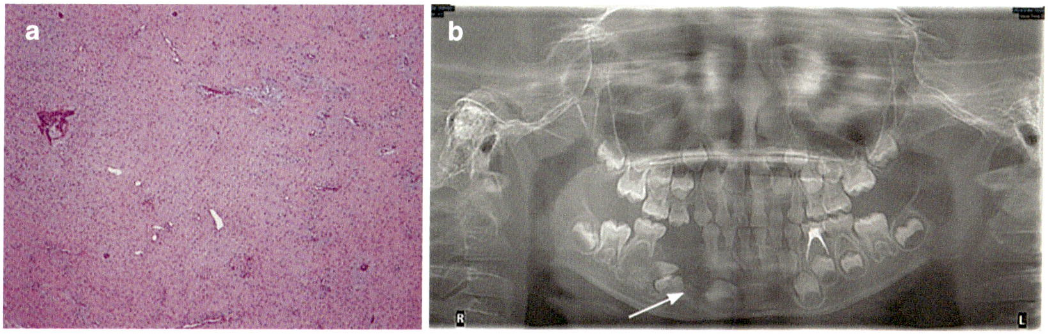

Fig. 29.2 (**a**) Odontogenic epithelial masses (100×) in the neoplastic fibrous tissue. (**b**) Postoperative changes of the right mandible

29.3 Peripheral Odontogenic Fibroma

29.3.1 Case 60

A 84-year-old woman suffered from a gradually growing right upper gingival mass for over 1 year.

[History of Present Illness] More than 1 year ago, the patient found a hard bean-size mass in the right upper anterior tooth region without rupture or pain symptoms, no obvious loosening of the teeth. The mass gradually enlarged and occasionally bled when brushing. Eight months ago, the patient was treated in at our outpatient department and was recommended to receive biopsy surgery if necessary. Recently, the mass increased significantly to about the size of quail egg, affecting the daily life, so the patient sought medical treatment our hospital again.

[Specialty Examination] The face was basically symmetrical, and an exophytic mass was observed on the right upper gum, causing the right upper lip to be raised and the mouth closing to be incomplete. There was no abnormality in the mouth opening range and the mouth opening pattern. Intraoral examination revealed permanent dentition, dental defect, multiple residual roots and crowns, poor periodontal hygiene, CI=II°-III°, DI=II°-III°, a large amount of food debris accumulation, gingival margin redness, and swelling. An exophytic mass with a pedicle on the 12–14 buccal gingiva was found, which was approximately 3.0 cm × 1.5 cm in size, with no obvious ulceration or bleeding, red, hard on palpation, tenderness (−), base involvement of 11–15 gums, 12 displacement, deep infiltration, poor base mobility, and no significant loosening of teeth (Fig. 29.3a). The tongue moved freely. No significant bilateral submandibular and cervical lymph node enlargement was observed.

[Auxiliary Examination]

1. Panoramic radiographs suggested multiple residual roots and crowns in the mouth, and incomplete bone formation in the upper anterior tooth region (Fig. 29.3b).
2. Maxillofacial enhanced CT scan suggested a circular mass shadow in the gingiva of the right upper anterior tooth region, with clear boundary and a size of approximately 2.1 cm × 1.2 cm × 1.3 cm, appearing to have a thin capsule, with uniform internal density, and a CT value of approximately 17 Hu. Mild enhancement was obtained for the lesion with a CT value of 27 Hu. The surrounding bone cortex of the lesion was rough and not smooth (Fig. 29.4).

[Preliminary Diagnosis] Right upper gingival mass (nature to be determined).

[Treatment] "Partial resection of the right maxilla" was performed under general anesthesia: a gingival and palate incision was made along the outer margin of the mass for 1–2 cm. The tumor was completely resected, 12–14 alveolar bone was

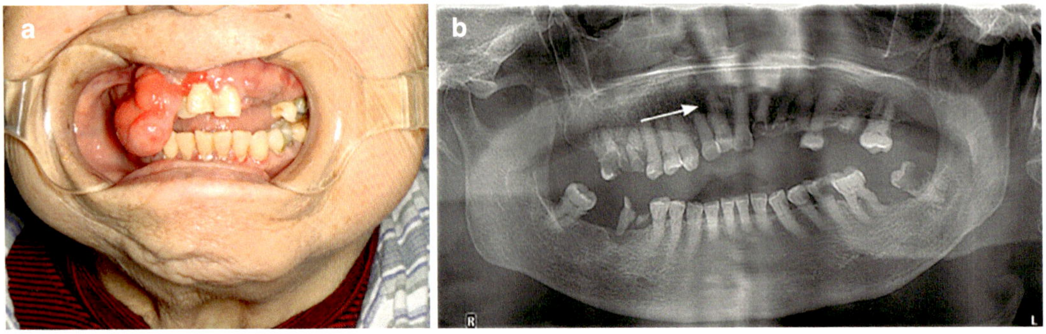

Fig. 29.3 (**a**) An exophytic mass with a pedicle on the 12–14 buccal gingiva was found, which was approximately 3.0 cm × 1.5 cm in size, with no obvious ulceration or bleeding, red, base involvement of 11–15 gums, and 12 displacement. (**b**) Multiple residual roots and crowns in the mouth, and incomplete bone formation in the anterior tooth region

removed, along with part of the maxilla. Intraoperative frozen pathological examination suggested peripheral odontogenic fibroma of the "right upper gum." Sharp bone tip and bone margin were trimmed. The wound was rinsed, hemostatic, and closed with transposition of local tissue flap.

[Pathological Examination] Gross pathological examination revealed tumor, 3 cm × 2.5 cm × 2 cm, nodular, and gray and grayish yellow. Microscopically, the mucosal subepithelial fibrous tissue showed significant tumor hyperplasia with light inflammation, scattered in the hyperplastic odontogenic epithelial mass (Fig. 29.5).

[Pathological Diagnosis] Peripheral odontogenic fibroma of the "right upper gum" ICD-O code: 9330/0.

[Follow-Up] The patient healed uneventfully. The postoperative 6-month follow-up exhibited no obvious postoperative reaction and no tumor relapse

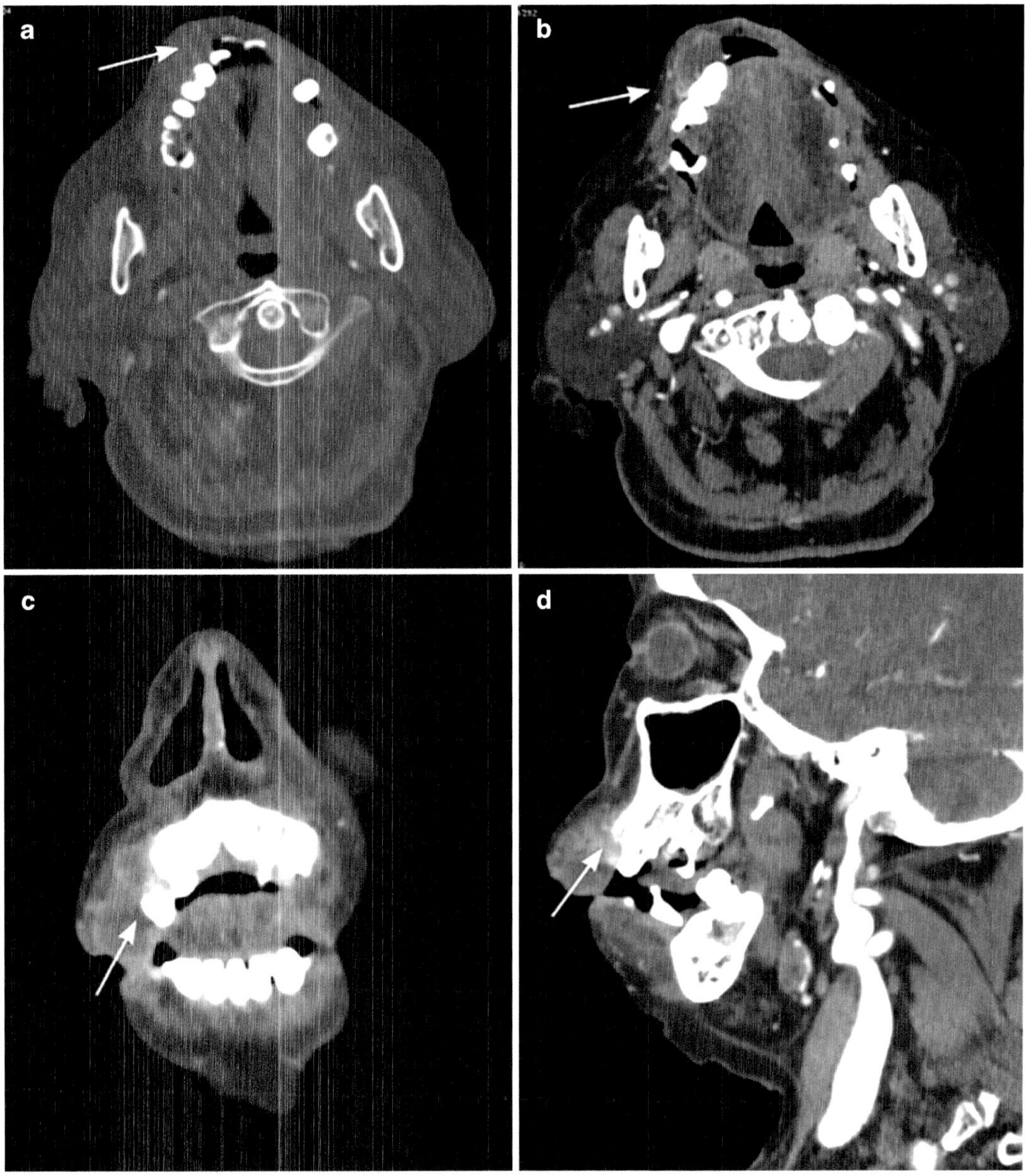

Fig. 29.4 (**a**) CT plain axial scan: A circular mass shadow in the gingiva of the right upper anterior tooth region, with clear boundary and a size of approximately 2.1 cm × 1.2 cm × 1.3 cm, appearing to have a thin capsule, with uniform internal density, and a CT value of approximately 17 Hu. (**b**) Enhanced CT axial scan: Mild enhancement of the lesion with a CT value of 27 Hu. (**c**, **d**) Enhanced CT coronal and sagittal scan: the surrounding bone cortex of the lesion was rough and not smooth

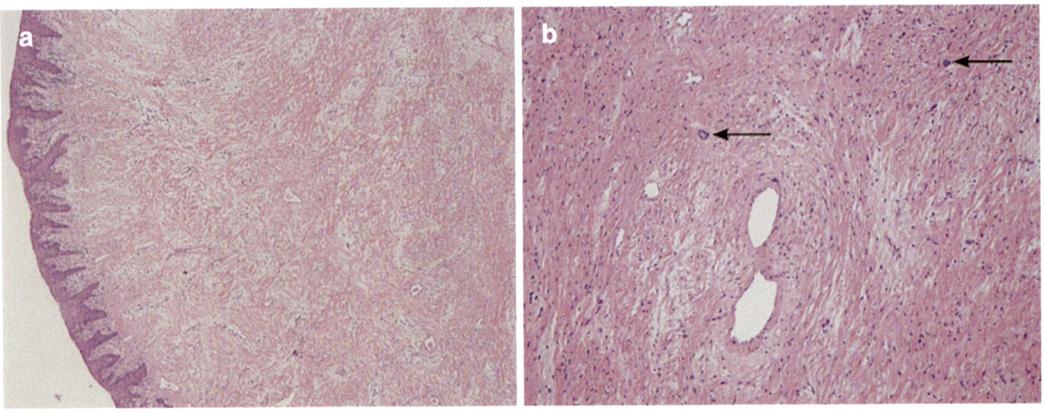

Fig. 29.5 (**a**) Submucosal fibrous tissue neoplasia similar to fibrous gingival tumor (40×). (**b**) Small odontogenic epithelial masses in fibrous tissue (arrow) (100×)

29.4 Granular Cell Odontogenic Tumor

29.4.1 Case 61

A 51-year-old woman suffered from left cheek mass for one and a half years with distension and pain for more than 10 days.

[History of Present Illness] A year and a half ago, the patient discovered a thumb tip-sized mass in the left vestibular groove and cheek mucosa, without obvious symptoms such as redness, pain, fever, lower lip numbness, and facial paralysis. One year ago, the patient received anti-inflammatory symptomatic treatment at our hospital, but without remission; 3 months ago, the patient realized that the tumor significantly increased, and repeatedly cut it off with scissor, causing a small amount of bleeding; More than 10 days ago, the patient felt that the left cheek was swollen and painful. Panoramic radiographs showed space-occupying of multiple low-density shadows in the left mandible.

[Specialty Examination] The face was asymmetrical, and the left cheek was obviously swollen, with intact surface skin, and normal color and skin temperature (Fig. 29.6a, b). There was no abnormality in mouth opening range and mouth opening pattern. There was a mass about 6 cm × 6 cm in size on the gum and cheek of the left mandible with a cauliflower surface. The mandible bone distention was hard with no obvious tenderness on palpation, unclear boundary with the surrounding tissue, and poor mobility. No significant bilateral submaxillary and cervical lymph node enlargement was observed.

[Auxiliary Examination]
Panoramic radiographs suggested multilocular low-density shadow of the left mandibular angle and ascending branch, with clear boundary and no obvious signs of root resorption (Fig. 29.6c).

[Preliminary Diagnosis] Mass of the left mandible (malignant to be ruled out).

[Treatment] "Left segmental mandibulectomy with resection of left cheek mass, left fibular flap transfer and tracheotomy" was performed under general anesthesia: an incision was made along the lower margin of the mandible for 1–2 cm, and the gingival flap was elevated for surgical exposure of the bone distention of the mandibular body and angle. Mandibular segment including mass was resected at 34 mesio-sigmoid incisure. Intraoperative frozen pathological reported granular cell odontogenic tumor of the left mandible. The left peroneal muscle flap was shaped and reconstructed to restore mandibular continuity and occlusal relationship. The vascular anastomosis of the fibula and facial arteriovenous vessels was performed.

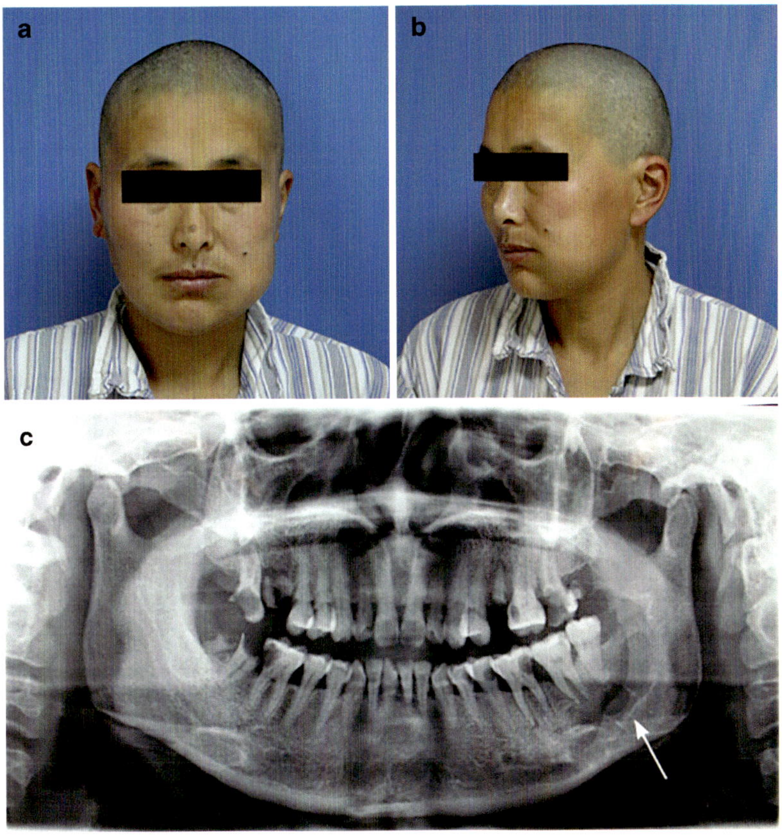

Fig. 29.6 (**a**, **b**) The maxillofacial region was asymmetrical, and the lower 1/3 of the left side was swollen and distended. (**c**) Panoramic radiograph suggested multilocular low-density shadow of the left mandibular body, angle and ascending branch, with clear boundary and no obvious signs of 35–38 root resorption

The wound was rinsed and tightly hemostatic, the negative pressure drainage tube was indwelled, and the wound was closed in layers with sutures (Fig. 29.7).

[Pathological Examination] Gross pathological examination revealed a part of maxillary bone structure, 9 cm × 5 cm × 4 cm, a gray brown swelling was found on the section, 4 cm × 4 cm × 3 cm, brittle. Microscopic examination showed the lesions were relatively confined and the tumor cells were large and proliferated in sheets, with abundant cytoplasm and eosinophilic particles, scattered in odontogenic epithelial cords and cementicle structures. Peripheral reactive new bone formation was observed (Fig. 29.8).

[Pathological Diagnosis] Granular cell odontogenic tumor of the "left mandible," a variant of the WHO Classification of Central Odontogenic Fibroma, ICD-O code: 9321/0.

[Follow-Up] The patient healed uneventfully. The postoperative 6-month follow-up exhibited no tumor relapse, with satisfactory reconstruction of the mandible and good recovery of mandibular functions (Fig. 29.9).

29.4.2 Case 62

A 38-year-old woman suffered from a relapse of left mandibular granular cell tumor 7 months after multiple operations at other hospital.

[History of Present Illness] About 2 years ago, the patient felt swollen in the left mandible and received surgery at a local hospital. Pathological diagnosis suggested ameloblastoma. The patient suffered from a relapse 3 months after surgery, and received "left segmental mandibulectomy with right fibular transfer. Postoperative pathology showed ameloblastoma. Seven months ago, the patient was again found to have left cheek soft tissue swelling and received "excision of left

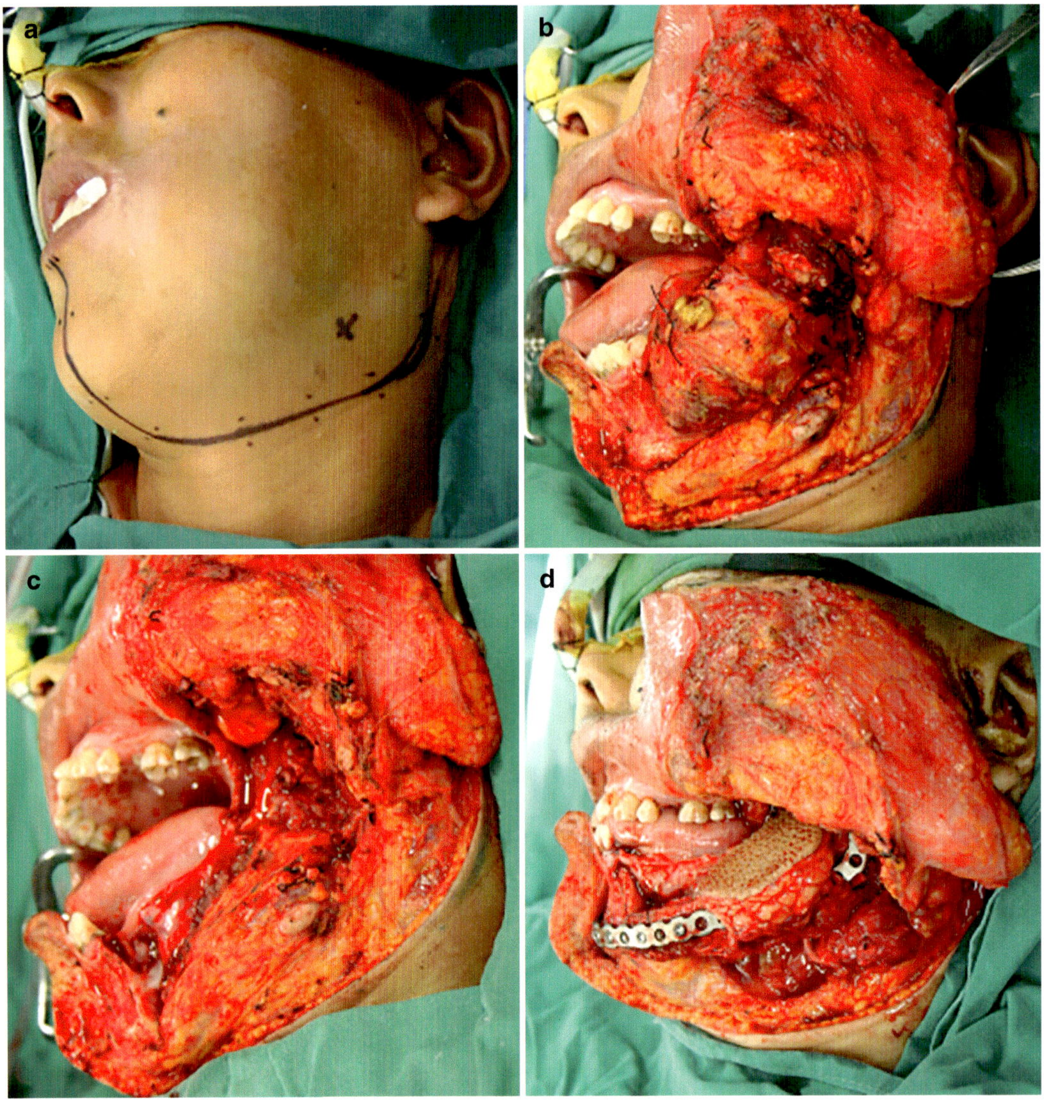

Fig. 29.7 (**a**) Incision design. (**b**) Exposure of mass. (**c**) Defect after left segmental mandibulectomy. (**d**) Fibular myocutaneous flap reconstruction to restore mandibular continuity

mandibular soft tissue lesion." Postoperative pathology suggested that granular cell ameloblastoma recurred and developed into malignant, accompanied by necrosis, showing highly malignant. The consultation in our oral pathology department a month ago reached the diagnosis conclusion that left mandibular granular cell odontogenic tumor (granular cell odontogenic tumor) was first considered. This time, it was recurrent and malignant, with focal odontogenic epitheliomatous hyperplasia.

[Specialty Examination] The face was asymmetrical. The left mandible and chin were obviously swollen, forming mass about 6.0 cm × 3.0 cm in size, with local skin redness and swelling, soft on palpation, and mild pain. The fibula of the left mandible body was repaired, making the bone continuous. An obvious mass on the lower part of the earlobe was found, which was about 2.5 cm × 2.5 cm in size, hard in texture, and mild tenderness. The mouth opening range was about three transverse fingers, and the

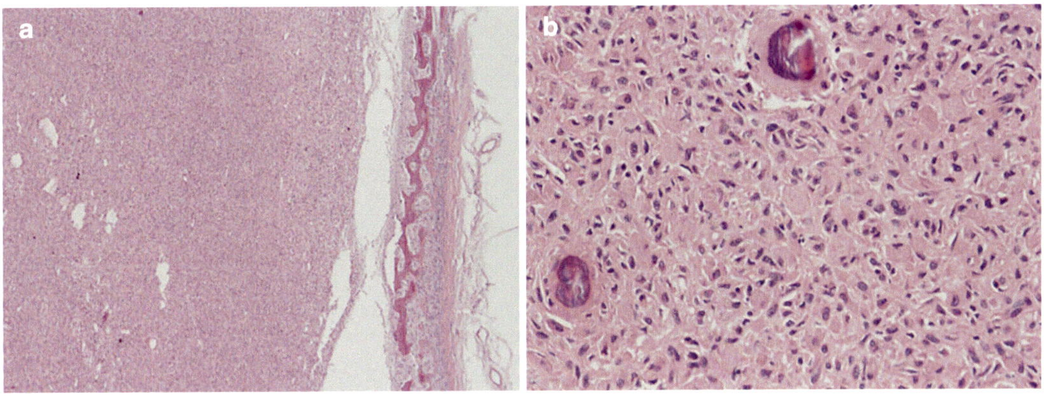

Fig. 29.8 (**a**) The lesions were confined without protrusion through the bone cortex (40×). (**b**) Tumor cells had abundant cytoplasm, eosinophilic particles, and obvious polymorphic nuclei, but mitosis was rare, and local calcifications were observed (400×)

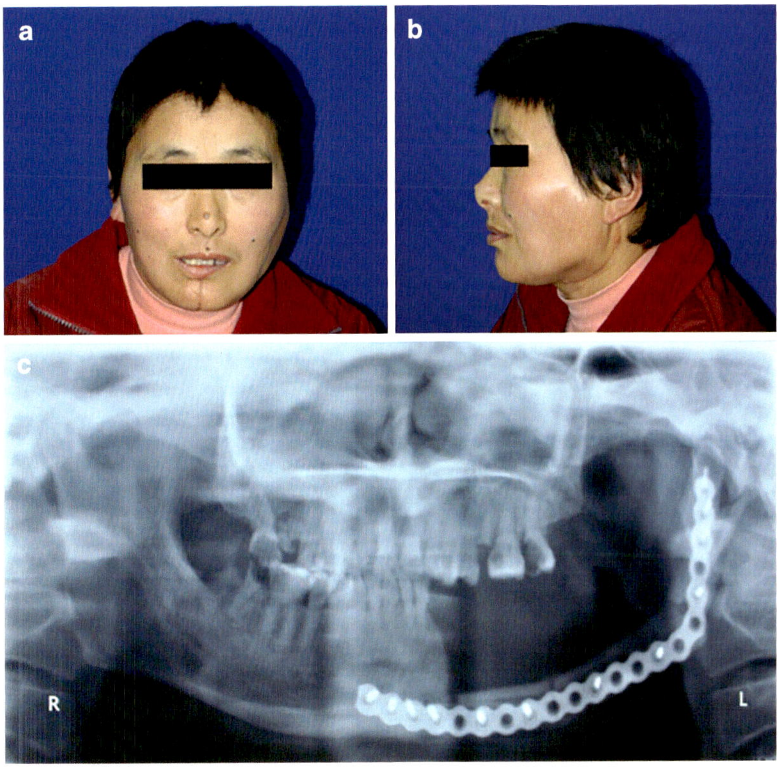

Fig. 29.9 (**a**, **b**) Postoperative follow-up showed no tumor recurrence and good recovery of mandibular shape. (**c**) Postoperative changes of mandible

mouth opening is skewed toward right. Oral hygiene was poor. The left buccal fibula flap was in place with normal color, shape, and quality. There was a gray mass between 31–42 labial gingiva and the mandible, with no obvious pain on palpation. Teeth 32–38 were missing. The lymph nodes in cervical region II were significantly enlarged, about 2.5 cm × 2.0 cm in size, with clear boundary and hard texture. Enlarged lymph node was observed in the left supraclavicular fossa, about 1.5 cm × 1.5 cm in size, with hard texture and obvious tenderness (Fig. 29.10a, b).

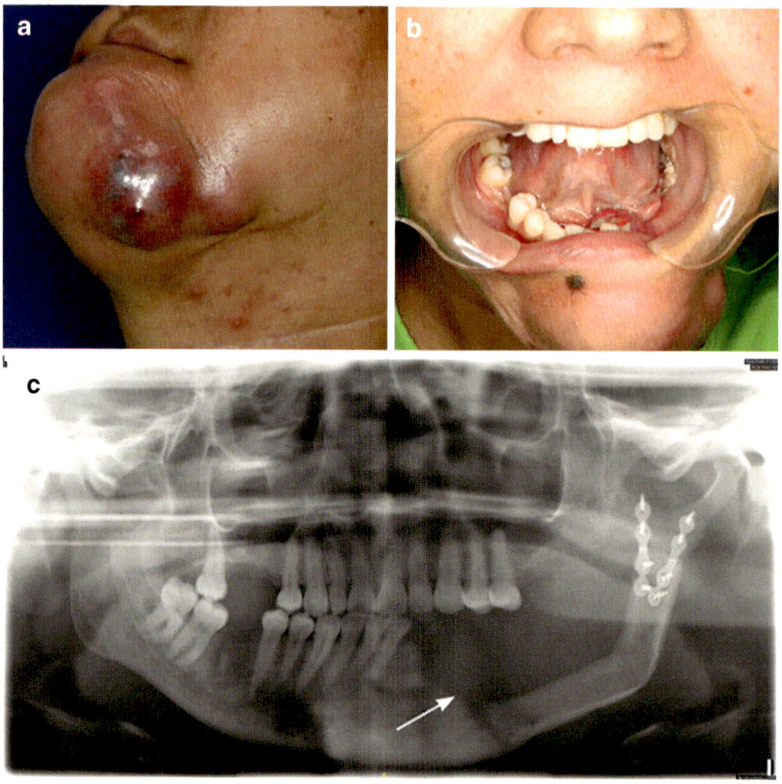

Fig. 29.10 (**a**) The left mandible and chin were obviously swollen, forming mass about 6.0 cm × 3.0 cm in size, with local skin redness. (**b**) A gray mass between 31–42 labial gingiva and the mandible, involving the lingual floor mucosa. (**c**) Postoperative change in the left mandible with internal fixation. The upper and lower teeth on both sides were not aligned, multiple teeth were missing, with local bone destruction in the mandible, and density attenuation (preoperative)

[Auxiliary Examination]

1. Panoramic radiographs suggested postoperative change in the left mandible with internal fixation. The upper and lower teeth on both sides were not aligned, multiple teeth were missing, with local bone destruction in the mandible, and density attenuation (Fig. 29.10c).
2. Maxillofacial enhanced CT scan suggested postoperative changes after multiple surgeries. In referring to previous histological report, left mandibular ameloblastic carcinoma, there is bony destruction in the symphysis, body, and ramus of the left mandible invaded into surrounding soft tissue. Coronal view showed that the recurrence malignant lesion involving temporomandibular joint the had entended into the infratemporal fossa; enlarged lymph nodes in level Ia and II, lymph node metastasis cannot be ruled out. After surgery for left mandibular ameloblastoma, there were irregular soft tissue shadows around the region, ranging from approximately 5.8 cm, with an average CT value of 42 Hu. After enhancement, there was uneven enhancement, with an arterial phase of 90 Hu and a venous phase of 103 Hu (Fig. 29.11).

[Preliminary Diagnosis] Relapse and malignant transformation of granular cell tumor of the left mandible after multiple surgeries at other hospital.

[Treatment] "Expanded resection of mandibular and skull base malignant tumors with radical neck lymph node dissection, anterolateral fibular flap transfer, and tracheotomy" was performed under general anesthesia: a combined incision was made along the lower margin of the mandible for 1~2 cm to the left ear under the eardrum, and an S-shaped incision from the posterior edge of the sternocleidomastoid muscle to the middle point of the clavicle. Besides, an incision was designed to extend 2 cm along the chin mass, downward to the cervical incision, and upper close to the red margin of the lower lip. The gingival flap was elevated for surgical exposure of

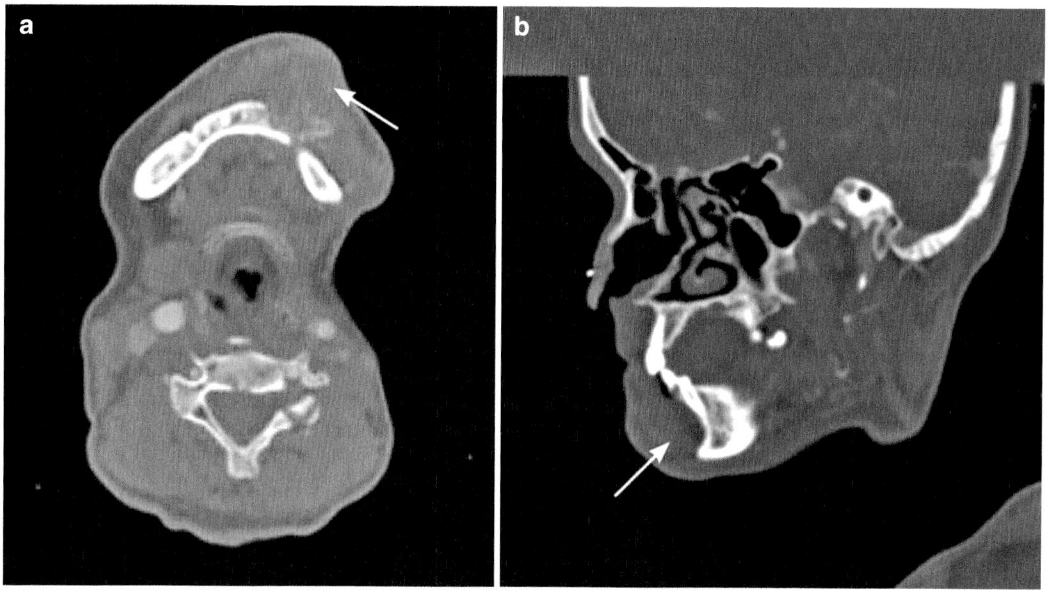

Fig. 29.11 (**a**) CT axial scan: Local bone destruction of the mandible. (**b**) CT sagittal reconstruction: multiple soft tissue mass shadows in the left parapharyngeal space, muscles of mastication space, and behind the parotid gland, with uneven enhancement after enhancement

the mandible. Radical cervical lymph node dissection was performed. Frozen pathology indicated that no epithelial malignant tumor metastasis was found in the lymph node examined (−). The cytoplasm of the "posterior cervical" tumor cells was rich in particles, with significant cell atypia and visible mitotic signs, which, combined with the medical history, considered as metastasis/recurrence of the original tumor (granular cell tumor, malignant). The mandible was amputated from the median of the mandible and the left condylar neck. The left parotid gland was completely removed, the zygomatic arch was severed, and the soft tissues around the zygomatic arch were isolated for continued upward separation to the skull base. Part of the temporal muscle, the soft tissues of the stem process and temporal, the lesion, and cervical lymph nodes were completely resected. Intraoperative frozen pathological examination revealed tumor in the zygomatic arch. The tissues around the temporal and skull base including zygomatic arch were further removed, and the incisal margin was removed again for frozen pathology examination, showing all incisal margins were negative (−). Bone of skull base, stylomastoid foramen, and mastoid process were removed. The anterolateral thigh flap was cut, with the size of about 33 cm × 8 cm. Peroneal arteriovenous anastomosis with superior thyroid artery and internal jugular vein branches was performed. The flap was shaped to repair the soft tissue defects of the chin, floor of the mouth, buccal, and intraoral regions. Skull base, temporal defect was repaired with temporal muscle flap. The wound was rinsed and thoroughly hemostatic, negative pressure drainage tube was indwelled, and layered suture was performed to close the wound (Fig. 29.12).

[Pathological Examination] Gross pathological examination revealed bilateral mandibular tissue, 13 cm × 6 cm × 5 cm, with six attached teeth. The chin buccolingual side of the mandible was swollen, and the section showed a diffuse mass, about 6.5 cm × 5 cm × 5 cm, grayish white, medium hard, and unclear in boundary. Microscopic examination indicated cellular plasma of tumor cells, with significant cell atypia, visible mitosis, some intranuclear pseudo-inclusion bodies, focal necrosis, and no odontogenic epithelium (Fig. 29.13).

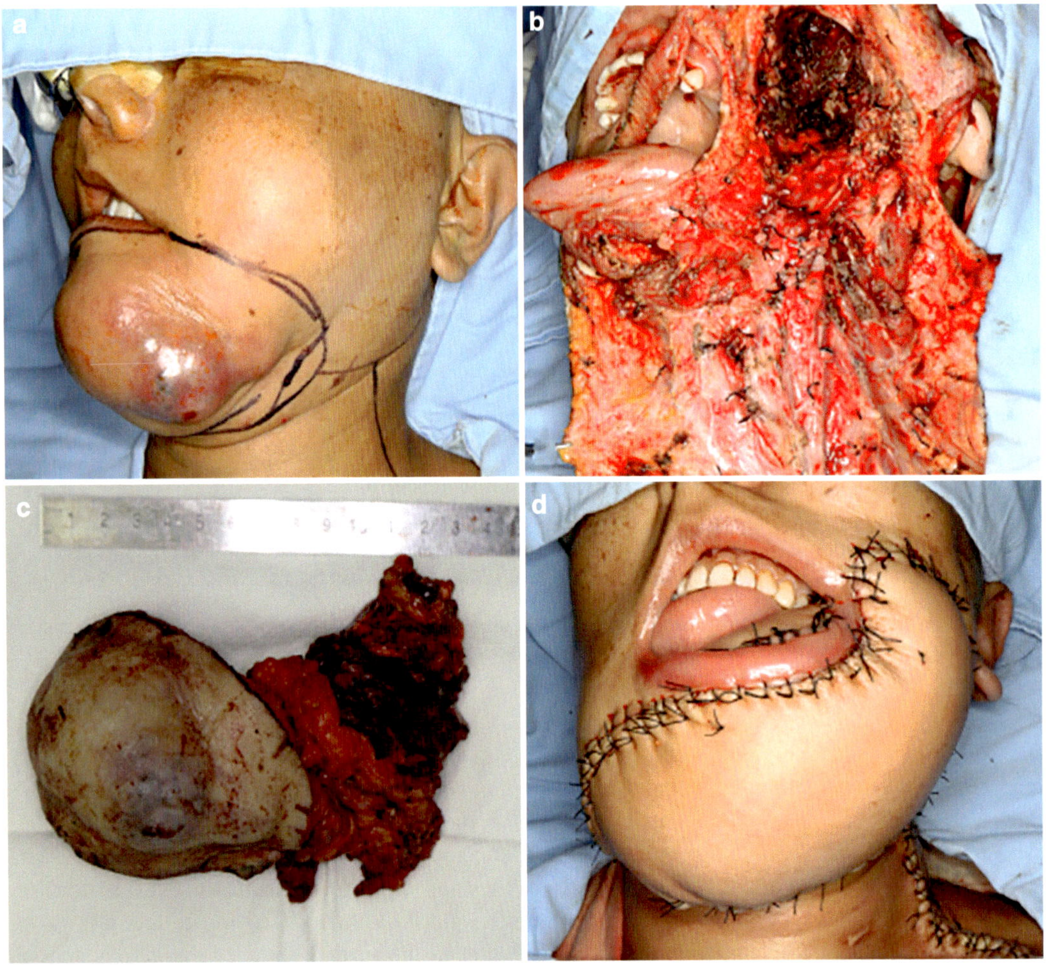

Fig. 29.12 (**a**) Incision design. (**b**) Large tissue defect after complete resection of the tumor. (**c**) Gross view of the tumor in vitro. (**d**) Anterolateral thigh flap for repair of the defect

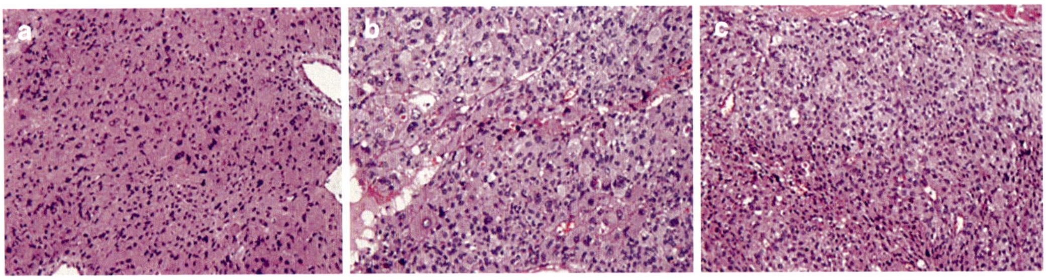

Fig. 29.13 (**a**) Cellular plasma of tumor cells, containing eosinophilic particles, nucleopytosis, obvious atypia, some intranuclear pseudo-inclusion bodies. (**b**) In some areas, the tumor cells are large, with cellular plasma, containing eosinophilic particles, vesicular nuclei, which may be multinuclear and have obvious atypia. (**c**) Relatively benign region of the lesion. The tumor cells and nuclei were uniform in size, with mild atypia (200×)

[Pathological Diagnosis] Malignant transformation of "mandibular" granular cell odontogenic tumor, ICD-O code: 9321/3.

[Follow-Up] The patient healed uneventfully. The postoperative follow-up exhibited good healing of flap with no special postoperative reaction in the operative area.

29.5 Key Points of Diagnosis and Treatment

The WHO defines odontogenic fibroma as "a benign odontogenic tumor of fibroblast origin, characterized by relatively mature collagen fibrous tissue and varying amounts of odontogenic epithelium, which may occur in the center of the jaw or in an extrasolar location." Central odontogenic fibroma (COF) is a rare odontogenic tumor, accounting for about 4–5% of all odontogenic tumors [2, 7, 9, 14]. COF clinically manifests as painless swelling, slow growth, and ultimately causes jawbone bone swelling. In addition, some patients may experience clinical symptoms such as increased tooth space, pain, and paresthesia due to tooth displacement, which are not common.

COF Imaging Characteristics Small COF radiographically presents as a well-circumscribed, unicapsular radioparent shadow, while large COF shows as scalloped or multicapsular radioparent shadow. Most of the lesions have sclerotic bone lines around them, and root resorption could be seen in the relevant teeth. It is often difficult to diagnose COF by imaging, especially when the lesion is associated with the crown of unerupted tooth. COF should be distinguished from odontogenous cyst. Kaffe and Buchner pointed out that most small tumors often appear as unicystic and tend to become polycystic during growth. In addition, root resorption is observed in 29 percent of cases. Although the maximum diameter of COF rarely exceeds 3 cm on imaging, many cases show invasive clinical and radiographic features, including cortical bone dilation with perforation, adjacent tooth displacement, and significant root resorption. Therefore, COF needs to be differentiated from other odontogenic tumors, such as odontogenic keratocyst, ameloblastoma, odontogenic myxoma, and odontogenic squamous cell tumor [6].

COF Pathological Characteristics Some scholars divided central odontogenic fibroma into two tissue types, simple COF (epithelial-poor type) and complex COF (epithelial-rich type) because of the great changes in its histopathological manifestations. Complex COF, also known as WHO type, is mainly different in its histological characteristics. The amount of remaining small, inactive odontogenic epithelium is an important evaluation indicator. The simple COF is composed of stellate reticular fibroblasts, sometimes with inconspicuous scattered calcifications in a background of fine collagen fibers and a large matrix. Complex or WHO type COF is usually composed of fibrous connective tissue between collagen fibers, with hypercellular feature, and residual odontogenic epithelium in the shape of long cords or isolated nests can be seen in the lesion, which can be used as the main component of the tumor. Calcification can be observed in some cases, such as bone, dentin, and cementoid material. Histopathological differential diagnosis includes adjacent enlarged dental sacs and odontogenic myxoma. In addition, Ikeshima and Utsunomiya et al. believe that the differential diagnosis of COF should include multiple fibrous tissue tumors, especially fibromyxoma and fibroproliferatory fibroma, as such lesions are associated with a significant recurrence rate, but the recurrence rate of COF is not high.

COF Treatment Now, the common treatment methods of COF are surgical excision and thorough curettage. If properly treated, COF has a less recurrence and good prognosis. Although COF may appear invasive on imaging, good prognosis can be achieved in most cases if conservative resection of the tumor is performed with adjacent tooth retained.

In rare cases, COF is composed of varying numbers of large granular cells, formerly known as "granular cell ameloblastoma" or "granular cell odontogenic fibroma." It is now defined as granular cell odontogenic fibroma (GCOT), which is considered as COF subtype and is one of the rarest odontogenic tumors in the jaw bone. GCOT has not yet been included in the 2017 World Health Organization (WHO) Classification of Odontogenic Tumors. GCOT is more common in middle-aged women, which often occurs in the posterior dental area of the mandible, and generally only occurs in the tooth bearing area of the jaw, which can be manifested as painless swelling. Radiographically, GCOT is mostly manifested as well-circumscribed radioparent shadow or mixed radioparent—radiopaque lesion. Extraosseous and granulosa cell odontogenic sarcomas have also been reported. Histopathological examination revealed that the tumor is composed of lamellar and lobular macroeosinophilic granulosa cells, interspersed with long, narrow cords or odontogenic epithelium islands. Occasionally, cementoid substances or dystrophic calcifications associated with granulosa cells can be observed. Differential diagnosis includes soft tissue granulosa cell tumor, ameloblastoma granulosa cell variation, and congenital gingival tumor. Most GCOT tumors are benign, with curettage as the effective treatment method. Nonetheless, close follow-up is indispensable.

POF Characteristics Peripheral odontogenic fibroma is also a rare benign ectodermal mesenchymal lesion that is clinically manifested as hard, painless, smoot-surfaced gingival nodules. A few POFs present as multifocal or diffuse lesions in the literature. POF mainly occurs in the buccal gingiva of the mandible, with incisor, cusp, and premolar as the most common sites. Patients are usually asymptomatic, while a few patients may have tooth displacement. Its clinical manifestations are indistinguishable from other proliferative lesions in the gingiva. Differential diagnosis should include peripheral giant cell granuloma, suppurative granuloma, focal fibroplasia of the gingiva, peripheral ossifying fibroma, peripheral ameloblastoma, and peripheral calcifying epithelial odontogenic tumor. POF is now considered to be a mucosal analogue of central odontogenic fibroma, which may exhibit similar pathological features to COF, including fibrous connective tissue matrix of varying densities and scattered odontogenic epithelial residue, sometimes with dentin, cementum, or osteoid calcification foci. In a few cases, granulosa cell changes and giant cell granulomatous regions can be observed in the connective tissue components. Soft tissue mass is seen on imaging, with calcification present in a few areas. COF generally does not involve deep bone tissue.

POF Treatment Local surgical resection is adopted for the treatment of peripheral odontogenic fibroma, which leads to good prognosis. Only a few cases of recurrence have been reported. Incomplete resection may be the main cause for recurrence. However, it is not easy to distinguish diseased connective tissue from normal connective tissue in most histopathologic sections, making it difficult to determine whether the tumor is completely removed based on the pathological section. In addition, the lesion located between the roots of the tooth is hard to completely resect, which is also an important cause for its recurrence. Therefore, complete surgical resection is vital to preventing recurrence, and postoperative long-term follow-up should also be conducted.

References

1. Daniels JS. Central odontogenic fibroma of mandible: a case report and review of the literature [J]. Oral Surg Oral Med Oral Pathol Oral Radiol Endod. 2004;98(3):295–300.
2. Gardner DG. Central odontogenic fibroma current concepts [J]. J Oral Pathol Med. 1996;25(10):556–61.
3. Daskala I, Kalyvas D, Kolokoudias M, et al. Central odontogenic fibroma of the mandible: a case report [J]. J Oral Sci. 2009;51(3):457–61.
4. Cicconetti A, Bartoli A, Tallarico M, et al. Central odontogenic fibroma interesting the maxillary sinus: a case report and literature survey [J]. Minerva Stomatol. 2006;55(4):229–39.
5. Günhan O, Erseven G, Ruacan S, et al. Odontogenic tumours: a series of 409 cases [J]. Aust Dent J. 1990;35(6):518–22.

6. Kaffe I, Buchner A. Radiologic features of central odontogenic fibroma [J]. Oral Surg Oral Med Oral Pathol. 1994;78(6):811–8.
7. Upadhyaya JD, Cohen DM, Islam MN, et al. Hybrid central odontogenic fibroma with giant cell granuloma like lesion: a report of three additional cases and review of the literature [J]. Head Neck Pathol. 2018;12(2):166–74.
8. Roza A, Sousa EM, Leite AA, et al. Central odontogenic fibroma: an international multicentric study of 62 cases [J]. Oral Surg Oral Med Oral Pathol Oral Radiol. 2020;131:549.
9. Sarode SC, Sarode GS, Vaidya K. Central granular cell odontogenic tumor: a systematic review [J]. J Oral Pathol Med. 2014;43(3):167–76.
10. Meer S, Altini M, Coleman H, et al. Central granular cell odontogenic tumor: immunohistochemistry and ultrastructure [J]. Am J Otolaryngol. 2004;25(1):73–8.
11. Rinaggio J, Cleveland D, Koshy R, et al. Peripheral granular cell odontogenic fibroma [J]. Oral Surg Oral Med Oral Pathol Oral Radiol Endod. 2007;104(5):676–9.
12. Piattelli A, Rubini C, Goteri G, et al. Central granular cell odontogenic tumour: report of the first malignant case and review of the literature [J]. Oral Oncol. 2003;39(1):78–82.
13. Atarbashi-Moghadam S, Saebnoori H, Shamloo N, et al. Granular cell odontogenic tumor, an extremely rare case report [J]. J Dent (Shiraz). 2019;20(3):220–3.
14. Buchner A, Merrell PW, Carpenter WM. Relative frequency of central odontogenic tumors: a study of 1, 088 cases from Northern California and comparison to studies from other parts of the world [J]. J Oral Maxillofac Surg. 2006;64(9):1343–52.
15. Daley TD, Wysocki GP. Peripheral odontogenic fibroma [J]. Oral Surg Oral Med Oral Pathol. 1994;78(3):329–36.
16. Weber A, van Heerden WF, Ligthelm AJ, et al. Diffuse peripheral odontogenic fibroma: report of 3 cases [J]. J Oral Pathol Med. 1992;21(2):82–4.
17. Baiju CS, Rohatgi S. Peripheral odontogenic fibroma: a case report and review [J]. J Indian Soc Periodontol. 2011;15(3):273–5.

Part X

Malignant Odontogenic Tumors

Ameloblastic Carcinoma

30

Jing Song Hou, Hui Shan Ong, Zhen Tian, Lin Zhu, and Xing Zhou Qu

30.1 Introduction

Ameloblastic carcinoma is a rare malignant odontogenic tumor, accounting for 1–3% of all maxillary tumors and cysts [1–4]. It mainly occurs in the mandible, with an aggressive clinical course and poor prognosis. The clinical manifestations can be cystic lesion with benign clinical features, while larger mass presented as ulcer with obvious bone resorption, and mobile teeth or loss of partial teeth, accompanied by regional lymph node metastasis or distant metastasis [5–21]. Ameloblastic carcinoma has atypical clinical features, resulting in a high rate of clinical misdiagnosis [10–21]. The treatment for ameloblastic carcinoma is radical resection with simultaneous regional lymph node dissection [15–23]. Moreover, due to its high relapse rate, close and regular follow-up is prerequisite.

J. S. Hou (✉)
Hospital of Stomatology, Guanghua College of Stomatology, Sun Yat-sen University, Guangdong, China
e-mail: houjs@mail.sysu.edu.cn

H. S. Ong · Z. Tian · X. Z. Qu
Department of Oral Maxillofacial-Head & Neck Oncology, Shanghai Ninth People's Hospital, Shanghai Jiao Tong University School of Medicine, Shanghai, China

L. Zhu
Department of Radiology, Ninth People's Hospital Affiliated to Shanghai Jiao Tong University, Shanghai, China

30.2 Case 63

A 49-year-old gentleman suffered from a painless but gradually growing mass in his left mandible for 1 year.

[History of Present Illness] The patient happened to see a hard bean-size mass on the buccal side of the left mandibular bone 1 year ago. The mass grew gradually but with no discomfort symptoms such as tooth pain and lower lip numbness. Without seeking for treatment, the mass grew gradually, and then developed into an egg-size swelling at the buccal side.

[Specialty Examination] The face was asymmetrical, obviously bone protrusion over the left mandibular body, with a size of about 4.0 cm × 3.0 cm. The overlying facial skin was intact with normal color and no obvious ulceration. The lesion was hard upon palpation, and was well circumscribed with no obvious adhesion with the skin. There was no abnormality in mouth opening range and mouth opening pattern. Intraoral examination revealed permanent dentition, crowded mandibular dentition. There was buccal expansion over the 33–37; however, the overlying mucosa was intact with no obvious rupture, sinus tract, or fistula. The buccal sulcus was shallow. 34–36 teeth were tender to percussion and I° mobile. The 31–33 had mild expansion over the lingual plate, 46 was having dental cav-

Y. He (ed.), *Inflammatory and Neoplastic Diseases of Craniofacial Bones*,
https://doi.org/10.1007/978-981-97-4155-7_30

ity but not mobile and not tender to percussion (−) (Fig. 30.1a, b). Multiple small lymph nodes were palpable in the submandibular (Level Ib) and Level II bilaterally. The palpable lymph nodes were not tender to palpation, they are otherwise not clinically significant.

[Auxiliary Examination]

1. Panoramic radiographs suggested a hypodense bone destruction (radiolucency) in the symphysis and bilateral parasymphysis and mandibular body, in which the margins were not well circumscribed (Fig. 30.1c).
2. Maxillofacial enhanced CT scan suggested a hypodense bone destruction in the symphysis and bilateral parasymphysis and mandibular body. CT images suggested the mass protruding from the left buccal wall with center soft tissue density. The CT value of the mass was 37HU before enhanced and 82HU after enhanced, the CT value was 100HU at delayed phase of contrast enhanced CT. The CT images revealed multilocular lesion with cortical destruction (thinning and discontinuation of cortical bone) and bony partition within the nonmineralized radiolucent lesion. The margin of the lesion was poorly demarcated with periosteal reaction,; however, there was no sign of root resorption. The mucosa of the maxillary and ethmoid sinuses grew thickened bilaterally. No significant enlarged cervical lymph nodes were seen (Fig. 30.2).

[Preliminary Diagnosis] Mass of the left mandible, malignancy need to be ruled out.

[Treatment] "Radical resection of mandibular lesion included segmental mandibulectomy with simultaneous fibula flap reconstruction and tracheostomy" was performed under general anesthesia. An incision was made at 1–2 cm from the lower margin of the mandible, and the flap was elevated to expose the neoplastic cells which had infiltrated the cortical bone of the left mandibular body. Segmental mandibulectomy as per preoperative virtual planning (using the osteotomy

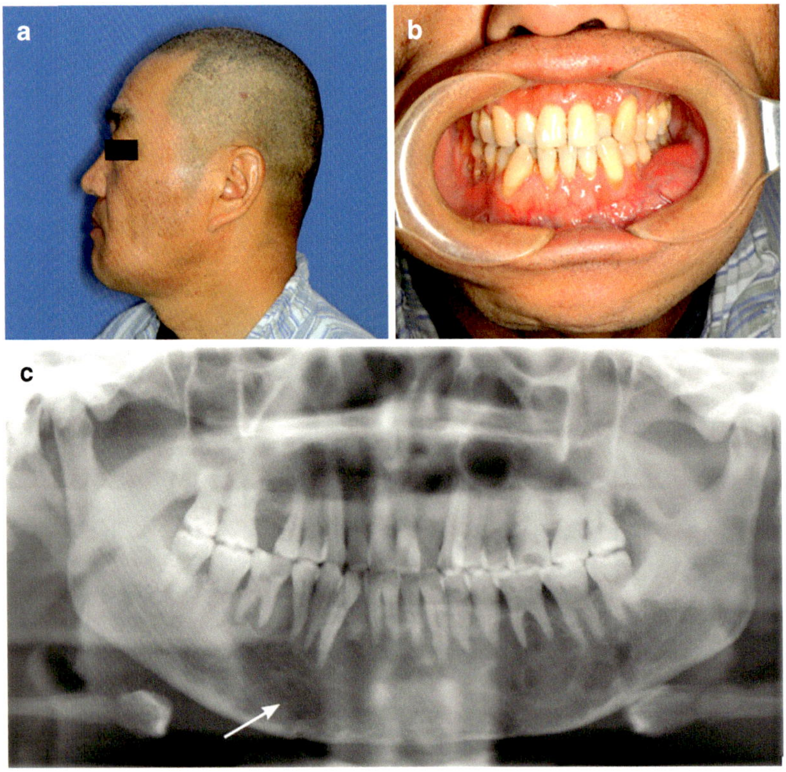

Fig. 30.1 (**a**) Left mandibular distension. (**b**) Intraoral mucosa intact, left mandibular distension. (**c**) Hypodense bone destruction in the mandible bilaterally at the chin and mandibular body, not well circumscribed (preoperative)

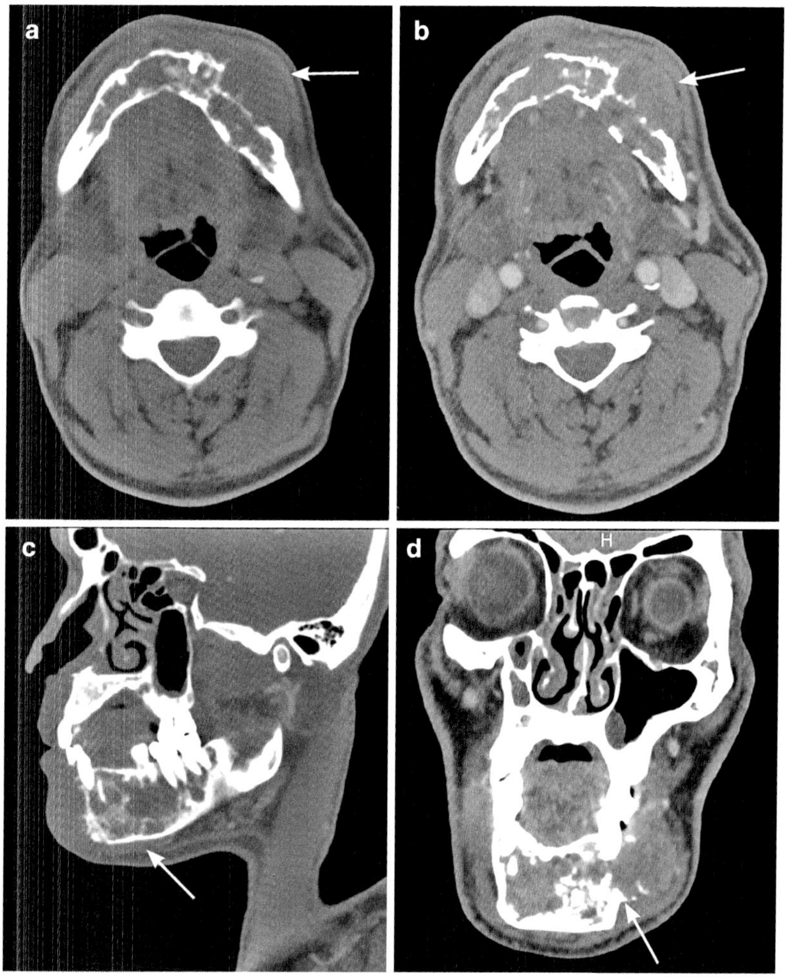

Fig. 30.2 (**a**) The axial and coronal views of CT images suggested a hypodense bony destruction of symphysis and bilaterally mandibular body and parasymphysis. Intraosseous lesion presented as soft tissue density (white arrow), protruding toward the left cheek with a CT value of 37 Hu. (**b**) The axial and coronal views of enhanced CT images showed that the lesion was significantly enhanced, with a CT value of 82 Hu. (**c**, **d**) The coronal and sagittal view of enhanced CT images: Bone partition was observed within the lesion, with no significant dental root absorption. Yet, presented with thinning and discontinuity of the cortical bone

guide). Region of the mandible osteotomy started from the left sigmoid notch and ended distally to 47. Radical resection of the mandibular lesion and bilateral submandibular region lymph nodes dissection were done and sent for frozen section pathological examination. The results showed the odontogenic epithelial islands and cords of ameloblastoma, hypercellular and pleomorphic changes of the odontogenic epithelial nest suggested malignancy could not be excluded. The left vascularized fibula flap was routinely harvested. The fibula was shaped as per preoperative virtual design to restore the continuity of the mandible. Routine microvascular anastomosis of the peroneal artery and vein to the right facial artery and vein. The skin paddle was trimmed to repair the intraoral defects such as floor of mouth and buccal mucosal. The wound was rinsed and thoroughly hemostatic, negative pressure drainage tube was placed and complete with wound closure (Fig. 30.3).

[Pathological Examination] Gross pathological examination revealed a mandible with surrounding soft tissues and teeth, 10 cm × 9 cm × 7 cm in size. A solid mass was seen in the left mandible body, 5 cm × 4 cm × 3 cm in size, grayish white, moderate hardness, and well circumscribed. The microscopic examination showed that the tumor was composed of both benign and malignant regions. In the benign region, the neoplastic cell nests were in network-like arrangement, with columnar cells with hyperchromatic nuclei at basal layer, exhibiting

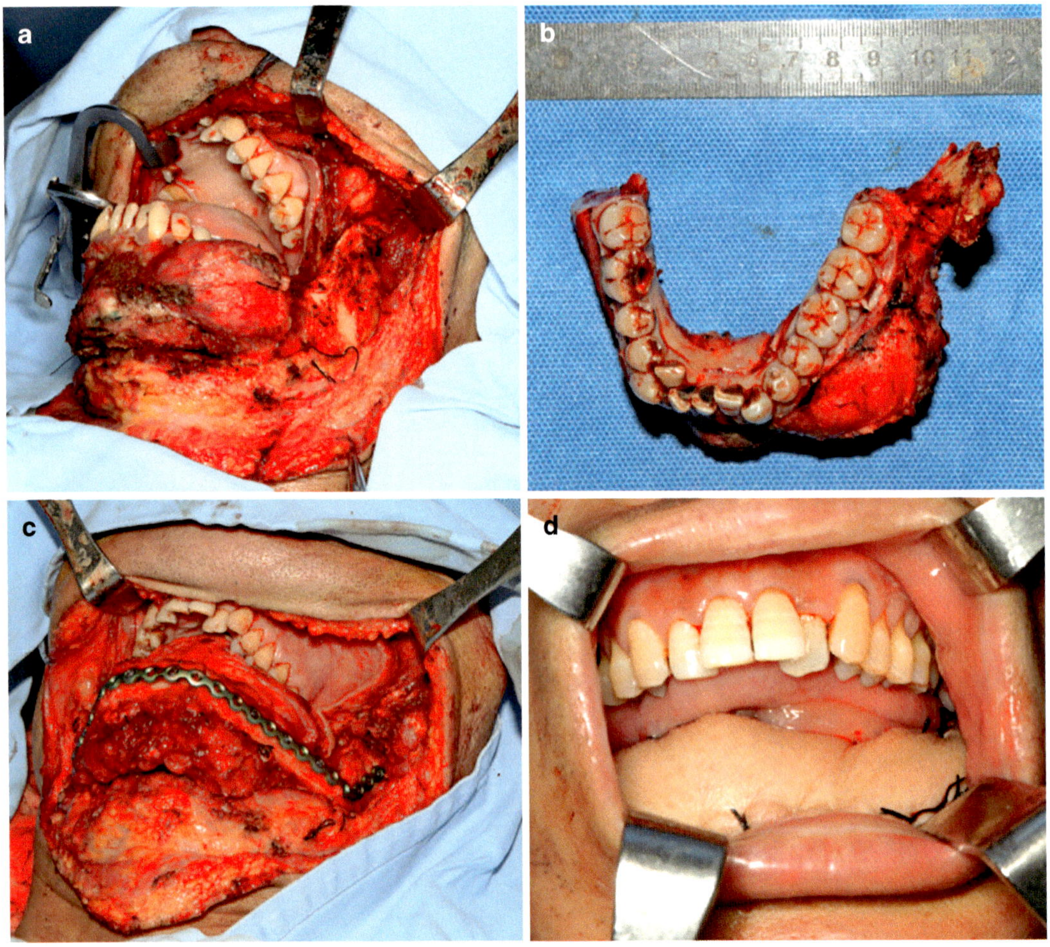

Fig. 30.3 (**a**) The mandibular body lesion was exposed using the submental-cervical crest horizontal incision and intraoral buccal sulcus incision. (**b**) Radical resection of tumor with segmental mandibulectomy. (**c**) Fibula osseocutaneous flap restored the continuity of the mandible. (**d**) Skin paddle to repair of intraoral mucosal defect

peripheral palisading, squamous differentiation, and sparse arrangement of central cells, supporting the diagnosis of ameloblastoma. The malignant region presented with diverse cell morphologies, nucleoplasm vacuolization, pleomorphism of nuclear cell, and stellate reticulum-like cells presented with granular eosinophilic cytoplasm. The mesenchymal cells were also accompanied with atypical hyperplasia. The tumor cells invaded the cortical bone and adjacent dental alveolar nerves (Fig. 30.4).

[Pathological Diagnosis] Odontogenic carcinoma of the "mandible," malignant ameloblastoma. Ameloblastic carcinoma, with ICD-O code: 9270/3.

[Follow-Up] The patient healed uneventfully. The postoperative 6-month follow-up exhibited no obvious postoperative reaction and ruled out tumor relapse, with satisfactory aesthetic and functional mandibular reconstruction (Fig. 30.5).

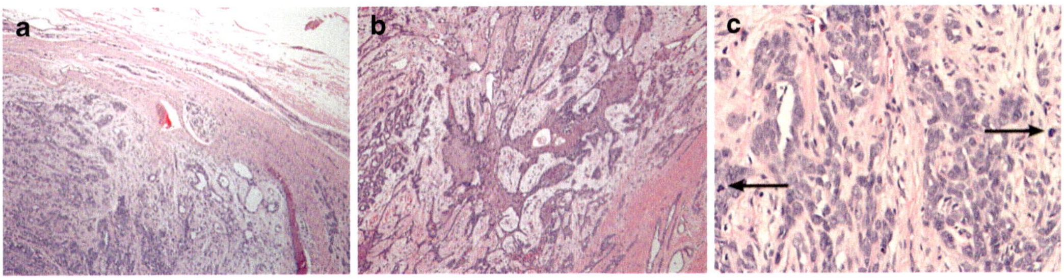

Fig. 30.4 (**a**) The tumor destroyed the bone cortex and invaded the inferior dental nerves (10×). (**b**) The benign tumor region showed ameloblastoma, with squamous differentiation of central stellate reticulum cells (100×). (**c**) The malignant tumor region presented with cell pleomorphism, with mitotic signs visible (arrow) (400×)

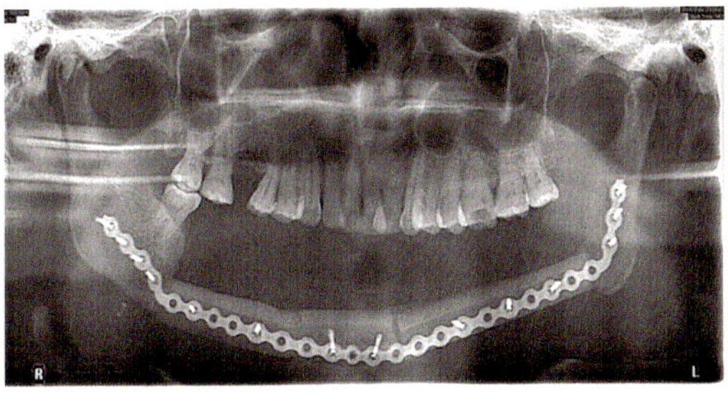

Fig. 30.5 Postoperative changes of the mandible, fibula free flap in restoring the mandibular shape and function. Criteria for functional mandibular reconstruction such as jaw continuity, facial symmetry, stable occlusion, and TMJ within condylar fossa were fulfilled

30.3 Key Points of Diagnosis and Treatment

Ameloblastic carcinoma was first described in 1974 by Shafer et al. The World Health Organization (WHO) classification for Head and Neck tumors (year 2005 version), ameloblastic carcinoma is categorized into three main subtypes; primary type, secondary type (dedifferentiated) intraosseous and secondary type (dedifferentiated) peripheral [24]. Primary tumors arise de novo, whereas the secondary type represents malignant transformation of a preexisting well-differentiated ameloblastoma or odontogenic cyst. In the updated World Health Organization (WHO) classification of odontogenic tumors (version 2017), ameloblastic carcinoma was defined as a rare odontogenic malignancy that contained both the histological features of well-differentiated ameloblastoma and histologic evidence of malignancy such as cellular atypia of ameloblastic carcinoma, regardless of the presence of metastasis. The distinction between ameloblastic carcinoma and malignant ameloblastoma are subjected to histological and clinical manifestations. Well-differentiated benign histology of ameloblastoma in both primary and metastatic sites are defined as malignant ameloblastoma. Ameloblastic carcinoma exhibited with cytological atypia. In summary, the diagnosis would be judged by the clinical behaviors rather than histological manifestations.

Ameloblastic carcinomas account for approximately 2% of odontogenic tumors [25]. Literature reviews show that the median age for ameloblastic carcinoma is 44 years old with the male-to-female gender ratio at1.75:1.The lesion is predilected at mandible in comparing to maxilla at the ratio of 2.14:1. Overall, the 5-year survival rate is approximately 69.1%.

Clinical Manifestations Ameloblastic carcinoma has diverse clinical manifestations. Swollen jaw is the most common symptom, invaded into mandibular ramus and condylar process. The maxilla ameloblastic carcinoma can be confined to the hard palate, and may also invade into the maxillary sinus, nasal floor, and orbital floor. Secondly, it can be manifested as swelling, pain, limited mouth opening, swollen gum, ulceration, and mobile teeth. In severe cases, subject can be presented with eye protrusion, fixed eye ball, diplopia and nasal congestion, nasal discharge, or loss of sense of smell. Compared with ameloblastoma, ameloblastic carcinoma exhibits as aggressive clinical features, such as rapid growth, perforation of the bone cortex, pain, and sensory disturbances. The metastasis rate of ameloblastic carcinoma is about 15%, mainly to regional lymph nodes. Lung is the common site of distant metastasis for ameloblastic carcinoma, but it can also spread to ribs, spine bone, skull, chest wall, small intestine, etc. The presence of distant metastasis suggested of poor prognosis.

Pathological Characteristics Ameloblastic carcinoma is a rare disease with atypical clinical features, so clinical diagnosis is difficult and the final diagnosis should be based on postoperative pathological diagnosis. Microscopic observation shows that ameloblastic carcinoma has the histological features of a typical ameloblastoma, i.e., the tumor masses or strips are composed of peripherally fenestrated columnar cells and central stellate reticulocytes; in addition, there are obvious cytological malignant manifestations, i.e., absence of stellate reticulum-like areas and replaced by malignancy features such as poorly differentiated fusiform epithelial cells, ovoid or short fusiform basal cells, with pleomorphic nuclei, hyperchromatism, deep staining, increased mitotic index, necrosis and calcification foci, and nerve and vascular invasion. A high proportion of p53, p63, and Ki-67 in the neoplastic cells of ameloblastic carcinoma shows significant cell proliferation activity, which could be distinguished from ameloblastoma.

Imaging Characteristics Ameloblastic carcinoma and ameloblastoma share the same X-ray manifestations with mostly indistinct transmissive lesions and cortical destruction; compared with other intraosseous malignancies, ameloblastic carcinoma has no specific radiographic and CT scan presentation. Case reports suggest that positron emission tomography (PET-CT) can be used to differentiate ameloblastic carcinoma from benign ameloblastoma; however, this needs to be verified by further studies.

Differential Diagnosis In the diagnosis of ameloblastic carcinoma, the differential diagnosis includes, but is not limited to, ameloblastoma, odontogenic keratocyst, primary intraosseous carcinoma, odontogenic sarcoma, ameloblastic carcinosarcoma, mucinous epidermoid carcinoma, and jaw metastatic carcinoma.

Treatment Now, there is a lack of consensus-based guideline for managing ameloblastic carcinoma. The preferred treatment is radical resection with extended surgical margin. Owing to its aggressive invasion behavior, the tumor should be resected at the normal tissue, and the literature suggests osteotomy performed at 2–3 cm safe margin en bloc resection along with cervical lymph node dissection, simultaneous jaw reconstruction will be optional. The available literature reports that radiotherapy has little effect on preventing relapse and metastasis of ameloblastic carcinoma, and McClary et al. [1] reported no statistical difference in relapse rate between subjects who only receive surgery for ameloblastic carcinoma compared to those who received postoperative adjuvant radiotherapy. However, radiotherapy is still recommended for unresectable lesion, positive surgical margin or presented with distance metastasis. No evidence has proved that chemotherapies are effective in managing ameloblastic carcinoma. Chemotherapies such as cyclophosphamide, carboplatin, paclitaxel, and 5-fluorouracil have not been reported in the literature to show satisfactory therapeutic effects. BRAF V600E inhibitors (such as Vemurafenib) and immune checkpoint inhibitors are expected targeted therapy in managing ameloblastic carcinoma; however, it is within clinical trials stage and have not yet been approved for clinical treatment. Ameloblastic carcinoma has a significant tendency to relapse after treatment. Multiple relapses and histological findings of clear cells suggest a poor prognosis, requiring long-term follow-up.

References

1. McClary AC, West RB, McClary AC, et al. Ameloblastoma: a clinical review and trends in management [J]. Eur Arch Otorrinolaringol. 2016;273(7):1649–61.
2. Benlyazid A, Lacroix-Triki M, Aziza R, et al. Ameloblastic carcinoma of the maxilla: case report and review of the literature [J]. Oral Surg Oral Med Oral Pathol Oral Radiol Endod. 2007;104(6):e17–24.

3. Routray S, Majumdar S. Ameloblastic carcinoma: sometimes a challenge [J]. J Oral Maxillofac Pathol. 2012;16(1):156–8.
4. Ganjre AP, Sarode G, Sarode S. Molecular characterization of metastasizing ameloblastoma: a comprehensive review [J]. J Cancer Res Ther. 2019;15(3):455–62.
5. Fujita S, Anami M, Satoh N, et al. Cytopathologic features of secondary peripheral ameloblastic carcinoma: a case report [J]. Diagn Cytopathol. 2011;39(5):354–8.
6. Dutta M, Kundu S, Bera H, et al. Ameloblastic carcinoma of mandible: facts and dilemmas [J]. Tumori. 2014;100(5):e189–96.
7. Gawande PD, Khande K, Agrawal G, et al. Ameloblastic carcinoma: a rare malignant tumour in maxillofacial region [J]. J Maxillofac Oral Surg. 2017;16(3):377–81.
8. Kikuta S, Furukawa Y, Hino K, et al. Huge ameloblastic carcinoma of the mandible with metastases treated in several different ways [J]. Br J Oral Maxillofac Surg. 2019;57(2):182–4.
9. Yoon HJ, Hong SP, Lee JI, et al. Ameloblastic carcinoma: an analysis of 6 cases with review of the literature [J]. Oral Surg Oral Med Oral Pathol Oral Radiol Endod. 2009;108(6):904–13.
10. Gunaratne DA, Coleman HG, Lim L, et al. Ameloblastic carcinoma [J]. Am J Case Rep. 2015;16:415–9.
11. Hu JA. Pathological diagnosis of odontogenic malignant tumor [J]. Chinese J Pract Stomatol. 2010;3(12):705–8.
12. Coulibaly B, Le Hemon A, Sorbier C, et al. Ameloblastic carcinoma: primary or secondary? [J]. Ann Pathol. 2009;29(1):28–31.
13. Matsuzaki H, Katase N, Hara M, et al. Ameloblastic carcinoma: a case report with radiological features of computed tomography and magnetic resonance imaging and positron emission tomography [J]. Oral Surg Oral Med Oral Pathol Oral Radiol Endod. 2011;112(1):e40–7.
14. Makiguchi T, Yokoo S, Miyazaki H, et al. Treatment strategy of a huge ameloblastic carcinoma [J]. J Craniofac Surg. 2013;24(1):287–90.
15. Kar IB, Subramanyam RV, Mishra N, et al. Ameloblastic carcinoma: a clinicopathologic dilemma — report of two cases with total review of literature from 1984 to 2012 [J]. Ann Maxillofac Surg. 2014;4(1):70–7.
16. Slootweg PJ, Muller H. Malignant ameloblastoma or ameloblastic carcinoma [J]. Oral Surg Oral Med Oral Pathol. 1984;57(2):168–76.
17. Li J, Du H, Li P, et al. Ameloblastic carcinoma: an analysis of 12 cases with a review of the literature [J]. Oncol Lett. 2014;8(2):914–20.
18. Roy Chowdhury SK, Ramen S, Chattopadhyay PK, et al. Ameloblastic carcinoma of the mandible [J]. J Maxillofac Oral Surg. 2010;9(2):198–201.
19. Angiero F, Borloni R, Macchi M, et al. Ameloblastic carcinoma of the maxillary sinus [J]. Anticancer Res. 2008;28(6B):3847–54.
20. Kallianpur S, Jadwani S, Misra B, et al. Ameloblastic carcinoma of the mandible: report of a case and review [J]. J Oral Maxillofac Pathol. 2014;18(Suppl 1):S96–S102.
21. Saluja TS, Hosalkar R. Reconnoitre ameloblastic carcinoma: a prognostic update [J]. Oral Oncol. 2018;77:118–24.
22. Brown NA, Betz BL. Ameloblastoma: a review of recent molecular pathogenetic discoveries [J]. Biomark Cancer. 2015;7(Suppl 2):19–24.
23. Kennedy WR, Werning JW, Kaye FJ, et al. Treatment of ameloblastoma and ameloblastic carcinoma with radiotherapy [J]. Eur Arch Otorrinolaringol. 2016;273(10):3293–7.
24. Sciubba JJ, Eversole LR, Slootweg PJ. Odontogenic/ameloblastic carcinomas. In: Barnes L, Eveson JW, Reichart P, et al., editors. World Health Organization classification of tumours pathology and genetics of head and neck tumours. Lyon: IARC Press; 2005. p. 287–9.
25. Gunaratne DA, Coleman HG, Lim L, Morgan GJ. Ameloblastic Carcinoma. Am J Case Rep. 2015;16:415–9.

31 Odontogenic Ghost Cell Carcinoma

Jing Song Hou, Hui Shan Ong, Zhen Tian, Lin Zhu, and Min Ruan

31.1 Introduction

Ghost cell odontogenic carcinoma (GCOC) is a rare odontogenic tumor with both features of calcifying odontogenic cyst containing unequal quantities of ghost cells and malignant cytologic features with unpredictable biological behaviors and difficult clinical and imaging diagnosis [1–6]. Radical resection with a negative surgical margin is the pivotal treatment, nevertheless more studies are required to verify the benefit of postoperative adjuvant therapy [7–13]. As GCOC has a high rate of local relapse, thereby long-term postoperative follow-up is recommended.

J. S. Hou (✉)
Hospital of Stomatology, Guanghua College of Stomatology, Sun Yat-sen University, Guangdong, China
e-mail: houjs@mail.sysu.edu.cn

H. S. Ong · Z. Tian · M. Ruan
Department of Oral Maxillofacial-Head & Neck Oncology, Shanghai Ninth People's Hospital, Shanghai Jiao Tong University School of Medicine, Shanghai, China

L. Zhu
Department of Radiology, Ninth People's Hospital Affiliated to Shanghai Jiao Tong University, Shanghai, China

31.2 Case 64

A 61-year-old gentleman suffered from a relapse of mandibular mass for 1 year after incomplete surgery at other hospital.

[History of Present Illness] A year ago, the patient was diagnosed as having gingival mass in other hospital and underwent marginal mandibulectomy. Postoperative pathology findings revealed mandibular ameloblastoma with positive surgical margins. One month ago, he complained a walnut-size swelling over the chin, with moderate hardness and average mobility. But, the mass expanded rapidly within a month, about 8 cm in diameter. Their pathological consultations reported gingival basaloid squamous cell carcinoma; however, our oral pathology consultants revised the pathological slides and reported ghost cell odontogenic carcinoma.

[Specialty Examination] An obvious protruding swelling was seen in the chin, about 8.0 cm × 5.0 cm × 5.0 cm in size, moderate hardness, well circumscribed, poor mobility, local skin redness, normal high skin temperature, no obvious ulcer, tenderness, or fluctuation. The mouth opening was normal, the intraoral mucosa was normal, and the lower anterior teeth were extracted during previous surgical resection. Submandibular and submental lymph nodes were palpable with moderate consistency and tender upon palpation (Fig. 31.1a, b).

Y. He (ed.), *Inflammatory and Neoplastic Diseases of Craniofacial Bones*,
https://doi.org/10.1007/978-981-97-4155-7_31

[Auxiliary Examination]

1. Panoramic radiographs suggested a bony destruction in the symphysis and parasymphysis of the mandible and occupied by hypodense soft tissue lesion extended beyond the lower border of mandible (Fig. 31.1c).
2. Maxillofacial enhanced CT scan suggested a mandibular bony destruction crossing midline, the soft tissue mass within the bony destruction area extended into the mouth floor and submental region with a size of about 6.7 cm × 6.3 cm; soft tissue mass invaded into the overlying skin as per subcutaneous fatty tissue layer is not visible, with a CT value of 24 Hu. Heterogeneous enhancement occurred after enhancement, with a CT value of 50 Hu in the arterial phase and a CT value of 66 Hu in the venous phase (Fig. 31.2).

[Preliminary Diagnosis] Relapse of mandibular mass after incomplete surgical resection.

[Treatment] Segmental mandibulectomy with radical resection of surrounding soft tissue in ensuring a 1 cm surgical margin. Radical resection resulting in large soft tissue defect and a segment of bony defect. The reconstruction planning was Anterior Lateral Tight Flap and the mandibular continuity was maintained using simple titanium plate. **Delayed bone flap reconstruction was planned.**

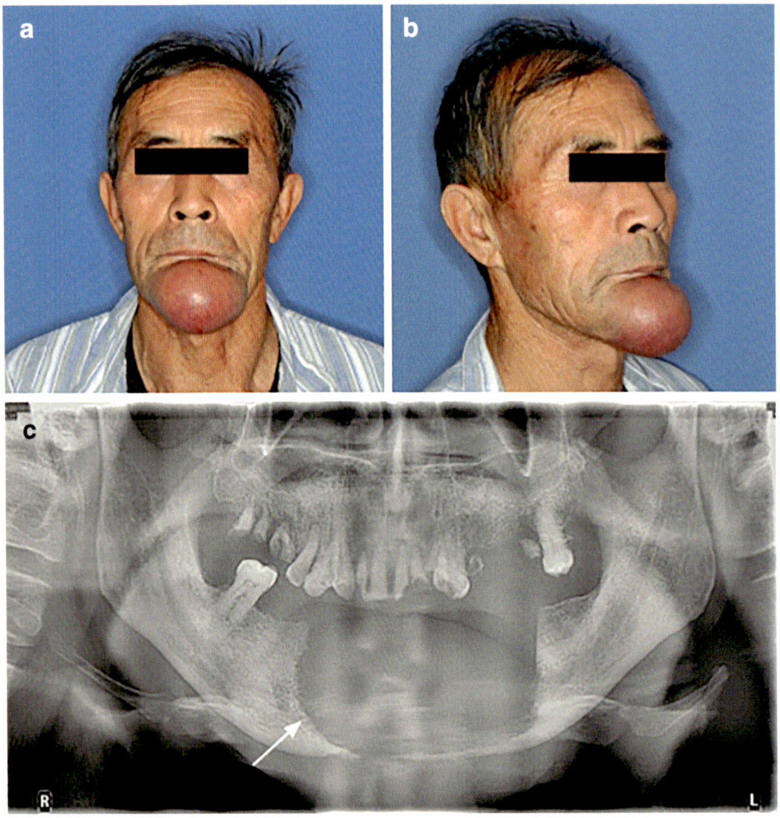

Fig. 31.1 (**a**, **b**) Prominent protruding mass in the chin, approximately 8.0 cm × 5.0 cm × 5.0 cm, with local skin redness and no obvious ulcer. (**c**) Panoramic radiographs suggested a bony destruction in the symphysis and parasymphysis of the mandible and occupied by hypodense soft tissue lesion extended beyond the lower border of mandible

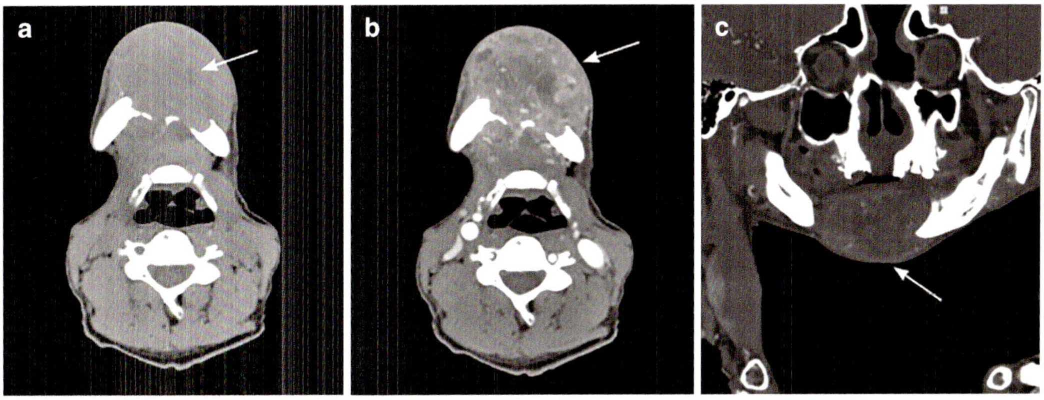

Fig. 31.2 (**a**) CT axial plus coronal scan manifested the destruction of the mandibular body and the extent of the mass, with linear bone ridge visible within the mass. (**b**) Enhanced CT axial plus coronal scan: heterogeneous enhancement of the mass. (**c**) Enhanced CT coronal scan: the mass extended beyond the lower border of mandible

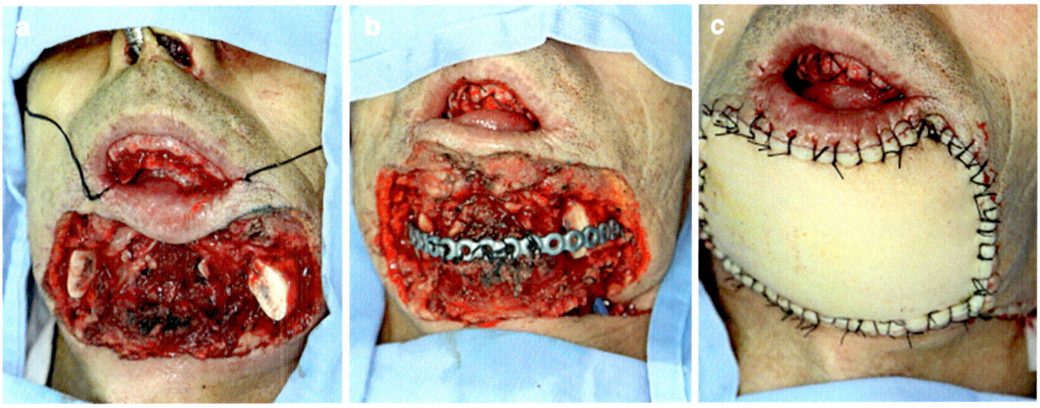

Fig. 31.3 (**a**) Surgical defect after radical resection of mandible and neoplastic mass. (**b**) Reconstructed titanium plate to restore mandibular continuity. (**c**) Anterolateral thigh flap was wrapped around the reconstructed titanium plate to repair mandibular defect

Upon surgical resection, an incision was designed at the normal tissue which is 1–1.5 cm away from the mandibular mass. Vermillion border of the lower lip was retained, the mandible was segmented at the 38 and 48 distally along with part of mouth floor.

The mass and mandible were radically resected, and the surgical margin and submandibular lymph nodes were taken and sent for intraoperative frozen pathology examination. Intraoperative frozen section reported as the "mandibular mass," a relapse of ghost cell odontogenic carcinoma with negative surgical margin. The left anterolateral thigh flap was prepared, and vascular anastomosis was performed with the superior thyroid artery and external jugular vein respectively. The flap was reshaped and wrapped around the reconstructed titanium plate to repair the chin defect. After thorough hemostatic control, the negative pressure drainage tube was indwelled, and the wound was closed in layers with sutures (Fig. 31.3).

[Pathological Examination] Gross pathological examination revealed the skin tissue 11 cm × 7 cm × 7.5 cm, with an expanded mass. There was a dark red solid mass, 7 cm × 7 cm × 6.8 cm in size, with hard consistency accompanied by internal hemorrhage. The microscopic examination showed that basal cells were densely arranged in nests or patches. The peripheral cells of some nests were arranged in

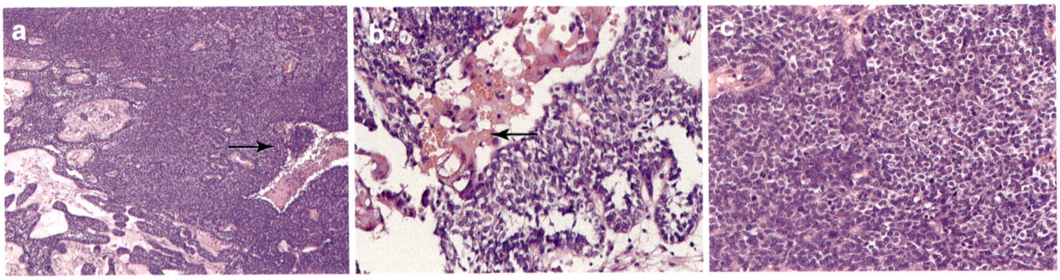

Fig. 31.4 (**a**) Tumor cells grew in nests and patches, with local necrosis (arrow) (100×). (**b**) A few ghost cells with missing nuclei could be observed (400×). (**c**) Increased nucleo-plasma ratio of tumor, obvious heteromorphism, and visible mitosis (400×)

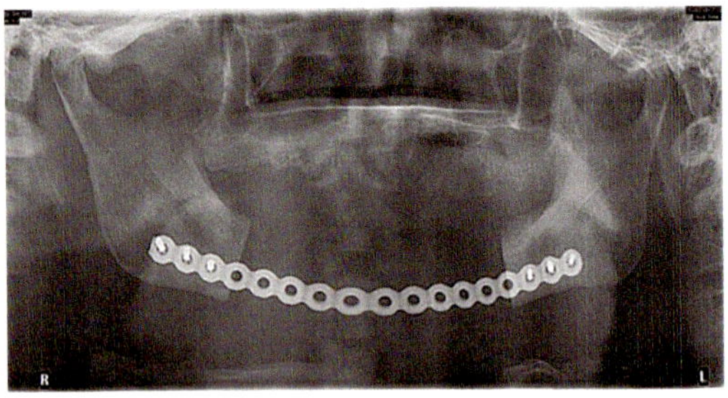

Fig. 31.5 Postoperative changes of the mandible, bone defects were reconstructed with simple titanium plate, bilateral condyle remained within the glenoid fossa

order while the central cells were sparsely arranged. The neoplastic cells were significantly heteromorphic, with mitosis and necrosis. A small number of ghost cells with red cytoplasm and missing nuclei can be seen locally (Fig. 31.4).

[Pathological Diagnosis] Ghost cell odontogenic carcinoma of the mandible, ICD-O code: 9302/3.

[Follow-Up] The patient healed uneventfully after the operation. The postoperative 6-month follow-up exhibited no tumor relapse, no adverse reactions such as titanium plate exposure or fracture. Range of mouth opening was normal without deviation (Fig. 31.5).

31.3 Key Points of Diagnosis and Treatment

Ghost cell odontogenic carcinoma (GCOC) is a rare odontogenic tumor, accounting for about 0.37–2.1% of odontogenic tumors and 3% of all jaw ghost cell lesions [1–8]. It has both features of calcifying odontogenic cyst containing unequal quantities of ghost cells and malignant cytologic features. GCOC can arise de novo or malignancy transformation from a preexisting calcifying odontogenic cyst (COC) or dentinogenic ghost cell tumor (DGCT).

The first case of GCOC was reported by Gorlin et al. in 1962. GCOC is an exceptional rare malignant odontogenic neoplasm with a significant aggressive behavior with high rate of local relapse. It is gender predilection with male–female ratio of 3.2:1. It is more frequent in the maxilla than in the mandible (2.1:1), with a mean age of about 40 years, and a 5-year survival rate of about 73%.

Clinical Manifestations GCOC mostly presents as painless swollen jaw, which can progress slowly or appear as rapid destructive growth, with pain for a few cases. Some patients may also suffer local sensory abnormalities, tooth loss, and mucosal ulcers. Distant metastases may occur, hardly presented with cervical lymph node metastases.

Imaging Characteristics GCOC lacks of characteristic imaging features and presents as translucent areas with clear or indistinct margins, which may be unicystic or multicystic, with radiolucent masses inside, mostly with root displacement and varying degrees of bone destruction, and rarely with dental root resorption.

Pathological Characteristics Gross pathological observation indicates that GCOC is solid or cystic, with a hard solid nature and a yellowish gray profile. The cutting section is gritty.

Microscopic observation reveals the presence of epithelial components with malignant features and calcifying odontogenic cyst separately or mixed together. The neoplastic cells are small round undifferentiated basal cells, with vesicular nuclei in larger cells. The neoplastic cells are arranged in clusters or cords, while their peripheral cells are arranged in a fenestrated pattern, with necrosis visible in the center and localized calcification. Many ghost cells may appear between cells or emerge in a large number of necrotic tissues in clusters. Ghost cells are round or ovoid microscopically, with red staining of the cytoplasm, disappearance of the nucleus without coloration, and hollow bright area in the nucleus. The interstitium is fibrous connective tissue that maybehyalineormucinous.Immunohistochemical staining shows strong positive keratin, positive P53, and negative vimentin, junctional protein, SMA and CD34. In addition, the expression of Ki-67 and MMP-9 is considered to be related to the proliferation, invasion, and poor prognosis of GCOC.

Differential Diagnosis The diagnosis of GCOC is supported by the histopathology presentation rather than clinical symptoms or radioimaging alone. The differential diagnosis is not limited to COC, DGCT, ameloblastic carcinoma, primary jaw sarcoma, and jaw metastatic carcinoma.

Treatment GCOC patients who received local curettage alone show a higher rate of local relapse. Studies reveal a relapse rate of 56.2% during the first 3 months to 7 years. Most scholars agreed that radical resection with negative surgical margins must be adopted for GCOC, that is, extended maxillectomy for maxilla and segmental mandibulectomy or total mandibulectomy for mandible. The need for sequential postoperative adjuvant therapy such as radiation and/or chemotherapy remains controversial. So far, no studies have proved that radiotherapy and chemotherapy are effective for GCOC. Owing to its highly invasive biological behavior, study reported a high relapse rate after radical resection, thereby long-term follow-up is recommended to track and evaluate the changes in patients' conditions.

References

1. Kasahara K, Iizuka T, Kobayashi I, et al. A recurrent case of odontogenic ghost cell tumour of the mandible [J]. Int J Oral Maxillofac Surg. 2002;31(6):684–7.
2. Goldenberg D, Sciubba J, Tufano RP. Odontogenic ghost cell carcinoma [J]. Head Neck. 2004;26(4):378–81.
3. Nel C, Robinson L, van Heerden WFP. Ghost cell odontogenic carcinoma arising in the background of a calcifying odontogenic cyst [J]. Oral Radiol. 2020;37:537.
4. de Arruda JAA, Monteiro J, Abreu LG, et al. Calcifying odontogenic cyst, dentinogenic ghost cell tumor, and ghost cell odontogenic carcinoma: a systematic review [J]. J Oral Pathol Med. 2018;47(8):721–30.
5. Jia MQ, Jia J, Wang L, et al. Ghost cell odontogenic carcinoma of the jaws: report of two cases and a literature review [J]. World J Clin Cases. 2019;7(3):357–65.
6. Martos-Fernandez M, Alberola-Ferranti M, Hueto-Madrid JA, et al. Ghost cell odontogenic carcinoma: a rare case report and review of literature [J]. J Clin Exp Dent. 2014;6(5):e602–6.
7. Tarakji B, Ashok N, Alzoghaibi I, et al. Malignant transformation of calcifying cystic odontogenic tumour - a review of literature [J]. Contemp Oncol (Pozn). 2015;19(3):184–6.
8. Martos-Fernández M, Alberola-Ferranti M, Hueto-Madrid JA, et al. Ghost cell odontogenic carcinoma: a rare case report and review of literature [J]. J Clin Exp Dent. 2014;6(5):e602–6.
9. Remya K, Sudha S, Nair RG, et al. An unusual presentation of ghost cell odontogenic carcinoma: a case report with review of literature [J]. Indian J Dent Res. 2018;29(2):238–43.
10. Gomes da Silva W, Ribeiro Bartholomeu Dos Santos TC, Cabral MG, et al. Clinicopathologic analysis and syndecan - 1 and Ki - 67 expression in calcifying cystic odontogenic tumors, dentinogenic ghost cell tumor, and ghost cell odontogenic carcinoma [J]. Oral Surg Oral Med Oral Pathol Oral Radiol. 2014;117(5):626–33.
11. Arashiyama T, Kodama Y, Kobayashi T, et al. Ghost cell odontogenic carcinoma arising in the background of a benign calcifying cystic odontogenic tumor of the mandible [J]. Oral Surg Oral Med Oral Pathol Oral Radiol. 2012;114(3):e35–40.
12. Qin Y, Lu Y, Zheng L, et al. Ghost cell odontogenic carcinoma with suspected cholesterol granuloma of the maxillary sinus in a patient treated with combined modality therapy: a case report and the review of literature [J]. Medicine (Baltimore). 2018;97(7):e9816.
13. Ledesma-Montes C, Gorlin RJ, Shear M, et al. International collaborative study on ghost cell odontogenic tumours: calcifying cystic odontogenic tumour, dentinogenic ghost cell tumour and ghost cell odontogenic carcinoma [J]. J Oral Pathol Med. 2008;37(5):302–8.

Ameloblastic Fibrosarcoma

32

Jing Song Hou, Hui Shan Ong, Zhen Tian, Lin Zhu, and Wen Jun Yang

32.1 Introduction

Odontogenic sarcoma (OS) is a group of mixed odontogenic tumors with cytologically benign ameloblastic epithelium and malignant mesenchyma stroma [1, 2]. Ameloblastic fibrosarcoma (AFS) is by far the most common type and is often considered to be the malignant counterpart of ameloblastic fibroma (AF) [3]. Aameloblastic fibrodentinosarcoma produces dentin/dentin-like, while ameloblastic fibro-odontosarcoma generates enamel/ enamel-like and dentin. AFS can be divided into primary (de novo) and secondary types (secondary to AF) [1–3].

J. S. Hou (✉)
Hospital of Stomatology, Guanghua College of Stomatology, Sun Yat-sen University, Guangdong, China
e-mail: houjs@mail.sysu.edu.cn

H. S. Ong · Z. Tian · W. J. Yang
Department of Oral Maxillofacial-Head & Neck Oncology, Shanghai Ninth People's Hospital, Shanghai Jiao Tong University School of Medicine, Shanghai, China

L. Zhu
Department of Radiology, Ninth People's Hospital Affiliated to Shanghai Jiao Tong University, Shanghai, China

32.2 Case 65

A 53-year-old gentleman suffered from a painless left mandibular mass that had been gradually increasing in size for 9 months.

[History of Present Illness] Nine months ago, the patient discovered a painful tooth in the left posterior mandible and a gradually growing gingival mass. He was treated at the local dental clinic, but the mandibular lesion did not resolve. Six months ago, he went to the hospital for radiography examination and reported space-occupying lesions in the left mandible. He was recommended to be transferred to a tertiary hospital for diagnosis and treatment. After the relevant outpatient examinations, biopsy was performed. Pathological findings suggested the consideration of "ameloblastoma of the mandible," and surgical resection in hospital was recommended.

[Specialty Examination] The patient presented as facial asymmetry, and expansile lesion over the left mandible extended from the midline to the posterior edge of the mandible ramus, with egg shell crackling sensation upon palpation. The overlying skin is normal. There was no abnormality in the range of mouth opening and mouth opening pattern. The teeth in the left posterior mandibular area were displaced and loose, and an ulceroproliferative growth lesion was observed in the buccal gingival mucosa of 37. The left mandibular vestibular groove was swollen, with a

Y. He (ed.), *Inflammatory and Neoplastic Diseases of Craniofacial Bones*,
https://doi.org/10.1007/978-981-97-4155-7_32

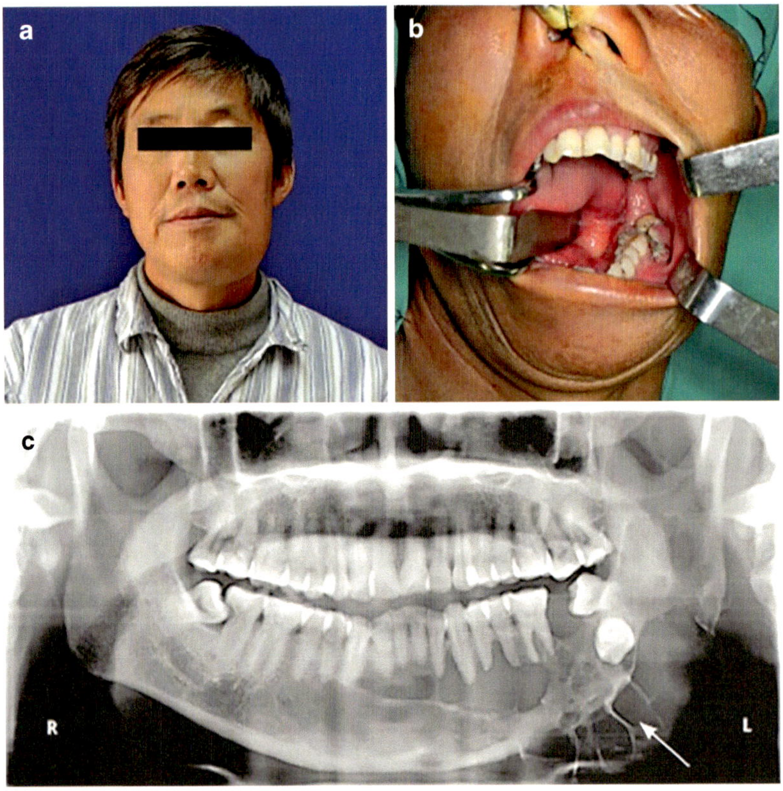

Fig. 32.1 (**a**) Facial asymmetry, with swelling over the left mandible. (**b**) Displacement and loosening of teeth in the left posterior mandibular area, ulceroproliferation soft tissues in the buccal gingival mucosa of 37, and swelling in the left mandibular buccal sulcus. (**c**) Bony destruction in the mandibular chin, the left mandibular body, the mandibular angle, and the ramus

sense of fluctuation upon palpation. The pharynx had no redness or swelling, the tonsils were not enlarged, and the tongue was centered and can move freely. Progressive paresthesia over the skin of the left cheek and mouth angle. Several enlarged lymph nodes could be palpated under the left jaw, which were soft and mobile (Fig. 32.1a, b).

[Auxiliary Examination]

1. Panoramic radiographs suggested a hypodensity bony destruction in the mandibular chin, the left mandibular body, angle, and ramus (Fig. 32.1c).
2. Maxillofacial enhanced CT scan suggested an increase in the extent of bony destruction in the mandibular chin, the left mandibular body, the mandibular angle, and the ramus, with significant expansion, ranging from approximately 9.3 cm × 5.0 cm × 3.8 cm, within which the loculation and teeth were visible, with significant non-homogeneous enhancement, thinning of surrounding bone cortex, and disruption and discontinuation of local bony cortex. The lesion invades both bucally and lingually (Fig. 32.2).

[Preliminary Diagnosis] Mass of the left mandible, malignancy to be ruled out.

[Treatment] "Left mandible resection with fibular flap transfer and tracheotomy" was performed under general anesthesia: a horizontal incision was designed at 1–2 cm away from the lower margin of the mandible, and the gingival flap was elevated for surgical exposure of the mandibular body and angle. Segmental mandibulectomy was performed at the midline and distally to 46, radical resection of mandibular lesion with preservation of left condyle. The left fibular flap was harvested to restore mandibular continuity and occlusal relationship. Peroneal and facial vessels anastomosis was performed. The wound was rinsed and thoroughly hemostatic, negative pressure drainage tube was indwelled, and finalized with layered wound closure (Fig. 32.3).

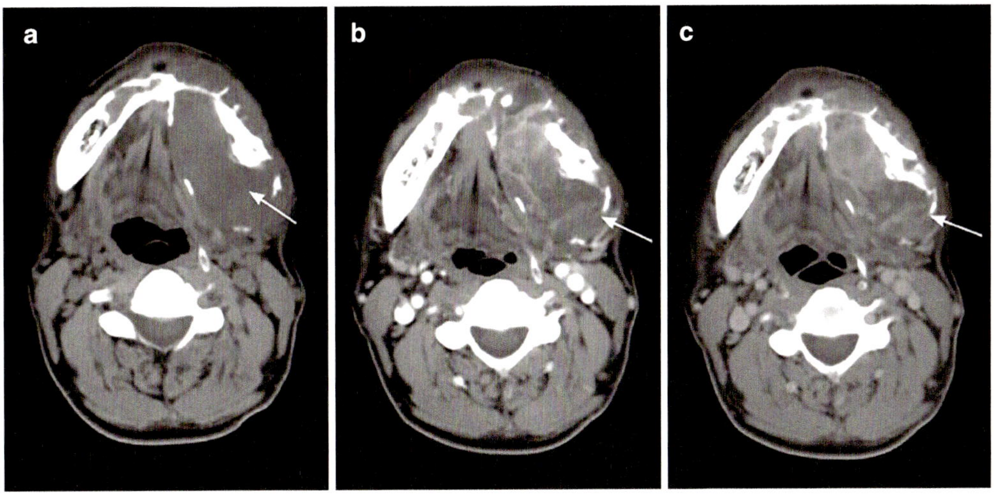

Fig. 32.2 (**a**) CT axial and coronal view show swollen bony destructive lesion accompanied with soft tissue mass, thinning of surrounding bone cortex, expansion toward the lingual side with disruption and discontinuation of bony cortex. (**b**, **c**) Enhanced CT axial plus coronal scan: heterogeneous enhancement of the mass

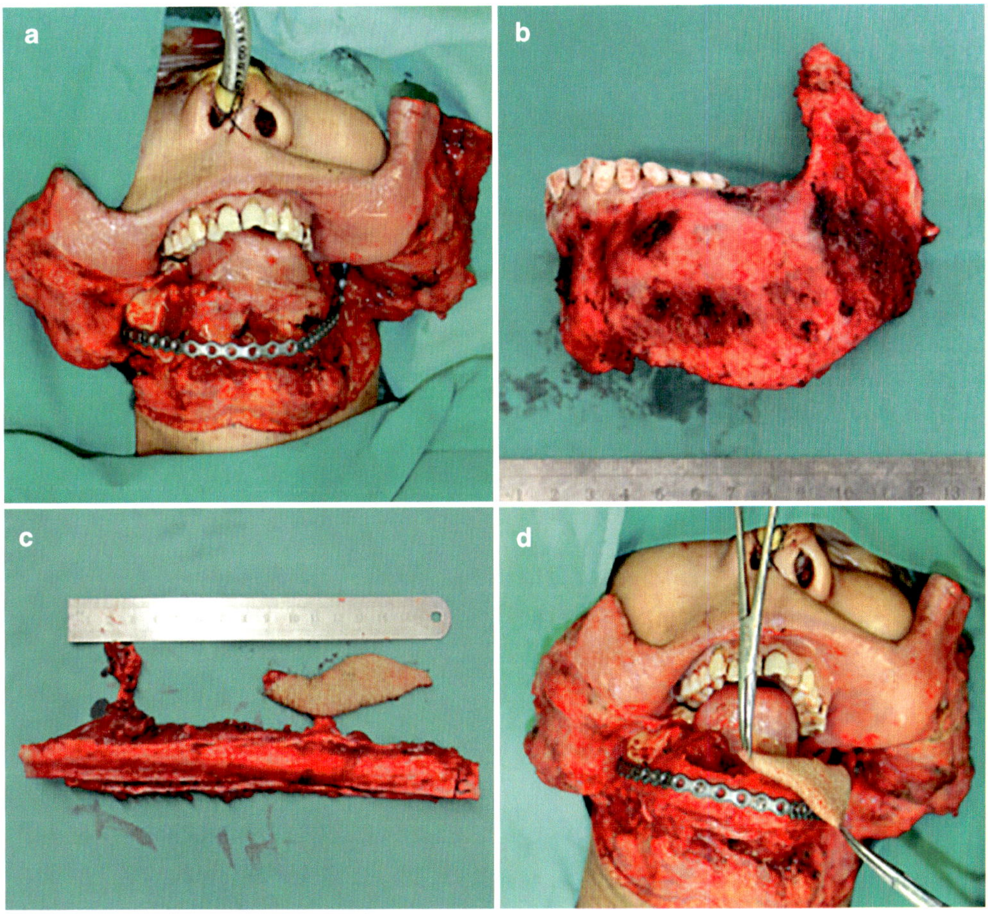

Fig. 32.3 (**a**) Prebending of reconstructed titanium plate after segmental mandibulectomy. (**b**) View of the mandible in vitro. (**c**) Fibula musculocutaneous flap (about 18 cm in length) prepared. (**d**) Fibula reconstruction to restore mandibular continuity

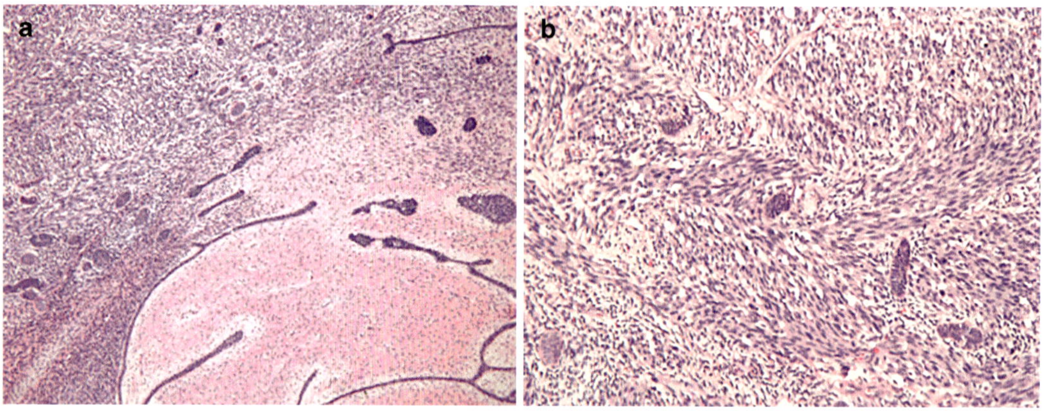

Fig. 32.4 (**a**) Well circumscribed between benign region (lower right) and malignant region (upper left). (**b**) The odontogenic mesenchymal cells were fusiform and locally interwoven, with obvious cell atypia and visible mitosis. Scattered odontogenic epithelial cells with atypical features (200×)

[Pathological Examination] Gross pathological examination revealed a part of the mandible and surrounding soft tissues, 13 cm × 7 cm × 6 cm in size, and a solid mass, 6 cm × 5 cm × 4 cm in size, grayish-yellow and tender. The microscopic examination showed that the tumor was composed of funiform and fungiform hyperplastic odontogenic epithelium and spindle cells between epitheliums. The odontogenic epithelium showed ameloblastoma, with partially insignificant polarity inversion of surrounding cells, many central cells, atypical cells, no stellate reticular stratification; The surrounding spindle cells were immature and hypercellular with obvious atypia and visible mitosis (Fig. 32.4).

[Pathological Diagnosis] Ameloblastic fibrosarcoma, a malignant transformation from ameloblastic fibroma of the "mandible," with active odontogenic epithelial growth (atypical hyperplasia). Odontogenic sarcoma, ICD-O code: 9330/3.

[Follow-Up] The patient healed uneventfully after the operation. The postoperative 6-month follow-up exhibited no tumor relapse. The patient can open and close his mouth normally, with good occlusal relationship of the right posterior teeth.

32.3 Key Points of Diagnosis and Treatment

Malignant odontogenic tumors account for about 10% of odontogenic tumors. Odontogenic sarcoma (OS), occupying about 5% of all reported sarcomas in the oral and maxillofacial region, generally appears in the mandible (80%) and maxilla (20%). Mandibular odontogenic sarcoma usually occurs in the molar area, involving the mandibular ramus and chin. Maxillary odontogenic sarcoma usually occurs in the posterior tooth area and may cause the destruction of the sinuses, nasal passages, and orbital floor. Ameloblastic fibrosarcoma can arise de novo or undergo stepwise malignant transformation from the preexisting ameloblastic fibroma. In the past, "ameloblastic dentinosarcoma" and "ameloblastic odontosarcoma" had been applied as subtypes of this neoplasms based on the histological appearance of enamel or dentin. However, ameloblastic odontosarcoma and dentinosarcoma are listed separately from ameloblastic fibrosarcoma in the new WHO classification.

Ameloblastic fibrosarcoma usually develops among people between the ages of 3 and 89, particularly among young people [4]. Radiographic examination reveals that odontogenic sarcoma usually presents an expansile change in the jaw with bony destruction and poorly demarcated boundary.

OS is considered to be a low-to-moderate malignancy with local aggressive nature. OS has a 37% relapse rate, with rare metastasis. Radical resection with negative surgical margins is the primary therapeutic decision. Cervical lymph node dissection is usually not required as the sarcoma extends through the vascular channels and hardly via the lymphatic metastasis. Neoadjuvant and/or adjuvant chemotherapy are indicated. Adjuvant radiotherapy with a total dose of 50–60 Gy to minimize the risk of local recurrence. Recurrence rate for ameloblastic fibrosarcoma is 24–37%, hence the need for radical treatment and regular follow-up. Thereby, the tretament strategy for ameloblastic fibrosarcoma is radical resection followed by adjuvant therapies.

References

1. Ramani P, Krishnan RP, Karunagaran M, et al. Odontogenic sarcoma: first report after new who nomenclature with systematic review [J]. J Oral Maxillofac Pathol. 2020;24(1):157–63.
2. Bregni RC, Taylor AM, García AM. Ameloblastic fibrosarcoma of the mandible: report of two cases and review of the literature [J]. J Oral Pathol Med. 2001;30(5):316–20.
3. Al Shetawi AH, Alpert EH, Buchbinder D, et al. Ameloblastic fibrosarcoma of the mandible: a case report and a review of the literature [J]. J Oral Maxillofac Surg. 2015;73(8):1661.e1–7.
4. Ramakrishnan DS, Gouthaman SS, Muthusekhar MR. Ameloblastic fibrosarcoma transformation from ameloblastic fibroma. Natl J Maxillofac Surg. 2022;13(Suppl 1):S145–S149. https://doi.org/10.4103/njms.NJMS_100_20. Epub 2022 Aug 20. PMID: 36393933; PMCID: PMC9651257.

33 Odontogenic Carcinosarcoma

Jing Song Hou, Hui Shan Ong, Zhen Tian, Lin Zhu, and Jie He

Odontogenic carcinosarcoma (OCS) is an extremely rare malignant tumor that was included in the WHO classification of jaw lesions in 1992 [1–3]. It shares similar overall structure with ameloblastic fibroma (AF) with both epithelial and mesenchymal components showing the morphological parameters of malignant neoplasm. The histopathological findings reflected a distinct biphasic neoplasm with well-demarcated islands and cords of invasive malignant epithelial cells embedded in pleomorphic, hyperchromatic, and hypercellular mesenchymal cells [3–5].

This malignant tumor may arise de novo that originates from an embryological process of odontogenesis, or develop from the preexisting odontogenic lesion. OCS presents with clinically aggressive behavior with a high relapse rate and frequent metastasis. Some OCS cases are easily misdiagnosed as ameloblastic carcinoma owing to failure in identifying malignant mesenchymal component.

J. S. Hou (✉)
Hospital of Stomatology, Guanghua College of Stomatology, Sun Yat-sen University, Guangdong, China
e-mail: houjs@mail.sysu.edu.cn

H. S. Ong · Z. Tian · J. He
Department of Oral Maxillofacial-Head & Neck Oncology, Shanghai Ninth People's Hospital, Shanghai Jiao Tong University School of Medicine, Shanghai, China

L. Zhu
Department of Radiology, Ninth People's Hospital Affiliated to Shanghai Jiao Tong University, Shanghai, China

33.1 Case 66

A 9-year-old boy suffered from a cervical metastasis for more than 2 months after postoperative radiotherapy for carcinosarcoma of the left maxilla.

[History of Present Illness] The patient was diagnosed as "left maxillary cyst" and received marsupialization surgery. Two weeks after the surgery, the mass grew excessively into the oral cavity via the marsupialization opening, the subject subsequently underwent maxillary curettage. The first postoperative pathology analysis revealed the consideration of cyst, but the second postoperative pathologic findings exhibited inconclusive evidence. Oral pathology and radiographic findings revealed as cyst for the primary lesion, but the diagnosis upon relapse was undefined, they suggested a complete resection to confirm the pathology.

[Specialty Examination] The patient's face was symmetrical with no obvious swollen submandibular and cervical lymph nodes bilaterally. A large exogenous mass with ulcerative surface and bleeding upon palpation was visible in the left maxillary anterior tooth area. Intra-oral

Y. He (ed.), *Inflammatory and Neoplastic Diseases of Craniofacial Bones*,
https://doi.org/10.1007/978-981-97-4155-7_33

examination was difficult as it was blocked by the large lesion.

[Auxiliary Examination] Maxillofacial enhanced CT scan suggested that the 21 was missing, the alveolar bone was discontinued at the left center and lateral incisal owing to previous surgical resection of left maxillary mass. A soft tissue mass located labially indicated a relapse, was seen labially to previous surgical area, about 1 cm × 2.5 cm in size and discontinuous labial bony cortex, with a CT− value of 67 Hu. Enhanced CT scan suggested heterogeneous enhancement, with a CT+ value of 82 Hu. Small lymph node shadows were observed in the cervical IB area on both sides (Fig. 33.1).

[Preliminary Diagnosis] Incomplete resection of left maxillary mass at other hospital

[Treatment]

1. The biopsy was performed under general anesthesia, and the pathologic findings suggested that the mucosal epithelium of the "left upper gingiva" was found to have odontogenic epi-

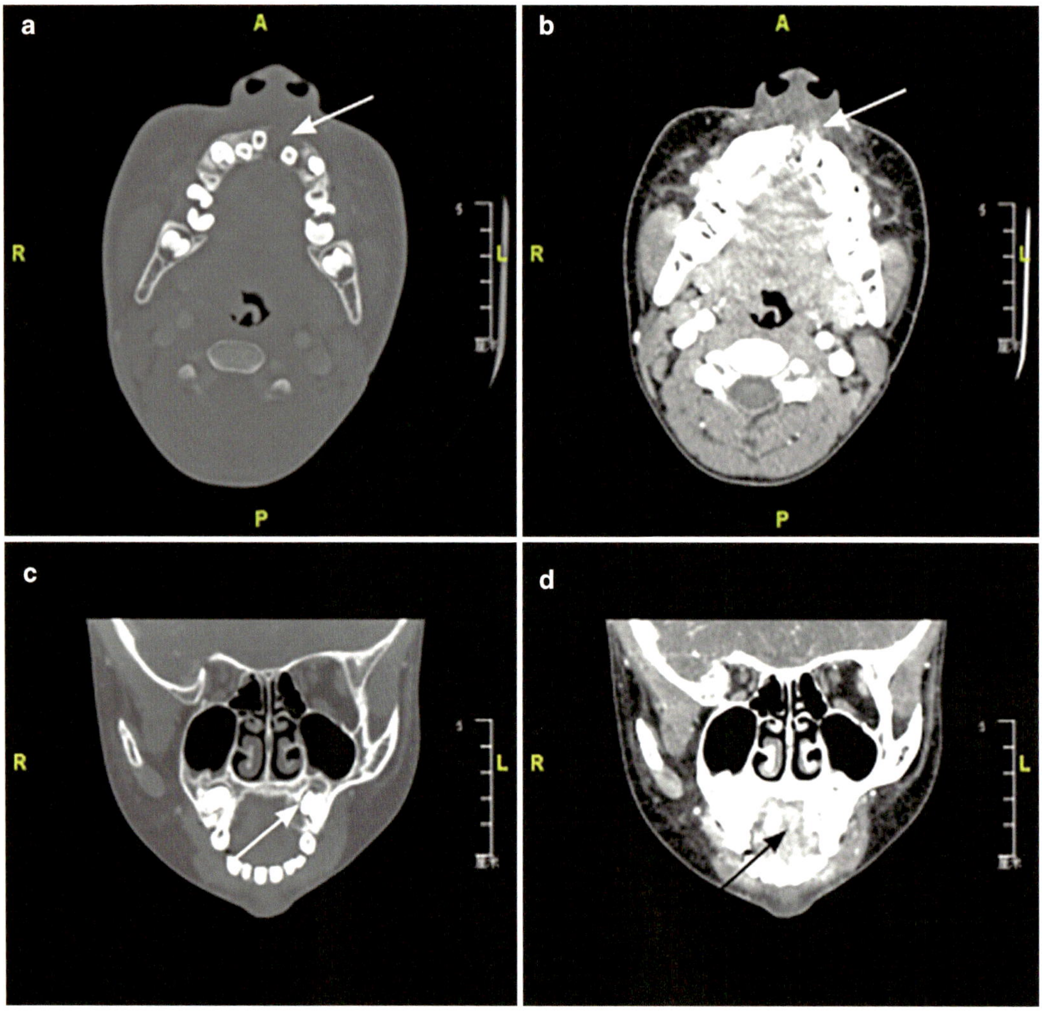

Fig. 33.1 (**a**) Enhanced CT axial plus coronal scan (bone window) suggested an incomplete alveolar bone at the left upper center and lateral incisor positions, and a discontinuity in the labial bony cortex. (**b**) Enhanced CT axial plus coronal scan (soft-tissue window) suggested a soft tissue mass in the left upper jaw and labial sulcus, about 1 cm × 2.5 cm in size. Enhanced scan showed heterogeneous enhancement, with a CT+ value of 82 Hu. (**c**, **d**) Coronal scan

thelial and odontogenic mesenchymal components, with moderate-to-severe abnormal hyperplasia, hyperchromasia of nuclei and atypical mitotic figures. Combined with the imaging findings, the mass was considered to be a malignant odontogenic tumor, with low or low-moderate malignancy. Complete resection of the tumor was performed.

2. "Bilateral partial maxillectomy and packing with iodoform gauze" was performed under general anesthesia: a Weber incision was designed, an intraoral incision was made from 11 to 25 and the gingival flap was elevated for surgical exposure of the anterior wall of the maxilla, and the mass could be seen growing from 23 gingival and extend posteriorly to the molar area. The left maxilla and the anterior portion of the right maxilla were resected. The rupture of maxillary sinus floor was observed, thereby Caldwell-Luc operation was performed. Frozen section of surgical margin reported "right and left maxillary sinus" is positive (+), the rest are negative (−), so extended resection was performed until we obtained a negative safe margin. The intraoral wound was hemostatic, rinsed, and packing with iodoform gauze.

[Pathological Examination] Gross pathological examination revealed part of the left maxilla tissue, 4 cm × 4 cm × 3 cm in size, with 4 teeth. The jaw bone was ruptured, soft tissue mass within the incision area, 3 cm × 2.5 cm × 2 cm in size, grayish white, tender, and containing fragmentation of osseous tissues. The microscopic examination demonstrated invasive growth of the tumor interspersed with osseous tissues. The tumor was composed of odontogenic epithelium and mesenchyme. Mesenchymal cells were spindle-shaped and sparsely arranged. Odontogenic epithelial cells presented as nests, with large nucleo-plasma ratio and deep chromatin. The two types of cells showed atypical features, active proliferation, and visible mitotic signs (Fig. 33.2).

[Pathological Diagnosis] Odontogenic tumor of epithelial and mesenchymal origin in the "maxilla" suggested an ameloblastic fibroma with malignant transformation, and presented as an odontogenic carcinosarcoma, ICD-O code: 8980/3, moderate grade.

[Follow-Up] At 1 month postoperative follow-up, the patient's MRI showed relapse of odontogenic carcinoma, apatinib targeted therapy was performed for 1 week followed by postoperative adjuvant radiotherapy. After radiotherapy, the patient received seven cycles of chemotherapy at another hospital. The chemotherapy response was evaluated as progressive disease (PD) and showed possible metastasis to the left submandibular region (Fig. 33.3). Then, the left total maxillectomy with left supramohyoid neck dissection (SOND) was performed under general anesthesia. Postoperative pathological analysis revealed a relapse of odontogenic carcinosarcoma (sarcomatous relapse) (Fig. 33.4).

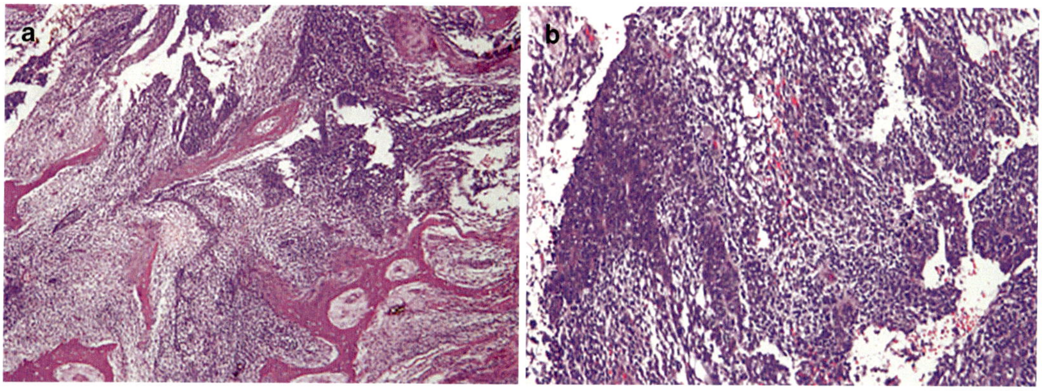

Fig. 33.2 (**a**) Invasive growth of the tumor composed of sparsely arranged mesenchymal cells with epithelial cells arranged in nests (100×). (**b**) Mesenchymal cells and epithelial cells showed atypical features, larger nucleus/cytoplasm ratio with active proliferation and visible mitotic signs (200×)

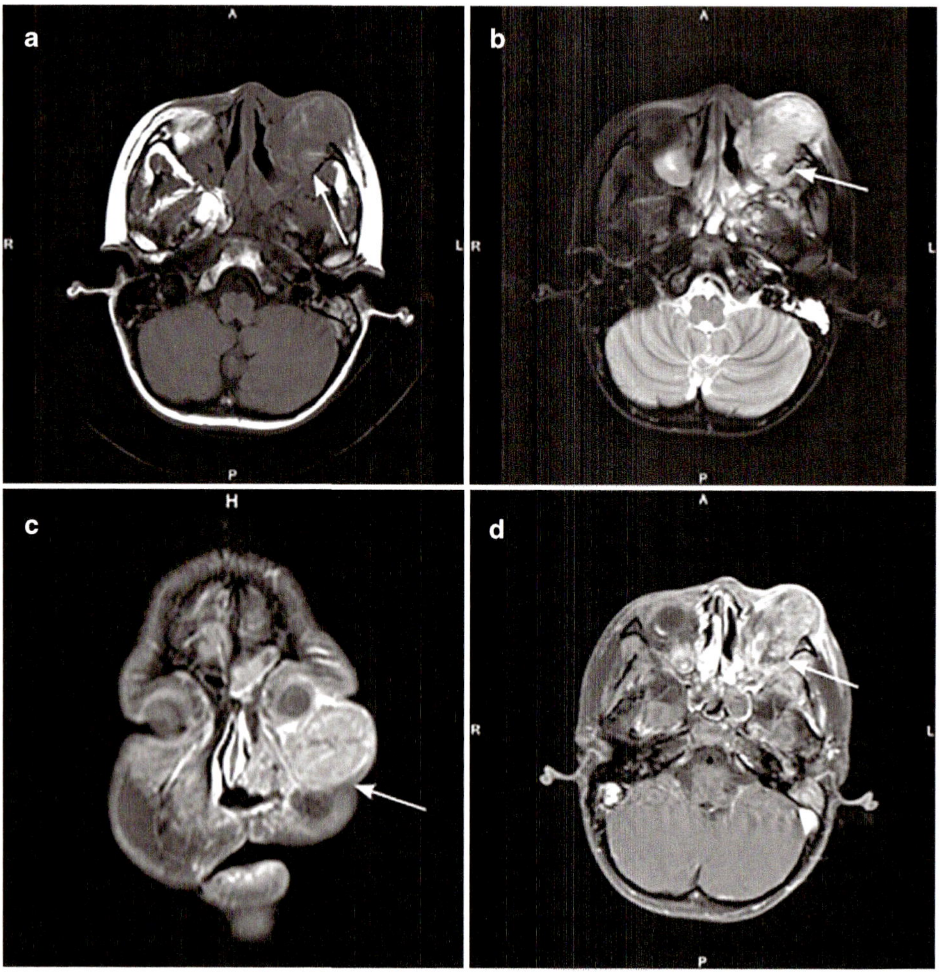

Fig. 33.3 (**a**, **b**) CT axial plus coronal scan on T1WI and T2WI revealed that the tumor invaded the left nasolacrimal duct, paranasal, left infraorbital fissure, and pterygopalatine fossa. (**c**, **d**) Enhanced CT of coronal and axial view on T1WI and T2WI showed heterogeneous enhancement mass

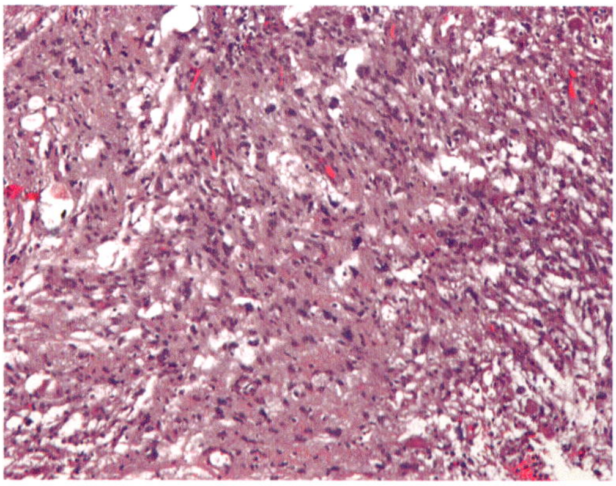

Fig. 33.4 The tumor contained fusiform cells with cellular atypia and visible mitosis, up to a relapse of odontogenic carcinosarcoma (sarcomatous component) compared to pathological section after the first surgery (200×)

33.2 Key Points of Diagnosis and Treatment

Till now, only 9 OCS cases have been reported in the literature, including 2 tumors that arose de novo and 7 tumors that malignantly transformed from ameloblastoma. OCS often develops from the malignant transformation of ameloblastic fibroma or ameloblastoma. Malignant transformation to OCS often occurs after multiple surgical recurrences. OCS usually presented as slow swelling, pain, ulceration, and tooth loosening in the posterior portion of the mandible, similar to ameloblastic carcinoma, primary intraosseous carcinoma, clear cell odontogenic carcinoma, and odontogenic sclerosing carcinoma, etc. Due to the oddity of cases, it is unlikely to conclude the imaging features of OCS, which has the imaging manifestations similar to most osteolytic lesions. The available reports indicate that the average lesion of OCS is 6 cm, and not well circumscribed, often with bony cortical destruction and dental root resorption. Biphasic malignant odontogenic neoplasm shows abundant large cells, hyperchromasia of the nuclei, and atypical mitotic figures. Immunohistichemical is an important tool to determine concurrent of both epithelial and mesenchymal components to determine the definitive diagnosis. The epithelial components showed positivity for cytokeratin and pan-cytokeratin (AE1/AE3), whereas sarcomatous elements demonstrated positivity for vimentin.

OCS is treated mainly by radical resection, while adjuvant treatment remains controversial. OCS has a tendency to metastasis which appears in the lymph node, lung, rib, and pelvis in the 4 reported cases. OCS has a poor prognosis. Follow-up results showed that only 3 out of 7 patients survive, with a mean follow-up time of 21 months. The mean survival time for patients is 42.7 months. It is important to highlight that OCS may be misdiagnosed due to the rarity of the clinical presentation or difficulty in identification of the malignant features in both mesenchymal and epithelial components. Oral health care providers must remain vigilant to the possibility of the malignancy. Unawareness may result in late diagnosis, delayed treatment, and increased need of aggressive management with associated increased morbidity and mortality.

References

1. Kramer IR, Pindborg JJ, Shear M. The World Health Organization histological typing of odontogenic tumours. Introducing the second edition [J]. Eur J Cancer B Oral Oncol. 1993;29B(3):169–71.
2. Kim IK, Pae SP, Cho HY, et al. Odontogenic carcinosarcoma of the mandible: a case report and review [J]. J Korean Assoc Oral Maxillofac Surg. 2015;41(3):139–44.
3. da Silva KD, Flores IL, Etges A, et al. Unusual osteolytic lesion of the jaw [J]. Oral Surg Oral Med Oral Pathol Oral Radiol. 2017;124(5):443–8.
4. Schuch LF, de Arruda JAA, Silva LVO, et al. Odontogenic carcinosarcoma: a systematic review [J]. Oral Oncol. 2018;85:52–9.
5. Kunkel M, Ghalibafian M, Radner H, et al. Ameloblastic fibrosarcoma or odontogenic carcinosarcoma: a matter of classification [J]. Oral Oncol. 2004;40(4):444–9.

Part XI

Benign Tumors of Craniomaxillofacial Bones and Cartilage

34 Osteoma

Yue He, Hui Shan Ong, Zhen Tian, Lin Zhu, and Wei Wei Deng

34.1 Introduction

Osteoma is a benign tumor composed of differentiated and mature bone tissue. It can occur at any age, with a predication for males over females, ranging from 10 to 49 years old. It is common in the mandible, mostly in the condyle process, the lingual side of the mandibular body and the lower margin of the mandibular angle. It typically occurs unilaterally, but can also be bilateral [1–8].

34.2 Case 67

A 37-year-old woman suffered from a painless but gradually growing mass in her left submandibular region for more than 10 years.

[History of Present Illness] The patient found a left submandibular swelling of bean size 10 years ago, which grew slowly without pain or other discomfort. The swelling lesion enlarge (about "yolk" size) with time without undergo any treatment.

[Specialty Examination] The patient's maxillofacial region was asymmetrical, with obvious mass in the left submandibular region, about 2 cm in diameter, round, hard, well circumscribed, immobile, and not tender to percussion (−). There was no abnormality in mouth opening range and mouth opening pattern. Intraoral examination revealed permanent dentition, with no obvious abnormality of teeth and gums. No submandibular or cervical lymph node enlargement was observed.

[Auxiliary Examination] Maxillofacial CT scan suggested a bony protrusion on the left mandible with a size of about 15 mm × 17 mm × 14 mm and a CT value of 1100 Hu. The rest of the mandibular cortex was continuous, no obvious bone abnormalities were observed, and the temporomandibular joint was in place. No significant swelling was seen in the surrounding soft tissues. The epiglottic mucosa was rough (Fig. 34.1).

[Preliminary Diagnosis] Osteoma of the left mandible

[Treatment] Under general anesthesia, "left mandibular osteoma resection" was performed: an incision was made along the lower margin of the mandible for 1~2 cm, and the gingival flap

Y. He (✉) · H. S. Ong · Z. Tian
Department of Oral Maxillofacial-Head & Neck Oncology, Shanghai Ninth People's Hospital, Shanghai Jiao Tong University School of Medicine, Shanghai, China

L. Zhu
Department of Radiology, Ninth People's Hospital Affiliated to Shanghai Jiao Tong University, Shanghai, China

W. W. Deng
Hospital of Stomatology Wuhan University, Hubei, China

Y. He (ed.), *Inflammatory and Neoplastic Diseases of Craniofacial Bones*,
https://doi.org/10.1007/978-981-97-4155-7_34

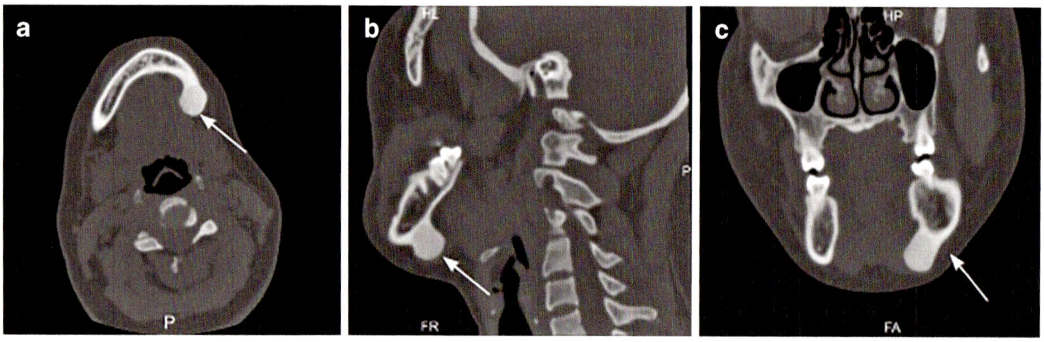

Fig. 34.1 (**a**) CT axial scan suggested a bony protrusion on the left mandible with a well-demarcated margin and uniform density. (**b**, **c**) CT axial scan sagittal and coronal views

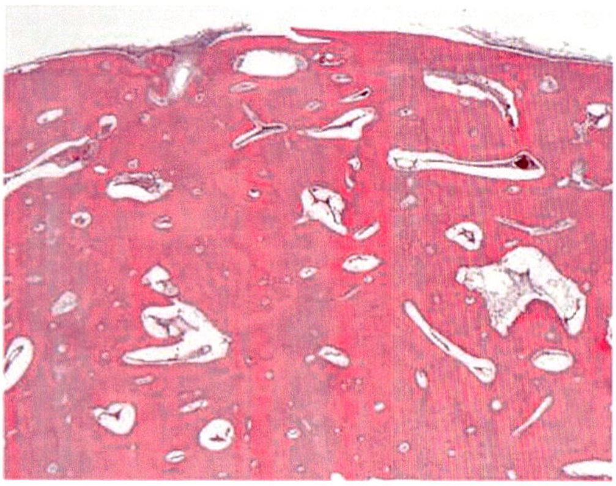

Fig. 34.2 Significant hyperplasia of lamellar bone tissues, with a small amount of bone marrow tissues (40×)

was elevated for surgical exposure of the mass. Then, the mass was resected and sent for pathological examination. The surrounding bone was trimmed and smoothened. Finally, the wound was thoroughly rinsed and hemostatically controlled, and layered suture was performed.

[Pathological Examination] Gross pathological examination revealed two bony tissues, 3 cm × 2 cm × 1.2 cm in size, grayish yellow and grayish red. The microscopic examination showed that bone tissues were hyperplasia and dense, and fused into a tumor-like mass with lamellar structure, and the bone marrow cavity was narrowed and lined with fatty bone marrow with vascular tissue (Fig. 34.2).

[Pathological Diagnosis] Osteoma of the "left mandible", ICD-O code: 9180/0.

[Follow-up] The patient healed uneventfully. The postoperative 6-month follow-up exhibited no recurrence.

34.3 Key Points of Diagnosis and Treatment

The prevailing view is that osteoma is a benign tumor. Osteomas are slow-growing, well-defined osteogenic lesions developing from mature bone. Typical histological presentation shows the proliferation of compact or cancellous bone. The etiology of osteomas remains unknown. But some scholars argue that osteoma is a malformation tumor that is easily confused with reactive bone hyperplasia caused by trauma and inflammation, odontogenic-ossifying fibroma with progressive ossification, and osteochondroma, is not significantly different from developmental abnormalities such as bony protuberance and exostosis [1–8]. The continuation of growth after adulthood is the most characteristic feature that differentiates these lesions from other bony exostoses. Contunuating slow growing rate feature had signified the benign nature of the lesion.

Osteomas that occur in the bone are called central type while those that occur in the subperiosteal are called peripheral type. Peripheral osteoma has well-defined margin, it can be growing on a broad base or a stalk on the cortex. The lesion neither causes destruction of the adjacent bone tissue nor grows invasively. In rare cases, osteomas may also occur in soft tissues [6–11].

Clinical Manifestations The clinical manifestations of maxillofacial osteoma depend on the location. Osteomas are usually asymptomatic, they are usually detected upon routine checkup. The common clinical manifestations are slow growing, hard, non-tender, immobile, and well-demarcated mass in the oral and maxillofacial region, often manifesting as a bulging jaw, which may cause numbness or pain, if the nerve canal is involved or the mass compresses the nerve. Limited mouth opening if the condyle is involved. Multiple osteoma of the jaw and skull is accompanied by (1) colonic manifestations such as gastrointestinal tract polyps; (2) cutaneous lesions such as dermatofibroma, epidermoid cysts and desmoid; and (3) dental abnormalities such as impacted teeth, or odontoma, hypodontia, or abnormal tooth morphology, which shall be associated to Gardner syndrome. For Gardner syndrome, the interstinal polyps carry a 100% risk of malignant transformation, an early diagnosis is essential, thereby Gardner syndrome needs to be ruled out in subjects with multiple osteotoma. X-rays show dense and coarse trabeculae of dense bone, and well-circumscribed protruding lesion with increased density.

Pathological Characteristics Pathologically, the central osteoma is visually surrounded by a periosteum with a section of spongy bone or dense bone, while the peripheral osteoma is round or ovoid with a smooth or nodular surface and a broad base attached to the host bone surface. Microscopically, it is seen to consist of mature bone trabeculae with irregular arrangement with marked osteoblastic activity [11–13]. There are fibers, blood vessels, and adipose tissue between the trabeculae, and sometimes hematopoietic components are visible. Osteomas can be divided into dense osteomas and spongy osteomas subtypes depending on the ratio of bone/fiber,

Treatment The slow and continuous growth pattern of osteoma is symtomless. Facial asymmetry and functional impairment usually present in very large size osteotma. Thereby, surgical excision from the base of the lesion is usually preferred. Owing to the benign nature of osteoma, if the osteoma does not grow significantly nor has any accompanying clinical discomfort, a delayed surgical resection with close follow-up is allowed. Recurrence of osteoma after surgical resection is rare. To date, there have been no reports of osteoma malignancy.

References

1. Valente L, Tieghi R, Mandrioli S, et al. Mandibular condyle osteoma [J]. Ann Maxillofac Surg. 2019;9(2):434–8.
2. Ostrofsky M, Morkel JA, Titinchi F. Osteoma of the mandibular condyle : a rare case report and review of the literature [J]. J Stomatol Oral Maxillofac Surg. 2019;120(6):584–7.
3. Ata-Ali J, Ata-Ali F. Giant peripheral osteoma of the mandible simulating a parotid gland tumor [J]. Braz J Otorhinolaryngol. 2019;85(3):393–5.
4. Nilesh K, Vande AV, Veerabhadrappa SK. Solitary peripheral ivory osteoma of the mandible presenting with difficulty in deglutition: a case report [J]. J Dent Res Dent Clin Dent Prospects. 2017;11(1):56–60.
5. Debta P, Debta FM, Bussari S, et al. Cancellous osteoma of maxilla: a rare case report [J]. J Int Soc Prev Community Dent. 2016;6(3):261–4.
6. Ragupathy K, Priyadharsini I, Sanjay P, et al. Peripheral osteoma of the body of mandible: a case report [J]. J Maxillofac Oral Surg. 2015;14(4):1004–8.
7. Kshirsagar K, Bhate K, Pawar V, et al. Solitary peripheral osteoma of the angle of the mandible [J]. Case Rep Dent. 2015;2015:430619.
8. Nojima K, Niizuma-Kosaka F, Nishii Y, et al. Multidisciplinary treatment of peripheral osteoma arising from mandibular condyle in patient presenting with facial asymmetry [J]. Bull Tokyo Dent Coll. 2014;55(1):39–47.
9. Batra N, Batra R, Singh G, et al. Peripheral osteoma of maxilla: a case report [J]. Natl J Maxillofac Surg. 2014;5(2):240–2.
10. Prabhuji ML, Kishore HC, Sethna G, et al. Peripheral osteoma of the hard palate [J]. J Indian Soc Periodontol. 2012;16(1):134–7.
11. Panjwani S, Bagewadi A, Keluskar V, et al. Gardner's syndrome [J]. J Clin Imaging Sci. 2011;1:65.
12. Kaplan I, Nicolaou Z, Hatuel D, et al. Solitary central osteoma of the jaws: a diagnostic dilemma [J]. Oral Surg Oral Med Oral Pathol Oral Radiol Endod. 2008;106(3):e22–9.
13. Lew D, DeWitt A, Hicks RJ, et al. Osteomas of the condyle associated with gardner's syndrome causing limited mandibular movement [J]. J Oral Maxillofac Surg. 1999;57(8):1004–9.

35 Chondroma

Yue He, Hui Shan Ong, Zhen Tian, Lin Zhu, and Wei Wei Deng

35.1 Introduction

Chondroma is composed of mature hyaline cartilage tumor (mostly isolated, occasionally involving more than one bone or multiple parts of one bone), which often occurs in the limb bones, but rarely in the jaws, with different sites of onset and clinical features [1–4]. It usually has limited growth potential and is not locally aggressive. Chondroma may occur in the central part of bones (enchondroma) or on the periosteal surface (periosteal/juxtacortical chondroma), and occasionally in oral and maxillofacial soft tissues in the tongue and buccal (soft tissue chondroma) [5–8]. Subject with multiple enchondromas (joint disease), along with skeletal deformities and hemangiomas (vascular disease) over the skin, it shall be considered as Maffucci syndrome [8, 9]. Enchondroma associated with Maffucci syndrome usually begins as benign, but it may turn cancerous. Likewise, Maffucci syndrome has increased risk of other cancers such as ovarian and liver cancer.

35.2 Case 68

A 24-year-old man had pain in the left preauricular region for 5 years.

[History of Present Illness] The patient complained of pain and discomfort after a trauma in the left temporomandibular joint 5 years ago, and the symptoms were improved but not cured after physiotherapy in the hospital. One year ago, he felt that the pain in the left preauricular area was aggravated without numbness, but there was a restriction in his range of mouth opening. There was no improvement with his local treatment. Temporal mandibular joint MRI examination showed an abnormal bone structure of the left condyle with ankylosis to be ruled out.

[Specialty Examination] The patient's face was basically symmetrical, and there was no clicking when opening and closing the mouth in the bilateral temporomandibular joint area. However, the motion of the left condyle was significantly reduced, and the left anterior auricular condyle area was tender. The mouth opening range was about 1 cm without deviation upon opening and closing. Intraoral examination revealed permanent dentition, the mandibular

Y. He (✉) · H. S. Ong · Z. Tian
Department of Oral Maxillofacial-Head & Neck Oncology, Shanghai Ninth People's Hospital, Shanghai Jiao Tong University School of Medicine, Shanghai, China

L. Zhu
Department of Radiology, Ninth People's Hospital Affiliated to Shanghai Jiao Tong University, Shanghai, China

W. W. Deng
Hospital of Stomatology Wuhan University, Hubei, China

Y. He (ed.), *Inflammatory and Neoplastic Diseases of Craniofacial Bones*, https://doi.org/10.1007/978-981-97-4155-7_35

midline was shifted 1 mm to the right with deep overbite, and the posterior teeth had a fair occlusal relationship.

[Auxiliary Examination]

1. Panoramic radiographs suggested abnormally reduced bone density in the left condyle (Fig. 35.1a).
2. MRI of temporomandibular joint: (1) Right TMJ: sagittal scan showed the disc-condylar relationship was normal in both open and closed mouth condition; coronal scan showed the articular disc was displaced medially, and the anterior oblique surface of the condyle was hypoplastic. (2) Left TMJ: The bone morphology of the condylar crest was abnormal, it is hyperintense in the T2 signal, and the articular disc was unclear and appeared to be adhering to the lesion (Fig. 35.2). Isointensed mass as compared to muscle in T1 signal.

[Preliminary Diagnosis] Left condylar mass (probably a chondroma).

[Treatment] Under general anesthesia, "left condyle/articular disc/mass radical resection + simultaneous joint reonstrcution with costal cartilage and temporalis fascia flap" was performed. A modified auriculotemporal incision was made. The skin flap was elevated and the parotid gland was dissected for surgical exposure and protection of temporal branch of facial nerve. The T-shaped incision was made between the articular capsule and the periosteum and the superior and inferior discotemporal cavities were opened to expose the uneven surface of the condyle and a cartilage-like expanded mass. The condylar process was osteotomized at the neck of the condyle which is 1.5 cm below the condylar apex, and the specimen was taken and sent for pathological examination; the bone graft was prepared. Intermaxillary fixation was performed to maintain the occlusal relationship. The anchorage of articular disc was performed. The ipsilateral temporalis fascial flap sized 2 cm × 3 cm with a medial temporal artery and venous were harvested and transferred to occupy the anterior space of the articular disc. The contralateral 6th rib of 6 cm with 0.5 cm of cartilage portion was implanted as neo-condyle; arthroscope-assisted strong internal fixation was performed with the aid of a buccal penetrator. The wound was rinsed and thoroughly hemostatic. A rubber drainage strip was placed and sutured in layers; the intermaxillary fixation was removed and local pressure dressing was applied.

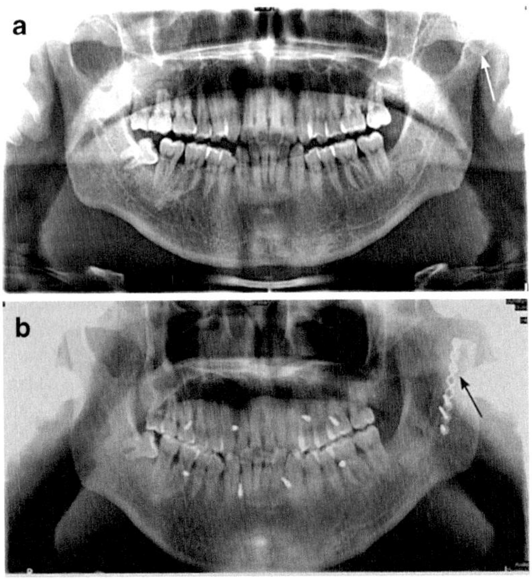

Fig. 35.1 (**a**) Abnormally reduced bone density in the left condyle (preoperative). (**b**) Postoperative changes in the left mandibular condylar region with internal fixation (postoperative)

[Pathological Examination] Gross pathological examination revealed a piece of white chondroid tissue 1.5 cm × 1 cm × 1 cm. Microscopically, the soft tissue on the surface of the condyle showed tumor-like and lobulated hyperplasia, which was well circumscribed with the surrounding tissues. A large number of chondrocytes were distributed in patches in the basophilic hyaline cartilage matrix, with abundant cells, mild atypia, and multinucleated cells (Fig. 35.3). The principal diagnostic difficulty is distinguishing chondroma from well-differentiated chondrosarcoma. Well-differentiated chondrosarcoma usually presents with heterogeneous pattern of cytological atypia and irregular spaced chondrocytes.

[Pathological Diagnosis] Osteochondromatous proliferation on the condylar surface of the "left temporomandibular joint," consistent with chon-

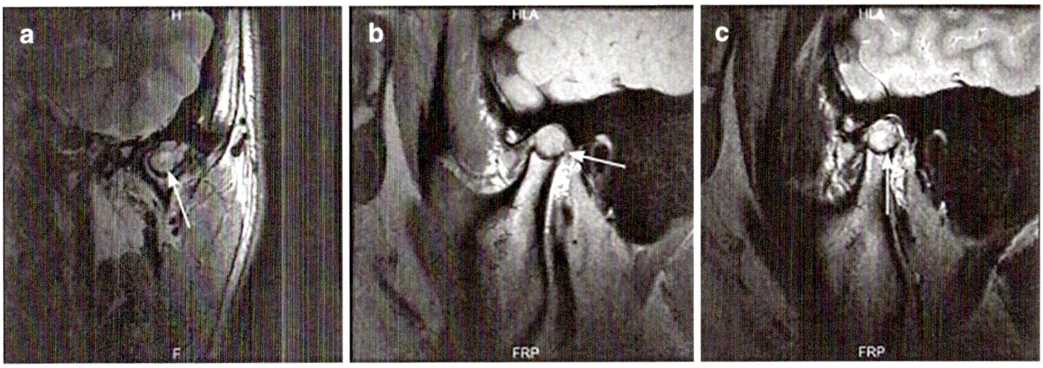

Fig. 35.2 (**a**) MRI coronal view of the temporomandibular joint: the left condylar crest was occupied with abnormal mass. (**b**, **c**) MRI sagittal views of the temporomandibular joint in the close and open mouth position respectively

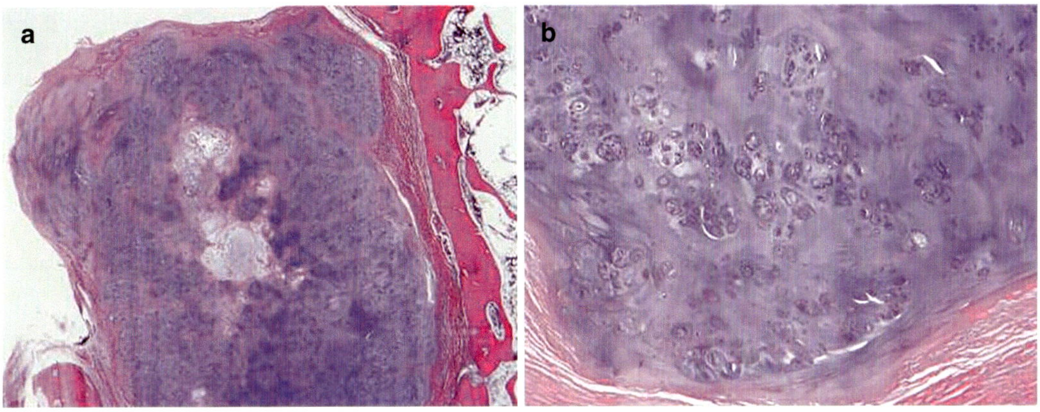

Fig. 35.3 (**a**) The tumor is well circumscribed, with lobulated growth (20×). (**b**) The chondrocytes vary in size, some of them are large and may be multinucleated. The cells are mildly atypical, with a large amount of basophilic cartilage stroma between the cells (100×)

droma. ICD-O code: 9220/0, some cells are mildly heteromorphic.

[Follow-up] The patient healed uneventfully. The postoperative 6-month follow-up exhibited no recurrence and normal range of mouth opening and stable occlusion. (Fig. 35.1b).

35.3 Key Points of Diagnosis and Treatment

Chondroma usually occurs in the 40s to 60s, with no gender predilection [1–6]. In the maxilla, chondroma occurs mainly in the alveolar bone of the anterior region, nose, molar region, and hard palate; while in the mandible, chondroma occurs mainly in the molar region, symphysis, condyle, and coronoid process. The location and clinical characteristics of chondroma vary greatly. The chondroma occurring in the central part of bone is usually referred to as central chondroma, while the chondroma occurring in the periosteal surface is referred to as periosteal chondroma. The clinical manifestations are pain and swelling of the jaws, loosening and loss of teeth due to bone destruction. The condyle chondroma can cause maxillofacial asymmetry, facial deformation, and mandibular movement disorders [1–4].

Imaging Characteristics X-ray shows central chondromas are usually well-circumscribed translucent to mineralized masses, and the matrix mineralization can be characterized in a punctate or endosteal scalloping. Pertinent negatives (none aggressive) features such as no gross bony destruction, no periosteal reaction and no soft tissue involvement. Periosteal chondromas appear as clear or mineralized surface tumors with well-circumscribed butterfly-shaped depressions in the bone cortex, often with thickened basal bone cortex and covered with hyperplastic periosteum. In Maffucci's syndrome, a spot-like high-density shadow is seen on radiographs due to soft tissue calcification caused by hemangioma phlebiolith formation. Chondroma requires differential diagnosis from osteoma, osteoblastoma, osteochondroma, chondrosarcoma, and osteosarcoma.

Pathological Characteristics Chondromas are generally grayish or milky white in color, with yellow or red gravel-like lesions representing areas of calcification or ossification. Histologically, chondromas appear as mature hyaline chondrocytes with abundant chondrocyte cytoplasm and vacuoles inside. Chondroma contains few cellular components. The cells are visibly pleomorphic and may be multinucleated. There is a shortage of vascularity but abundant hyaline cartilage matrix exists, and the degree of mineralization within chondroma varies greatly.

Treatment The main therapy for maxillofacial chondroma is surgical resection. It is generally believed that recurrence after surgical resection is rare, as evidenced by the report on the single case of postoperative recurrence of chondroma in condyle and maxilla.

References

1. Nao EE, Ndiaye M, Tall A, et al. Chondroma of the tongue: about a case [J]. Rev Stomatol Chir Maxillofac Chir Orale. 2014;115(6):e47–8.
2. Marchetti C, Mazzoni S, Bertoni F. Chondroma of the mandibular condyle-relapse of a rare benign chondroid tumour after 5 years5 follow-up: case report [J]. Br J Oral Maxillofac Surg. 2012;50(5):e69–71.
3. Heitz C, Vogt BF, Bergoli RD, et al. Chondroma in temporomandibular region — case report and therapeutic considerations. Oral Maxillofac Surg. 2012;16(1):75–8.
4. Kiralj A, Ilic M, Markov B, et al. Chondroma of the skull base and maxilla [J]. Med Pregl. 2007;60(11–12):649–51.
5. Onodera K, Xu H, Kimizuka S, et al. Chondroma of the cheek: a case report [J]. Int J Oral Maxillofac Surg. 2005;34(8):924–6.
6. Rico Niria R, Perez Mejia R, Galvez G. Chondroma of the soft tissues of the oral cavity: report of two cases [J]. Pract Odontol. 1987;8(2):212–24.
7. Carnelutti S, Mantero F. On a case of recurrent chondroma of the maxilla [J]. Stomatologica (Genova). 1965;9(3):241–54.
8. Bardach J, Pruszczynski A. An exceptionally large chondroma of the maxilla: case report [J]. Br J Plast Surg. 1965;18:105–8.
9. Cimino A. Clinical and developmental aspects of chondroma of the superior maxilla [J]. Boll Mal Orecch Gola Naso. 1960;78:158–75.

36 Osteoblastoma

Yue He, Hui Shan Ong, Zhen Tian, Lin Zhu, and Jin Song Li

36.1 Introduction

Osteoblastoma is a rare benign neoplasm of bone, also known as chondroblastoma, osteoblastic giant cell tumor, or giant osteoid osteoma [1–5]. Clinically, osteoblastoma occurs mostly in the spine and long bones, it rarely occurs in the oral and maxillofacial regions [6–8]. In about 15% of the patients, it occurs in the jaw.

36.2 Case 69

A 48-year-old woman suffered a right mandibular mass for more than 1 month.

[History of Present Illness] Panoramic radiographs at other hospital 1 month ago showed a hypodense shadow at the patient's right mandible. The patient denied the history of swelling and pain, the history of bleeding, the history of restricted mouth opening, the history of trauma, and the history of local injection.

[Specialty Examination] Facial symmetry was observed, and a cortical expansion of about 1.5 cm × 1.0 cm was detected in the buccal side of lower right premolar and molar region, with no cortical defects, no tenderness, and good continuity of bilateral mandibles. The mouth opening and pattern were normal, and the intraoral mucosa was intact with no abnormal redness or exudation. No submandibular or cervical lymph node enlargement was observed.

[Auxiliary Examination]

1. Panoramic radiographs suggested an abnormal hypodense shadow between teeth 45 and 46 at the right mandible, with ill-defined boundaries (Fig. 36.1).
2. Maxillofacial enhanced CT scan suggested a cystic hypodense shadow at the buccal side of right mandible (the 45 and 46 dental apical region) with a cross-section of 8 mm × 10 mm and a CT value of 120 Hu. The rest of the mandible and zygomatic arch bones were cortically intact with no obvious signs of dislocation or fracture, the temporomandibular joint was intact, and no sign of swelling of the surrounding soft tissues. No effusion was seen in the maxillary sinus and pterygoid sinus. The mucosa

Y. He (✉) · H. S. Ong · Z. Tian
Department of Oral Maxillofacial-Head & Neck Oncology, Shanghai Ninth People's Hospital, Shanghai Jiao Tong University School of Medicine, Shanghai, China

L. Zhu
Department of Radiology, Ninth People's Hospital Affiliated to Shanghai Jiao Tong University, Shanghai, China

J. S. Li
Sun Yat-Sen Memorial Hospital, Sun Yat-Sen University, Guangdong, China

Y. He (ed.), *Inflammatory and Neoplastic Diseases of Craniofacial Bones*,
https://doi.org/10.1007/978-981-97-4155-7_36

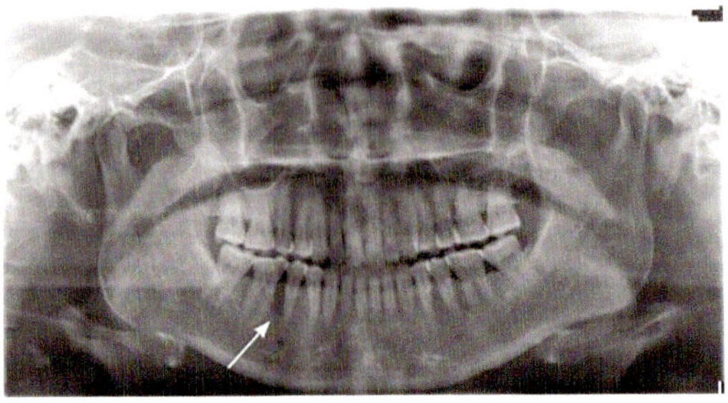

Fig. 36.1 The preoperative panoramic radiograph showed an abnormal hypodense shadow between teeth 45 and 46 at the right mandible, with ill-defined boundaries (arrow)

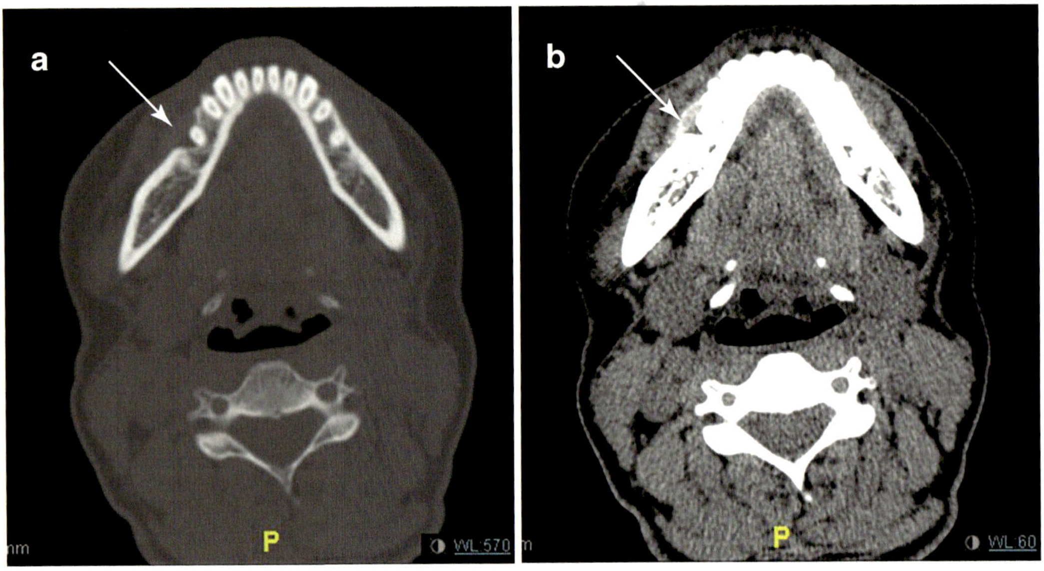

Fig. 36.2 (**a**) CT axial scan (bone): Cystic hypodense shadow at the buccal side of the right mandible (between 45 and 46 root apex area). (**b**) CT axial scan (tissue): No obvious swelling of the surrounding soft tissues

of the septal sinus was thickened and the inferior turbinate was hypertrophied (Fig. 36.2).

[Preliminary Diagnosis] Mass of the right mandible.

[Treatment] "Right mandibular resection" was performed under general anesthesia: An incision was made from 44 to 46, and the gingival flap was elevated for surgical exposure of 45 and 46 dental root mass on the buccal side after partial bone abrasion. The mass was completely resected and sent for intraoperative frozen pathological examination. Histoathology indicated as "right mandible" osteoblastoma; the wound was rinsed and thoroughly hemostatic, and wound closure.

[Pathological Examination] Gross pathological examination revealed the tumor was 1.2 cm × 0.8 cm × 0.4 cm in size, grayish-yellow in color with hard consistency. Microscopically, the tumor was relatively limited, with woven bone trabeculae formation, abundant surrounding osteoblasts, no obvious cellular atypia, and few mitosis (Fig. 36.3).

[Pathological Diagnosis] Osseogenic lesion of the "right mandible" with abundant osteoblasts. Combined with imaging findings, it was considered as osteoblastoma. ICD-O code: 9200/0.

[Follow-up] The patient healed uneventfully. The postoperative 6-month follow-up exhibited no obvious postoperative reaction.

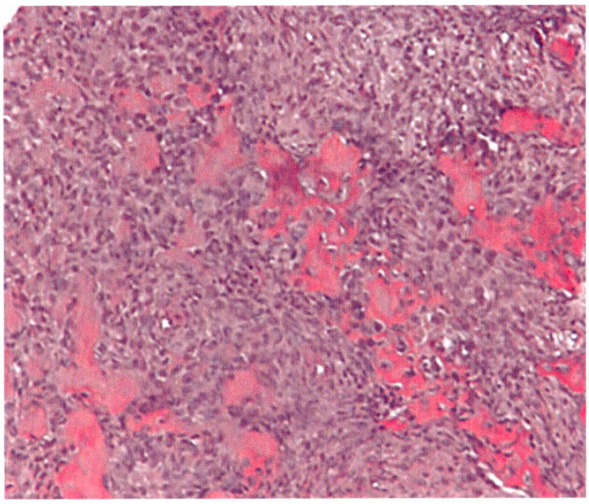

Fig. 36.3 The tumor consisted of a large number of proliferative woven bones and osteoblasts (200×)

36.3 Key Points of Diagnosis and Treatment

Osteoblastoma rarely occurs in the jaw. The etiology is associated to trauma, inflammation, and an abnormal local response of the jawbone. Osteoblastoma of the jaw is commonly found in the mandible than in the maxilla, especially at the mandibular ramus, the condyle, or the temporomandibular joint. Most patients are male and below 30 years old.

Clinical Manifestations The main clinical symptom is nocturnal pain, which can be relieved using aspirin. Osteoblastoma of the jaw often manifests as tooth pain and swelling, tooth displacement, tooth resorption, or tooth disorder. In some cases, it may involve the maxillary sinus and eyes, resulting in narrowing of the eye cavity, eye displacement, vision disturbance, etc. In a few cases, there is numbness of the inferior alveolar nerve.

Imaging Characteristics X-ray shows that osteoblastoma appears as round or oval osteolytic defect with well-defined borders. In subperiosteal cases, a thin reactive bone shell remains at the border. 1/3 of patients show localized ossification, indicating calcification of the tumor bone. A mixture of opacification and translucency, as well as the absence of a sclerotic rim around the lesion, are common radiological manifestations of osteoblastoma.

Pathological Characteristics Histologically, osteoblastoma is a bone-forming tumor characterized by the presence of osteoid and woven bone deposits and a large number of osteoblasts, which are often closely associated with newly formed bones. Pathologic examination reveals a tumor lesion with needle-like, woven bone surrounded by distinctive osteoblasts, and osteoblasts with visible mitosis, but without atypical mitosis. This type is called benign osteoblastoma. In some cases, some osteoblasts appear large and hypertrophic with distinct nucleus and visible mitosis. This type is called epithelioid osteoblastoma, which has the characteristics of osteoblastoma on X-ray and tissue structure, but shows remarkable atypia, local invasive growth, and a tendency of local recurrence. Distant metastases to the lung and liver have been reported, characterized by low-grade malignancy. This particular type is called invasive osteoblastoma.

[Differential Diagnosis] Osteoblastoma of the jaw is a rare benign tumor, but it may become malignant. Osteoblastoma of the jaw should be differentiated from osteoma, ossifying fibroma, and fibrous dysplasia of bone.

[Treatment] The most widely accepted therapy for osteoblastoma is surgical excision, and scaling is not recommended because of the high probability of recurrence. Osteoblastoma enjoys a sound prognosis, with a recurrence rate of 13.6%. In invasive epithelioid osteoblastoma, an extended maxillary resection with postoperative radiotherapy and/or chemotherapy is recommended.

References

1. Sahu S, Padhiary S, Banerjee R, et al. Osteoblastoma of mandible: a unique entity [J]. Contemp Clin Dent. 2019;10(2):402–5.
2. Khokhar S, Mumtaz S, Liggins S. Osteoblastoma of the mandible: a rare locally aggressive benign tumour [J]. Oral Oncol. 2018;82:198–9.

3. Caltabiano R, Serra A, Bonfiglio M, et al. A rare location of benign osteoblastoma: case study and a review of the literature [J]. Eur Rev Med Pharmacol Sci. 2012;16(13):1891–4.
4. Bokhari K, Hameed MS, Ajmal M, et al. Benign osteoblastoma involving maxilla: a case report and review of the literature [J]. Case Rep Dent. 2012;2012:351241.
5. Manjunatha BS, Sunit P, Amit M, et al. Osteoblastoma of the jaws: report of a case and review of literature [J]. Clin Pract. 2011;1(4):e118.
6. Jones AC, Prihoda TJ, Kacher JE, et al. Osteoblastoma of the maxilla and mandible: a report of 24 cases, review of the literature and discussion of its relationship to osteoid osteoma of the jaws [J]. Oral Surg Oral Med Oral Pathol Oral Radiol Endod. 2006;102(5):639–50.
7. Angiero F, Mellone P, Baldi A, et al. Osteoblastoma of the jaw: report of two cases and review of the literature [J]. In Vivo. 2006;20(5):665–70.
8. Weinberg S, Katsikeris N, Pharoah M. Osteoblastoma of the mandibular condyle: review of the literature and report of a case [J]. J Oral Maxillofac Surg. 1987;45(4):350–5.

Osteoid Osteoma

37

Yue He, Hui Shan Ong, Zhen Tian, Lin Zhu, and Wen Jun Yang

37.1 Introduction

Osteoid osteoma is a benign, slow growing osteogenic tumor with over-formation of unmineralized bone matrix [1–4]. It occurs mostly in the long bones of the spine and lower extremities, but may also occur in atypical sites such as the jaw bone [5–8]. The typical clinical features are small size, a tendency to self-limiting growth, and disproportionate pain.

37.2 Case 70

A 15-year-old girl suffered from a painless mass in her left mandible for half a year.

[History of Present Illness] Panoramic radiographs at other hospital half a year ago showed a hyperdense shadow at the patient's left mandible. But no treatment was performed. CT examination in another tertiary hospital 4 months ago indicated a possibility of left mandible mass or cementoma.

[Specialty Examination] The face was symmetrical and the mouth opening was normal. No submandibular or cervical lymph node enlargement was found. There were no obvious inflammatory secretions from the parotid and submandibular gland ducts, normal tongue movement, and no obvious lower lip numbness.

[Auxiliary Examination]

1. Panoramic radiographs suggested a round hyperdense shadow at the 35th and 36th teeth root apex.
2. Maxillofacial CT scan suggested an anomalous round shadow, about 11 mm in diameter, with a slightly distensible, ground glass-like lesion, and a clear border with radio-opaque ring, in resembling a tooth density shadow. The adjacent mandibular bone was intact, and no soft tissue mass was seen (Fig. 37.1).

[Preliminary Diagnosis] Mass of the left mandible.

[Treatment] "Left mandibular excision" was performed under general anesthesia: an incision was designed along the gingival margin, and the gingival flap was elevated for surgical exposure of the mass at buccal side of apical region of 34. Part of the mandible was removed, and the mass was com-

Y. He (✉) · H. S. Ong · Z. Tian · W. J. Yang
Department of Oral Maxillofacial-Head & Neck Oncology, Shanghai Ninth People's Hospital, Shanghai Jiao Tong University School of Medicine, Shanghai, China

L. Zhu
Department of Radiology, Ninth People's Hospital Affiliated to Shanghai Jiao Tong University, Shanghai, China

Y. He (ed.), *Inflammatory and Neoplastic Diseases of Craniofacial Bones*,
https://doi.org/10.1007/978-981-97-4155-7_37

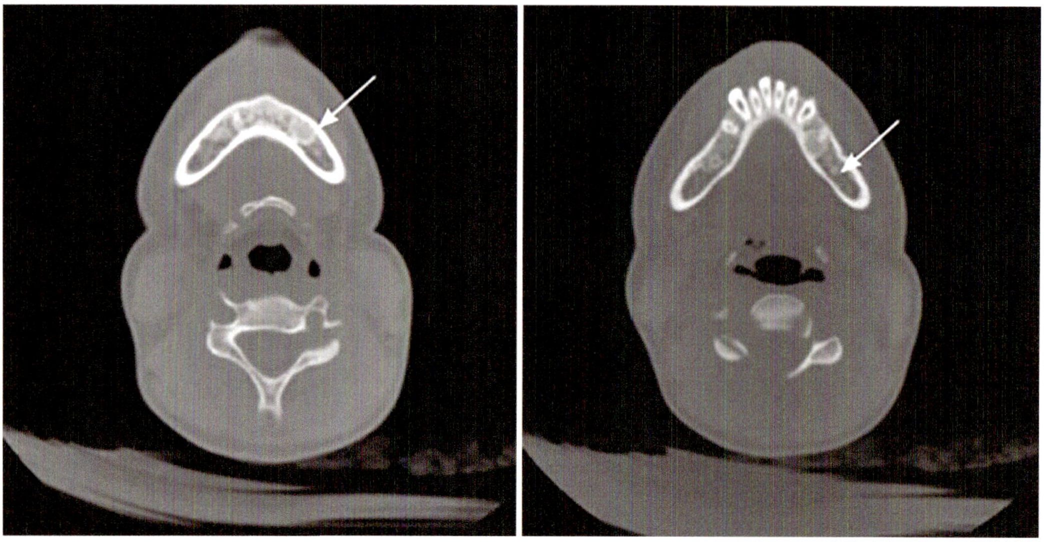

Fig. 37.1 Well-circumscribed, round, ground glass-like sclerotic lesion at teeth 34 root apex in the left mandible. The lesion is slightly distensible

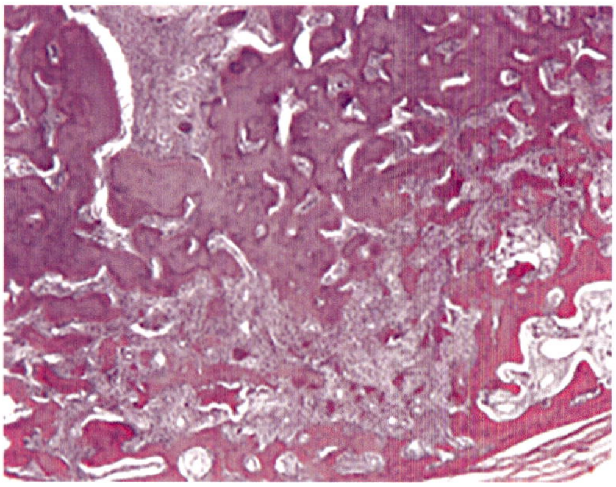

Fig. 37.2 The tumor was composed of bony trabeculae with disordered arrangement and varying degree of calcification and abundant osteoblasts around (200×)

pletely excised and sent for pathological examination. The sharp edges were trimmed, followed by rinsing, hemostatic control, and wound closure.

[Pathological Examination] Gross pathological examination revealed three pieces of hard tissue, 1.2 cm × 0.8 cm × 0.5 cm in size and grayish yellow in color. Microscopic observation indicated immature trabecular neoplastic hyperplasia

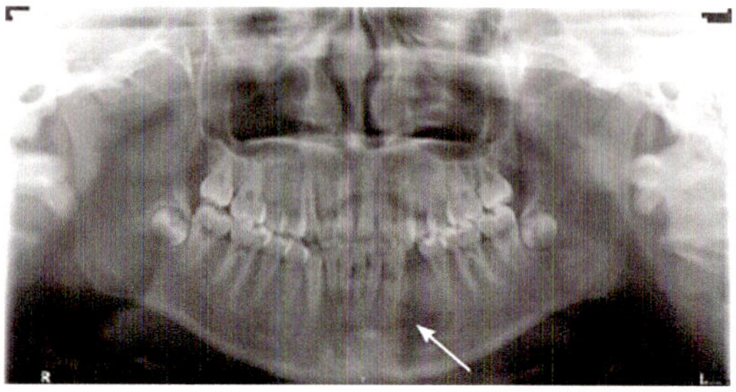

Fig. 37.3 Panoramic radiograph shows the postoperative changes. Loss of teeth 34 in the left mandible, with reduced mandibular bone density at the apical region

with varying degrees of calcification and abundant surrounding osteoblasts without obvious cellular anomalies. Proliferative bone tissues existed around the lesion, and fibrovascular bone marrow was present in the marrow cavity (Fig. 37.2).

[Pathological Diagnosis] Osteoid osteoma of the "left mandible", ICD-O code: 9191/0.

[Follow-up] The patient healed uneventfully. The postoperative 6-month follow-up exhibited no recurrence (Fig. 37.3).

37.3 Key Points of Diagnosis and Treatment

Osteoid osteoma is a benign bone tumor that leads to osteoid unmineralized bone. It strikes mainly in adolescents and young adults, and is common in males. It occurs usually in vertebrae and long bones such as the femur and tibia, while osteoid osteoma of the jaw is currently reported to be rare (less than 1%) in the literature and is mainly seen in the mandible [5–8].

Clinical Manifestations The main clinical manifestations of osteoid osteoma is less than 1 cm in diameter and severe pain. In the early stage, the pain is mild, intermittent, and dull but worsens at night, and later progresses into severe pain that affects sleep and can last for weeks or years. Oral aspirin or non-steroidal anti-inflammatory drugs can completely relieve the pain for several hours. The pain is generally thought to be related to elevated prostaglandins in the tumor. Physical examination often shows local tenderness and redness at the site of the lesion.

Imaging Characteristics X-ray shows that osteoid osteoma is characterized by dense cortical sclerotic rim encircling the ray-penetrating nests of the tumor, especially by eccentric spindle sclerosis. CT is the most effective imaging modality to detect osteoid osteoma and should be scanned at an interval of 1 mm. As osteoid osteoma lesion may be very small and therefore not be detected on panoramic radiographs or CT scans. CBCT presented with thin slices of images and is therefore more valuable in the diagnosis of osteoid osteoma of the jaw. The differential diagnosis includes osteoblastoma, odontogenic osteoblastoma, sclerosing osteomyelitis, and ossifying fibroma.

Pathological Characteristics Histologically, osteoid osteoma is located mainly in the bone cortex. The center area of osteoid osteoma is highly vascularized connective tissues stroma superimposed with differentiated osteoblasts forming an osteoid matrix or woven bone. Sometimes, ossification is visible, with no cellular atypia, and it is surrounded by reactive sclerotic bone, with a clear boundary. In addition, the immunohistochemical staining is similar in both osteoid osteoma and osteoblastoma.

Treatment Osteoid osteoma of the jaw is mainly treated through surgical complete resection. Postoperatively, the clinical symptoms of pain can be improved immediately. Osteoid osteoma enjoys a sound prognosis, rare recurrence, and sometimes self-limiting disappearance. In addition, radiofrequency ablation may be an alternative therapy for patients with extensive surgical damage, which is less invasive but unable to provide histological specimens. However, both techniques have shown similar long-term clinical outcomes in terms of recurrence.

References

1. Matthies L, Rolvien T, Pakusa TJ, et al. Osteoid osteoma of the mandible — clinical and histological findings [J]. Anticancer Res. 2019;39(1):291–6.
2. Diaz-Rengifo IA, Diaz-Caballero AJ, Oro KR, et al. Painless osteoid osteoma in the maxilla of an elderly female patient [J]. J Oral Maxillofac Pathol. 2019;23(2):280–3.
3. Bajpai M, Pardhe N. Osteoid osteoma of jaw in a 54-year male [J]. J Coll Physicians Surg Pak. 2018;28(6):498.
4. Singh A, Solomon MC. Osteoid osteoma of the mandible: a case report with review of the literature [J]. J Dent Sci. 2017;12(2):185–9.
5. Infante-Cossio P, Restoy-Lozano A, Espin-Galvez F, et al. Mandibular osteoid osteoma [J]. J Emerg Med. 2017;52(3):e83–4.
6. Weber MA, Sprengel SD, Omlor GW, et al. Clinical long-term outcome, technical success and cost analysis of radiofrequency ablation for the treatment of osteoblastomas and spinal osteoid osteomas in comparison to open surgical resection [J]. Skeletal Radiol. 2015;44(7):981–93.
7. Rahsepar B, Nikgoo A, Fatemitabar SA. Osteoid osteoma of subcondylar region: case report and review of the literature[J]. J Oral Maxillofac Surg. 2009;67(4):888–93.
8. Kransdorf MJ, Stull MA, Gilkey FW, et al. Osteoid osteoma [J]. Radiographics. 1991;11(4):671–96.

38 Chondroblastoma

Yue He, Hui Shan Ong, Zhen Tian, Lin Zhu, and Xing Zhou Qu

38.1 Introduction

Chondroblastoma (CB) is a relatively rare chondrogenic primary bone tumor, commonly found in the epiphysis and apophysis of the long limbs, such as the trochanter major of the femur, the tibial tuberosity, and the greater tuberosity of the humerus, but rarely in the maxillofacial region [1–4]. For maxillofacial region, chondroblastoma may found in the squamous portion of the temporomandibular joint (TMJ) and in the temporal bone. Due to its low incidence rate, chondroblastoma is not easy to be recognized by clinicians. Most chondroblastomas are benign, but a few lesions are locally invasive, leading to a high rate of local recurrence and malignancy [5, 6].

38.2 Case 71

A 20-year-old gentleman suffered from a growing facial swelling for more than 4 years.

Y. He (✉) · H. S. Ong · Z. Tian · X. Z. Qu
Department of Oral Maxillofacial-Head & Neck Oncology, Shanghai Ninth People's Hospital, Shanghai Jiao Tong University School of Medicine, Shanghai, China

L. Zhu
Department of Radiology, Ninth People's Hospital Affiliated to Shanghai Jiao Tong University, Shanghai, China

[History of Present Illness] About 4 years ago, the patient found a swelling on the right face accompanied by slight discomfort, and was once treated in hospital. Since the patient was still in the growing stage, they suggested to postpone the operation until after puberty age. Last year, the patient complained of blurred vision. The enhanced maxillofacial CT showed a space occupying in the right maxillary zygomatic region. Thereby, it was primitively diagnosed as calcifying epithelial odontogenic tumor, in which low grade malignancy to be excluded.

[Specialty Examination] The patient's face was asymmetrical, with an obvious swelling in the right mid-face region with an extrusion of right eye. The swelling was hard and no obvious tenderness upon palpation, and about 6 cm × 6 cm in the size. Eye movement was normal and without sign of double vision. There was no abnormality in mouth opening range and pattern. Intraoral examination revealed permanent dentition, normal occlusal relationship, and intact mucosa (Fig. 38.1a, b). No submandibular or cervical lymph node enlargement was found.

[Auxiliary Examination]

1. Panoramic radiographs suggested an abnormal dense shadow at the right maxilla, and bone destruction, which appeared as not well circumscribed (Fig. 38.1c).

Y. He (ed.), *Inflammatory and Neoplastic Diseases of Craniofacial Bones*,
https://doi.org/10.1007/978-981-97-4155-7_38

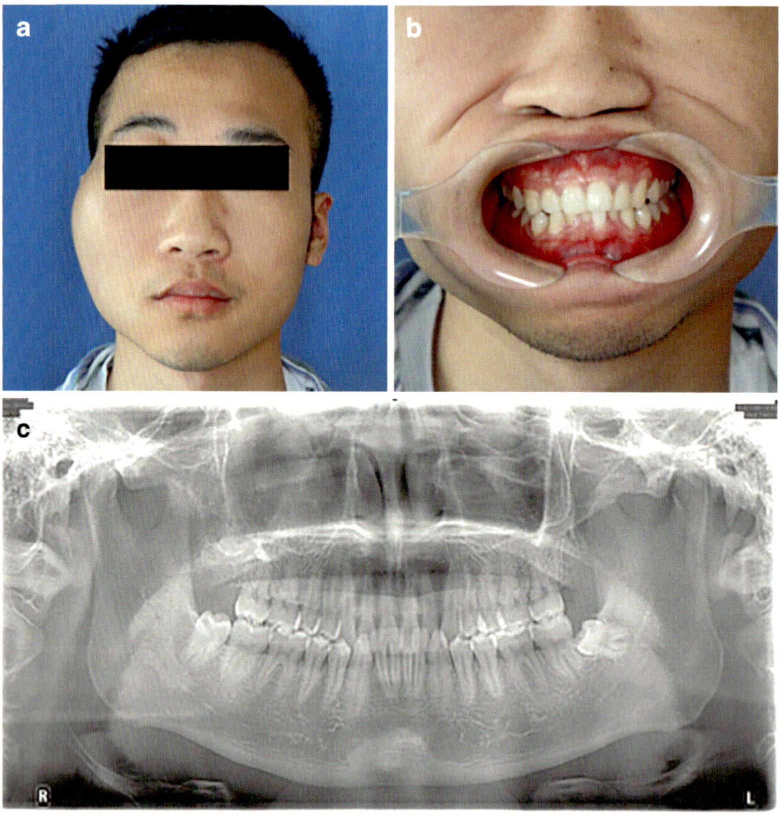

Fig. 38.1 (**a**) Asymmetrical face with obvious swelling at the right facial region. (**b**) Normal intra-oral occlusal relationship. (**c**) Abnormal dense shadow of the right maxilla with bone destruction and indistinct borders

2. Maxillofacial enhanced CT scan suggested a swelling bone destruction in the right maxillary zygomatic region, approximately 59 mm × 48 mm × 60 mm in size, with heterogeneous density and speckled hyperdense shadow. The bone cortex became thinned and interrupted, and the lesion involved the right lateral orbital wall superiorly, the right zygomatic arch posteriorly, and the right lateral maxillary sinus wall and anterior wall anteroinferiorly. The CT scan showed 56 Hu over the lesion (non-enhanced), but the enhancement was inhomogeneous with C+ 91 Hu. No significant thickening of the surrounding soft tissues was seen (Fig. 38.2).

[Preliminary Diagnosis] Mass of the right midface region

[Treatment] "Right maxilla resection and simultaneous reconstruction with fibular flap and tracheotomy" was performed under general anesthesia: a Weber incision was made, and the gingival flap was elevated for surgical exposure of the tumor. The zygomatic arch, lateral orbital rim, and lateral nasal bone were preserved. Osteotomy was performed along the Le Fort I fracture line, preserving the alveolar process and complete excision of the mass. The left fibula was harvested at about 15 cm. The orbital floor and anterolateral wall of the maxilla and the zygomatic process were reconstructed, and the peroneal arteriovenous anastomosis was performed with the superficial temporal vessels. The wound was rinsed and thoroughly hemostatic, negative pressure drainage tube was indwelled, and layered suture was performed to close the wound (Fig. 38.3).

[Pathological Examination] Gross pathological examination revealed a part of maxillary bone tissue, 7.5 cm × 6 cm × 5 cm in size, with a grayish white mass inside, 6 cm × 5 cm × 4 cm in size. Microscopic examination demonstrated chondroblast hyperplasia, eosinophilic or trans-

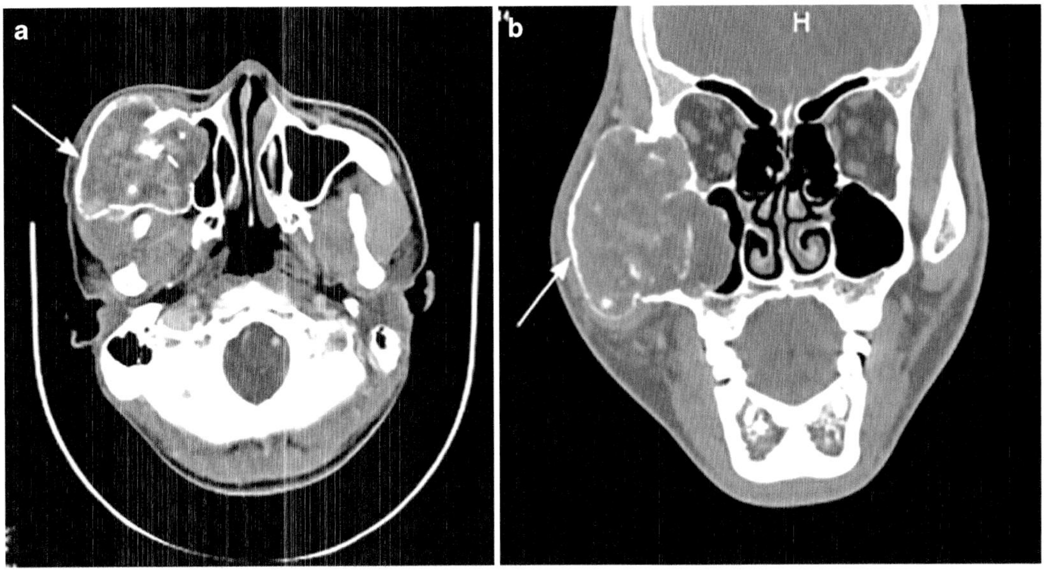

Fig. 38.2 (**a**) Enhanced CT axial scan: expansile bony lesion in the right maxillary zygomatic region. (**b**) Enhanced CT coronal scan: Mass involving lateral wall of maxillary sinus

parent cytoplasm, nuclear grooves, mild atypia, and few mitosis. The pink cartilage matrix between the tumor cells increased the cell spacing, and the characteristic pane-shaped calcification was seen, with scattered multinucleated giant cells (Fig. 38.4).

[Pathological Diagnosis] Chondroblastoma of the "right maxillary", ICD-O code: 9230/1.

[Follow-up] The patient healed uneventfully. The postoperative 6-month follow-up exhibited no recurrence.

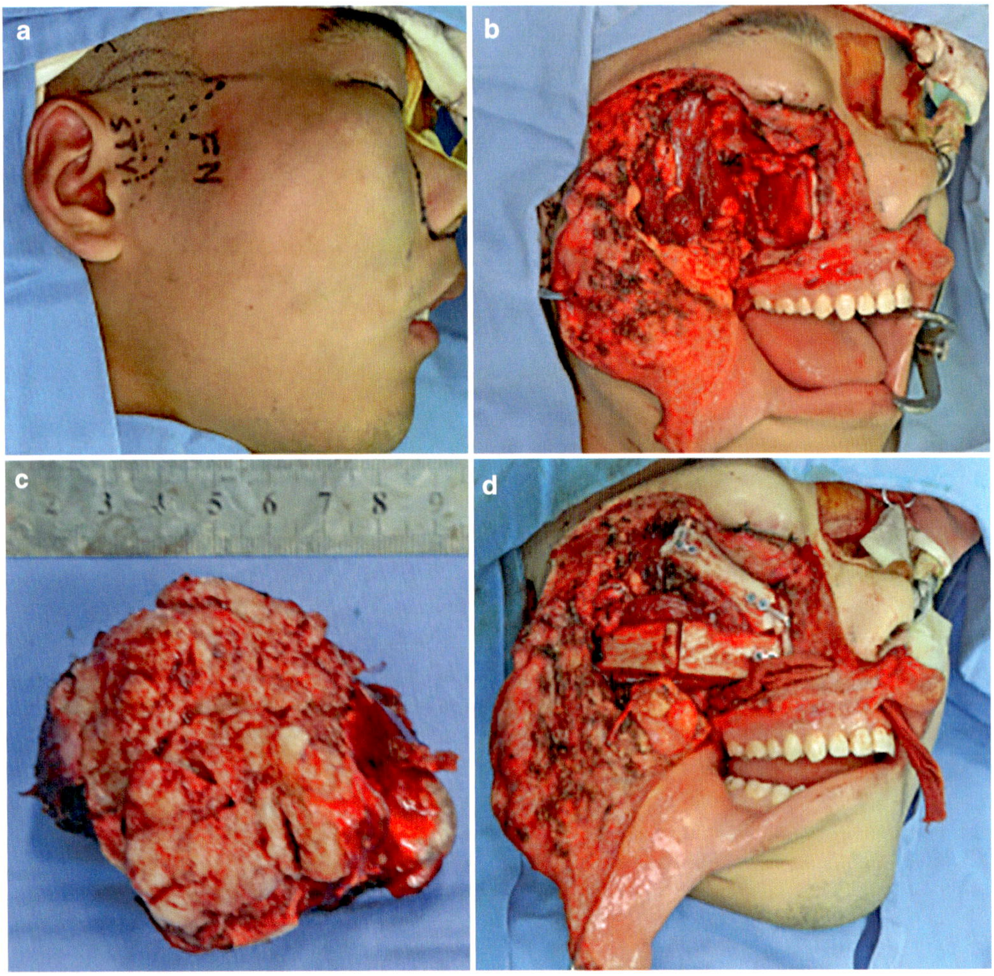

Fig. 38.3 (**a**) Incisional design with the superficial temporal artery as the recipient vessel. (**b**) Preservation of the alveolar process and complete excision of the mass. (**c**) Isolated cartilage mass from maxilla and zygomatic regions. (**d**) Reconstruction of the maxilla with a three-segmenteds fibula

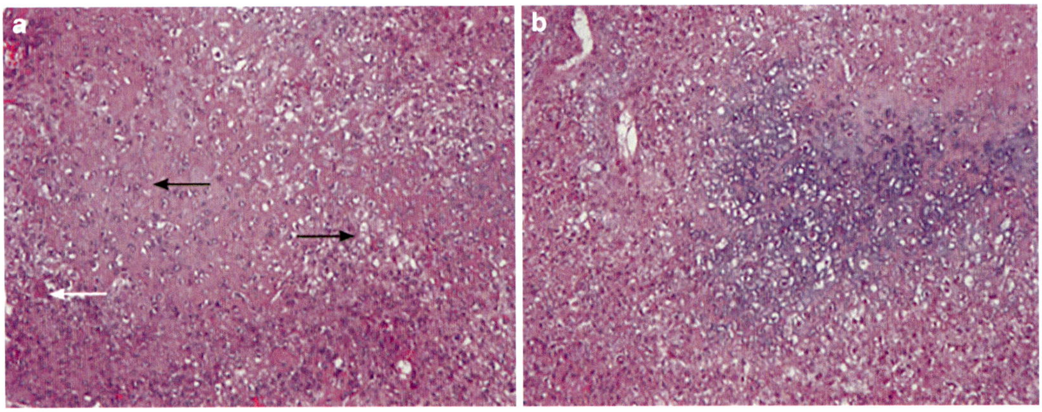

Fig. 38.4 (**a**) Chondrogenic tissue differentiation was visible uder 200× magnification. The chondroblasts are surrounded by pink cartilage matrix (indicated by black arrows), which is distinct from the light blue matrix of other cartilage tumors. Multinucleated giant cell infiltration is seen locally (indicated by yellow arrows). (**b**) Obvious chondrogenic tissue differentiation (200×)

38.3 Key Points of Diagnosis and Treatment

Chondroblastoma occurs mostly in males than females (approximately 2:1) between the ages of 5 and 25 years. Chondroblastoma has no characteristic clinical manifestations, and is common in maxilla. The main clinical manifestations of chondroblastoma are swelling, bulging, and dysfunction of the jaw, sometimes accompanied with pain.

Imaging Characteristics Chondroblastoma appears on X-ray as a round or oval osteolytic lesion with clear borders and a central or eccentric distribution in the lesion area. Some of the lesions are surrounded by sclerotic bands, and there are speckles of calcification within lesions, and the lesions are usually 2–6 cm in diameter.

Pathological Characteristics Chondroblastoma resembles granulation tissue and is blue-gray to dark red in color, with a gritty appearance due to calcification of some tissues. Microscopically, the tumor consists of diffuse or patchy distribution of chondroblasts and scattered multinucleated giant cells. Interstitial cells vary in number and may contain immature cartilage matrix, and myxoid lesions or small focal necrotic areas. Calcium salts deposited around the chondroblasts can form "pane-shaped calcification," which is the clinical characteristic of chondroblastoma.

Differential Diagnosis The differential diagnosis of chondroblastoma requires differentiation from giant cell tumor, aneurysmal bone cyst, and chondrosarcoma. Chondroblastoma commonly develops at the age of 20–40 years, and the lesion is large in extent with blurred margins, often without calcification, surrounded by a sclerotic zone of bone, and without bone marrow edema or periosteal reaction. Chondrosarcoma has a shorter disease course. The lesion is osteolytic, not well circumscribed with no sclerotic rim, and is associated with a distinct soft tissue mass. Annular, semi-annular, and mottled calcifications less than 1 cm in diameter were observed in the tumor and soft tissue mass. The final diagnosis of the disease requires pathological clarification.

Treatment Chondroblastoma is not sensitive to radiotherapy or chemotherapy, so the main therapy is surgical resection. For small lesions, the recurrence rate of surgical enucleation alone is about 10%. It is recommended that the tumor wall treated by enucleation required cauterization with carbolic acid, alcohol, hydrogen peroxide, or liquid nitrogen to completely inactivate the tumor and reduce the probability of recurrence. Although chondroblastoma is a benign lesion, it may exhibit aggressive behavior, it can be with bone infiltration and invasion into articular space, and malignant transformation of chondroblastoma can present with distant hematigenous spread of tumor with the lung as the most common metastatic site [5, 6].

References

1. Limaiem F, Tafti D, Rawla P. Chondroblastoma. In: StarPearls [Intemet]. Treasure Island: StatPearls Publishing; 2020.
2. Chen W, DiFrancesco LM. Chondroblastoma: An Update [J]. Arch Pathol Lab Med. 2017;141(6):867–71.
3. Deventer N, Deventer N, Gosheger G, et al. Chondroblastoma: is intralesional curettage with the use of adjuvants a sufficient way of therapy? [J]. J Bone Oncol. 2021;26:100342.
4. Muhammed A, Meshneb M, Saro H, et al. Management of cranial chondroblastoma in adults : a pooled analysis [J]. Am J Otolaryngol. 2020;41(4):102486.
5. Kyriakos M, Land VJ, Penning HL, Parker SG. Metastatic chondroblastoma. Report of a fatal case with a review of the literature on atypical, aggressive, and malignant chondroblastoma. Cancer. 1985;55(8):1770–89.
6. Kahn LB, Wood FM, Ackerman LV, Malignant chondroblastoma. Report of two cases and reviw of the literature. Arch Pathol. 1969;88(4):371–6.

Osteochondroma

39

Yue He, Hui Shan Ong, Zhen Tian, Lin Zhu, and Jun Shi

39.1 Introduction

Osteochondroma is a bony apophysis with a cartilaginous cap occurring on the outer surface of bone. The tumor contains a medullary cavity that connects to the medullary cavity of the basal bone. It is also known as osteochondral exostosis. So far, the pathogenesis is unknown. According to the location, osteochondroma can be divided into: (1) solitary osteochondroma, most common; (2) multiple osteochondroma, autosomal dominant inheritance [1–5].

39.2 Case 72

A 42-year-old woman suffered from mandibular deviation to the left for the past 3 years, accompanied with restricted mouth opening for 3 months.

Y. He (✉) · H. S. Ong · Z. Tian · J. Shi
Department of Oral Maxillofacial-Head & Neck Oncology, Shanghai Ninth People's Hospital, Shanghai Jiao Tong University School of Medicine, Shanghai, China

L. Zhu
Department of Radiology, Ninth People's Hospital Affiliated to Shanghai Jiao Tong University, Shanghai, China

[History of Present Illness] The patient found mandibular deviation to the left for the past 3 years, which gradually worsened and then developed pain and numbness over the right temporomandibular joint region for 6 months. But, no improvement was achieved after self-administration of painkillers (details unknown). Three months ago, the patient developed restricted mouth opening and right joint clicking, which progressively worsened. The patient received panoramic radiography in the hospital without treatment. CT examination showed a right condylar osteochondroma. The patient denied the history of left-sided joint clicking, trauma, bruxism, and lateral chewing.

[Specialty Examination] The bilateral maxillofacial region was asymmetrical, the lower jaw was deviated to the left about half a finger, the right temporomandibular joint area was slightly expanded, and the left joint area was slightly shunkened inward. A mass was found in the right joint area, about 4 cm × 2.5 cm, hard, poorly defined, fixed, and mild tenderness. No tenderness existed in the left condyle, bilateral posterior disc area, the bilateral temporalis, and occlusal muscles. The motion of the right condyle disappeared, and the motion of the left condyle was reduced, and there was a clicking upon mouth closing. The mouth opening pattern was deviated to the left, and the mouth opening was limited, about 17 mm. There was no tenderness in the bilateral extrinsic pterygoid and intrinsic ptery-

Y. He (ed.), *Inflammatory and Neoplastic Diseases of Craniofacial Bones*,
https://doi.org/10.1007/978-981-97-4155-7_39

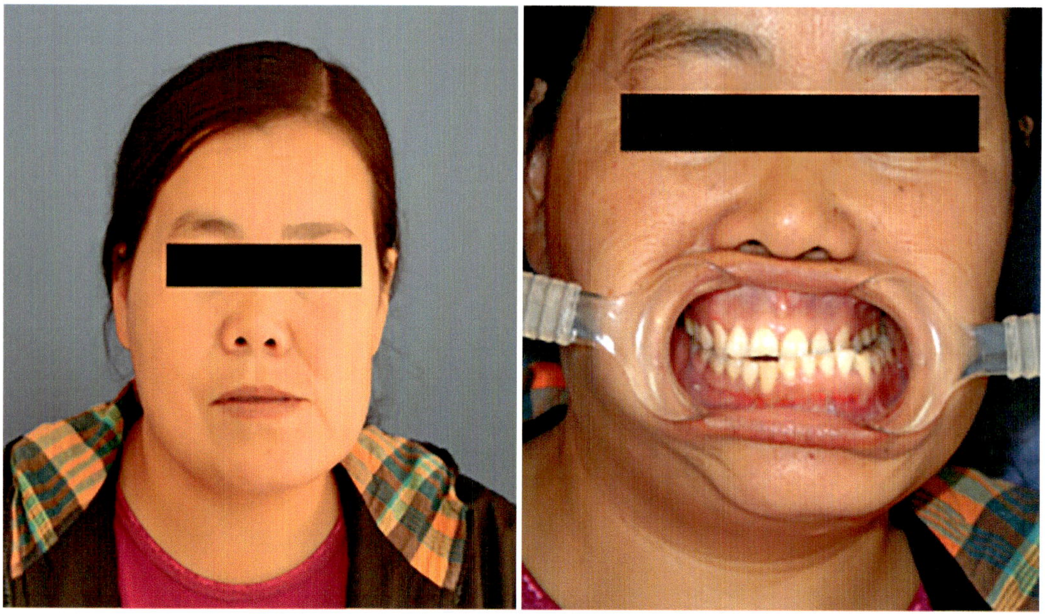

Fig. 39.1 Asymmetrical facial shape, the mandible skewed to the left, and disturbed occlusal relationship

goid muscles. Intraoral examination revealed permanent dentition, cross bite of 38–45 and significantly worn anterior teeth (Fig. 39.1). No abnormalities were found in buccal, lingual, palatal and oral base mucosa, bilateral submandibular glands, parotid glands and sublingual glands. No submandibular, submental, or cervical lymph node enlargement was found.

[Auxiliary Examination]

1. Panoramic radiographs suggested an expanded condylar head of the right mandible with inhomogeneous bone density, continuous bone cortex, and no obvious periosteal reaction (Fig. 39.2a).
2. Maxillofacial enhanced CT scan suggested an expansile change of bone at the medial margin of the condylar process with inhomogeneous bone density, glassy hyperintensities and cystic hypodensities, continuous bone cortex, no obvious periosteal reaction, no abnormalities in the surrounding soft tissues, and no enlargement of cervical lymph nodes (Fig. 39.2b, c).

[Preliminary Diagnosis] Osteochondroma of the right condyle

[Treatment] Excision of the right condylar lesion was performed under general anesthesia: a transcervical incision was made along the lower margin of the mandible and extended to the mastoid region, and the gingival flap was elevated for surgical exposure of the right mandibular ramus. The joint capsule was incised to expose the chondroid mass located on the surface of the condyle. Osteotomy was performed over the neck of the condyle for complete removal of the mass. The tumor was completely separated from the condyle in vitro, and the condyle was reduced and fixed firmly (Fig. 39.3). The wound was rinsed and thoroughly hemostatic, negative pressure drainage tube was indwelled, and layered suture was performed to close the wound.

[Pathological Examination] Gross pathological examination revealed condylar tissue, 5 cm × 3 cm × 3 cm in size, grayish yellow in color. Microscopically, fibrous tissue hyperplasia was observed on the surface of the lesion, and the cartilage cap was uneven in thickness, with well-differentiated hyaline cartilage and the underlying cancellous bone formed by chondrogenic bone, which was connected to the condylar medullary cavity (Fig. 39.4).

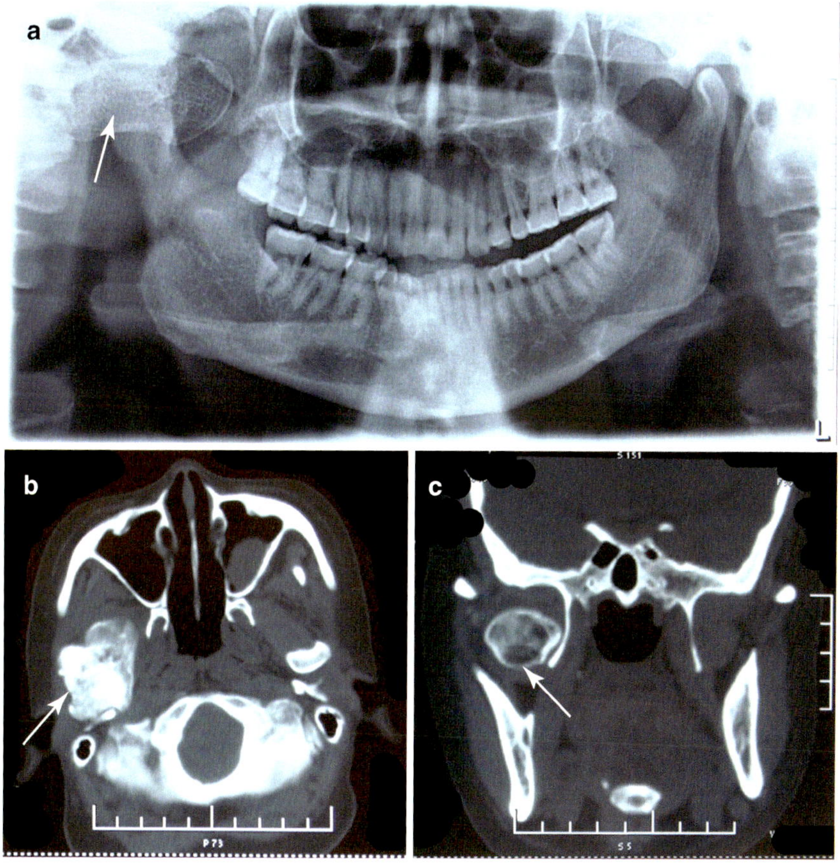

Fig. 39.2 (**a**) Expansile change in the condylar bone of the right maxilla with inhomogeneous bone density, continuous bone cortex, and no obvious periosteal reaction. (**b**, **c**) Bone dilatant change at the medial margin of the lateral maxillary condylar process with inhomogeneous bone density, glassy hyperintensities and cystic hypodensities, continuous bone cortex, no obvious periosteal reaction, and no abnormalities in the surrounding soft tissues

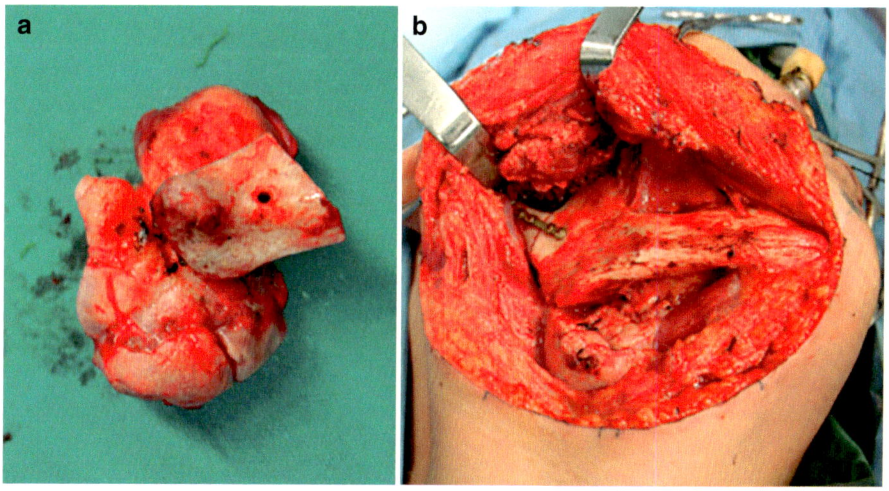

Fig. 39.3 Isolated osteochondroma of condyle bonex. (**a**) Condylectomy was performed, the osteochondroma could be isolated of condylar head. (**b**) Ex vivo complete separation of the tumor from the condyle, condylar repositioning, and rigid internal fixation

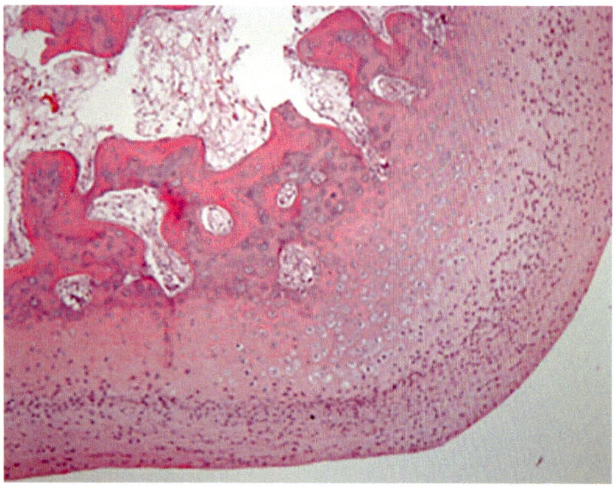

Fig. 39.4 Superficial fibrous tissue hyperplasia, well-differentiated hyaline cartilage in the middle, thickened cartilage cap, perichondral bone in the inner layer, connected with the medullary cavity which is filled with normal adipose tissues (100×)

[Pathological Diagnosis] Osteochondroma of the "right condyle," ICD-O code: 9210/0.

[Follow-up] The patient healed uneventfully, and the stable occlusal relationship was restored without premature contact. No recurrence of the tumor upon follow-ups.

39.3 Key Points of Diagnosis and Treatment

Osteochondroma mostly occurs in the distal femur, proximal humerus, proximal tibia, and proximal epiphysis of the fibula, and rare in the maxillofacial region. In most cases, there are no obvious clinical symptoms, but in some cases, the symptoms may be related to the corresponding complications, including restricted mouth opening, asymmetric facial deformity, and in severe cases, the symptom disturbs occlusal relationship. Osteochondroma grows slowly. Progressive pain and mass enlargement may suggest malignancy, with a malignancy rate of less than 1% for solitary osteochondromas and about 1–3% for multiple osteochondromas.

Imaging Characteristics On X-ray, osteochondroma generally presents as high-density mass shadow, while solitary osteochondroma is an extensive lesion with pedicle or base, and irregular calcification is often observed. When ossification appears in the tumor cartilage focus, cancellous bone and cartilage coexist within the tumor, which is a mass shadow with clear boundaries and inhomogeneous density. When most or all of the cartilaginous foci of the tumor are ossified, it is a well-defined, uniform, high-density image containing bone trabeculae. When the cartilaginous cap calcifies, irregular blotchy or annular shadows with increased density are seen around the tumor. In addition, excessive intracondral flocculent calcification suggests the possibility of malignant transformation.

Pathological Characteristics Histopathologic al findings show that the lesion is divided into three layers, cartilage membrane on the surface of the tumor, cartilage, cells and stroma below, and bone composed of mature bone trabeculae in the deeper part. Loss of cartilage structure, widening of cartilage membrane fibers, mucus-like changes, increased chondrocyte density, increased division activity, chondrocyte heterotypy, and necrosis are indicative of malignancy.

Treatment Surgery is currently considered to be the main treatment for osteochondroma, and radiotherapy is not advisable to prevent induction of malignant changes. Chondrosarcoma can recur after incomplete surgery, and develop into malignant fibrosarcoma and malignant fibrous histiocytoma. Therefore, complete resection is recommended, and the clinical course should be observed and followed up for a long time.

References

1. Alabdullrahman LW, Byerly DW. Osteochondroma. In: StatPearls [Internet]. Treasure Island: Stat Pearls Publishing; 2020.
2. Patel R, Obeid G. Osteochondroma of the zygomatic arch: a case report and review of the literature [J]. J Oral Maxillofac Surg. 2018;76(9):1912–6.
3. Baumhoer D. Bone-related lesions of the jaws [J]. Surg Pathol Clin. 2017;10(3):693–704.
4. Peroz I. Osteochondroma of the condyle: case report with 15 years of follow-up [J]. Int J Oral Maxillofac Surg. 2016;45(9):1120–2.
5. Chen MJ, Yang C, Qiu YT, et al. Local resection of the mass to treat the osteochondroma of the mandibular condyle: indications and different methods with 38-case series [J]. Head Neck. 2014;36(2):273–9.

Ossifying Fibroma

40

Yue He, Hui Shan Ong, Zhen Tian, Lin Zhu, and Zhe Shao

40.1 Introduction

Ossifying fibroma, named by Montgomery in 1927, is a well-circumscribed neoplastic lesion originating from periodontal membrane consisting of cellulous fibrous tissue and diverse mineralized tissue. According to the 2005 WHO Classification of Head and Neck Tumors, ossifying fibroma is divided into three types, i.e., cementa-ossifying fibroma, juvenile trabecular ossifying fibroma (JTOF), and juvenile psammomatoid ossifying fibroma (JPOF) [1–6]. In addition, peripheral ossifying fibroma refers to the ossifying fibroma that occurs in the soft tissues surrounding the jaw bone [2–5, 7–10].

Y. He (✉) · H. S. Ong · Z. Tian
Department of Oral Maxillofacial-Head & Neck Oncology, Shanghai Ninth People's Hospital, Shanghai Jiao Tong University School of Medicine, Shanghai, China

L. Zhu
Department of Radiology, Ninth People's Hospital Affiliated to Shanghai Jiao Tong University, Shanghai, China

Z. Shao
Hospital of Stomatology Wuhan University, Hubei, China

40.2 Cementa-Ossifying Fibroma

40.2.1 Case 73

A 31-year-old woman suffered from progressively increasing swelling for 3 years after surgery for a right mandibular mass.

[History of Present Illness] The patient underwent "right mandibular lesion excision" in the hospital 3 years ago due to "right mandibular mass." Intraoperative frozen section examination and postoperative histopathology indicated a mandibular cyst. The swelling in the right mandible continued after surgery and gradually increased in size, with occasional slight pain upon mouth opening, no numbness or discomfort, no limited mouth opening, no occlusal discomfort, and no bleeding or rupture.

[Specialty Examination] Maxillofacial asymmetry was observed with significant bulging of the right mandible. A hard mass was palpable in the middle of the right mandible, with absence of tenderness, and no sense of crackling of ping-pong ball. The mass was about 5 cm × 4 cm in size, with clear boundaries, no mobility, and no bleeding or ulceration of the surface skin. There was no abnormality in mouth opening range and mouth opening pattern. Intraoral examination revealed permanent dentition, loss of teeth 46–48 and 36, and caries of

Y. He (ed.), *Inflammatory and Neoplastic Diseases of Craniofacial Bones*,
https://doi.org/10.1007/978-981-97-4155-7_40

the proximal anterior teeth. Surgical scar was seen in the gingival mucosa of the right lower missing tooth area, the buccal side was significantly enlarged, and the mass was palpable, hard and nonmobile. No obvious rupture and bleeding happened in the remaining mucosa. No maxillofacial or cervical lymph node enlargement was found.

[Auxiliary Examination]

1. Panoramic radiographs suggested an extensive hypointense shadow of the right mandibular angle and ramus, affecting the tooth apices of 47 and 48, with no root resorption and proximally displaced root of 48. The density is heterogeneous and glassy. The borders are undefined and without sclerotic rim, and the cortex of bone was thinner at the lower margin of the right mandible (unknown transcervical surgical approach was performed in a primary hospital). One year ago, the right mandibular posterior and ramus were swollen, the bone trabeculae disappeared, and there was a wide range of inhomogeneous density shadow with unclear borders, some of which had multilocular cystic shadow areas. No sclerotic rim was seen, and teeth 47 and 48 were missing (Fig. 40.1).
2. Maxillofacial enhanced CT scan suggested a protuberance of the right mandibular posterior and ramus, with thinning of the bony cortex, center soft tissue density shadow, and low-density cystic shadow (Fig. 40.2).

[Preliminary Diagnosis] Fibrous structural malformation of the right mandible.

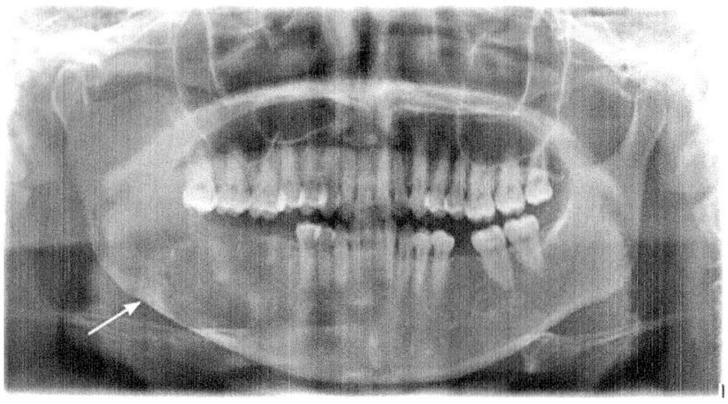

Fig. 40.1 Inhomogeneous bone density reduced in the body, angle, and ramus of the right mandible, bony expansion with center ground-glass attenuation, bone cortex incontinuity, no obvious periosteum reaction (preoperative)

[Treatment] "Right mandibular segmental mandibulectomy with simultaneous fibular osseocutaneous flap reconstruction and tracheotomy" was performed under general anesthesia: transcervical incision was made along the lower margin of the mandible, and the gingival flap was elevated at the right mental foramina for segmental mandibulectomy. The mandible along with the mass, including the condyle were completely excised. The intraoperative frozen section examination and pathological examination suggested fibrous lesion of the "right mandible," consistent with ossifying fibroma. The left fibula osseocutaneous flap was harvested, shaped, and reconstructed to restore mandibular continuity. Vascular anastomosis of the fibula and facial artery and vein were performed. The wound was rinsed and thoroughly hemostatic, negative pressure drainage tube was indwelled, and layered suture was performed to close the wound.

[Pathological Examination] Gross pathological examination revealed a part of the mandible and surrounding tissues, 9 cm × 5 cm × 4.5 cm, with local bony protuberance, approximately 6.5 cm × 4 cm × 3.5 cm in extent. The lesion was well circumscribed from the surrounding normal bone tissue in the section, and was grayish yellow, slightly hard, and gritty. Microscopically, a large amount of mineralization was seen in the fibrous tissue, and the lesion was well circumscribed from the surrounding normal bone tissue. The fusiform fibroblasts were locally sparse, locally abundant and closely arranged, and the mineralization is acellular cementoid with eosinophilic brush-like margins. Multiple cystic cavities of varying sizes are seen locally, with hyperplastic fibrous tissue in the walls and blood in the cavities. (Fig. 40.3)

[Pathological Diagnosis] Cementa-ossifying fibroma of the "right mandible," ICD-O code: 9274/0, with abundant cells and focal arterial aneurysmal bone cyst formation.

[Follow-up] The patient healed uneventfully. The postoperative 6-month follow-up exhibited satisfactory mandibular reconstruction and good occlusal relationship.

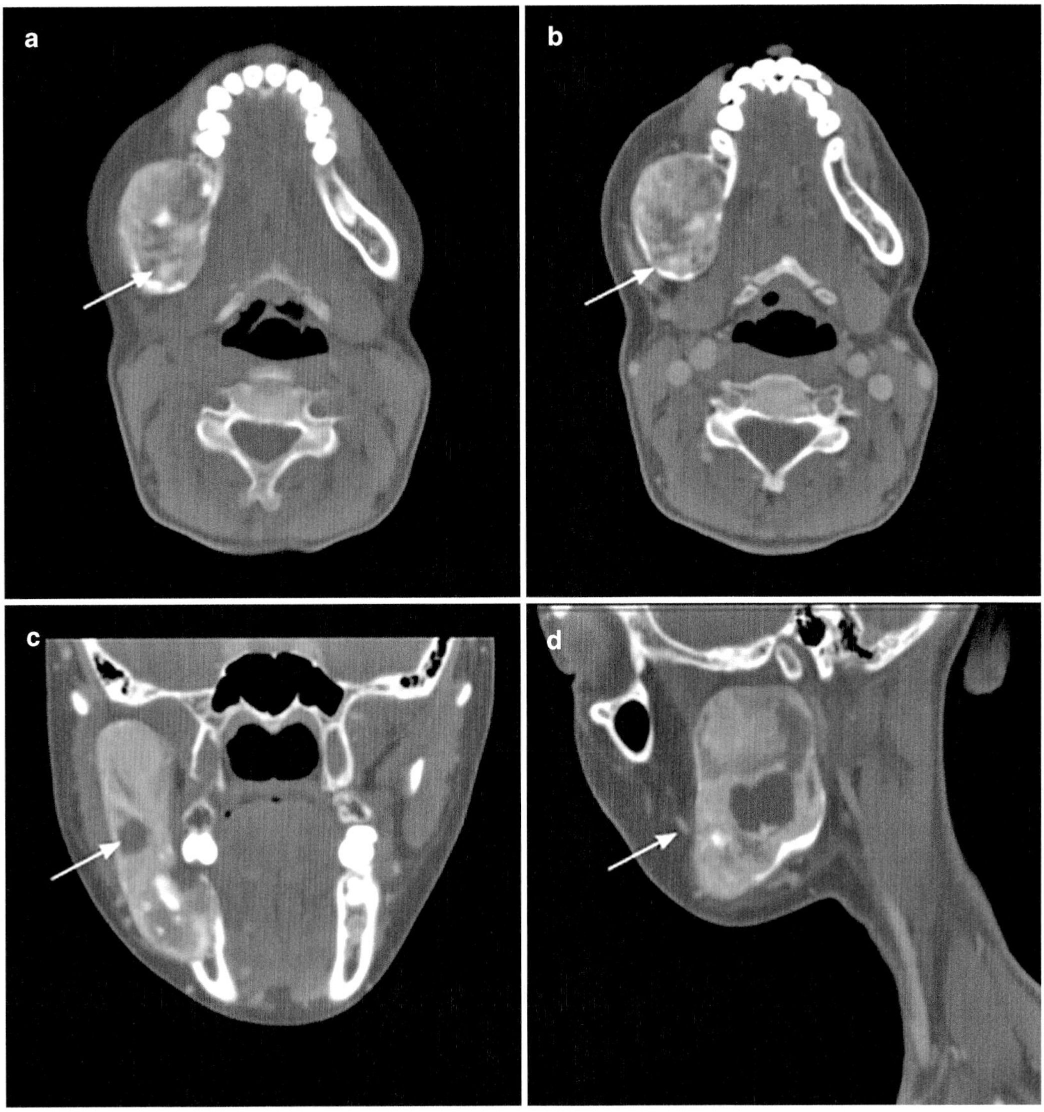

Fig. 40.2 (**a**) CT axial scan: Bony protuberance in right mandible and ramus, density layout, frosted glass-like high-density shadow. (**b**) Enhanced CT axial scan: no significant enhancement. (**c**) Enhanced CT coronal scan: continuous bone cortex, no obvious periosteal reaction. (**d**) Enhanced CT sagittal scan: no abnormalities in surrounding soft tissues

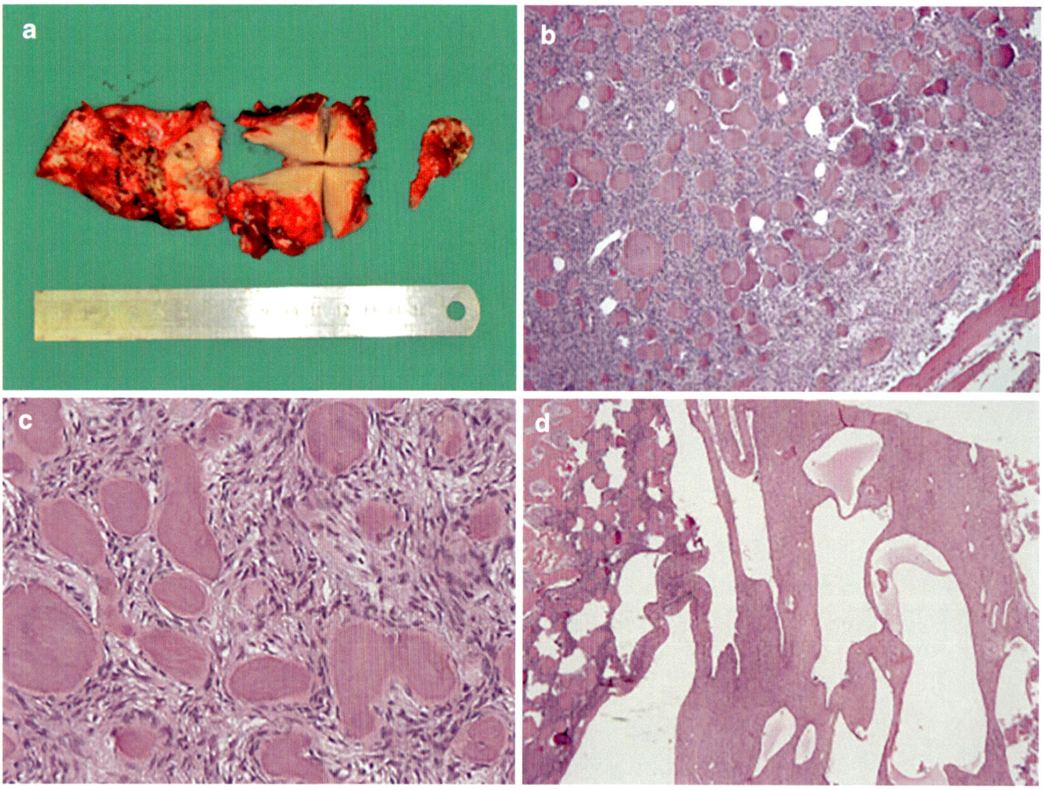

Fig. 40.3 (**a**) Isolated mass of the right mandible. The lesion was well circumscribed from the surrounding normal bone tissue in the section, and was grayish yellow, slightly hard, and gritty. (**b**) A large amount of cementoid calcification formation in the background of fibrous tissue with abundant cells and a clear boundary between the lesion and the lower right host bone (100×). (**c**) Abundant fusiform fibroblasts, and cementoid formation inside, with eosinophilic red brush border visible at the margin (400×). (**d**) Aneurysmal bone cyst formation locally in the lesion (40×)

40.3 Peripheral Ossifying Fibroma

40.3.1 Case 74

A 30-year-old man had a left upper gingival swelling for more than 5 months.

[History of Present Illness] The patient found a left upper gingival swelling 5 months ago with unknown pathogenesis, no obvious spontaneous or provoked pain, no spontaneous bleeding; the patient denied the history of toothache, denied the history of trauma, denied the history of special medication. During this period, the swelling slowly increased in size, with no history of obvious growth and decline.

[Specialty Examination] The face was symmetrical. There was no abnormality in mouth opening range and mouth opening pattern. Intraoral examination revealed permanent dentition. A protrusion reached the labial curve of teeth 22 and 23, and was about 1.5 cm × 1 cm in size, pink in color, soft in hardness, with pedicle possibly, and without obvious bleeding once palpation; tooth 22 presented with grade 1° morbility, and its lingual side was found with two prominent small lumps, about the size of rice and in pink color. The mouth was in poor sanitary condition, with dental calculus I°-III°, and soft scale deposits on the neck of multiple teeth. No obvious cervical lymph node enlargement was observed.

[Auxiliary Examination]

1. Panoramic radiographs suggested residual crowns of teeth 18 and 28, low horizontal impacted crowns of teeth 38 and 48, impacted teeth in bone, and no obvious bone destruction in the maxillary anterior teeth (Fig. 40.4).

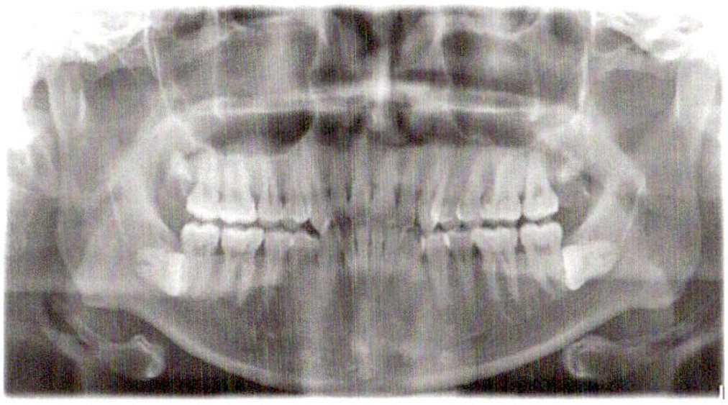

Fig. 40.4 Residual crowns of teeth 18 and 28, low horizontal impacted crowns of teeth 38 and 48, impacted teeth in bone, no obvious bone destruction in the maxillary anterior teeth

[Preliminary Diagnosis] Left upper gingival mass.

[Treatment] "Left upper gingival mass resection" was performed under local anesthesia: a fusiform incision was made along 0.5 cm outside the gingival mass, and the mass was completely excised. Intraoperative frozen pathological examination suggested peripheral ossifying fibroma with infection in the "left upper gingiva." Extraction of tooth 22 and curettage were performed, and the wound was rinsed, thoroughly hemostatic, and closed with suturing.

[Pathological Examination] Gross pathological examination revealed tumor-like tissue, 1.2 cm × 0.8 cm × 0.4 cm in size, grayish white in color, and medium in hardness. Microscopically, the lesion was seen to have no capsule, but it was still clearly demarcated from the surrounding tissue. The mucosal subepithelial fibrous tissue had neoplastic hyperplasia with inflammatory cell infiltration and abundant local fibroblasts, accompanied by osteoid mineralization formation (Fig. 40.5).

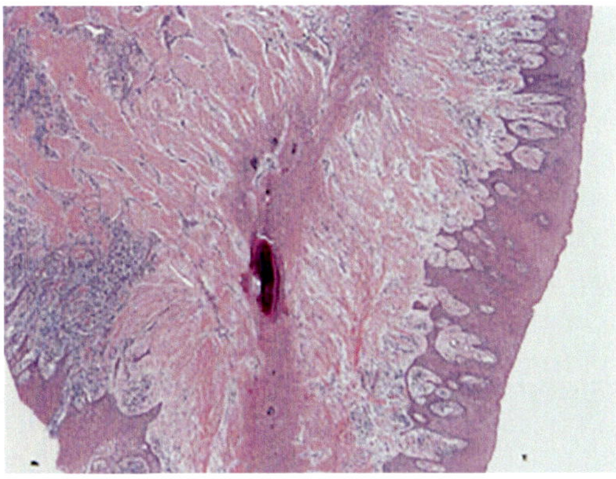

Fig. 40.5 The lesion was confined to the gingiva, with fibroblast proliferation, abundant cells, dark staining, and clear demarcation from the surrounding mature collagen fibers, accompanied by osteoid calculus formation (40×)

[Pathological Diagnosis] Peripheral ossifying fibroma of "upper left gum," ICD-O code: 9262/0, with secondary infection.

[Follow-up] The patient healed uneventfully with no recurrence of tumor.

40.4 Juvenile Trabecular Ossifying Fibroma

40.4.1 Case 75

A 4-year-old-boy suffered from a left mandibular mass for 4 years after incomplete surgery in other hospital.

[History of Present Illness] The patient underwent "mandibular revision" in the hospital 4 years ago due to "left mandibular mass," and the pathological findings showed poor bone fibrous structure. In recent years, the left mandible was found to be gradually enlarged without discomfort or numbness of the lower lip and chin. The outpatient CT indicated a left mandible mass, suspected of juvenile ossifying fibroma.

[Specialty Examination] The face was asymmetrical with left mandibular mass. The surface skin was intact, with normal color and skin temperature. The mass was hard upon palpation, with no obvious boundaries and not tender to percussion. There was no abnormality in mouth opening range and mouth opening pattern. Intraoral examination revealed permanent dentition with optimal oral hygiene. In teeth 31~38 buccolingual expansion of the mandible was observed. The mucosa showed no obvious redness, swelling, and exudation, and was hard upon palpation without tenderness (Fig. 40.6). No redness and swelling in intraoral salivary ducts, and the secretion was clear. The tongue was stretched out in the middle, with free movement and normal taste sensation. No significant enlarged submandibular or cervical lymph nodes were observed.

[Auxiliary Examination]

1. Panoramic radiographs suggested a bone destruction in the left mandibular body with soft tissue mass, irregular in shape, poorly defined, continuous cortical bone, no obvious periosteal reaction, no abnormal swelling in the adjacent soft tissue (Fig. 40.7).
2. Maxillofacial enhanced CT scan suggested a bone distension of the mandible along 31–38 teeth, with smooth margins and inhomogeneous density (96 Hu for C− and 132 Hu for C+, approximately 5.9 cm × 4.6 cm). There

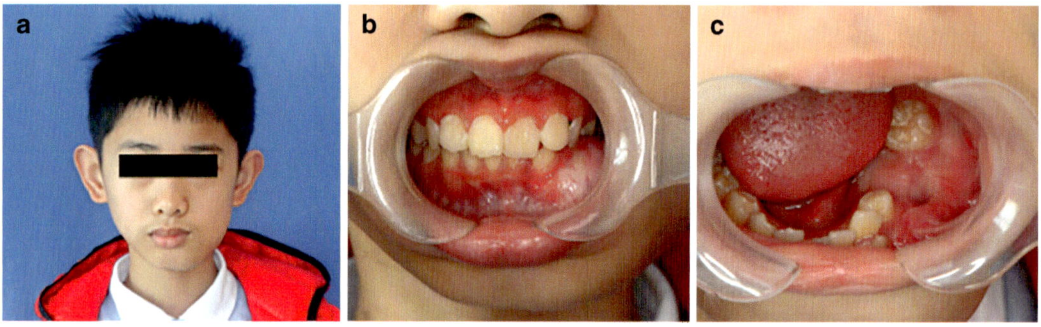

Fig. 40.6 (**a**) Asymmetrical face with left mandibular mass. (**b**) Buccolingual expansion of the left mandible, and intact mucosa, with no obvious abnormal exudation

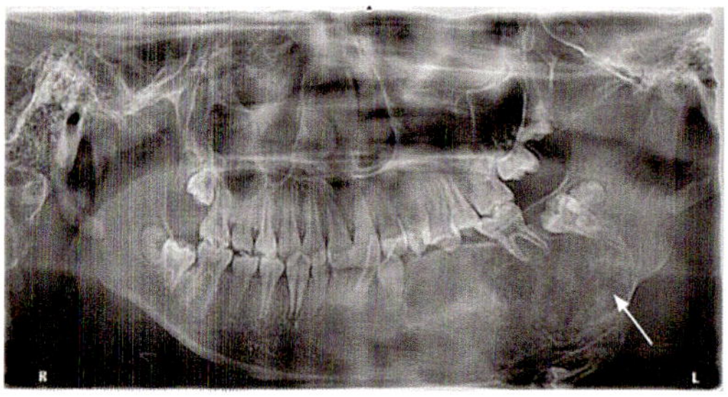

Fig. 40.7 Bone destruction in the left mandibular body with soft tissue mass, irregular in shape, poorly defined, continuous cortical bone, no obvious periosteal reaction, no abnormal swelling in the adjacent soft tissue

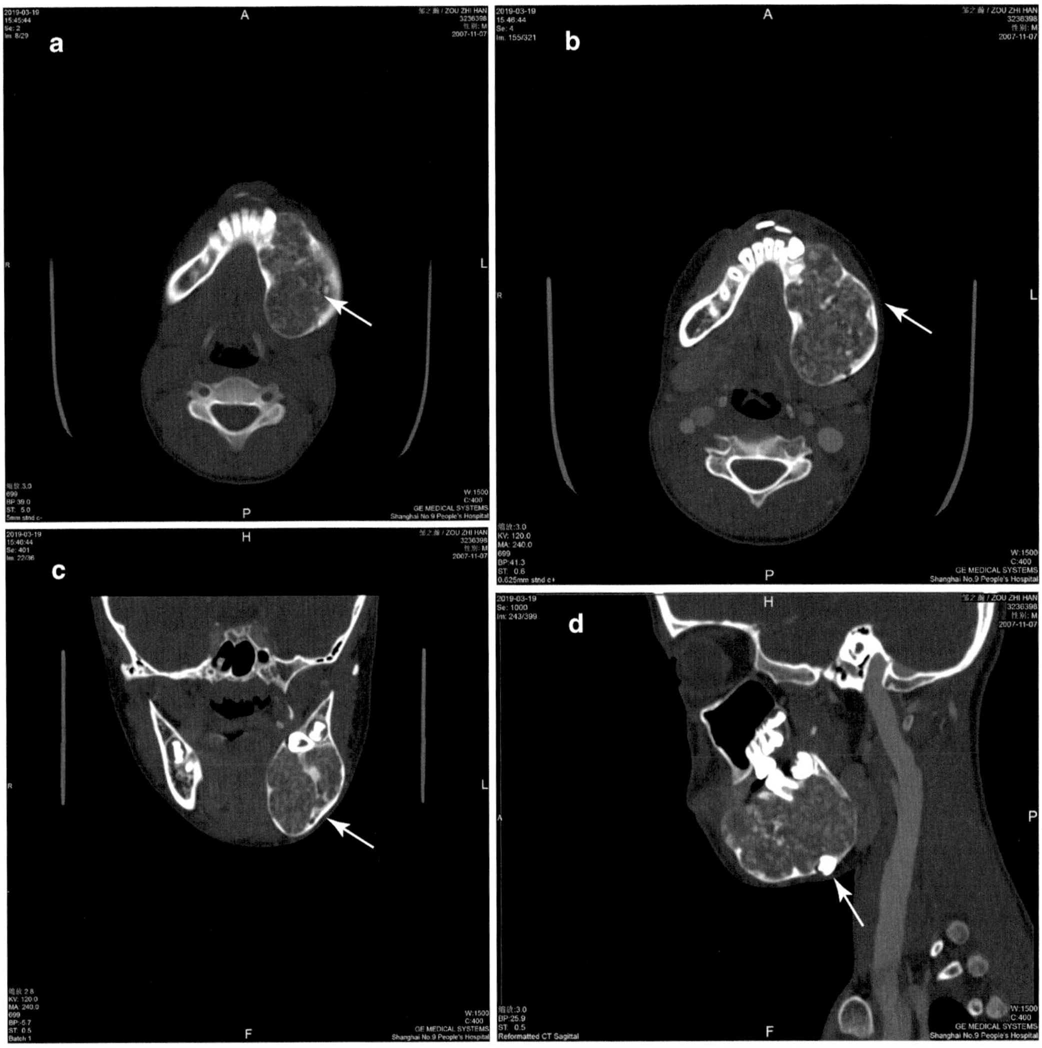

Fig. 40.8 CT axial scan: (**a**) distended bone destruction in the body and angle of the left mandible with a soft tissue mass of abnormal density. (**b**) Enhanced CT axial scan: no significant enhancement. (**c**) Enhanced CT coronal scan: continuous bone cortex, no obvious periosteal reaction. (**d**) Enhanced CT sagittal scan: no destruction of the left inferior alveolar nerve canal

were no abnormalities in the surrounding soft tissues. No significant enlarged cervical lymph nodes were seen. It was considered as a left mandible mass, possibly juvenile ossifying fibroma (Fig. 40.8).

[Preliminary Diagnosis] Mass of the left mandible.

[Treatment] "Extensive mandible resection and reconstruction with fibular flap followed by tracheotomy" was performed under general anesthesia: a transcervical incision was made along the lower margin of the mandible, the gingival flap was elevated for surgical exposure to excise the mandible in the middle of the mandible and at the midpoint of the left sigmoid notch. The intra-

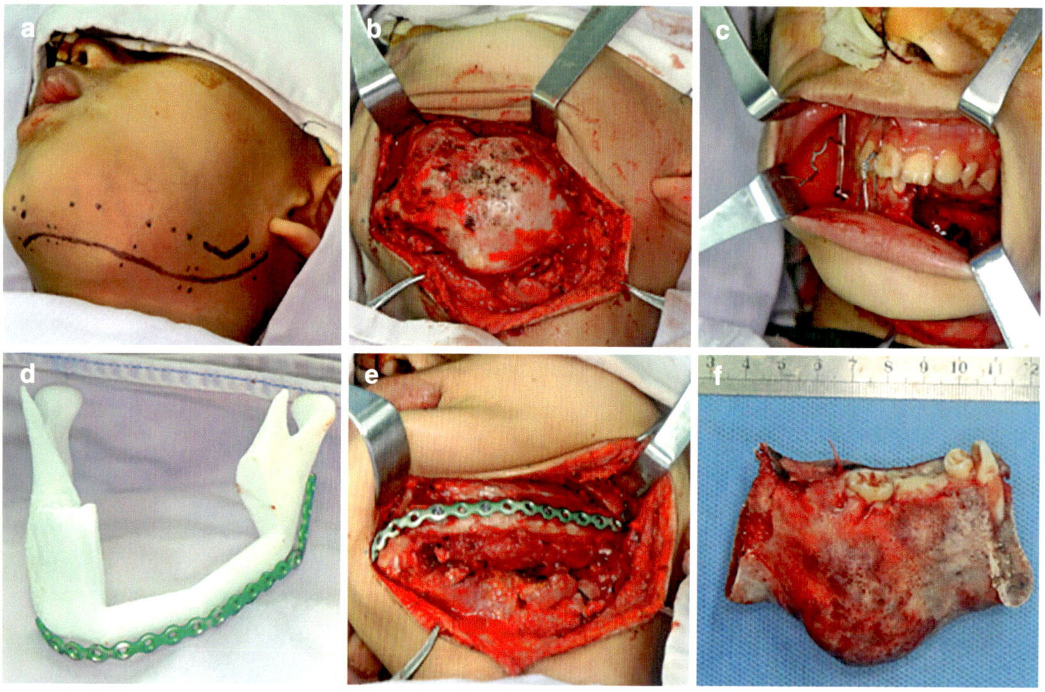

Fig. 40.9 (**a**) Incision design. (**b**) Exposure of the mandibular mass. (**c**) Temporary intermaxillary ligation with truncation of the mandible. (**d**) Digital model applied for titanium plate prebend. (**e**) Fibular reconstruction to restore mandibular continuity. (**f**) Isolated mandibular mass

operative frozen pathology showed fibrotic bone lesion of the right mandible, consistent with ossifying fibroma. The right fibula osseocutaneous flap was harvested, shaped according to the digital planning, and reconstructed to restore mandibular continuity and occlusal relationship, and vascular anastomosis of the fibula and facial artery and vein vessels was performed. The wound was rinsed and thoroughly hemostatic, negative pressure drainage tube was indwelled, and layered suture was performed to close the wound (Fig. 40.9).

[Pathological Examination] Gross pathological examination revealed a part of the mandible tissue, 8 cm × 5 cm × 4 cm in size, with local bone distension. The lesion was well circumscribed from the surrounding tissues, grayish white, grayish red, and slightly hard. The microscopic examination showed slender, naive bone trabeculae in a background of cell-rich fibrous tissue, which anastomoses into a meshwork surrounded by osteoblasts (Fig. 40.10).

[Pathological Diagnosis] Fibro-osseous lesion of the "mandible," considered to be an adolescent trabecular ossifying fibroma according to imaging diagnosis, ICD-O code: 9262/0, with abundant cells and blood vessels in some areas.

[Follow-up] The patient healed uneventfully. The postoperative 6-month follow-up exhibited satisfactory mandibular reconstruction and well-restored occlusal relationship (Fig. 40.11).

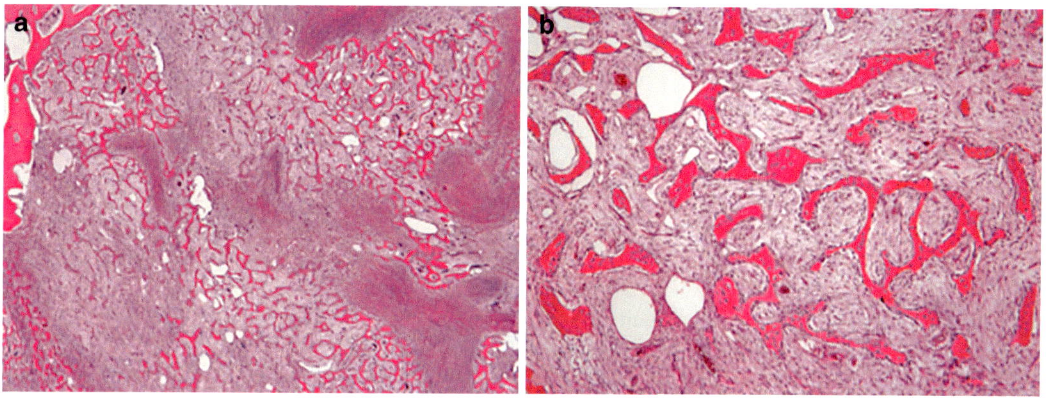

Fig. 40.10 (**a**) The lesion was well circumscribed from the normal bone tissue on the upper left side, mainly showing woven bone trabeculae formation in the background of proliferating fibrous tissue, with sparse and dense fibroblasts (20×). (**b**) Woven bone trabeculae were slender, without obvious calcification, with osteoblasts arranged around the trabeculae in a rim-like pattern, with fibroblasts proliferating between the woven bone and abundant blood vessels (100×)

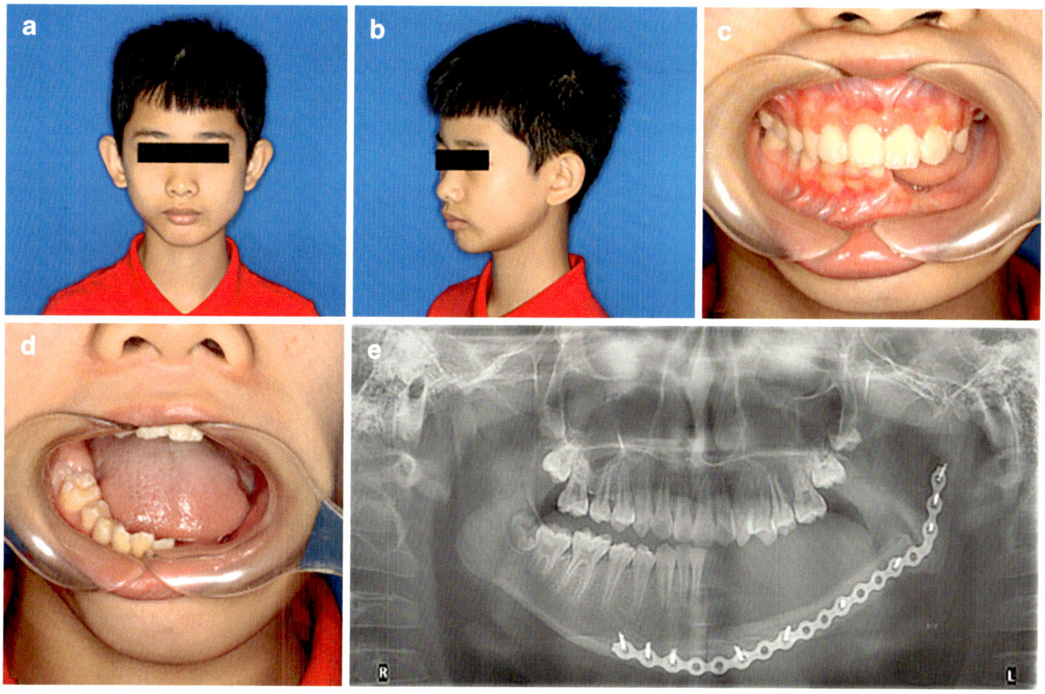

Fig. 40.11 (**a**, **b**) Both frontal and lateral view showed facial symmetry at postoperative 6-month. (**c**) The occlusal relationship of the teeth on the right side was well restored. (**d**) The mouth opening range and mouth opening pattern were normal, and the mucosa of the operative area was intact. (**e**) Good healing of the bone stump after the left mandible surgery

40.5 Juvenile Psammomatoid Ossifying Fibroma

40.5.1 Case 76

A 12-year-old boy suffered from a left facial swelling for more than 2 years, which gradually worsened.

[History of Present Illness] The patient suffered left facial swelling more than 2 years ago, which progressively worsened. He was admitted to the hospital and underwent biopsy in the otolaryngology department. Pathological findings showed juvenile psammomatoid ossifying fibroma.

[Specialty Examination] The face was asymmetrical, with scar at left lower eyelid and left nasal alar crest. Left facial swelling and extruded left eyeball were observed, with no diplopia and no visual impairment. There was no abnormality in mouth opening range and mouth opening pattern. Intraoral examination revealed permanent dentition, maxillary midline left deviation, lower maxillary plane. No significant submandibular or cervical lymph node enlargement was observed.

[Auxiliary Examination]

1. Panoramic radiographs suggested an expanded bony destruction of the left maxilla, with unclear boundaries, heterogeneous density, partially ground glass-like changes and cystic changes, intact adjacent bone cortex, no obvious periosteal reaction, and no abnormal soft tissue mass (Fig. 40.12).
2. Maxillofacial enhanced CT scan suggested an absence of soft and hard tissue (after left maxillary surgery) in the surgical area, expansion of the left sieve bone and maxillary bone, heterogeneous density inside, partially ground glass-like changes and cystic changes, with a horizontal scan of about 22-216 Hu and enhanced scan of C+ 25-239 Hu. Compared with the previous panoramic radiographs, the lesion area increased. There was no obvious abnormality in the surrounding soft tissues. The left maxillary sinus, ethmoid sinus, and frontal sinus were filled with soft tissue density shadow, and the left maxillary sinus was narrowed. No significant abnormality was seen in the bone of the skull base. An oblong low-density shadow was observed at the root of the neck, about 2.5 cm × 1.2 cm, with a CT value of 30 Hu. No significant enlarged cervical lymph nodes were seen (Fig. 40.13).

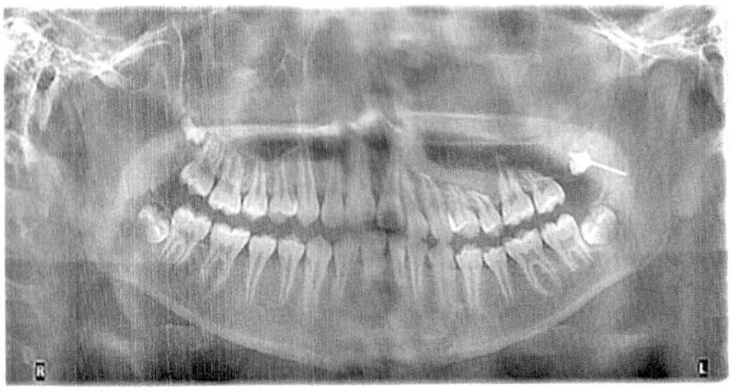

Fig. 40.12 Distended bone destruction of the left maxilla, with unclear boundaries, heterogeneous density, partially ground glass-like changes and cystic changes, continuous adjacent bone cortex, no obvious periosteal reaction, and no abnormal soft tissue mass (preoperative)

[Preliminary Diagnosis] Ossifying fibroma of the left maxilla.

[Treatment] "Left maxillary mass resection with PEEK implant repair" was performed under general anesthesia: a modified Weber incision was made on the left upper lip and the gingival flap was elevated for surgical exposure of the left maxillary mass superiorly to the orbital floor, inferiorly to the alveolar process, posteriorly to the zygomatic alveolar ridge, anteriorly to the nasal wing, and internally to the skull base. The left maxilla and skull base mass were resected using an osteotomy guide plate. Intraoperative frozen pathology suggested fibro-osseous lesion of the left maxilla, considered to be juvenile psammomatoid ossifying fibroma according to imaging diagnosis. The wound was tightly hemostatic, the individualized PEEK was inserted and fixed in place, the maxillary sinus cavity was filled with iodoform to drain from the nasal cavity, and the skin and subcutaneous tissue were tightly sutured in alignment.

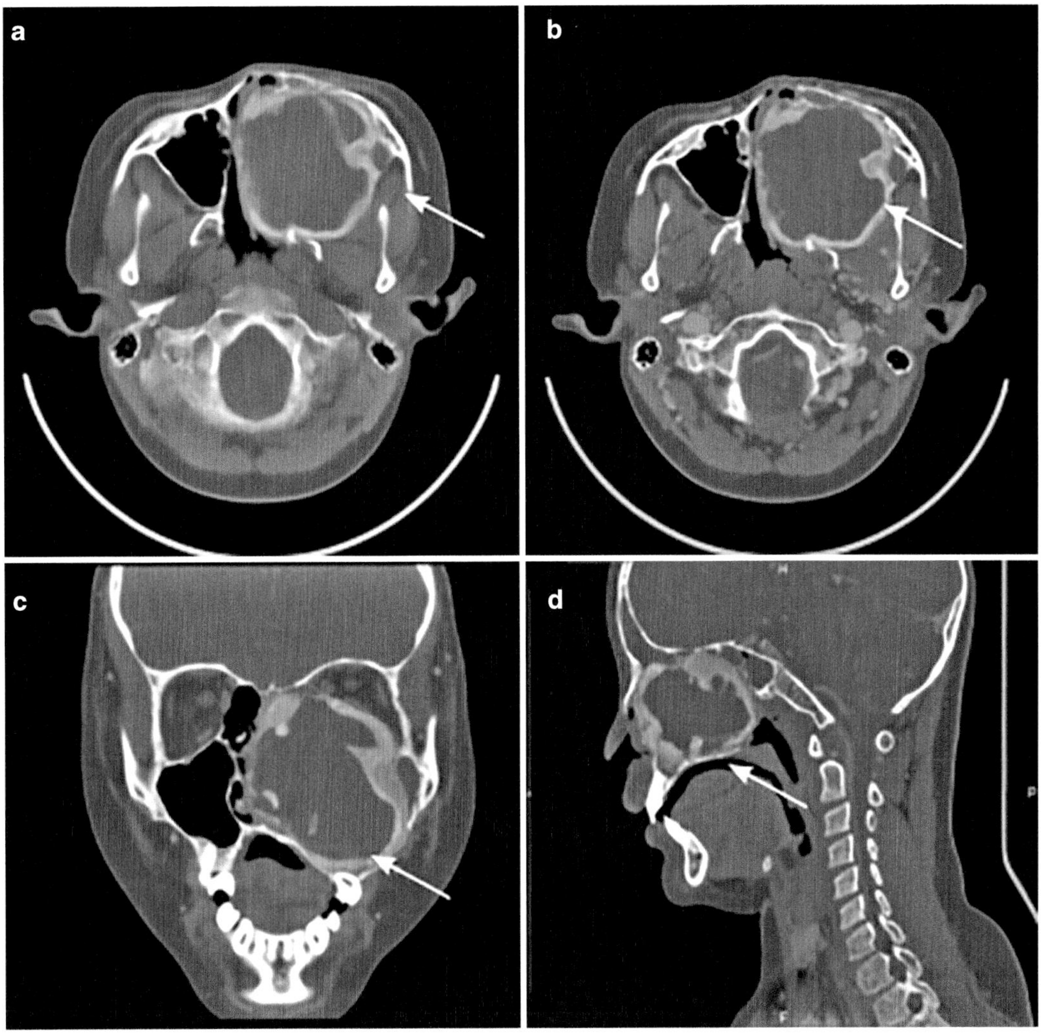

Fig. 40.13 (**a**) Non-enhanced CT scan: Axial view showed a distended bone destruction of the left ethmoid bone and the maxillary bone, with inhomogeneous internal density, partially ground glass-like changes and cystic changes. (**b**) Enhanced CT axial scan: no significant enhancement. Continuous bone cortex, no obvious periosteal reaction, and left nasal cavity compression stenosis (**c**) Enhanced CT coronal scan: the left orbital floor wall was compressed upward. (**d**) Enhanced CT sagittal scan: bone thinning of the maxilla

[Pathological Examination] Gross pathological examination revealed gray white tissue of cystiform and bone tissue in the shape of an eggshell, 6 cm × 3.5 cm × 2.5 cm in size. The thickness of the cyst wall varied from 0.2 to 1.5 cm, and a few blood clot-like tissues were seen inside the cyst. The microscopic examination showed fibrous connective tissue hyperplasia, abundant fibroblasts, and a large number of cementoid structures, with clear boundaries between surrounding tissues. Some areas were cystic and contained blood with abundant peripheral vascularity and multinucleated giant cell infiltration (Fig. 40.14).

[Pathological Diagnosis] Juvenile psammomatoid ossifying fibroma the "left maxilla," ICD-O code: 9262/0, with abundant cells and aneurysmal bone cyst formation.

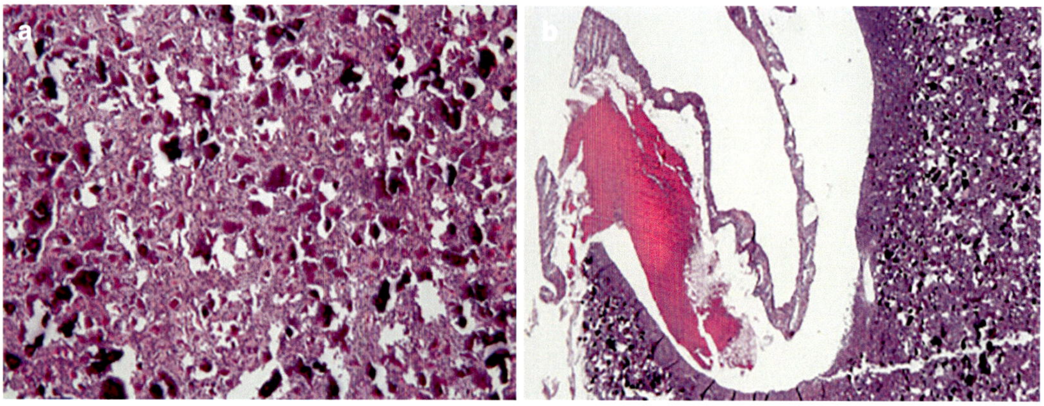

Fig. 40.14 (**a**) A large number of sarcoma-like vesicles formation in the background of abundant fibroblasts (100×). (**b**) Localized aneurysmal bone cyst formation in the lesion, containing blood (40×)

[Follow-Up] The patient healed uneventfully. The postoperative 6-month follow-up exhibited no reoccurrence.

40.6 Key Points of Diagnosis and Treatment

Ossifying fibroma occurs more in women than men between 10 and 40 years of age, mostly as a solitary mass. It happens in the upper and lower jaws, but is more common in the mandible. Histological subtypes vary from age of onset. JTOF has a younger age of onset (8–12 years old), in contrast with the average age of around 20 years for JPOF patients, 35 years for classical ossifying fibroma patients, and between 30 and 40 years for peripheral ossifying fibroma patients. Classic ossifying fibroma occurs mainly in the posterior mandible, JTOF in the maxilla, JPOF in the sinus bone wall, and peripheral ossifying fibroma in the soft tissue of the maxilla.

Clinical Manifestations Ossifying fibroma has no obvious symptoms in the early stage, making it difficult to be detected. With tumor growth, it may cause tooth displacement, disturbed occlusal relationship and maxillofacial deformity due to the expansion of jaw bone. The ossifying fibroma that occurs in the maxilla is prone to spread to the zygomatic bone, and possibly to the maxillary sinus and palate, causing orbital deformation, protrusion or displacement of the eyeball, or even diplopia. In addition to facial deformity, the ossifying fibroma that occurs in the mandible can lead to disruption of the occlusal relationship and sometimes to secondary infection with osteomyelitis. On X-ray, ossifying fibroma is presented as well-circumscribed, monolocular reduced-density area. Due to the formation of hard tissue, opaque areas are common in the center of the lesion.

Pathological Characteristics Microscopic examination shows that classic ossifying fibroma is microscopically rich in fibroblast-rich connective tissue, with trabecular woven bone commonly surrounded by rows of osteoblasts. JTOF consists of cell-rich fibrous tissue with cellular bands of osteoid, and slender, naive bone trabeculae filled with bone traps and osteoblasts and surrounded by rows of larger osteoblasts with mitosis in the cell-rich areas. JPOF is characterized by the presence of abundant sarcoma-like vesicles within the fibroblastic mesenchyme, which are not surrounded by radial collagen fibers.

Differential Diagnosis Ossifying fibroma is mainly distinguished from fibrous dysplasia, which is difficult to diagnose histologically alone and often requires a combination of radiographic and clinical features. Ossifying fibroma is a benign tumor that happens mostly to young people, and is often solitary, and most likely to occur in the lower jaw. It appears on X-ray as a limited expansion of the jaw bone with well-defined, round or oval-shaped, hypodense images in all directions. Fibrous dysplasia is a developmental deformity with an early age of onset and a long course, which mostly occurs in the maxilla and is often multiple; the X-ray shows widespread or limited expansion of the maxillofacial bones to varying degrees, along the long axis of the bone, with no clear boundary between the lesion and the normal bone. The density varies according to the amount of bone contained in the lesion, with some shadows of varying density, others appearing as ground glass, and a few appearing as multifocal cystic shadows. Histologically, rows of osteoblasts are common around the trabeculae in ossified fibroma, but not in fibrous dysplasia.

Treatment Ossifying fibroma is generally considered as a true tumor of periodontal origin that can continue to grow if left untreated. It should be treated by complete excision. Juvenile ossifying fibromas are extremely active morphologically, with no recurrence generally through surgical resection but a high recurrence rate by scaling. A review of the literature reported a high recurrence rate of 8–20% with conservative local surgical excision of peripheral ossifying fibromas. Local recurrence may be attributable to residual periodontal tissue around the periphery of the peripheral ossifying fibroma, and therefore it is recommended that resection should include the periodontal ligament and periosteal tissue at the base of the lesion, and that patients should be followed up long after discharge. In addition, the higher the content of odontoblastic bone within the tumor and the less mature bone trabeculae, the higher the probability of tumor recurrence.

References

1. Chrcanovic BR, Gomez RS. Juvenile ossifying fibroma of the jaws and paranasal sinuses: a systematic review of the cases reported in the literature [J]. Int J Oral Maxillofac Surg. 2020;49(1):28–37.
2. Lazare H, Peteiro A, Perez Sayans M, et al. Clinicopathological features of peripheral ossifying fibroma in a series of 41 patients [J]. Br J Oral Maxillofac Surg. 2019;57(10):1081–5.
3. Nadimpalli H, Kadakampally D. Recurrent peripheral ossifying fibroma: case report [J]. Dent Med Probl. 2018;55(1):83–6.
4. Mainville GN, Turgeon DP, Kauzman A. Diagnosis and management of benign fibro-osseous lesions of the jaws: a current review for the dental clinician [J]. Oral Dis. 2017;23(4):440–50.
5. Franco-Barrera MJ, Zavala-Cerna MG, Fernandez-Tamayo R, et al. An update on peripheral ossifying fibroma: case report and literature review [J]. Oral Maxillofac Surg. 2016;20(1):1–7.
6. Ranganath K, Kamath SM, Munoyath SK, et al. Juvenile psammomatoid ossifying fibroma of maxillary sinus: case report with review of literature [J]. J Maxillofac Oral Surg. 2014;13(2):109–14.
7. Triantafillidou K, Venetis G, Karakinaris G, et al. Ossifying fibroma of the jaws: a clinical study of 14 cases and review of the literature [J]. Oral Surg Oral Med Oral Pathol Oral Radiol. 2012;114(2):193–9.
8. Trasad VA, Devarsa GM, Subba Reddy VV, et al. Peripheral ossifying fibroma in the maxillary arch [J]. J Indian Soc Pedod Prev Dent. 2011;29(3):255–9.
9. Yadav R, Gulati A. Peripheral ossifying fibroma: a case report [J]. J Oral Sci. 2009;51(1):151–4.
10. MacDonald-Jankowski DS. Ossifying fibroma: a systematic review [J]. Dentomaxillofac Radiol. 2009;38(8):495–513.

41 Chondromyxoid Fibroma

Yue He, Hui Shan Ong, Zhen Tian, Lin Zhu, and Wen Jun Yang

41.1 Introduction

Chondromyxoid fibroma is a benign tumor characterized by lobulated growth with mucinous and cartilaginous differentiation [1–7]. It originates from the connective tissue that forms cartilage, and is a relatively rare cartilaginous tumor. Although chondromyxoid fibroma has been classified as a benign tumor, it carries a certain risk of recurrence.

41.2 Case 77

A 41-year-old woman suffered from facial deformity with pain for more than 2 years.

[History of Present Illness] The patient was found to have right facial swelling with pain 2 years ago. She was admitted to the hospital, but didn't receive special treatment, so there was no significant improvement in symptoms. The outpatient CT examination 1 month ago indicated space occupying of the right zygomatic bone.

[Specialty Examination] The face was asymmetrical and the right zygomatic region was more elevated than the contralateral one, ranging from the infraorbital rim to the root of the zygomatic arch and up to the zygomatic frontal suture, about 5 cm × 3 cm in size, unclear in boundary, inactive, hard and obvious tenderness. Neither diplopia nor facial palsy happened. There was no abnormality in mouth opening range and mouth opening pattern. Intraoral examination revealed permanent dentition, normal occlusal relationship, no obvious redness or swelling at the parotid gland duct, free tongue movement, no obvious abnormality in the remaining mucosa of the mouth, and no obvious enlarged cervical lymph nodes.

[Auxiliary Examination] Maxillofacial enhanced CT scan suggested distended bone attenuation of the right zygomatic bone, with fine osteoid shadow inside. After enhancement, the enhancement was mild and no obvious soft tissue swelling was observed. It was considered as benign vascular malformation, with giant cell lesion to be excluded (Fig. 41.1).

[Preliminary Diagnosis] Right zygomatic mass.

[Treatment] "Resection of right zygomatic mass" was performed under general anesthesia: a transconjuctival incision was made at the right

Y. He (✉) · H. S. Ong · Z. Tian · W. J. Yang
Department of Oral Maxillofacial-Head & Neck Oncology, Shanghai Ninth People's Hospital, Shanghai Jiao Tong University School of Medicine, Shanghai, China

L. Zhu
Department of Radiology, Ninth People's Hospital Affiliated to Shanghai Jiao Tong University, Shanghai, China

Y. He (ed.), *Inflammatory and Neoplastic Diseases of Craniofacial Bones*, https://doi.org/10.1007/978-981-97-4155-7_41

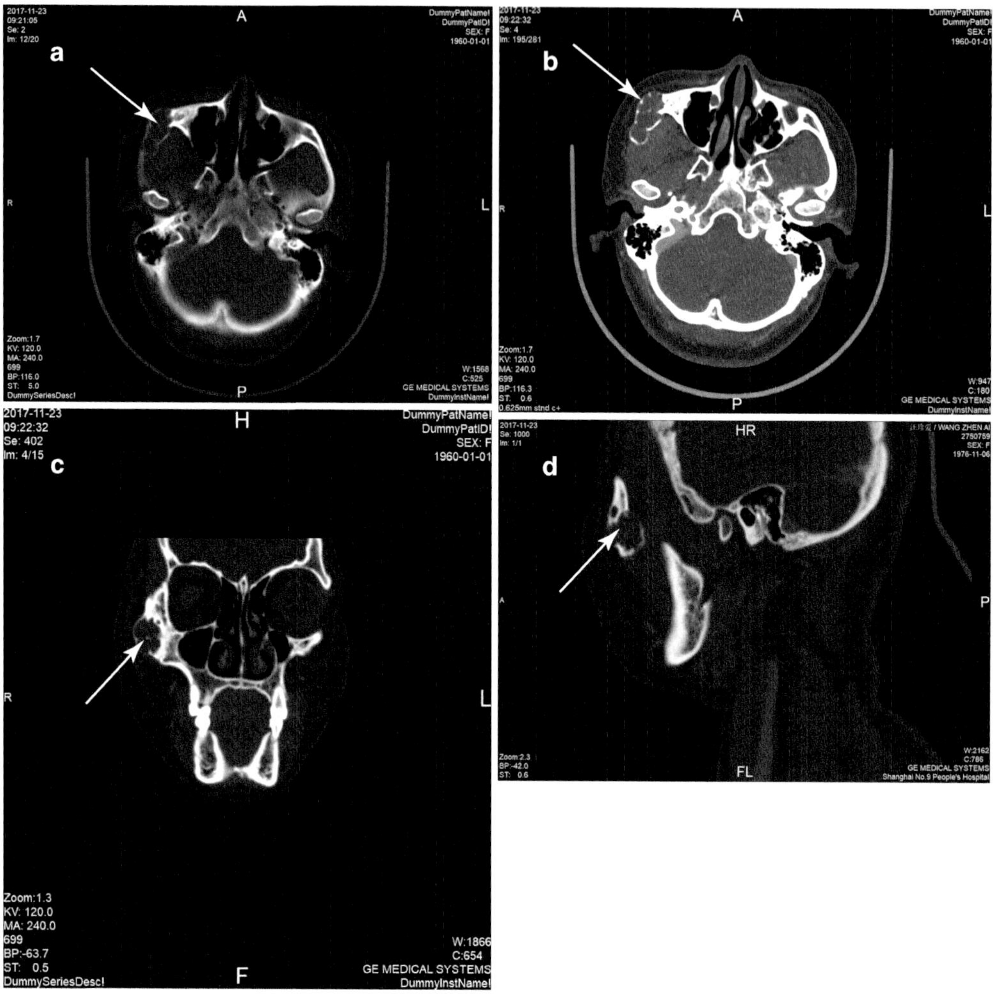

Fig. 41.1 (**a**) CT axial scan: distended bone attenuation of the right zygomatic bone, with fine osteoid shadow inside. (**b**) Enhanced CT axial scan: partial enhancement of the lesion. (**c**, **d**) Enhanced CT coronal and sagittal views

orbital region, extending laterally for exposure of zygomatic arch. Skin flap was elevated to expose a localized mass occupying the zygomatic bone from the inner to the infraorbital margin and from the outer to the zygomatic arch. The mass was irregularly bordered, hyaline solid and brittle. The mass was excised completely. Intraoperative frozen pathological examination suggested a mesenchymal tumor of the "right zygomatic bone" with fibrous, mucinous tissue predominating, and partially cellular prone to be borderline. The wound was irrigated, tightly hemostatic, negative pressure drainage tube was left in place, and the wound was closed with layered sutures.

[Pathological Examination] Gross pathological examination revealed a part of tumor-like tissue, 2.5 cm × 2 cm × 1.8 cm in size, grayish white and red, and tender, surrounded by hard bone tissue. Microscopically, the tumor was well circumscribed from the surrounding tissues, and the tumor cells were arranged in a lobular pattern, with sparse cells in the center of the lobules, which could show chondrocyte differentiation. The denser cells in the periphery were spindle-shaped or star-shaped, with abundant mucus-like or cartilage-like matrix between the cells (Fig. 41.2).

[Pathological Diagnosis] Chondromyxoid fibroma of the "right zygomatic bone," ICD-O code: 9241/0.

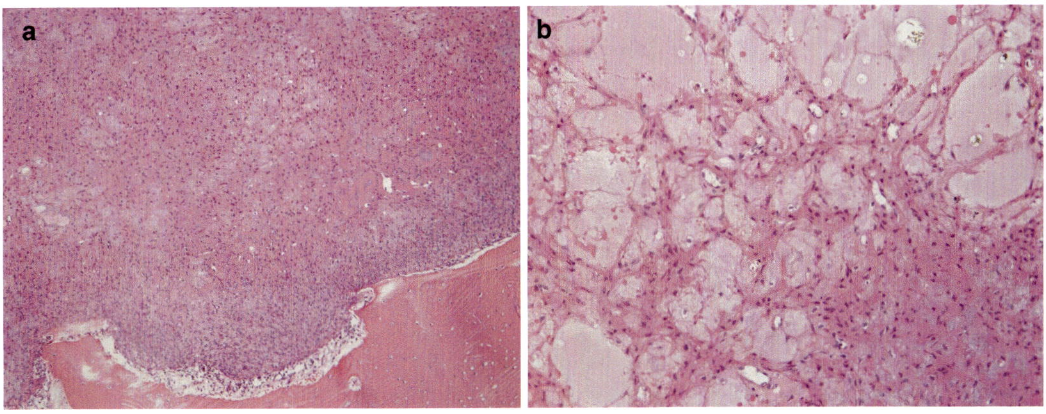

Fig. 41.2 (**a**) The tumor was well circumscribed from the surrounding tissues (100×). (**b**) The tumor presented a characteristic lobular arrangement, with sparse cells in the center of the lobule and dense cells in the periphery, and abundant mucus-like or cartilage-like matrix between the cells (200×)

[Follow-Up] The patient healed uneventfully. The postoperative 6-month follow-up exhibited no reoccurrence.

41.3 Key Points of Diagnosis and Treatment

Chondromyxoid fibroma is more common in males than females between the ages of 10 and 30 and can occur in any bone, mostly in the long bones, especially in the proximal tibia and distal femur, followed by the ilium, but rare in the vertebrae and craniofacial bones of the head and neck. The literature at home and abroad mainly report on individual cases.

Clinical Manifestations Chondromyxoid fibroma is slow in onset but long in course, up to several years. The systemic symptoms are not obvious, mainly manifested as local pain or swelling. Patients with oral and maxillofacial chondromyxoid fibroma may present with facial swelling, disturbed occlusal relationship, mouth opening restriction, and diplopia.

Imaging Characteristics Chondromyxoid fibroma contains a low proportion of cartilage and has characteristic imaging findings. X-ray shows that the classic lesions are characterized by eccentric, well-circumscribed, round-like osteolytic destruction. The lesion may be divided from bony septa of varying thickness into single or multilocular clear areas, and periosteum reaction is rarely observed. Sclerotic or fan-shaped edge can be seen around the lesion, with few calcification within the lesion. However, it has been reported that periosteal reaction, calcification, and ossification are common in cases occurring in the bone cortex.

Pathological Characteristics Chondromyxoid fibroma histologically presents a characteristic lobulated structure, with fusiform or stellate cells in a rich myxoid or chondroid matrix.

Differential Diagnosis Chondromyxoid fibroma requires differentiation from chondrosarcoma and odontogenic myxofibrosarcoma. Chondromyoma, as a common tumor in adults and the elderly, is characterized by large lesion volume, invasive destruction of bone cortex, unclear boundary, no sclerotic zone, and calcification inside. Odontogenic myxofibrosarcoma also presents as unicellular or multilocular projection, but sometimes as a "soap bubble" or "bee chamber," and is usually well circumscribed with bony sclerotic margin, which can cause periosteum reaction.

Treatment Chondromyxoid fibroma is a benign cartilaginous tumor, and the main therapy is surgical resection. There is a tendency to recurrence after simple curettage of lesion bone, with the recurrence rate between 12.5% and 25%. Follow-up should be strengthened after local curettage. Extensive focal excision or complete excision of intralesional bone may reduce recurrence and is the recommended therapy.

References

1. Elsamanody A, den Aardweg MV, Smits A, et al. Chondromyxoid fibroma of the mastoid: a rare entity with comprehensive literature review [J]. J Int Adv Otol. 2020;16(1):117–22.
2. El-Kouri N, Elghouche A, Chen S, et al. Sinonasal chondromyxoid fibroma: case report and literature review [J]. Cureus. 2019;11(10):e5841.
3. Zambo I, Vesely K. WHO classification of tumours of soft tissue and bone 2013: the main changes compared to the 3rd edition [J]. Cesk Patol. 2014;50(2):64–70.
4. McClurg SW, Leon M, Teknos TN, et al. Chondromyxoid fibroma of the nasal septum: case report and review of literature [J]. Head Neck. 2013;35(1):E1–5.
5. Khatana S, Singh V, Gupta A. Unilocular anterior mandibular swelling [J]. Int J Pediatr Otorhinolaryngol. 2013;77(6):964–71.
6. De Mattos CB, Angsanuntsukh C, Arkader A, et al. Chondroblastoma and chondromyxoid fibroma [J]. J Am Acad Orthop Surg. 2013;21(4):225–33.
7. Wu CT, Inwards CY, O'Laughlin S, et al. Chondromyxoid fibroma of bone: a clinicopathologic review of 278 cases [J]. Hum Pathol. 1998;29(5):438–46.

Desmoplastic Fibroma

42

Yue He, Hui Shan Ong, Zhen Tian, Lin Zhu, and Zheng Wu Liu

42.1 Introduction

Desmoplasmic fibroma, also known as ligamentous fibroma and invasive fibroma, is a rare locally invasive bone tumor of myofibroblastic origin [1–5]. It has the age of onset mostly less than 30 years old, and is most common in jaw bone. The clinical and imaging findings are lack of characteristics, so diagnosis by disease examination is required [6–10]. Currently, there is no unified treatment standard, and surgical resection is the main therapy in clinic. Long-term postoperative follow-up is recommended due to its high recurrence rate [7–12].

Y. He (✉) · H. S. Ong · Z. Tian
Department of Oral Maxillofacial-Head & Neck Oncology, Shanghai Ninth People's Hospital, Shanghai Jiao Tong University School of Medicine, Shanghai, China

L. Zhu
Department of Radiology, Ninth People's Hospital Affiliated to Shanghai Jiao Tong University, Shanghai, China

Z. W. Liu
The Second Nanning People's Hospital (the Third Affiliated Hospital), Guangxi Medical University, Guangxi, China

42.2 Case 78

A 20-year-old man suffered from left maxillofacial distension for more than 4 months.

[History of Present Illness] The patient was found to have left maxillofacial swelling without obvious cause 4 months ago. His self-examination showed that the thumb-sized swelling had no obvious pain on palpation, with facial numbness and restricted opening of mouth. With no treatment, he felt that the mass grew significantly. He was admitted to the hospital 2 months ago. CT examination suggested a space occupying of the left mandible, considered to be ameloblastoma of the left mandible.

[Specialty Examination] The face was asymmetrical with left maxillofacial mass deformity. The mass was palpated from below the pretragal zygomatic arch, down to the lower margin of the mandible, anteriorly from the anterior edge of the parotid gland, and posteriorly to the posterior edge of the ramus, approximately 6 cm × 5 cm in size, with a hard texture, a little ping-pong-like sensation, no pulsation, no tenderness, and no mobility (Fig. 42.1a). There was no abnormality in mouth opening range and mouth opening pattern. The intraoral opening was mild. The buccal and lingual side of the ascending rami of the left mandible was distended. The mucosa of the posterior

Y. He (ed.), *Inflammatory and Neoplastic Diseases of Craniofacial Bones*,
https://doi.org/10.1007/978-981-97-4155-7_42

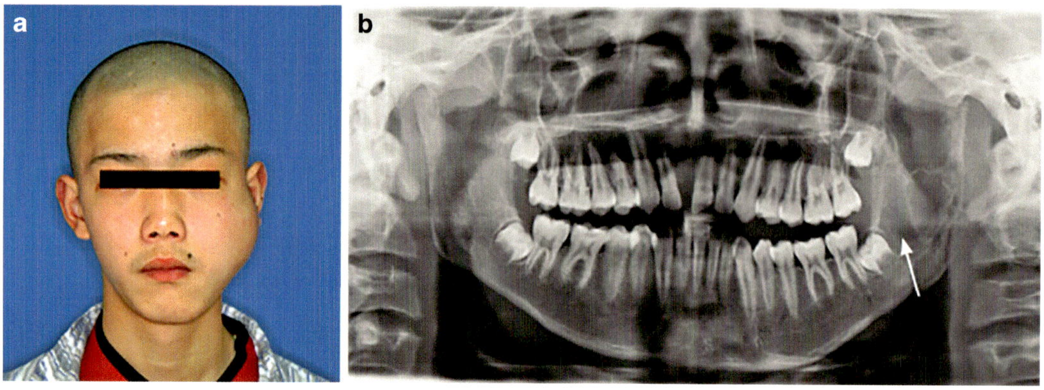

Fig. 42.1 (**a**) Asymmetrical face, with obvious swelling deformity on the left face. (**b**) Swelling of the left mandibular ramus, disorganized bone cortex, and bone density attenuation

molar area to the lateral wall of the pharynx was swollen without tenderness, the tonsils were enlarged bilaterally, and the suspensory pendulum was displaced to the left. No significant submandibular or cervical lymph node enlargement was observed.

[Auxiliary Examination]

1. Panoramic radiographs suggested a distensible change in the left mandibular ramus, with discontinuous bone cortex, and bone density attenuation (Fig. 42.1b).
2. Maxillofacial enhanced CT scan suggested a bone destruction in the left mandibular ramus accompanied by abnormal soft tissue mass with clear boundary and inhomogeneous density, and mild enhancement was observed after enhancement (Fig. 42.2).

[Preliminary Diagnosis] Mass of the left mandible.

[Treatment] "Left mandible resection and reconstruction with free iliac crest" was performed under general anesthesia: a transcervical incision was made along the lower margin of the mandible, and the gingival flap was elevated for surgical exposure of the mass in the molar region, retromolar, and mandibular ramus. The mandible was segmented at the distal 36 for radical resection of the mandible including the condyle and the mass. The left free iliac graft was harvested, shaped, and restore the mandibular continuity and maintain the origical occlusal relationship. The wound was rinsed and thoroughly hemostatic, negative pressure drainage tube was indwelled, and layered suture was performed to close the wound

[Pathological Examination] Gross pathological examination revealed a mass of the mandible, 7 cm × 6 cm × 5 cm in size, and gray and gray red in the section surface, with woven texture and visible bone destruction. Microscopically, the tumor was poorly circumscribed, with localized destruction of bone tissue. The tumor was composed of proliferating fibroblasts/ myofibroblasts and collagen fibers of varying size. The tumor cells were spindle-shaped and arranged in bundles, with no obvious anomalies and no nuclear division (Fig. 42.3).

[Pathological Diagnosis] Desmoplasmic fibroma of the "left mandible," ICD-O code: 8823/1.

[Follow-Up] The patient healed uneventfully. The postoperative 6-month follow-up exhibited no recurrence of the tumor (Fig. 42.4), normal mouth opening and closing, well-recovered occlusal relationship, and satisfactory mandible appearance.

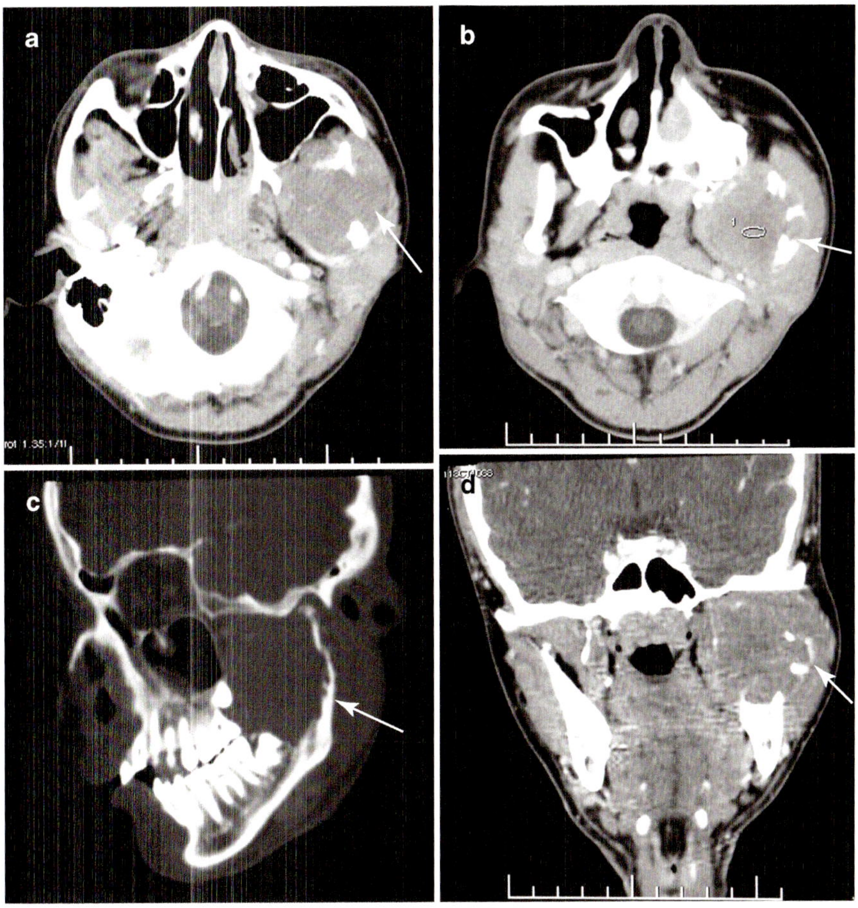

Fig. 42.2 (**a**, **b**) Enhanced CT axial scan: Bony destruction in the left mandibular ramus with abnormal soft tissue mass, clear boundary, inhomogeneous density, and mild enhancement after enhancement. (**c**) Enhanced CT sagittal scan. (**d**) Enhanced CT coronal scan

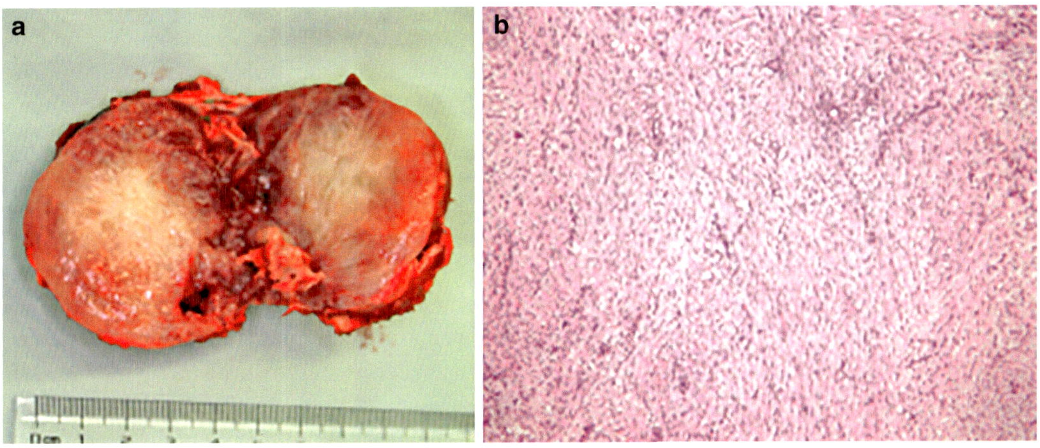

Fig. 42.3 (**a**) The sectional surface of the mass was gray and gray red, partially woven. (**b**) Spindle tumor cell fascicular hyperplasia with intercellular collagen fibers (100.00×)

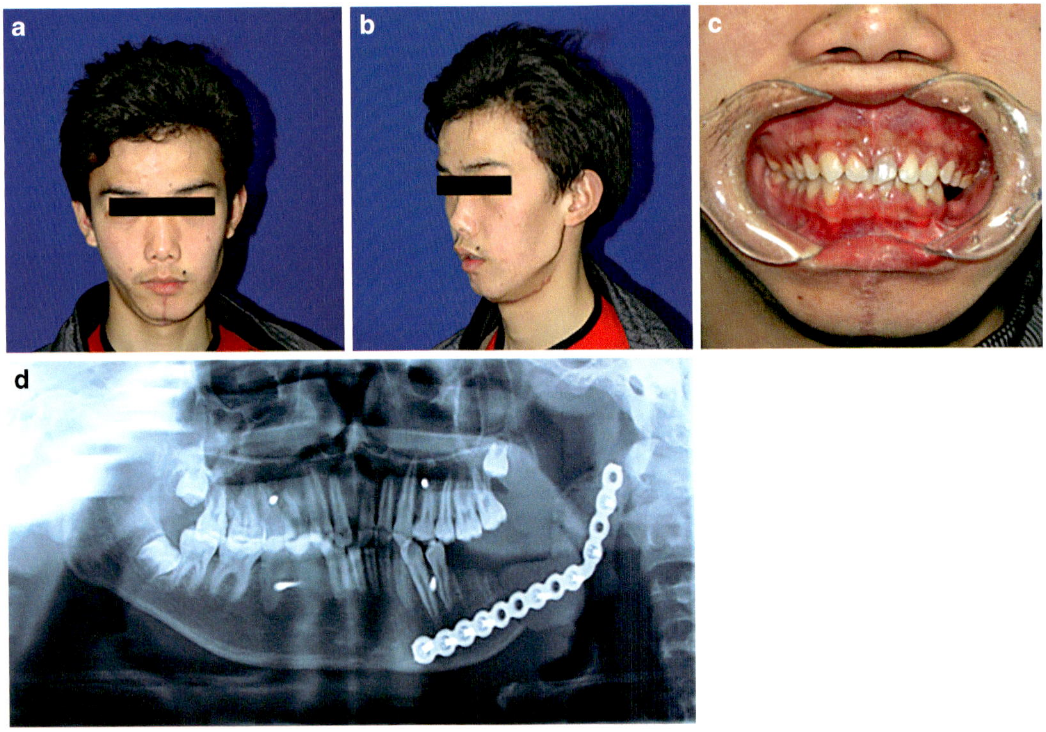

Fig. 42.4 (**a**, **b**) Both frontal and lateral view showed a significant postoperative changes of mandible, it is now facial symmetry. (**c**) The occlusal relationship between anterior teeth and left posterior teeth recovered well. (**d**) Panoramic radiograph suggested good healing of the bone stump

42.3 Case 79

A 13-year-old boy suffered from pain in the left preauricular region for more than 6 months when he opened his mouth, accompanied by swelling and protuberance for 3 months.

[History of Present Illness] Six months ago, the patient felt occasional pain in the left preauricular region for no apparent reason when opening the mouth, and was treated with oral anti-inflammatory medication (details unknown) after diagnosis as temporomandibular arthritis during a hospital visit. But, the symptoms were not significantly relieved. About 3 months ago, he developed the mandibular ramus and preauricular swelling with progressive restriction of mouth opening, and was treated in a superior hospital. CT examination suggested a bone destruction of the left mandibular ramus accompanied by surrounding soft tissue swelling.

[Specialty Examination] The face was asymmetrical, with left mandibular ramus and preauricular swelling. The skin was normal in color and texture, and a 4.0 cm diameter swelling was palpable with unclear borders and no mobility. The swelling was hard upon palpation, with no tenderness and no obvious sensation. The postural test was negative, with no obvious facial nerve involvement. The opening of the mouth was slightly to the left, and the degree of mouth opening was about two and a half fingers. Intraoral examination revealed permanent dentition, intact mucosa, and no obvious sensorimotor disorder of the tongue. Bimanual examination showed mass and bone distension of the mandibular ramus, but with no other abnormalities found. No significant submandibular or cervical lymph node enlargement was observed.

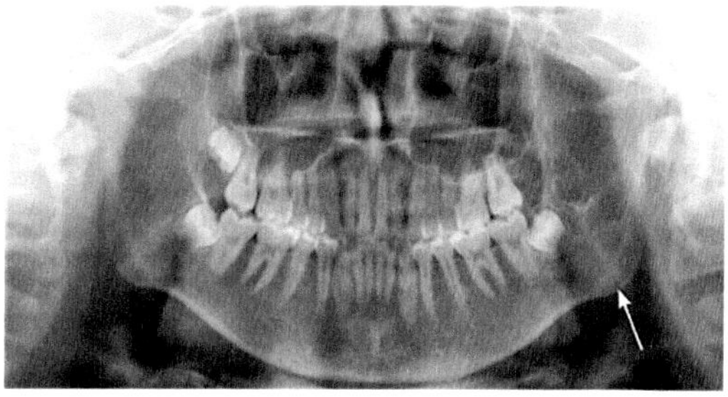

Fig. 42.5 Expansive bone destruction in the left mandibular ramus and condyle, with unclear boundary

[Auxiliary Examination]

1. Panoramic radiographs suggested an expansive bone destruction in the left mandibular ramus and condyle, with unclear boundary (Fig. 42.5).
2. Maxillofacial enhanced CT scan suggested an expansive bone destruction and soft tissue mass in the left mandibular ramus and condyle. The size was about 4 cm × 4.8 cm. CT value was 38 Hu. After enhancement, the lesion was inhomogeneous enhancement, with CT value of 59 Hu. The lesion involved the masticatory space. A radiolucent bone ridge was visible within the lesion, with interrupted peripheral bone cortex and a sclerotic margin (Fig. 42.6).

[Preliminary Diagnosis] Mass of the left mandibular ramus.

[Treatment] "Left mandibular tumor extracranial resection" under general anesthesia was performed: a transcervical incision was made along the lower margin of the mandible, and the gingival flap was elevated for surgical exposure of the mass in the left mandibular ramus. The mandibular ramus mass protruded from the bony cortex and involved the condyle without erosion of the skull base. A biopsy performed at the lower margin of the tumor. The tumor was found to be a spindle cell tumor in the left mandible with mild heterogeneity and no obvious nuclear division, and there was insufficient evidence for a direct diagnosis of malignancy. The tumor was carefully dissected from the skull base at the superior border of the tumor, and the condyle and articular disc were radically resected along with mandibular ramus and tumor. Frozen section pathology suggested spindle cell tumor of the "left mandible" with mild cellular atypia and eosinophilic collagen-like substance in some areas, malignancy to be excluded. The margins were negative (−).The wound was rinsed and thoroughly hemostatic, negative pressure drainage tube was indwelled, and layered suture was performed to close the wound (Fig. 42.7).

[Pathological Examination] Gross pathological examination revealed the mandibular ramus tissue, including condyle and coracoid process, 5.5 cm × 5 cm × 4 cm in size. The mass was 4 cm × 4 cm × 3.5 cm on the section of the ascending ramus. The section was gray and gray red, and the cortical bone was damaged. Microscopic examination showed fusiform fibroblasts and myofibroblasts hyperplasia with many collagen fiber components. The lesion destroyed the bone cortex and involved the surrounding soft tissues (Fig. 42.8).

[Pathological Diagnosis] Desmoplastic fibroma of the "left mandible," ICD-O code: 8823/1.

[Follow-Up] The patient healed uneventfully. The postoperative 6-month follow-up exhibited no recurrence and slight mandibular deviation after surgery, with good contralateral occlusal relationship (Fig. 42.9).

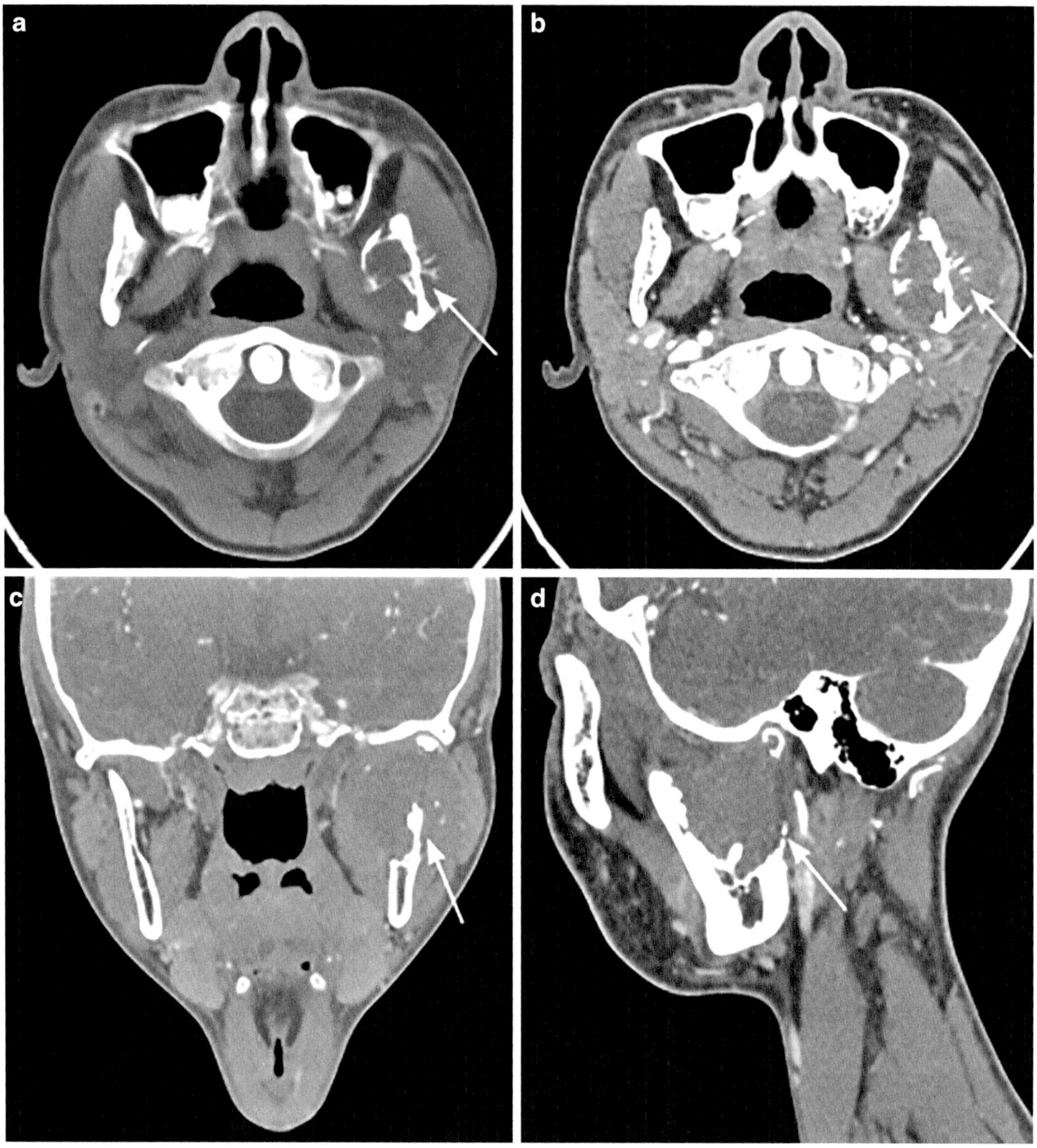

Fig. 42.6 (**a**) CT axial scan: expansive bone destruction and soft tissue mass in the left mandibular ramus and condyle with abnormal soft tissue mass, about 4 cm × 4.8 cm in size. (**b**) Enhanced CT axial scan: inhomogeneous enhancement of the lesion. (**c**, **d**) Enhanced CT coronal plus sagittal scan: lesion involving masticatory muscle space, radial bone ridge observed within lesion, peripheral bone cortex interrupted, and sclerotic edges seen at the margin

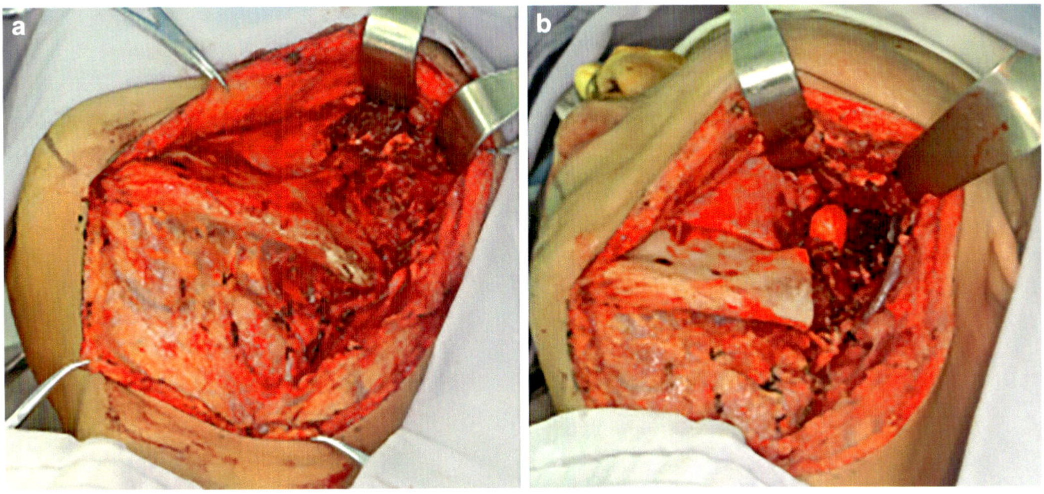

Fig. 42.7 (**a**) Exposed mandibular body and ascending ramus. Mandibular ramus distension and bone destruction were observed. (**b**) The mandible, including the condyle, was removed

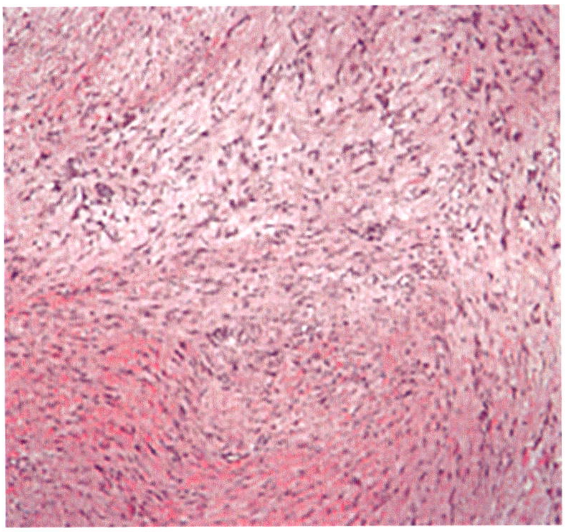

Fig. 42.8 Spindle/myofibroblast proliferation in the background of collagen fibers (100.00×)

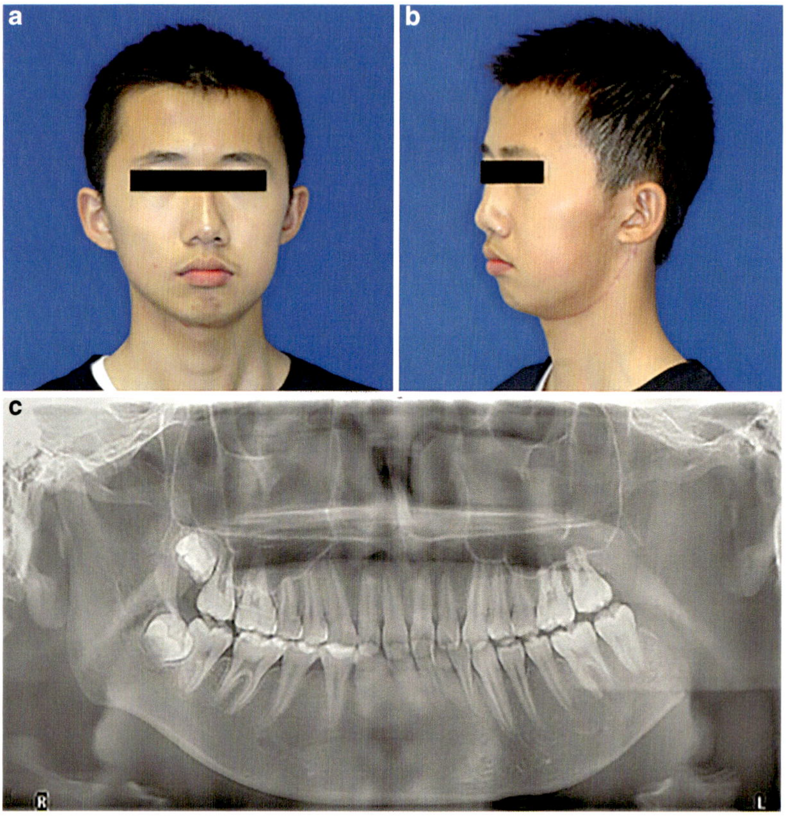

Fig. 42.9 (**a**, **b**) Left facial collapse, slight left deviation of the mandible. (**c**) Postoperative changes showed missing left mandibular ramus, and normal teeth occlusal relationship

42.4 Key Points of Diagnosis and Treatment

Desmoplastic fibroma (DF) is a rare locally aggressive bone tumor of myofibroblastic origin, also known as ligamentous fibroma of bone, intrasclerotic fibroma of bone, invasive fibroma of bone, and fibroblastic fibroma of bone because of its histologic similarity to soft tissue ligamentous fibroma. It is a dense fibrous tumor composed of fibroblasts rich in collagen fibers and accounts for approximately 0.1% of primary bone tumors. It can occur in any bone, with the jaw bone being the most common site (22–27%), followed by the femur (15%), pelvis (13%), radius (12%), and tibia (9%). DF occurring in the jaws, 84% of patients were younger than 30 years of age at the time of initial diagnosis, with slightly more female patients, 84% in the mandible and 16% in the maxilla.

Most of the tumors are located in the medullary cavity with thinning of the bone cortex, and the tumor may penetrate the buccal and lingual bone cortex to form soft tissue masses. Some patients have intermittent or persistent dull pain, and a few patients have pathological fracture as the first symptom.

Imaging Characteristics Slow growth and lack of specific imaging findings make it difficult to detect desmoplastic fibroma early. Radiographs and CT scans are characterized by single or multiple translucent distension areas, cystic distension destruction or lace-like, and multilocular mesh-like changes with clear or irregular boundaries composed of pseudobone trabeculae. The density of DF may be equal to or slightly higher than the soft tissue density of muscle because of the dense collagen fibrous tissue, and the high density reflects the dense connective tissue matrix and the relative lack of cellularity of the tumor. In a few cases, cystic degeneration and necrosis can be seen in the lesion area. MRI of DF is characterized by inhomogeneous isosignal or low signal in T1WI and inhomogeneous isosignal or high signal in T2WI. It is thought to be a typical MRI image of DF, with irregular cords or patches of matted

T1WI and T2WI low signal, similar in morphology and signal to ligaments, and incomplete calcification or ossification in the lesion area. It has been proposed by scholars that a low signal area greater than 50% within the lesion on T2WI is a characteristic manifestation of DF. The extent of the lesion on MRI is often greater than that on radiographs and CT examinations, and the extent of edema in the tumor and surrounding soft tissues can be shown more clearly, which is a reliable reference for the resection boundary during DF surgery.

Pathological Characteristics The gross specimen has a grayish-white, tough tissue appearance and is generally free of calcified or ossified tissue, although there are occasional areas of cystic softening. The microscopic findings are characteristic and consist of proliferating, mildly heterogeneous spindle cells and their production of large amounts of collagen. The proliferating fibroblasts are arranged in bundles and tangles, with heterogeneous cell density and few nuclear divisions. The interstitial matrix has varying degrees of hyaline degeneration, and when the collagen component is obvious, it is keloid-like. Some tumors may break through the bone cortex and infiltrate into the surrounding soft tissue, forming bone scabs and reactive bone. Immunohistochemical staining is positive for P-catenin and vimentin, and some cases express SMA to varying degrees, while desmin, S-100, CD34, and MDM2 are negative.

Differential Diagnosis The correct diagnosis of DF requires a combination of clinical and imaging findings and pathologic examination. The differential diagnosis includes, but is not limited to, enucleated cell tumor, neurofibroma, giant cell tumor, odontogenic mucinous tumor, aneurysmal bone cyst, mucinous fibroma of cartilage, central hemangioma of the jaws, eosinophilic granuloma, and intramedullary highly differentiated osteosarcoma.

Treatment Now, there is no unified treatment standard for DF, and surgical resection is the first choice for clinical treatment. The selection of surgical methods is still controversial, and tumor curettage, enucleation and osteotomy have all been reported. Due to the strong invasiveness of DF, complete tumor resection should be performed if possible; improper surgery may cause high recurrence rate. The recurrence rate after enucleation is 20–40%, while the recurrence rate after extensive excision is 15.4–17%. Chemotherapy, radiation, and/or hormone therapy are options for patients with no complete resection. DF does not metastasize and is rare for malignant changes. Proper treatment can lead to good prognosis. However, due to its high recurrence rate, it is recommended to follow up for at least 3 years.

References

1. Jaffe HL. Desmoplastic fibroma and fibrosarcoma [J]. Tumors and tumorous conditions of the bones and joints. Philadelphia: Lea & Febiger; 1958. p. 298–303.
2. Evans S, Ramasamy A, Jeys L, et al. Desmoplastic fibroma of bone: a rare bone tumour [J]. J Bone Oncol. 2014;3(3–4):77–9.
3. Apaydin M, Gelal F, Avci A, et al. Desmoplastic fibroma in humerus [J]. J Med Imaging Radiat Oncol. 2008;52(5):489–90.
4. Kim SY, Chung HW, Lee SY, et al. Cystic changes in desmoplastic fibroma of bone: a new MRI finding [J]. Clin Radiol. 2012;67(12):1170–4.
5. Vanhoenacker FM, Hauben E, De Beuckeleer LH, et al. Desmoplastic fibroma of bone: MRI features [J]. Skeletal Radiol. 2000;29(3):171–5.
6. Frick MA, Sundaram M, Unni KK, et al. Imaging findings in desmoplastic fibroma of bone: distinctive T2 characteristics [J]. AJR Am J Roentgenol. 2005;184(6):1762–7.
7. Callahan KS, Eberhardt SC, Fechner RE, et al. Desmoplastic fibroma of bone with extensive cartilaginous metaplasia [J]. Ann Diagn Pathol. 2006;10(6):343–6.
8. Yang W, Zhang FY, Sui FY. Desmoplastic fibroma in mandible : a case report [J]. Zhonghua Kou Qiang Yi Xue Za Zhi. 2019;54(10):696–8.
9. Madakshira MG, Bal A, Verma RK. Desmoplastic fibroma of the mandible : a rare gnathic bone tumor with a review of the literature [J]. Autops Case Rep. 2019;9(4):e2019091.
10. Tanwar YS, Kharbanda Y, Rastogi R, et al. Desmoplastic fibroma of bone: a case series and review of literature [J]. Indian J Surg Oncol. 2018;9(4):585–91.
11. Kahraman D, Karakoyunlu B, Karagece U, et al. Desmoplastic fibroma of the jaw bones: a series of twenty- two cases [J]. J Bone Oncol. 2021;26:100333.
12. Nedopil A, Raab P, Rudert M. Desmoplastic fibroma: a case report with three years of clinical and radiographic observation and review of the literature [J]. Open Orthop J. 2013;8:40–6.

43 Melanotic Neuroectodermal Tumor of Infancy

Yue He, Hui Shan Ong, Zhen Tian, Lin Zhu, and Wen Jun Yang

43.1 Introduction

Melanotic neuroectodermal tumor of infancy (MNTI) is a rare, rapidly growing, and locally aggressive tumor of neural crest origin. More than 90% of MNTI occurs in infancy, with a median age of about 5 months, slightly higher in males than females. With the anterior maxilla (>60%) being the most prevalent, followed by the skull, mandible, and brain, with occasional reports in the mediastinum, ovaries, uterus, testes and epididymis, limb bones, and soft tissues [1–11]. MNTI now has no clear treatment guidelines, and surgical resection is considered as the best therapy because the tumor rarely metastasizes to distant sites [12–15]. But, local recurrence is common, and the scope of surgical excision remains controversial.

Y. He (✉) · H. S. Ong · Z. Tian · W. J. Yang
Department of Oral Maxillofacial-Head & Neck Oncology, Shanghai Ninth People's Hospital, Shanghai Jiao Tong University School of Medicine, Shanghai, China

L. Zhu
Department of Radiology, Ninth People's Hospital Affiliated to Shanghai Jiao Tong University, Shanghai, China

43.2 Case 80

A 6-month-old infant boy suffered from maxillary mass 1 month ago.

[History of Present Illness] A round mass in the left maxilla was found unintentionally by the child's mother during feeding 1 month ago, which gradually increased in size.

[Specialty Examination] The size of the mass was about 2 cm × 2 cm, with a light blue-purple color, soft texture, no tenderness, immobility, no obvious rupture, and active bleeding.

[Auxiliary Examination]
Maxillofacial CT scan suggested a mass-like density shadow of soft tissue on the left maxilla, with a CT value of about 45 Hu, well-circumscribed, about 1.7 cm in diameter. The bone expanded and changed thinner, with local interruption, and teeth shadow visible inside; the soft tissue density of the maxillofacial region was uniform bilaterally, the fatty zone was clear, and the remaining bone structure of the maxilla was not significantly changed (Fig. 43.1).

[Preliminary Diagnosis] Left maxillary mass.

[Treatment] "Maxillary mass resection" under general anesthesia was performed: an incision was made along the gingival margin, and the gin-

Y. He (ed.), *Inflammatory and Neoplastic Diseases of Craniofacial Bones*,
https://doi.org/10.1007/978-981-97-4155-7_43

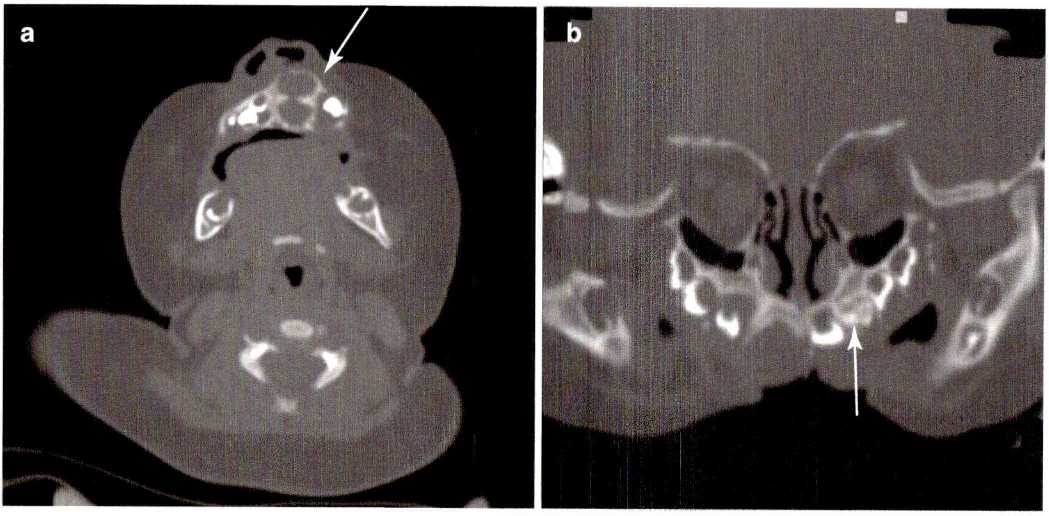

Fig. 43.1 (**a**) CT axial scan: space occupying of soft tissue density in the left maxilla, indicating bone expansion and thinning, local interruption, and tooth shadow. (**b**) CT coronal reconstruction: bone destruction at the lesion site with dental shadow

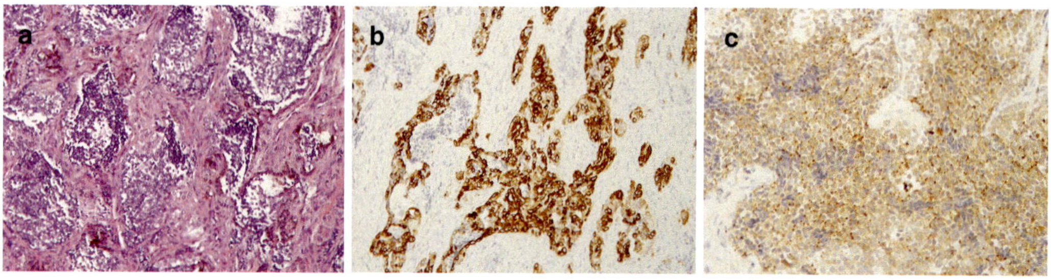

Fig. 43.2 (**a**) Tumor cells consist of epithelioid cells with brown-yellow pigment granules and small neuroblast-like cells (200×). (**b**) Epithelioid cytokeratin (AE1/AE3) positive (200×). (**c**) Tumor cells showed positive for neuron-specific enolase (NSE) paracarbonate (400×)

gival flap was elevated for surgical removal of the thin bone cortex above the mass, and the mass was seen to be cystic in nature and was completely removed along the cyst wall, along with the teeth surrounding the tumor. Curettage of wound surface was performed. Intraoperative frozen pathological examination suggested MNTI of the "maxilla." The wound was rinsed, hemostatic, and sutured.

[Pathological Examination] Gross pathological examination revealed tumor-like tissue, 2.7 cm × 1.8 cm × 1.6 cm in size, locally gray-black, with a small amount of white hard tissue inside. The microscopic examination showed that the submucosal tumor cells were arranged in nested clusters. Tumor cells consisted of large epithelioid cells with vacuolar nuclei and cytoplasm containing brown-yellow pigment granules, and small cells with dense chromatin in the lymphocytic or neuroblastoma-like appearance. Locally, dental embryonic tissue was seen (Fig. 43.2).

[Pathological Diagnosis] MNTI of the "maxilla," with ICD-O code: 9363/0.

[Follow-Up] The patient healed uneventfully. The postoperative follow-up exhibited no reoccurrence.

43.3 Key Points of Diagnosis and Treatment

Since MNTI was first reported by Krompecher in 1918, more than 500 cases have been reported worldwide. The relative infrequency of cases and related studies may lead to a lack of knowledge among clinicians about MNTI. However, MNTI is rapidly growing and locally aggressive, with a distinctive age of onset, so a proper understanding of MNTI by clinicians would be beneficial for prompt diagnosis and treatment.

Clinical Manifestations MNTI presents as a rapidly growing, painless mass with an average tumor size of about 3.5 cm, often accompanied by hyperpigmentation. MNTI usually has no obvious symptoms until the mass grows and causes facial asymmetry. Although MNTI is rare, MNTI should be included in the differential diagnosis when rapidly growing pigmentary masses in the head and neck are evaluated. Although neural criste-derived tumors may produce vanillaria amygdala (VMA), high urinary VMA levels vary and nevertheless support the diagnosis of MNTI.

Imaging Characteristics Radiologically, MNTI appears as a hypointense lesion on CT scan, but the melanin component of the soft tissue component of MNTI appears as a high-density shadow. The tumor invades and destroys the surrounding bone tissue, showing osteolytic, distending, or cystic bone destruction and osteophytes. Therefore, CT scan is a good option to determine the extent of the tumor and to plan the surgery. In a few cases, ultrasound is used to examine the surrounding lesions. Ultrasound shows heterogeneous and well-defined MNTI lesions with reduced vascularization. On magnetic resonance imaging (MRI), MNTI usually shows an enhanced T1 signal due to the presence of melanin. However, MNTI is commonly described on MRI as a T1-weighted and T2-weighted low-signal, well-defined mass.

Pathological Characteristics Eventually, biopsy and immunohistochemistry can be used to distinguish MNTI from other tumors with similar characteristics, leading to a definitive diagnosis. MNTI tumor cells showed obvious biphasic characteristics: large cuboidal epithelial cells, with empty cytoplasm and melanin, arranged in nests or cords, positive for NSE, Vimentin, CK, and S-100, and rarely positive for S-100; small round cells, similar to neuroblasts, often surrounded by fibers and epithelioid cells, positive for NSE, Vimentin, Synaptophysin, negative for CK, positive for GFAP in some cases, and positive for S-100 in only a few cases.

Differential Diagnosis MNTI generally presents as an asymptomatic, rapidly growing mass and therefore excludes other tumors that typically present with other concomitant symptoms. In the diagnosis of MNTI, the differential diagnosis includes, but is not limited to, neuroblastoma, malignant melanoma, Ewing sarcoma, neuroendocrine carcinoma, lymphoma, and soft tissue clear cell sarcoma.

Treatment Although MNTI is rapidly growing and locally aggressive, it has been considered a benign tumor. Now, there is a lack of clear treatment guidelines. Early diagnosis, complete surgical resection, and regular follow-up have been reported as the best treatment options for MNTI. A 2019 systematic evaluation suggests that resection appears to be the best option because it is associated with low recurrence and morbidity. The biggest controversy regarding surgical resection is the extent of resection. A small resection is associated with a high recurrence rate, while a large resection is associated with a high degree of defect, organ and functional destruction. In a few cases, preoperative neoadjuvant chemotherapy may reduce the need for extensive resection, thereby reducing the disfigurement caused by surgery. Nevertheless, the recurrence rate of resection with or without other treatments remains high (approximately 22%). We believe that the surgical plan should take into account not only the eradication of the tumor but also the postoperative growth and development of the child, minimizing surgical trauma and preserving organs and functions. When complete resection of the lesion would result in severe organ loss and/or dysfunction, a more conservative curettage may be chosen, with further management in the event of recurrence during follow-up.

A small number of MNTI cases can be successfully cured with chemotherapy alone without surgery. The chemotherapeutic agents used to treat MNTI are neuroblastoma-based regimens, including vincristine, adriamycin, etoposide, and cyclophosphamide. In one case report of MNTI, a 10-year-old female patient who presented with bilateral high-frequency hearing loss received a cisplatin-containing regimen at the age of 8 months. Radiotherapy was used as an adjunct to surgery or chemotherapy in only 6 case reports.

Prognosis Literature reports that local recurrence occurs in about 20% of MNTI cases after treatment, and the 5-year recurrence rate in women is slightly higher than that in men (25% vs. 22%). In a few cases, distant metastasis or even malignancy may occur. The prognosis and recurrence rate of MNTI are related to age of onset, lesion location, tumor size, and therapy, among which, age of onset less than 2 months is associated with a higher recurrence rate, while age of onset more than 12 months is associated with a higher mortality.

The very low incidence of MNTI is an impediment to differential diagnosis, and the lack of knowledge of MNTI leads to misdiagnosis, while delayed diagnosis results in local tissue infiltration. The diagnosis of MNTI requires a high degree of sensitivity, and any rapidly growing mass, especially in the head and neck, must be considered for the diagnosis of MNTI. A multidisciplinary collaborative model is preferred in the treatment of MNTI patients. Follow-up is necessary to detect possible recurrence and possible complications at an early stage and to avoid delays in treatment.

References

1. Krompecher E. Zur Histogenese und morphologie der adamantinoma und sonstiger kiefergeschewulste [J]. Beitr Pathol Anat. 1918;64:165–97.
2. Mengide JP, Jaimovich SG, Lubieniecki FJ, et al. Melanotic neuroectodermal tumor of infancy arising from the skull: report of an unusual case, review of the literature, and a diagnostic approach [J]. Childs Nerv Syst. 2020;36(3):469–75.
3. Pontes FSC, de Souza LL, Uchoa DCC, et al. Melanotic neuroectodermal tumor of infancy of the jaw bones: update on the factors influencing survival and recurrence [J]. Head Neck. 2018;40(12):2749–56.
4. Chrcanovic BR, Gomez RS. Melanotic neuroectodermal tumour of infancy of the jaws: an analysis of diagnostic features and treatment [J]. Int J Oral Maxillofac Surg. 2019;48(1):1–8.
5. Neven J, Hulsbergen-van der Kaa C, Groot-Loonen J, et al. Recurrent melanotic neuroectodermal tumor of infancy : a proposal for treatment protocol with surgery and adjuvant chemotherapy [J]. Oral Surg Oral Med Oral Pathol Oral Radiol Endod. 2008;106(4):493–6.
6. Rachidi S, Sood AJ, Patel KG, et al. Melanotic neuroectodermal tumor of infancy : a systematic review [J]. J Oral Maxillofac Surg. 2015;73(10):1946–56.
7. Soles BS, Wilson A, Lucas DR, et al. Melanotic neuroectodermal tumor of infancy [J]. Arch Pathol Lab Med. 2018;142(11):1358–63.
8. Chaudhary A, Wakhlu A, Mittal N, et al. Melanotic neuroectodermal tumor of infancy: 2 decades of clinical experience with 18 patients [J]. J Oral Maxillofac Surg. 2009;67(1):47–51.
9. Fowler DJ, Chisholm J, Roebuck D, et al. Melanotic neuroectodermal tumor of infancy: clinical, radiological and pathological features [J]. Fetal Pediatr Pathol. 2006;25(2):59–72.
10. Haque S, McCarville MB, Sebire N, et al. Melanotic neuroectodermal tumour of infancy: CT and MR findings [J]. Pediatr Radiol. 2012;42(6):699–705.
11. Maroun C, Khalifeh I, Alam E, et al. Mandibular melanotic neuroectodermal tumor of infancy: a role for neoadjuvant chemotherapy [J]. Eur Arch Otorrinolaringol. 2016;273(12):4629–35.
12. Kumari TP, Venugopal M, Mathews A, et al. Effectiveness of chemotherapy in melanotic neurectodermal tumor of infancy [J]. Pediatr Hematol Oncol. 2005;22(3):199–206.
13. Woessmann W, Neugebauer M, Gossen R, et al. Successful chemotherapy for melanotic neuroectodermal tumor of infancy in a baby [J]. Med Pediatr Oncol. 2003;40(3):198–9.
14. Emmerling MR, York TA, Caccamese JF. Melanotic neuroectodermal tumor of infancy : case report and review of management [J]. J Oral Maxillofac Surg. 2019;77(2):315–20.
15. Hojan-Jezierska D, Chomiak A, Czopor A, et al. Ototoxicity after platinum-based chemotherapy in the treatment of melanotic neuroectodermal tumour of infancy [J]. Oncol Lett. 2020;19(5):3411–6.

Part XII

Malignant Tumors of Craniomaxillofacial Bones and Cartilage

44 Osteosarcoma

Yue He, Hui Shan Ong, Zhen Tian, Lin Zhu, and Shan Liang Jin

44.1 Introduction

Osteosarcoma of jaws is a rare tumor with high malignancy, accounting for 1% of malignant tumors of head and neck and 5–13% of all osteosarcomas in the body [1–7]. It is more common in young adults between 20 and 50 years of age, and the incidence in males is generally more than that in females. The incidence in maxillary and mandibular bone is almost equal or predominant in the lower jaw. The clinical and imaging manifestations are complex and diverse, with a high rate of misdiagnosis and local recurrence, and a 5-year survival rate of 40–60% [4–11]. The diagnosis and treatment are challenging, and the first choice of treatment is radical surgical excision [8–11]. Postoperative adjuvant chemotherapy and close follow-up are recommended.

Y. He · H. S. Ong (✉) · Z. Tian · L. Zhu · S. L. Jin
Department of Oral Maxillofacial-Head & Neck Oncology, Shanghai Ninth People's Hospital, Shanghai Jiao Tong University School of Medicine, Shanghai, China

44.2 Conventional Osteosarcoma

44.2.1 Case 81

A 50-year-old woman suffered from a left inferior anterior dental mass for more than 3 months.

[History of Present Illness] Three months ago, the patient happened to find a mass in the left inferior anterior dental area, with no obvious symptoms at that time. CT examination in the hospital 2 months ago indicated multiple patellar dense shadow in the maxillary cusp area and adjacent soft tissue mass. "Maxillary mass biopsy" under local anesthesia 1 month ago indicated osteosarcoma in the left mandible. Oral pathology consultation 2 weeks ago: osteosarcoma considered.

[Specialty Examination] The face was asymmetrical, with swelling in the left chin. The overlying skin was intact, with no obvious congestion or increase in skin temperature. There was no abnormality in mouth opening range and mouth opening pattern. Buccal bone of 34–42 teeth was swollen. Post-biopsy sutures were visible locally, and the mass was hard upon palpation, well-circumscribed, and immobile. The corresponding teeth had grade 1° mobility, with no obvious pain. Submandibular lymph nodes with size less than 1cm in diameter were palpable, they are soft and tender upon palpation (Fig. 44.1a, b).

Y. He (ed.), *Inflammatory and Neoplastic Diseases of Craniofacial Bones*, https://doi.org/10.1007/978-981-97-4155-7_44

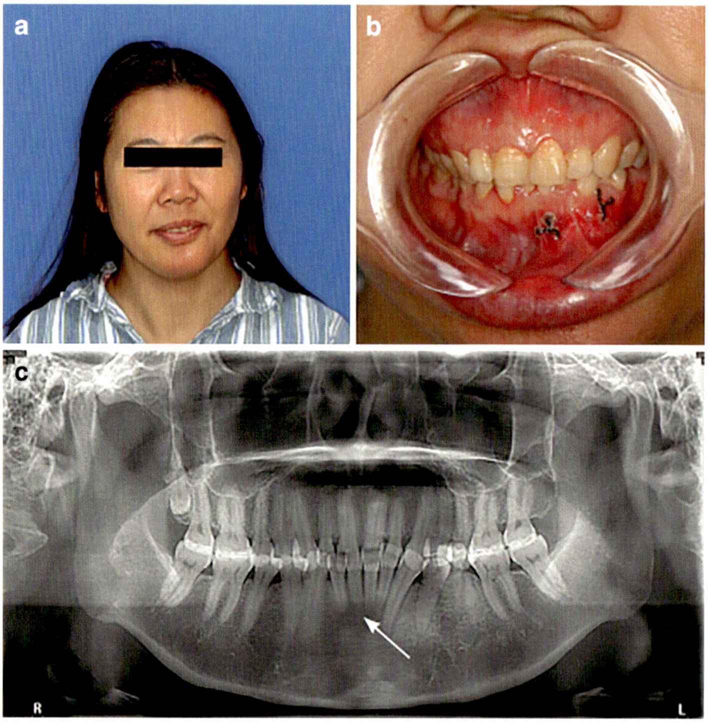

Fig. 44.1 (**a**) Facial asymmetry with left-sided chin expansion deformity. (**b**) Bone expansion in the left lower anterior region, post-biopsy view, sutures in place. (**c**) Inhomogeneous increase in bone density in the left mandibular body near the midline with unclear borders (preoperatively)

[Auxiliary Examination]

1. Panoramic radiographs suggested an inhomogeneous density increase in the left mandibular body near the midline, with indistinct borders (Fig. 44.1c).
2. Maxillofacial enhanced CT scan suggested a heterogeneous dense increase in bone density near the midline of the left mandibular body with unclear borders, anterior cortical destruction with soft tissue masses, 29 mm × 13 mm in size, heterogeneous density, CT value of about 72 Hu. After enhancement, the lesion was unevenly enhanced, with CT value of 90 Hu (Fig. 44.2).

[Preliminary Diagnosis] Osteosarcoma of the left mandible.

[Treatment] "Segmental mandibulectomy and reconstruction with fibular ossecutaneous flap and tracheotomy" was performed under general anesthesia: a transcervical incision was made along the lower margin of the mandible, and the gingival flap was elevated for surgical exposure of the mass located on the buccal side of 33~42 region, which was attached to the skin of the chin. The mandible was segmented from 46 to 37, and the mass was completely resected within the normal tissue, together with the overlying skin and the affected mucosa. Intraoperative frozen pathology suggested no tumor in the lymph nodes (−) and negative surgical margins (−). The 12 cm fibula ossecutaneous flap was harvested, shaped, and restored the continuity of the mandible and chin height. The wound was rinsed and thoroughly hemostatic, negative pressure drainage tube was indwelled, and layered suture was performed to close the wound (Fig. 44.3).

[Pathological Examination] Gross pathological examination revealed a part of mandibular bone tissue, 8 cm × 5.8 cm × 5 cm in size, with 11 teeth attached. Microscopic examination revealed that the tumor cells destroyed the bone cortex and involved the surrounding soft tissues, with hetero-

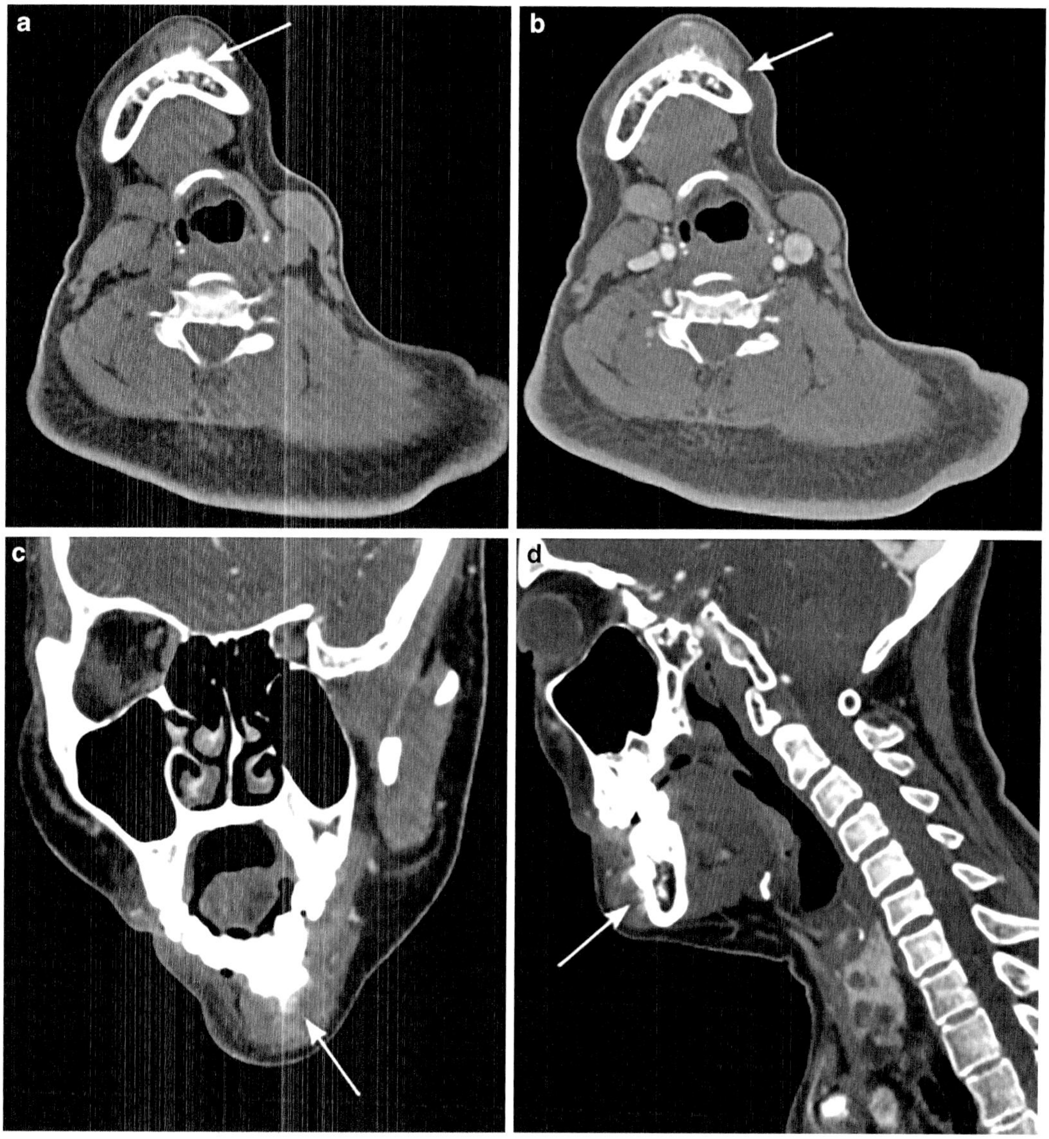

Fig. 44.2 (**a**) CT axial scan: heterogeneous increase in bone density of left mandible body near midline, unclear boundary, anterior bone cortical destruction with soft tissue mass shadow, 29 mm × 13 mm in size, inhomogeneous density, CT value about 72 Hu; (**b**) Enhanced CT axial scan: lesion inhomogeneously strengthened, CT value 90 Hu. (**c**, **d**) Coronal and sagittal scan views

geneous cells, fine and diffuse chromatin in the nucleus, obvious nucleoli, and more red-stained tumor-like bone tissue formation (Fig. 44.4).

[Pathological Diagnosis] Conventional osteosarcoma of the "mandible," with ICD-O code: 9180/3.

[Follow-Up] The patient healed uneventfully. The postoperative 6-month follow-up exhibited no recurrence of the tumor, with well-restored posterior occlusal relationship, and satisfactory mandibular appearance (Fig. 44.5).

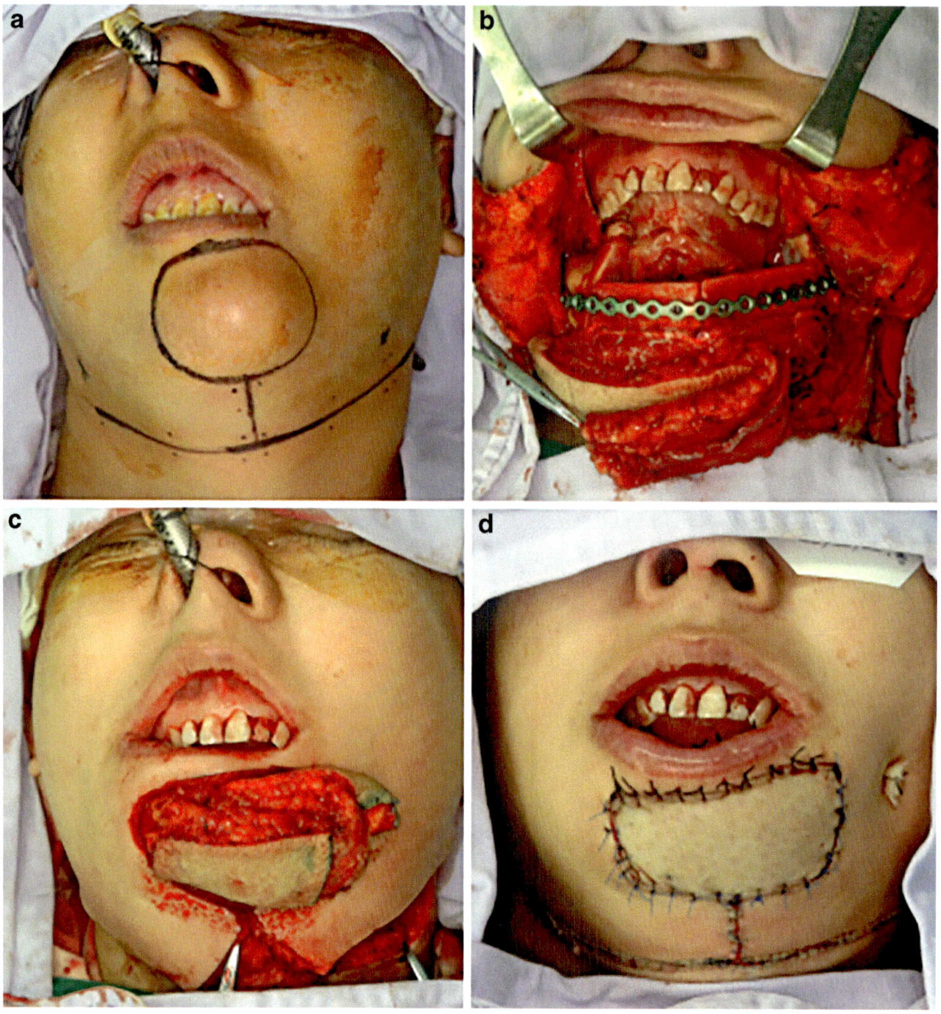

Fig. 44.3 (**a**) Incision design. (**b**) Fibula reconstruction to restore mandibular continuity. (**c**) Myoepithelial island revision to repair intraoral and extraoral defects, respectively. (**d**) Postoperative view

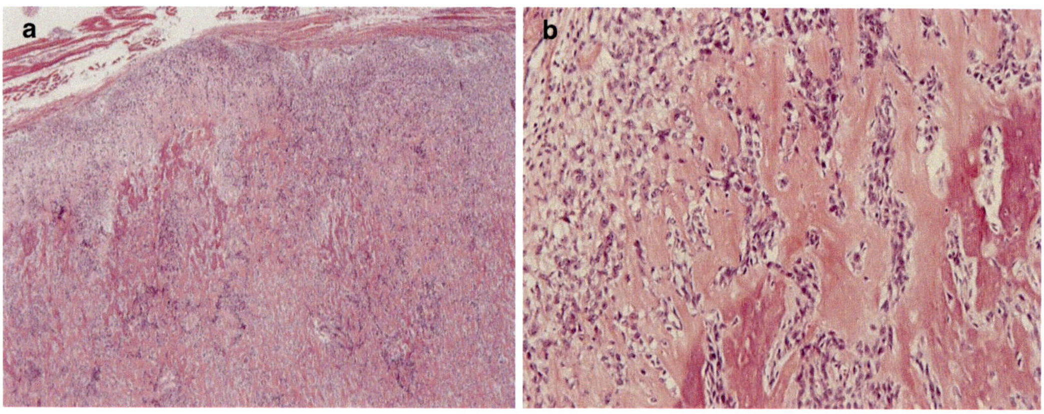

Fig. 44.4 (**a**) The tumor protruded from the bone cortex and involved muscle tissue (40x). (**b**) Tumor cells were consistent with atypia, obvious nucleoli, and paracellular neoplastic bone-like tissue formation (400x)

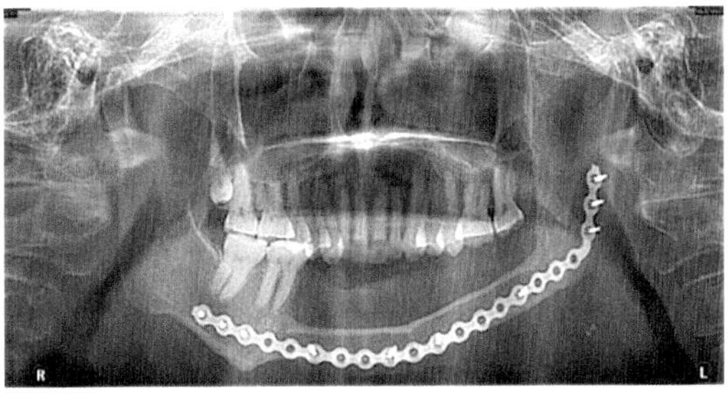

Fig. 44.5 Postoperative changes in the left mandible, good healing of the bone stump, and good restoration of the occlusal relationship of the right posterior teeth

44.3 Low-Grade Central Osteosarcoma

44.3.1 Case 82

A 28-year-old gentleman suffered from left lower lip numbness and discomfort for 1 month.

[History of Present Illness] The patient felt numbness in the red area near the left lower lip with unknown pathogenesis 1 month ago, without toothache, fever, and other discomforts. Under no treatment, the range of numbness in the posterior lip increased slowly. To improve the diagnosis and treatment, the patient was admitted to the hospital for CBCT examination, indicating the space occupying of the left mandible.

[Specialty Examination] The face was asymmetrical. The occlusal muscle attachment area of the left mandible was slightly distended. Palpation found that the bone surface was uneven, with no obvious swelling, no tenderness, or pulsation but presented with numbness of the left lower lip. There was no abnormality in mouth opening range and mouth opening pattern. Intraoral examination revealed permanent dentition, 37 was slightly lingually inclined without sign of loosening. Percussion (−) revealed that 37 distal lingual bone was slightly distended, the mucosa was intact, the bone surface was irregular, with no obvious tenderness, no mobility, or pulsatory sensation upon palpation. One lymph node was palpable under the left jaw, about 1 cm × 0.8 cm in size, medium in hardness, good mobility, and no tenderness. No abnormal enlarged cervical lymph nodes were observed.

[Auxiliary Examination]
CBCT suggested an inhomogeneous increase in the bone density of the left mandibular body, involving the mandible ramus, presenting an expansive change and bone destruction.

[Preliminary Diagnosis] Mass of left mandible.

[Treatment] "Left mandible resection with left superior hyoid cervical lymph node dissection + right iliac flap transfer reconstruction and repair + tracheotomy" was performed under general anesthesia: an incision was made along the lower margin of the mandible for 1–2 cm, and the gingival flap was elevated for surgical exposure of bony protuberance in the mandibular body and angle. Submandibular enlarged lymph nodes were found. Suprhaomohyoid neck dissection was performed together with en bloc removal of the mass and the affected mandible. Segmental mandibulectomy was performed distally to 34 and at the condylar neck. Intraoperative frozen pathological examination suggested osteosarcoma of the "left mandible." The right vascularized iliac flap (DCIA) was harvested, shaped, and restored the continuity of the mandible. The occlusal relationship of the right posterior teeth were well recovered, and vascular anastomosis of the fibula and facial artery and vein vessels was performed. The wound was rinsed and thoroughly hemostatic, negative pressure drainage tube was indwelled, and layered suture was performed to close the wound.

[Pathological Examination] Gross pathological examination revealed a pink fragment of the central lesion of the left mandible. Microscopically, the lesion was composed of atypically oval or spindle cells, distributed in sheets, and scattered within the osteoid matrix (Fig. 44.6).

[Follow-Up] The patient healed uneventfully. The postoperative 1-year follow-up exhibited that the bone stump of the mandible and the iliac

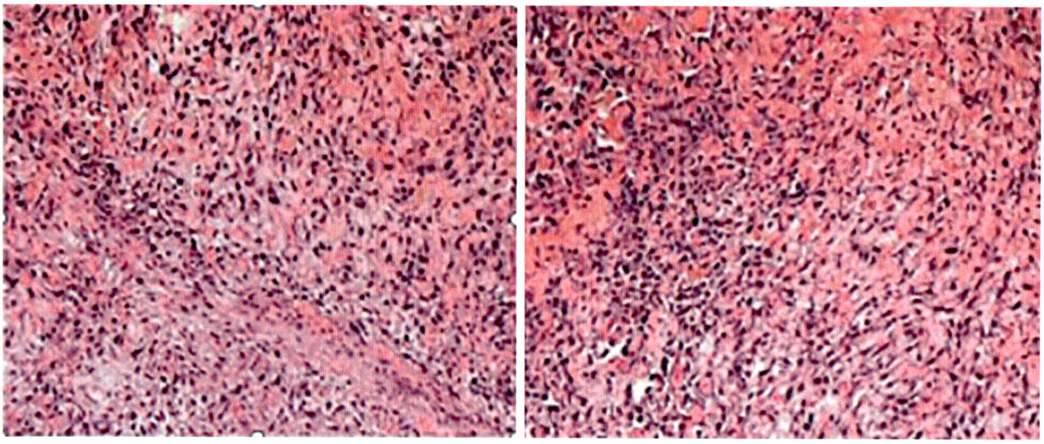

Fig. 44.6 Microscopically, the lesion was composed of atypically oval or spindle cells, distributed in sheets, and scattered within the osteoid matrix

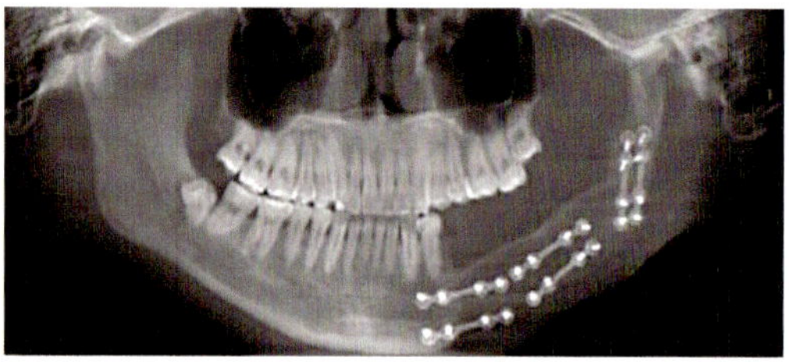

Fig. 44.7 Postoperative 1-year follow-up showed no reoccurrence of tumor, and the morphology and function of the mandible were well recovered

bone graft were well healed, and the morphology and function of the mandible were well recovered (Fig. 44.7).

44.4 Chondroblastic Osteosarcoma

44.4.1 Case 83

A 22-year-old gentleman suffered from right lower lip numbness for 5 months with facial swelling for 2 months.

[History of Present Illness] The patient had numbness and discomfort of the right lower lip with unknown pathogenesis 5 months ago, with no pain, swelling, bleeding, and other symptoms. The patient was given oral anti-inflammatory drugs, but there was no significant relief of numbness. Two months ago, the patient felt that her right face began to swell with pain, and was admitted to the hospital. CT examination indicated an abnormality in the right mandible. Pathological biopsy suggested chondroblastic osteosarcoma of the right mandible, with chondrosarcoma to be excluded. Surgical treatment was recommended.

[Specialty Examination] The patient's face was asymmetrical, with swelling in the right mandible. The overlying skin was intact, normal in color and temperature, with numbness in the skin of the right lower lip and chin. There was no abnormality in mouth opening range and mouth opening pattern. Oral hygiene was normal. The left posterior teeth were mildly open. The 44–47 buccal and lingual swelling covered 2/3 of the crown. The surface mucosa was intact, with medium hardness, mild tenderness, easy bleeding upon palpation. Patient complained of right lower gum numbness (41–44 teeth area). Multiple lymph nodes were found in the right submental and submandibular regions, with a maximum diameter of about 1.5 cm, medium hardness, clear boundaries, mobility, and no tenderness (Fig. 44.8a, b).

[Auxiliary Examination]

1. Panoramic radiographs suggested a heterogeneous change in bone density of the right mandible, involving the mandibular canal, and unclear boundary (Fig. 44.8c).

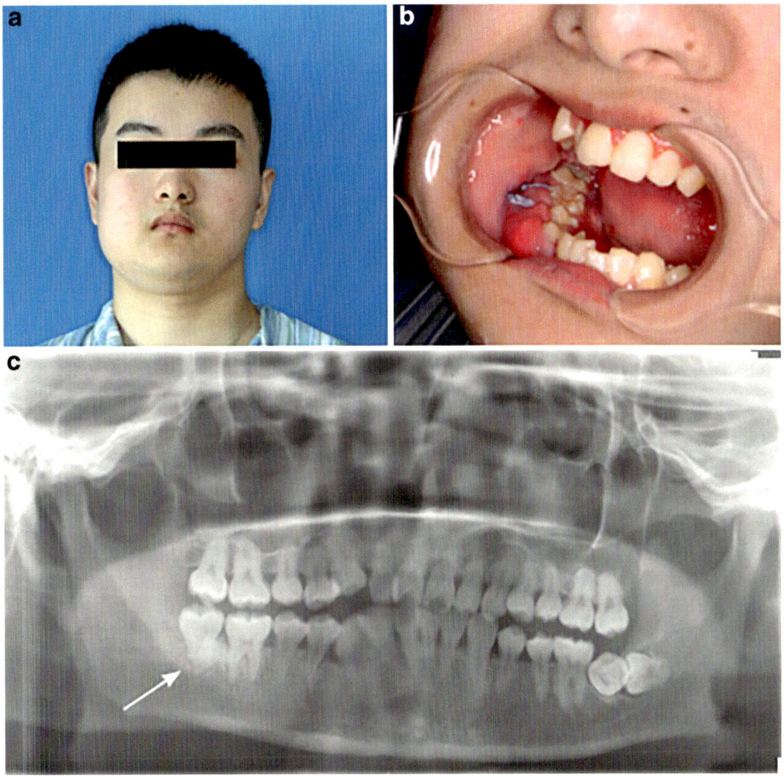

Fig. 44.8 (**a**) Asymmetrical face with maxillofacial swelling. (**b**) A distended mass in the posterior tooth area of the right mandible, covering 2/3 of the tooth crown. The surface mucous membrane was not broken or bleeding, and the suture was in place after biopsy. (**c**) Inhomogeneous changes in bone density of the right mandible involving the mandibular canal, with unclear boundaries (preoperative)

2. Maxillofacial enhanced CT scan suggested a heterogeneous change in bone density of the right mandible, irregular periosteal reaction at the edge, and abnormal soft tissue mass visible (Fig. 44.9). The lesion was approximately 4.3 cm × 6.1 cm × 4.1 cm in extent, with irregular morphology and unclear boundary, invading the surrounding occlusal muscle, internal pterygoid muscle, buccal muscle, mandibular hyoid muscle, and anterior belly of the diastasis. The lesion showed inhomogeneous enhancement after enhancement, with C− of 28 Hu, and C+ of 60 Hu and 63 H.

[Preliminary Diagnosis] Osteosarcoma of the right mandible.

[Treatment]

1. "Mandibulectomy and reconstruction with right anterolateral thigh flap and tracheotomy" was performed under general anesthesia: a transcervical incision was made along the lower margin of the mandible, and the gingival flap was elevated for surgical exposure of the buccal muscle, masseter muscle, mylohyoid muscle, medial pterygoid muscle, and temporalis muscle, as well as submental and submandibular triangle. Lymph nodes of submental triangle and submandibular triangle were dissected. The osteotomy was performed between the 32 and 33. All the attached muscles over the pathological mandible including condyle were completely resected. Intraoperative frozen pathological examination suggested that all incisional margins were negative (−). The anterolateral thigh flap was prepared to repair the defects of mandible and floor of mouth, and vascular anastomosis of the fibula and facial artery and vein vessels was performed. The wound was rinsed and thoroughly hemostatic, negative pressure drainage tube was indwelled, and layered suture was performed to close the wound (Fig. 44.10).
2. Postoperative adjuvant chemotherapy.

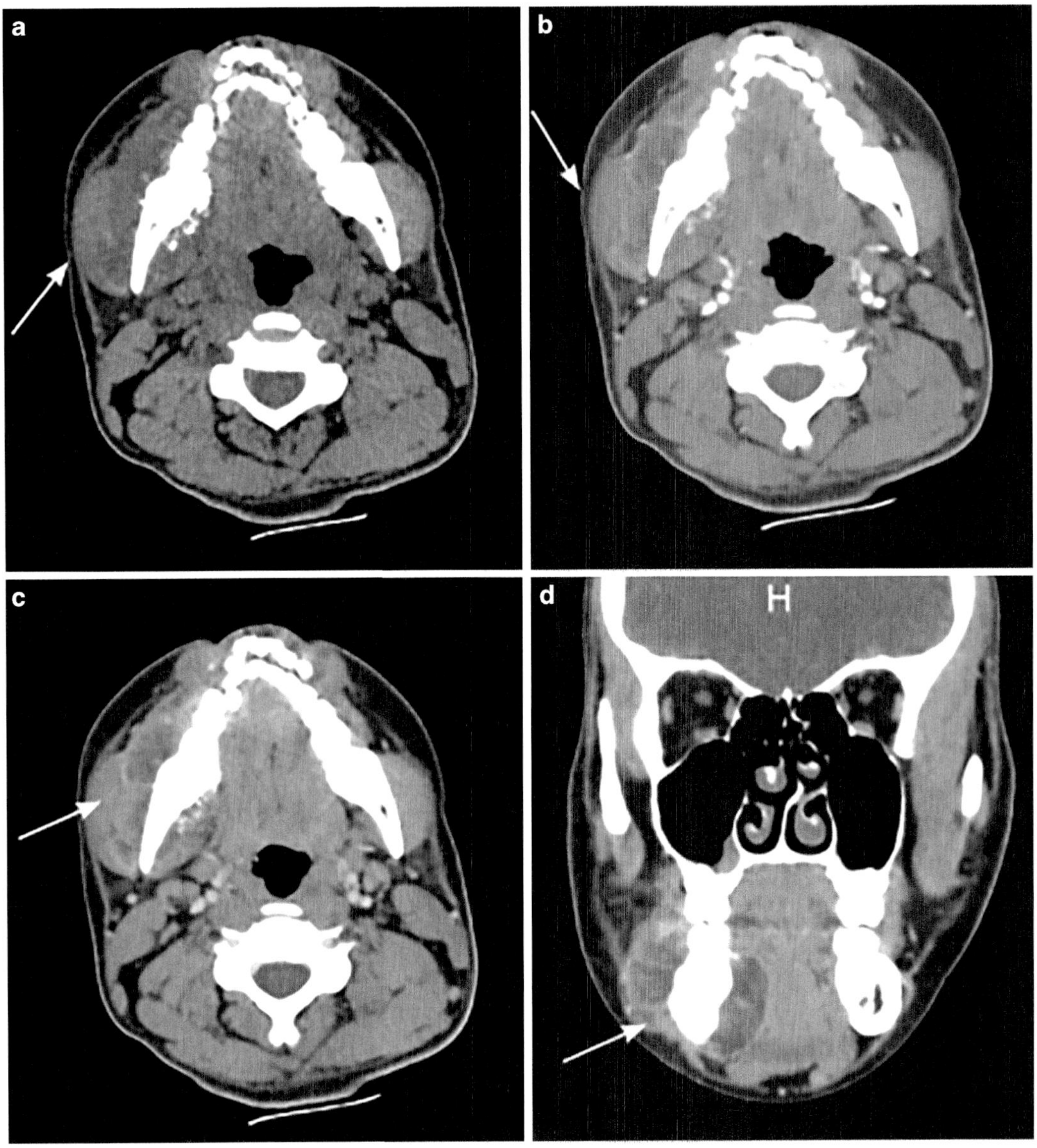

Fig. 44.9 (**a**) CT axial scan: right mandible bone abnormality, periosteal reaction and soft tissue mass. (**b**, **c**) Enhanced CT axial scan: inhomogeneous enhancement of the lesion. (**d**) Enhanced CT coronal reconstruction: lesions invaded the peripheral masseter, buccal and mandibular hyoid muscles

[Pathological Examination] Gross pathological examination revealed a part of the mandible and surrounding soft tissues, 11 cm × 10 cm × 6 cm in size. The section of the mandible showed a swollen mass, 8 cm × 5 cm × 5 cm in size, grayish white and poorly circumscribed. The microscopic examination indicated that the tumor was nodular and composed of spindle cells and polygonal cells, with obvious cell atypia, a small amount of osteoid tissue and a large amount of chondroid tissue formation, and local calcification. Chondroblast area contains blue-gray mucoid matrix, lacunae of varying sizes, and cell atypia (Fig. 44.11).

[Pathological Diagnosis] Chondroblast osteosarcoma of the mandible, ICD-O code: 9181/3.

[Follow-up] The patient healed uneventfully. The postoperative 3-month follow-up exhibited no recurrence of tumor.

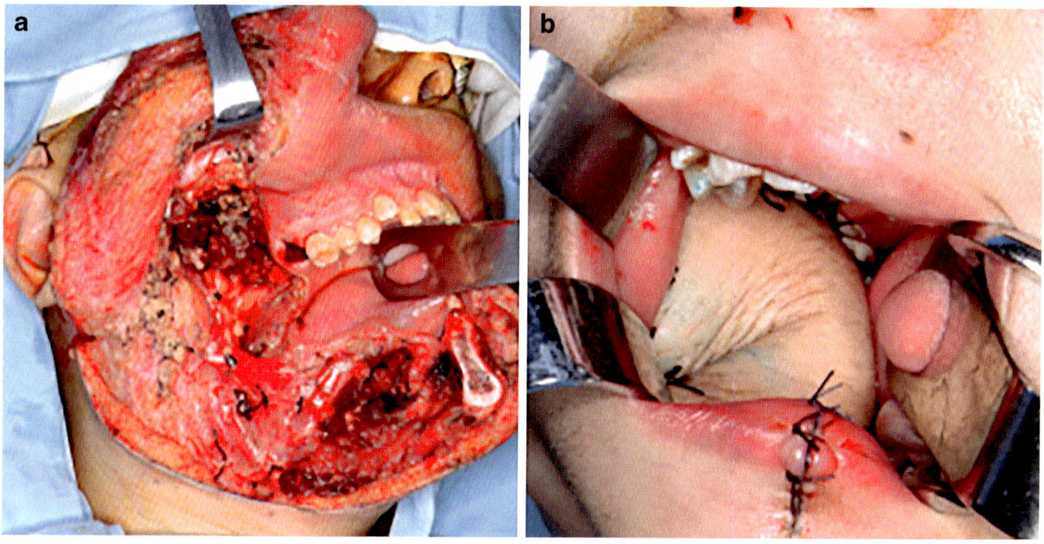

Fig. 44.10 (**a**) Wound defect after mandibular resection. (**b**) Anterolateral thigh flap to repair the defects of mandibular bone and oral floor

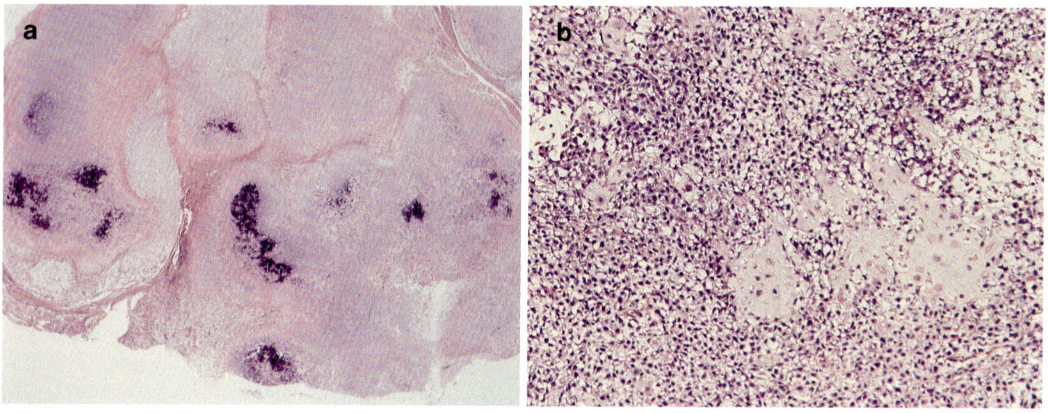

Fig. 44.11 (**a**) Nodular hyperplasia of chondroid tissue with calcification (20x). (**b**) Obvious tumor cells atypia, with light basophilic chondroid matrix formation, and cartilaginous lacunae of different sizes (20000x)

44.5 Parosteal Osteosarcoma

44.5.1 Case 84

A 55-year-old gentleman suffered from a left maxillary mass for more than 2 months.

[History of Present Illness] The patient was found to have a mass in the left maxillary gingival region 2 months ago without pain, discomfort, or bleeding. No significant improvement was observed after anti-inflammatory therapy.

[Specialty Examination] The face was basically symmetrical, with well-coordinated 1/3 proportion of upper, middle, and lower face. A swelling was seen in the left maxillary molar area, about 3 cm × 3 cm in size, hard and immobile, adherent to the surrounding tissues, and slight tenderness. The 26th and 27th teeth were missing. No obvious enlarged submandibular and cervical lymph nodes were observed.

[Auxiliary Examination]
Panoramic radiographs suggested a bone destruction from the left maxillary cusp region

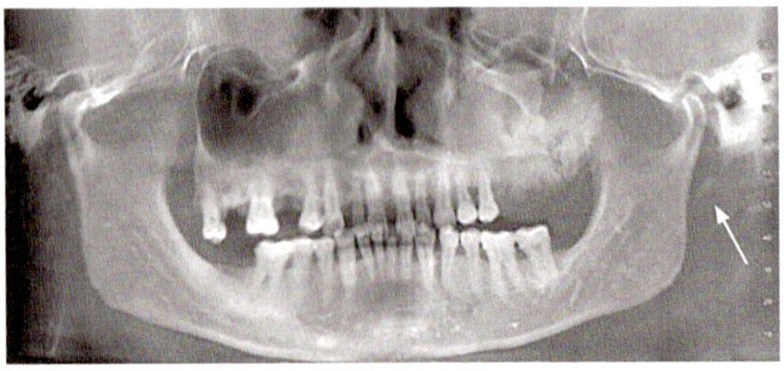

Fig. 44.12 Bone destruction from the left maxillary cusp region backward to the left maxillary tubercle with unclear boundary. There were a large number of inhomogeneous high-density shadows inside, and solar projection was observed. The lesions protruded into the left maxillary sinus cavity, causing bone destruction in the sinus wall and inward involvement of the hard palate

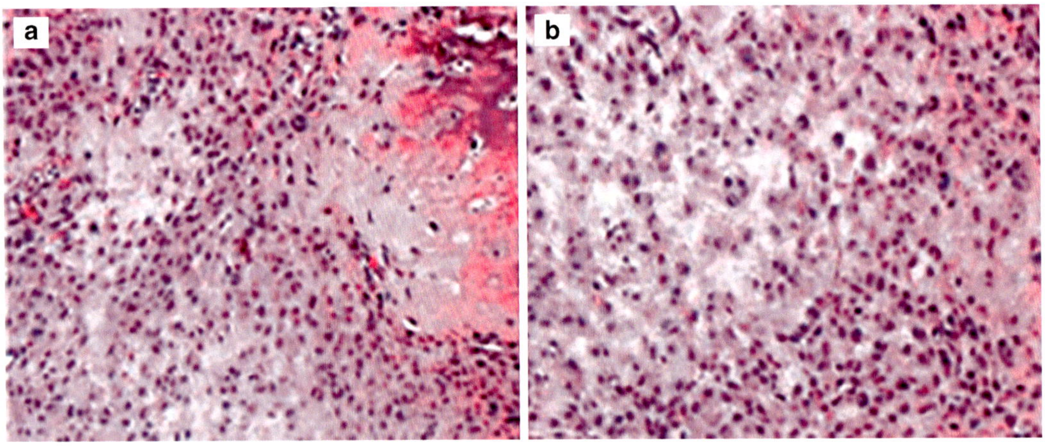

Fig. 44.13 (**a**) The tumor was composed of proliferative osteoblasts, accompanied by the formation of more immature osteoid matrix. (**b**) Chondroid differentiation was observed locally, and tumor cells were abundant with mild atypia, which invaded and destroyed alveolar bone. Locally fibrous connective tissue septa can be seen surrounding the tumor

backward to the left maxillary tubercle with unclear boundary. There were a large number of inhomogeneous high-density shadows inside, and solar projection was observed. The lesions protruded into the left maxillary sinus cavity, causing bone destruction in the sinus wall and inward involvement of the hard palate (Fig. 44.12).

[Preliminary Diagnosis] Mass of the left maxilla.

[Treatment] "Subtotal resection of the left maxilla" was performed under general anesthesia: a left Weber-Fergusson incision was made, and the gingival flap was elevated for surgical exposure. The palate and orbital floor were dissected, medially to the nasal concha and superiorly to the inferior orbital rim. The maxilla was excised along with the mass, and sent for examination, with negative result (−). Sharp bone tips and bone edges were trimmed. The surgical wound was rinsed and thoroughly hemostatic. The soft tissue wound was covered with artificial repair film, packed with iodoform oil gauze, and the extra-oral wound was closed in layers.

[Pathological Examination] Gross pathological examination revealed a part of the maxilla. A gingival mass was observed, which was 3 cm × 3 cm × 1.5 cm in size, solid, soft, and well circumscribed. One side of the mass was hard tissue, which was decalcified. The microscopic examination showed that the tumor was composed of proliferative osteoblasts accompanied by more immature osteoid matrix formation. Chondroid differentiation was observed in the local part, and tumor cells were abundant with mild atypia, which invaded and destroyed alveolar bone. Locally fibrous connective tissue septum was seen surrounding the tumor (Fig. 44.13).

[Pathological Diagnosis] The "left maxillary gingival area" tended to be a low-grade malignant tumor of osteogenic origin, considered to be a parosteal osteosarcoma in combination with imaging and clinical findings. ICD-O code: 9192/3.

44.6 Giant Cell-Rich Osteosarcoma

44.6.1 Case 85

A 68-year-old woman suffered from a bloody bulla mass on the wound surface of the left mandible after tooth extraction for more than 2 months.

[History of Present Illness] The patient had the residual root extracted for "residual root of the left mandible" in a local dental clinic 2 months ago. The patient complained of blood blisters after extraction, accompanied by slight pain and discomfort. Then, the patient received curettage of alveolar fossa under local anesthesia at oral surgery department, and a large amount of inflammatory granuloma was removed. The patient took oral amoxicillin, but granulation tissue reappeared in the extraction wound. The "left mandibular lesion curettage" was performed. The pathological examination suggested that "giant cell lesion in the left lower posterior region" tended to be giant cell reparative granuloma with active cell growth, and the MRI examination showed space occupying of the left lower posterior region ① possibility of reparative granuloma in combination with the clinical findings. ②Tumor to be excluded.

[Specialty Examination] The face was basically symmetrical. There was no abnormality in mouth opening range and mouth opening pattern. Teeth 35 and 36 were missing. A mass in tooth 33 buccolingual and distal middle, which was 2.5 cm × 2.0 cm in size, soft and unclear in boundary. Buccal side stretched over the vestibular groove and the lingual side extended to the floor of the mouth, with dark red surface (Fig. 44.14a). Multiple teeth were missing in the mouth, the residual mucosa was basically normal, with no lower lip numbness or distortion of commissure. The tongue could move normally. No enlarged lymph nodes were observed in the left submaxilla and neck.

[Auxiliary Examination]

1. Panoramic radiographs suggested an absence of teeth 35 and 36, mandibular bone destruction, unclear circumscription, involving the root of tooth 33 (Fig. 44.14b).
2. Maxillofacial enhanced CT scan suggested a bone destruction in the left mandible accompanied by abnormal soft tissue mass, with high signal on T2WI and marked enhancement on T1WI (Fig. 44.15).

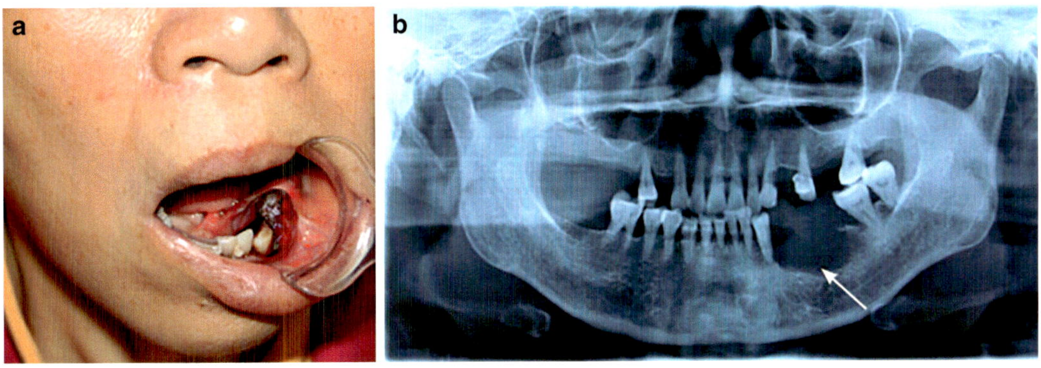

Fig. 44.14 (**a**) There was a mass in tooth 33 buccolingual and distal middle, which was 2.5 cm × 2.0 cm in size, soft and unclear in boundary. The mass had a dark red surface. (**b**) Absence of teeth 35 and 36, mandibular bone destruction, unclear circumscription, involving the root of tooth 33 (preoperative)

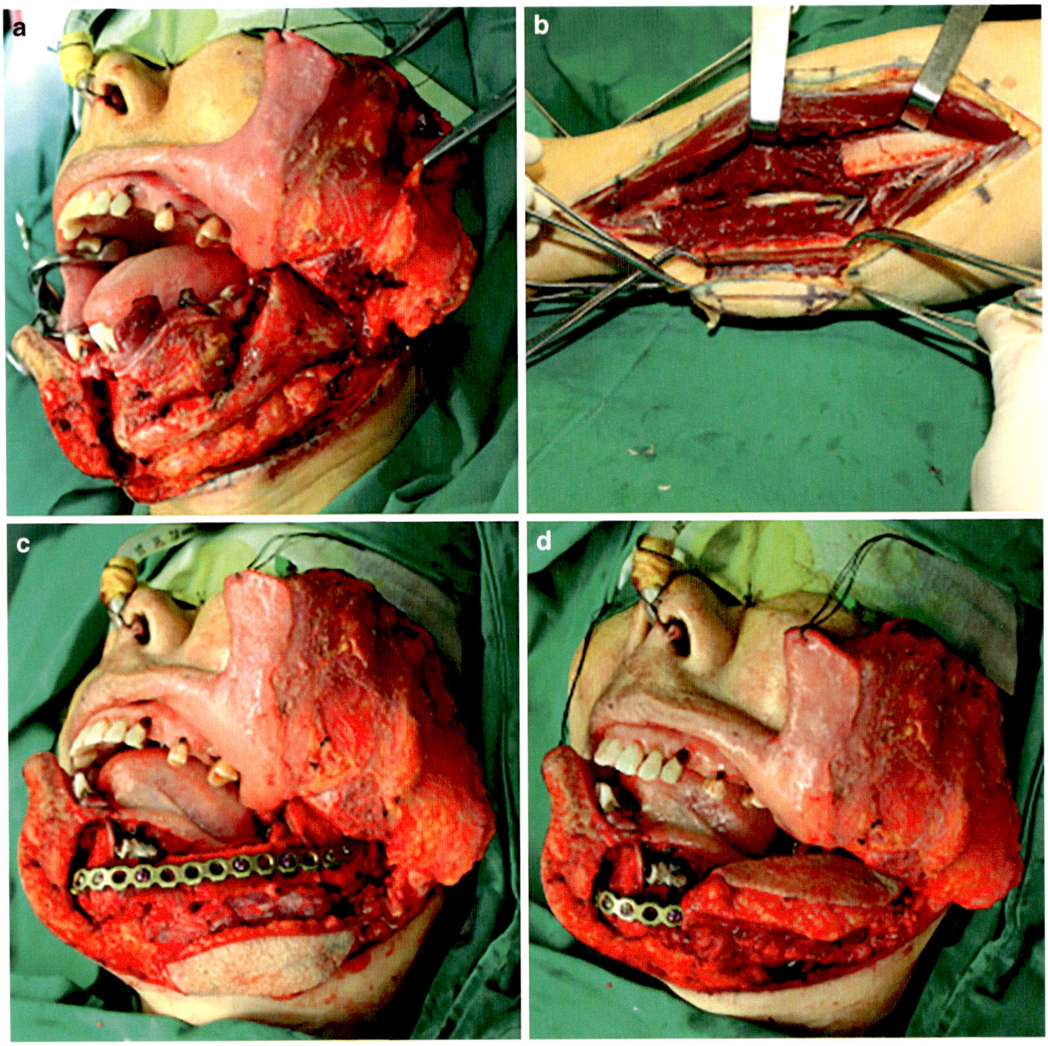

Fig. 44.15 (**a**) T1WI axial scan: left mandibular bone destruction with abnormal soft tissue mass. (**b**) T2WI axial scan: high signal for lesion. (**c**) T1W enhanced axial scan: marked lesion enhancement. (**d**) T1W enhanced coronal scan

[Preliminary Diagnosis] Giant cell reparative granuloma of the left mandible.

[Treatment] "Left mandibular segmentectomy with fibular flap transfer and tracheotomy" was performed under general anesthesia: an incision was made along the lower margin of the mandible for 1–2 cm, and the gingival flap was elevated to truncate the mandible from median mandible to left mandibular angle. The mass and mandible were removed completely within the normal tissue range. Intraoperative frozen pathological examination suggested giant cell-rich lesion of the "left mandible," with mitosis common, and malignancy to be excluded; all incisional margins were tested negative. The fibula flap with fibula about 9.0 cm long was prepared, shaped, and reconstructed to restore the continuity of the mandible and the occlusal relationship. Vascular anastomosis was performed. The wound was rinsed and thoroughly hemostatic, negative pressure drainage tube was indwelled, and layered suture was performed to close the wound (Fig. 44.16).

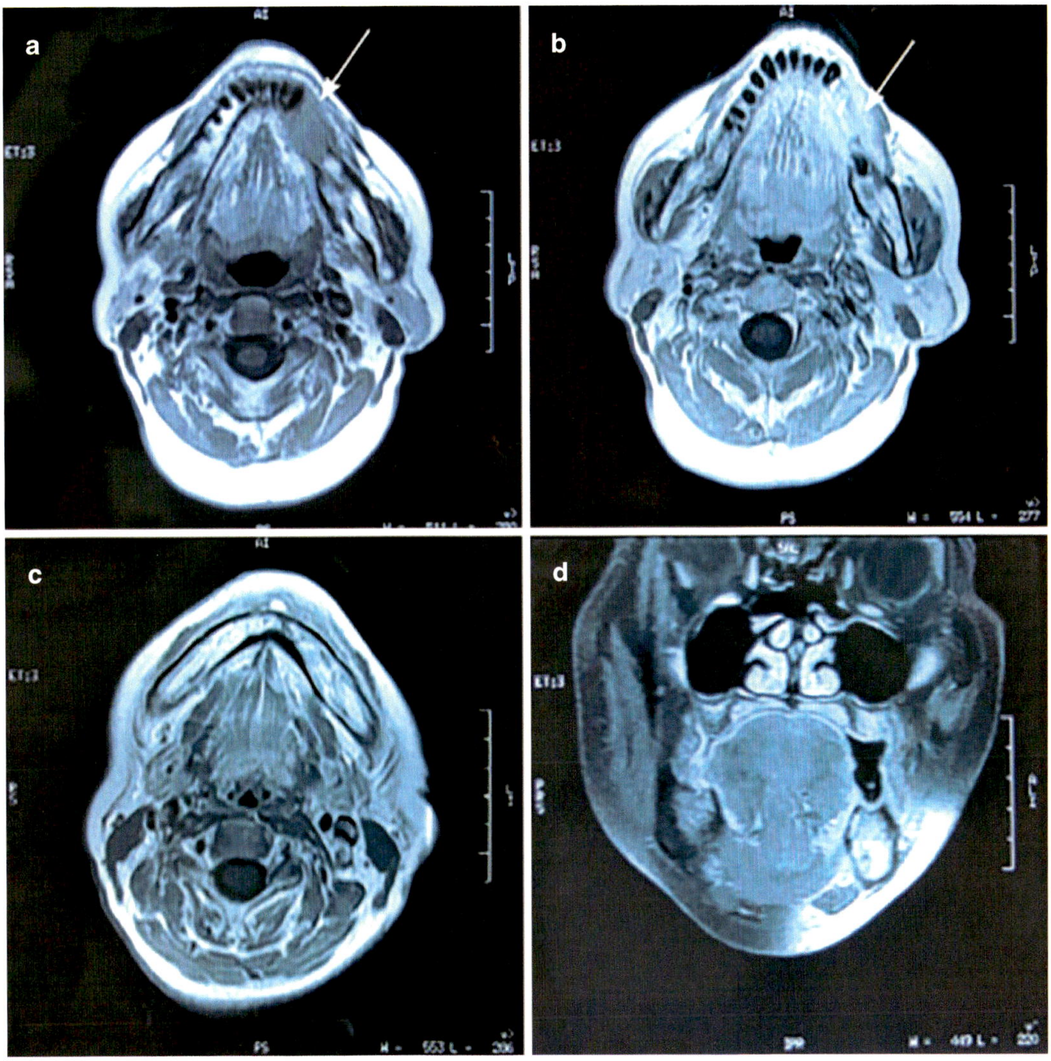

Fig. 44.16 (a) Exposure of the mandibular body and ramus. (b) Resection of fibular musculocutaneous flap. (c) Fibula reconstruction to restore mandibular continuity. (d) Myoepithelial island repair of intraoral defect

[Pathological Examination] Gross pathological examination revealed a part of the mandible and surrounding soft tissues, 6 cm × 4 cm × 2 cm in size, with 5 teeth attached. A mass of about 2 cm × 1.5 cm × 1 cm was found in the left inferior anterior tooth area, which was medium in hardness. Bone tissue resorption was observed. Microscopic examination suggested giant cell-rich lesion, with active growth of some cells, common mitosis, accompanied by bleeding and local osteoid tissue formation (Fig. 44.17).

[Pathological Diagnosis] Giant cell-rich osteosarcoma of the "left mandible."

[Follow-Up] The patient healed uneventfully. The postoperative 6-month follow-up exhibited no reoccurrence of tumor, with good recovery of the occlusal relationship between the posterior and lateral teeth, and satisfactory appearance (Fig. 44.18).

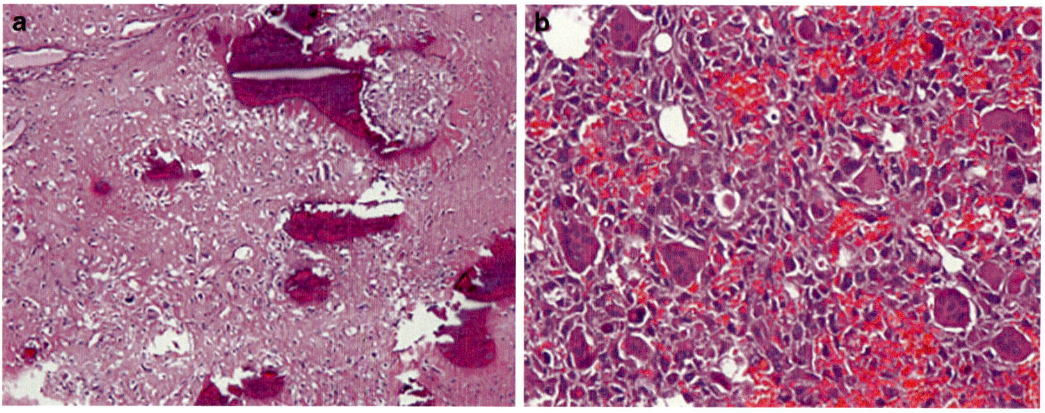

Fig. 44.17 (**a**) Osteoid tissue formation with calcification and surrounding tumor cells with atypia and sparse arrangement (100x). (**b**) More multinucleated giant cell infiltration was observed between tumor cells with obvious atypia, accompanied by bleeding (400x)

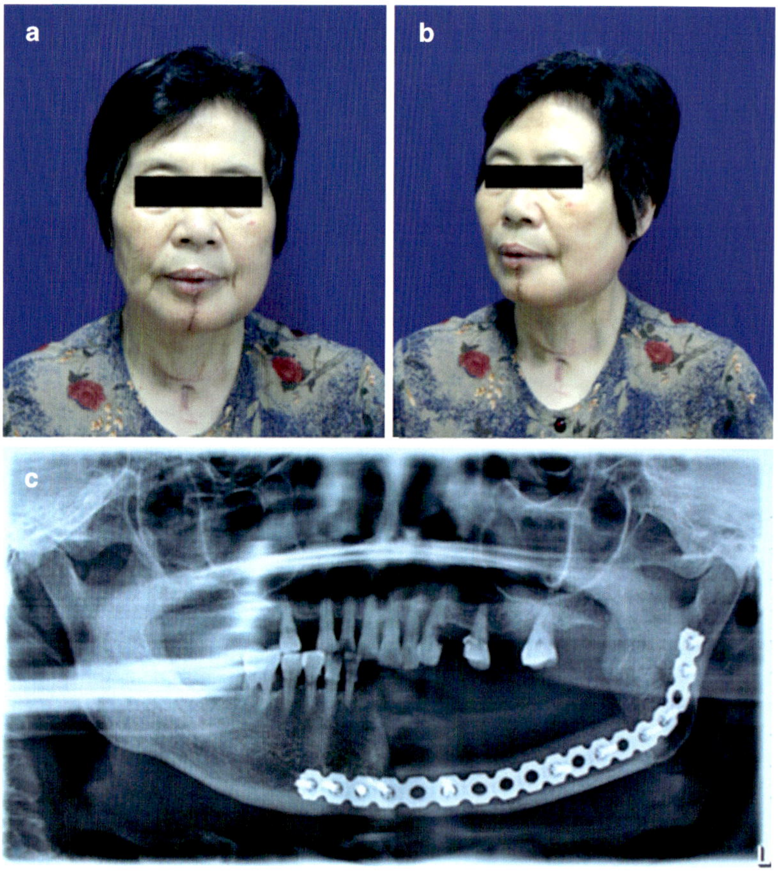

Fig. 44.18 (**a**, **b**) Postoperative changes of the mandible with basically symmetrical facial shape and no deviation of mandible. (**c**) Internal fixation of the left mandible, and well recovery of grafted fibular bone stump

44.7 Key Points of Diagnosis and Treatment

Osteosarcoma of the jaws is a rare and highly malignant tumor, accounting for 1% of head and neck malignancies, 5–13% of systemic osteosarcomas, and 86% of head and neck osteosarcomas. The prevalence of osteosarcoma in the jaws is significantly higher per unit volume than in other parts of the body, considering that the overall volume of the jaws accounts for only 0.86% of the whole body. Osteosarcoma of the jaws tends to occur in young adults between 20 and 50 years of age, with the age of onset 10–20 years older than that of osteosarcoma of the long bones. Osteosarcoma of the jaws is more common in male than female, with the incidence of upper and lower mandibles basically equal or more common. The pathogenesis remains unclear, but viral infection, trauma, history of radiation therapy, and multiple recurrences of benign bone lesions (e.g., osteofibrous dysplasia, osteochondromatosis, Paget's disease) may increase the risk of osteosarcoma of the jaws. Osteosarcoma of the jaws caused by implants has also been reported by foreign scholars.

Clinical Manifestations Unlike patients with osteosarcoma of the long bones with pain as initial symptom, most patients with osteosarcoma of the jaws present with progressive maxillofacial swelling as initial symptom, and some patients present with tooth pain, gum swelling, abnormal sensation or loose displacement of teeth as initial symptom. Distant metastases may occur, mainly to the lung, other bones, and liver, with rare regional lymph node metastases.

Imaging Characteristics Osteosarcoma of the jaws has a variety of conventional imaging findings, including bone destruction and soft tissue masses with blurred margins, often invading surrounding soft tissues. Bone destruction may be manifested as osteolytic lesion on X-ray or as osteosclerosis with increase in density, osteogenesis, or mixed bone destruction area. The circumscription of the tumor is often extremely irregular, typically shown as solar radiation. Marginal bone cortical and periosteum reactions are common.

Diagnosis The diagnosis of osteosarcoma of the jaws usually requires histopathological confirmation due to complex and diverse clinical and imaging manifestations. Its characteristic pathological change is the microscopic production of focal tumor-like bone tissue. The common pathological types are osteoblast osteosarcoma, chondroblast osteosarcoma, and fibroblast osteosarcoma, with osteoblast osteosarcoma being the most prevalent. The literature reports a high incidence of biopsy misdiagnosis of osteosarcoma of the jaws, ranging from 17% to 25%, because chondrosarcoma and conventional chondrosarcoma are often difficult to distinguish by standard morphologic analysis. As the clinical management of osteosarcoma differs significantly from that of chondrosarcoma, misdiagnosis will significantly reduce the prognosis of patients. Gomez-Brouchet A et al. suggested that Galactin-1 could be used as a diagnostic marker to differentiate chondroblast sarcoma from conventional chondrosarcoma and may help to reduce the rate of misdiagnosis of osteosarcoma. The commonly used immunohistochemical markers for osteosarcoma of the jaw are osteocalcin, osteomalacin, BMP, P53, Ki-67, PCNA, MDM2, CDK4, etc.

Differential Diagnosis In the diagnosis of osteosarcoma of the jaws, the differential diagnosis includes, but is not limited to, abnormal proliferation of bone fibers, ossifying fibroma, aggressive osteoblastoma, chondrosarcoma, fibrosarcoma, malignant fibrous histiocytoma, giant cell repair granuloma of bone, aneurysmal bone cyst, sarcomatoid carcinoma, or sarcoma of myogenic origin.

Treatment For osteosarcoma of the jaws, the first choice of treatment is radical surgical resection, with negative margins as an important condition to prevent recurrence. The incisal margin must be at least 1.5~2.0 cm away from the tumor. If it occurs in the maxilla, one side of the maxilla should be resected, and if it invades the orbit, the orbital contents can be removed together, and if the skull base is involved, brain surgery can be combined with resection of the affected bone at the skull base, and if necessary, some brain tissue should be removed. If it occurs in the mandible, mandibulectomy, segmental mandibulectomy, or hemimandibular resection can be performed. However, in some patients, surgical treatment is difficult to ensure negative margins due to the proximity of the lesion to vital structures and/or the significant cosmetic and functional impact. The postoperative recurrence rate of osteosarcoma of the jaws varies from 43% to 50%, and local recurrence is the main cause of death of patients. On the one hand, the adhesion of the original surgical area significantly increases the difficulty of surgery, and on the other hand, the formation of local scar also makes it difficult to judge the safety limit of tumor resection, thus affecting the effect of reoperation. Adjuvant chemotherapy after surgical treatment is recommended, which has been reported in the literature to be effective in improving local control and survival, especially in reducing the local recurrence rate with positive margins. Scholars have not reached a consensus on the role of radiotherapy in the treatment of osteosarcoma of the jaws, but it is generally believed that postoperative radiotherapy can be considered for patients with incomplete tumor resection to help improve the local control rate.

Prognosis The 5-year survival rate of osteosarcoma of the jaws after surgery is only 40–60%, and close follow-up is required. The prognosis of osteosarcoma of the jaw is generally considered to be influenced by the tumor size, pathologic staging, and grading. The fibroblastic osteosarcoma is generally considered to have the best prognosis, followed by chondroblastic osteosarcoma, while osteoblast osteosarcoma has the worst prognosis. In addition, osteosarcomas that occur in the maxilla are more likely to invade vital structures and less likely to be surgically complete than those in the mandible, resulting in a worse prognosis than osteosarcomas in the mandible.

References

1. Kumaravelu C, Sathya Kumar D, Chakravarthy C, et al. Chondroblastic osteosarcoma of maxilla: a case report and review of literature [J]. J Maxillofac Oral Surg. 2009;8(3):290–3.
2. McGuff HS, Heim-Hall J, Holsinger FC, et al. Maxillary osteosarcoma associated with a dental implant: report of a case and review of the literature regarding implant-related sarcomas [J]. J Am Dent Assoc. 2008;139(8):1052–9.
3. Santana L, Felix FA, de Arruda JAA, et al. A rare case of a metastatic giant cell-rich osteosarcoma of the mandible: update and differential diagnostic considerations [J]. Oral Surg Oral Med Oral Pathol Oral Radiol. 2021;131(5):e163–9.
4. Chindia ML. Osteosarcoma of the jaw bones [J]. Oral Oncol. 2001;37(7):545–7.
5. Nissanka EH, Amaratunge EA, Tilakaratne WM. Clinicopathological analysis of osteosarcoma of jaw bones [J]. Oral Dis. 2007;13(1):82–7.
6. Altuwairgi O, Papageorge MB, Karp DD. Maxillary chondroblastic sarcoma: presentation of two cases and a literature review [J]. J Oral Maxillofac Surg. 1996;54(11):1357–64.
7. Gomez-Brouchet A, Mourcin F, Gourraud PA, et al. Galectin - 1 is a powerful marker to distinguish chondroblastic osteosarcoma and conventional chondrosarcoma [J]. Hum Pathol. 2010;41(9):1220–30.
8. ElKordy MA, ElBaradie TS, ElSebai HI, et al. Osteosarcoma of the jaw: challenges in the diagnosis and treatment [J]. J Egypt Natl Canc Inst. 2018;30(1):7–11.
9. Guadagnolo BA, Zagars GK, Raymond AK, et al. Osteosarcoma of the jaw/craniofacial region: outcomes after multimodality treatment [J]. Cancer. 2009;115(14):3262–70.
10. Ferrari D, Codeca C, Battisti N, et al. Multimodality treatment of osteosarcoma of the jaw: a single institution experience [J]. Med Oncol. 2014;31(9):171.
11. Eder-Czembirek C, Moser D, Holawe S, et al. Osteosarcoma of the jaw-experience at the Medical University Vienna and comparative study with international tumor registries [J]. Clinics (Sao Paulo). 2019;74:e701.

Chondrosarcoma

45

Yue He, Hui Shan Ong, Zhen Tian, Lin Zhu, and Zhong Long Liu

45.1 Introduction

Chondrosarcoma is a rare malignant tumor. Chondrosarcomas in maxillofacial bone only account for 1–3% of chondrosarcomas in the whole body, with worse prognosis than that in other parts of the body [1–6]. The mean age of onset was about 30 years old, and there was no significant gender difference [7–9]. The incidence was more common in mandible than maxilla. Since chondrosarcoma is not sensitive to radiotherapy and chemotherapy, complete surgical resection is the main therapy. The median time to postoperative metastasis is more than 12 years, and long-term follow-up is recommended.

45.2 Grade I Chondrosarcoma

45.2.1 Case 86

A 40-year-old woman suffered from a right pretragal mass with numbness for 3 months.

[History of Present Illness] Three months ago, the patient found numbness and discomfort in the right face and was treated in hospital. Maxillofacial CT examination showed no obvious abnormalities. After 1 month of acupuncture in the Traditional Chinese Medicine Department, the symptoms showed no obvious relief. MRI examination revealed cystic solid mass of the right mandible, considered as ameloblastoma. Biopsy was performed under general anesthesia 3 weeks ago. Pathological examination revealed highly differentiated chondrosarcoma of the right condyle.

[Specialty Examination] The face was asymmetrical, with a right pretragal mass. The skin was normal in color. The mouth opening was restricted and downward, with no lower lip numbness. The right corner of the mouth was slightly oblique, with no puffing and leakage of air. An incision was found on the right pretragal anteriorly to the scalp, approximately 10 cm in length, with sutures in place. A right pretragal mass, approximately 3 cm × 3 cm in size, was palpable in the temporomandibular joint area, superiorly to the ala-tragus line, inferiorly to the lower margin of the earlobe by 1 cm, anteriorly to the anterior tragus by 2 cm, and posteriorly to the posterior edge of the earlobe, with tenderness and immobility. The tongue body can move freely. Intraoral examination revealed normal oral hygiene, no erosion of the oral mucosa, no redness or swelling of gland ducts, and no pus overflow. An

Y. He · H. S. Ong (✉) · Z. Tian · L. Zhu · Z. L. Liu
Department of Oral Maxillofacial-Head & Neck Oncology, Shanghai Ninth People's Hospital, Shanghai Jiao Tong University School of Medicine, Shanghai, China

Y. He (ed.), *Inflammatory and Neoplastic Diseases of Craniofacial Bones*, https://doi.org/10.1007/978-981-97-4155-7_45

enlarged lymph node was palpated under the right jaw, which was 1 cm × 1 cm in size, with good mobility and no tenderness.

[Auxiliary Examination] Maxillofacial enhanced CT scan suggested a bone destruction of the right mandible ramus and condyle, and unevenly increased and decreased density of the medullary cavity, surrounded by radiolucent periosteal reaction, and soft tissue mass. The mass was approximately 30 mm × 53 mm × 50 mm in size, with a blurred lateral border with the parotid gland and inhomogeneous density. Patchy, marginal, and compartmentalized enhancement presented with a CT value of 29 Hu in axial scan and 97 Hu after enhancement. The right temporomandibular joint space was widened and no abnormalities were seen on the bones of the temporal articular surface. The skull base structure was normal. Several submandibular and cervical lymph nodes less than 1 cm in diameter were observed (Fig. 45.1).

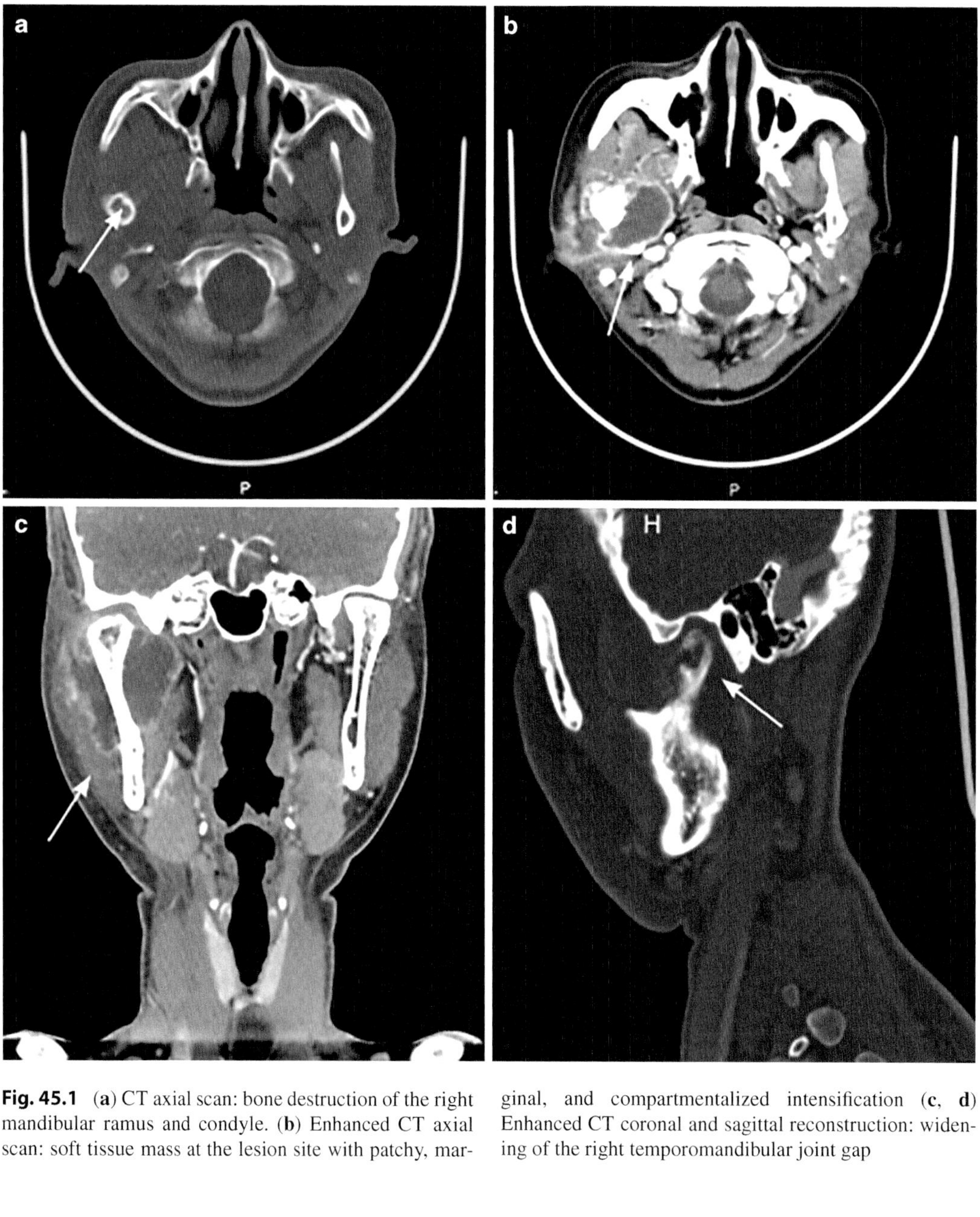

Fig. 45.1 (**a**) CT axial scan: bone destruction of the right mandibular ramus and condyle. (**b**) Enhanced CT axial scan: soft tissue mass at the lesion site with patchy, marginal, and compartmentalized intensification (**c**, **d**) Enhanced CT coronal and sagittal reconstruction: widening of the right temporomandibular joint gap

[Preliminary Diagnosis] Malignant tumor of the right condyle (chondrosarcoma).

[Treatment] "Right condylectomy and reconstrcuted with anterolateral thigh flap followed by tracheotomy" was performed under general anesthesia: a posterior temporal—pretragal—opisthotic—submandibular incision was made from and the gingival flap was elevated for surgical exposure of fascia parotidea masseterica and tumor. The tumor was located on the medial side of the mandibular ramus and was closely connected with the common trunk of the facial nerve. The temporal ramus was retained and the rest was cut off. The posterior margin of the mandibular ramus, including the condyle, was removed from the vertical line of the midpoint of the sigmoid notch, and dissected close to the skull base. Partial mandible, medial pterygoid, partial lateral pterygoid, the whole lobe of the parotid gland, and the tumor were completely removed. Intraoperative frozen pathological examination suggested cartilage-rich tumor of the "right condylar," tending to be grade I chondrosarcoma combined with the medical history. All incisional margins were negative (−).

[Pathological Examination] Gross pathological examination revealed tumor-like tissue, 8.5 cm × 7 cm × 5.8 cm in size. The tumor surrounded the mandibular ramus, the section was gray and white, and the bone was destroyed. Microscopic examination showed that the tumor was nodular and lobulated, involving surrounding tissues. A large amount of basophil cartilage matrix was formed in the tumor, in which the tumor cells were distributed with chondrocyte differentiation, small cells and dense nuclei. Some cells were located in lacunae and some were not. The cell atypia was not obvious, with rare mitosis (Fig. 45.2).

[Pathological Diagnosis] Grade I chondrosarcoma of the "right condylar process" combined with medical history, ICD-O code: 9222/1.

[Follow-Up] The patient healed uneventfully after surgery. The postoperative 2-month follow-up exhibited reoccurrence of tumor according to maxillofacial enhanced CT and MR (Figs. 45.3 and 45.4). Five courses of chemotherapy were performed in other hospital, with details unknown. Monthly maxillofacial enhanced CT revealed that no significant changes were observed in the tumor. So, the patient was admitted to the hospital for surgical treatment again, and

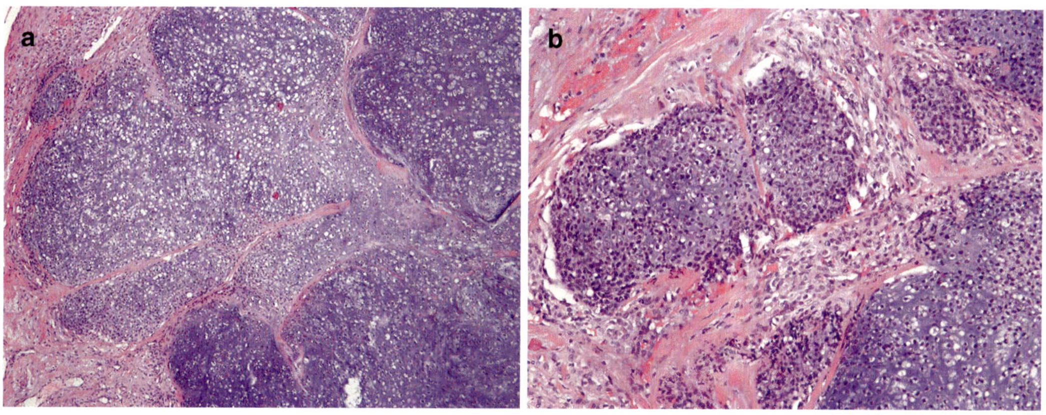

Fig. 45.2 (**a**) The lesion was irregularly lobulated, with fibrous tissue intervals between the lobules. The chondrolobules were composed of basophil myxoid matrix and tumor cells distributed inside (100x). (**b**) Small chondrocytes, partially located in cartilage lacunae, with no obvious cell atypia, and rare mitosis (200x)

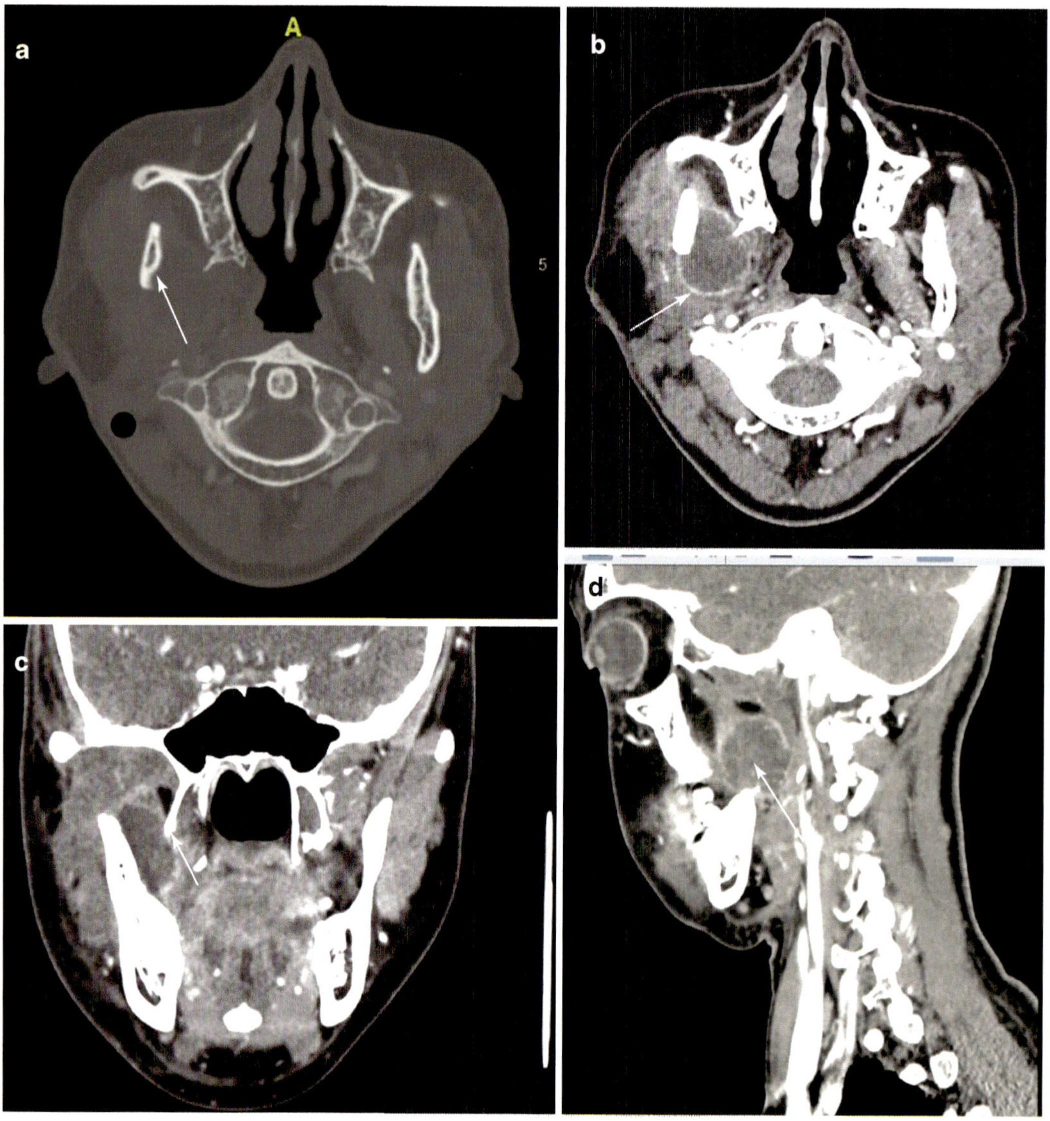

Fig. 45.3 (**a**) CT axial scan: Postoperative changes in the right mandibular ramus, with local bone destruction of the remaining bone, and marginal roughness. (**b**) Enhanced CT scan: Soft tissue mass in the medial of the mandibular ramus, patellar, enhanced edge and division, involving the pterygoid process. (**c**, **d**) Enhanced CT coronal and sagittal reconstruction: postoperative changes of the right temporomandibular joint, absence of condyle, and shadow of soft tissue mass in the mandible

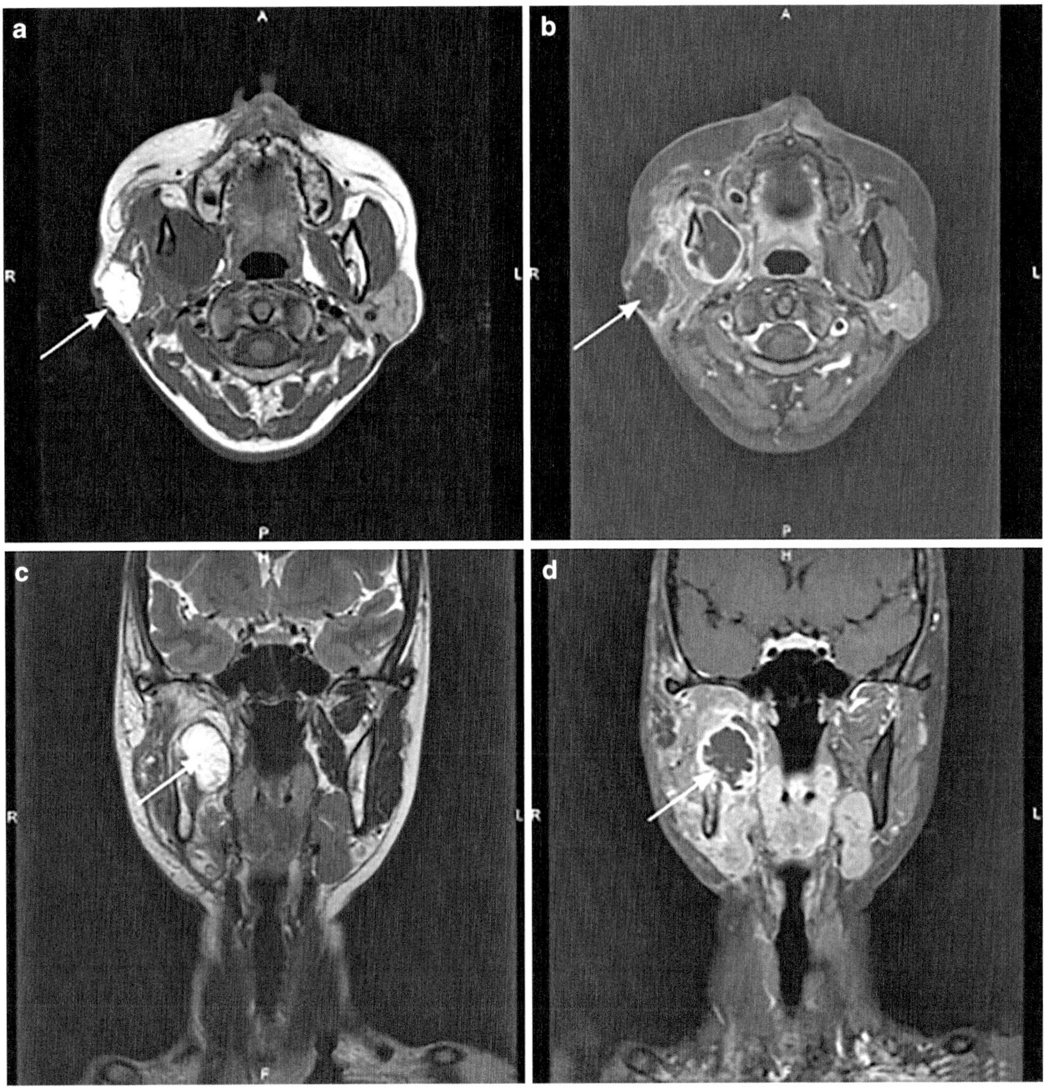

Fig. 45.4 (**a**) T1WI axial scan: abnormal soft tissue signal shadow inside the right mandibular ramus. (**b**) T1WI enhanced axial scan: annular enhancement of the lesion. (**c**) T2WI coronal scan. (**d**) T1WI enhanced coronal scan

underwent "extracranial extended radical operation" along with postoperative adjuvant chemotherapy.

45.3 Grade II/III Chondrosarcoma

45.3.1 Case 87

A 25-year-old woman suffered from a right mandibular mass which gradually grew in size for more than 6 months.

[History of Present Illness] Six months ago, the patient found a soybean-sized mass in the right mandibular premolar area without significant pain, and the mass slowly increased in size without treatment. The right mandibular mass grew significantly faster than before 3 months ago. The pathological biopsy 1 month ago suggested mucosal squamous epithelial hyperplasia with incomplete keratinization, with cartilage-like stroma locally, tending to be chondrogenic tumor. The pathology consultation at other hospital 2 weeks ago revealed a foliated cartilage with

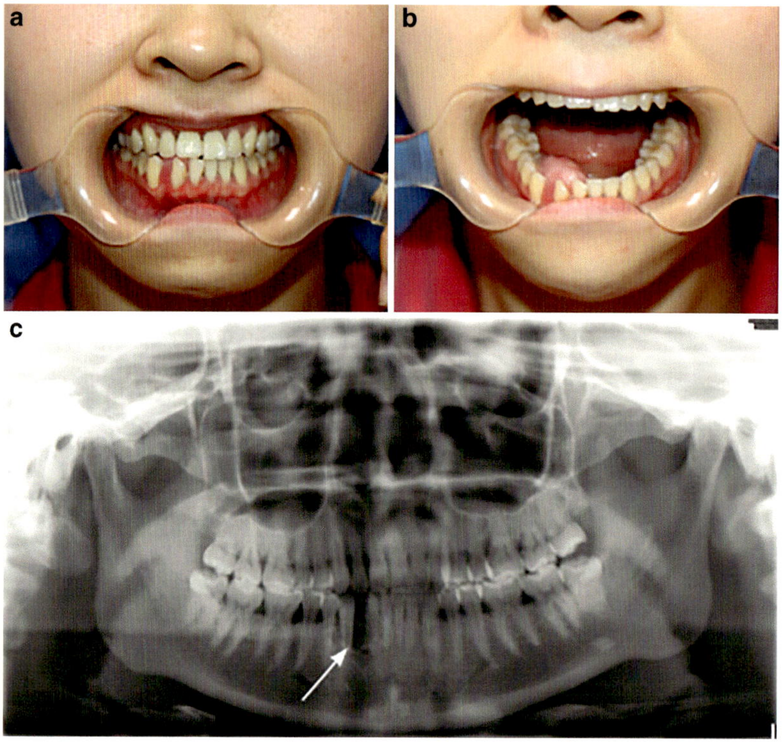

Fig. 45.5 (**a**) Normal occlusal relationship on the left side, lingual swelling in the right anterior region, displacement of teeth 41 and 42 caused by compression. (**b**) The mass clearly expanded lingually, and the mucosa was intact without rupture. (**c**) Bone destruction in the right mandibular anterior region, uneven density attenuation, poorly circumscribed

abundant chondrocytes and mild abnormalities, but no tumorigenic osteogenic or spindle cell sarcoma areas. The present mass was approximately the size of quail egg.

[Specialty Examination] The face was basically symmetrical, with well-coordinated 1/3 proportion of upper, middle, and lower face. There was no abnormality in skin color, mouth opening range, and mouth opening pattern. No obvious numbness existed in upper and lower lip. Intraoral examination revealed general oral hygiene. An exophytic mass (3.5 cm × 2.0 cm in size) was observed on the lingual side from teeth 31 to 45, with base infiltration, poor boundary definition, hard quality, no obvious tenderness, no obvious ulceration, and exudation on the mucosal surface. Buccal displacement started from teeth 41 to 43, with no obvious loosening or percussion tenderness (Fig. 45.5a, b). A part of teeth 38 and 48 protruded. The tongue could move freely, without numbness in the tip of the tongue. No significant enlargement of submandibular and cervical lymph nodes was observed.

[Auxiliary Examination]

1. Panoramic radiographs suggested a bone destruction in the right mandibular anterior region with inhomogeneous density attenuation and poorly circumscribed (Fig. 45.5c).
2. Maxillofacial enhanced CT scan suggested a distended bone change in the right mandibular anterior region (teeth 41–44), approximately 1.7 cm × 1.2 cm in size. The lesion was multifocal with a C− of 90 Hu and a C+ of 98 Hu. The lesion expanded lingually, and the adjacent bone cortex became thinning and partially disappeared, with no obvious periosteal reaction. No significant swelling of the surrounding soft tissues was seen. No significant enlargement of cervical lymph nodes was observed. (Fig. 45.6).

[Preliminary Diagnosis] Malignant tumor of the right mandible.

[Treatment] "Right mandible resection with fibular flap transfer and tracheotomy" was performed under general anesthesia: an incision was made along the lower margin of the mandi-

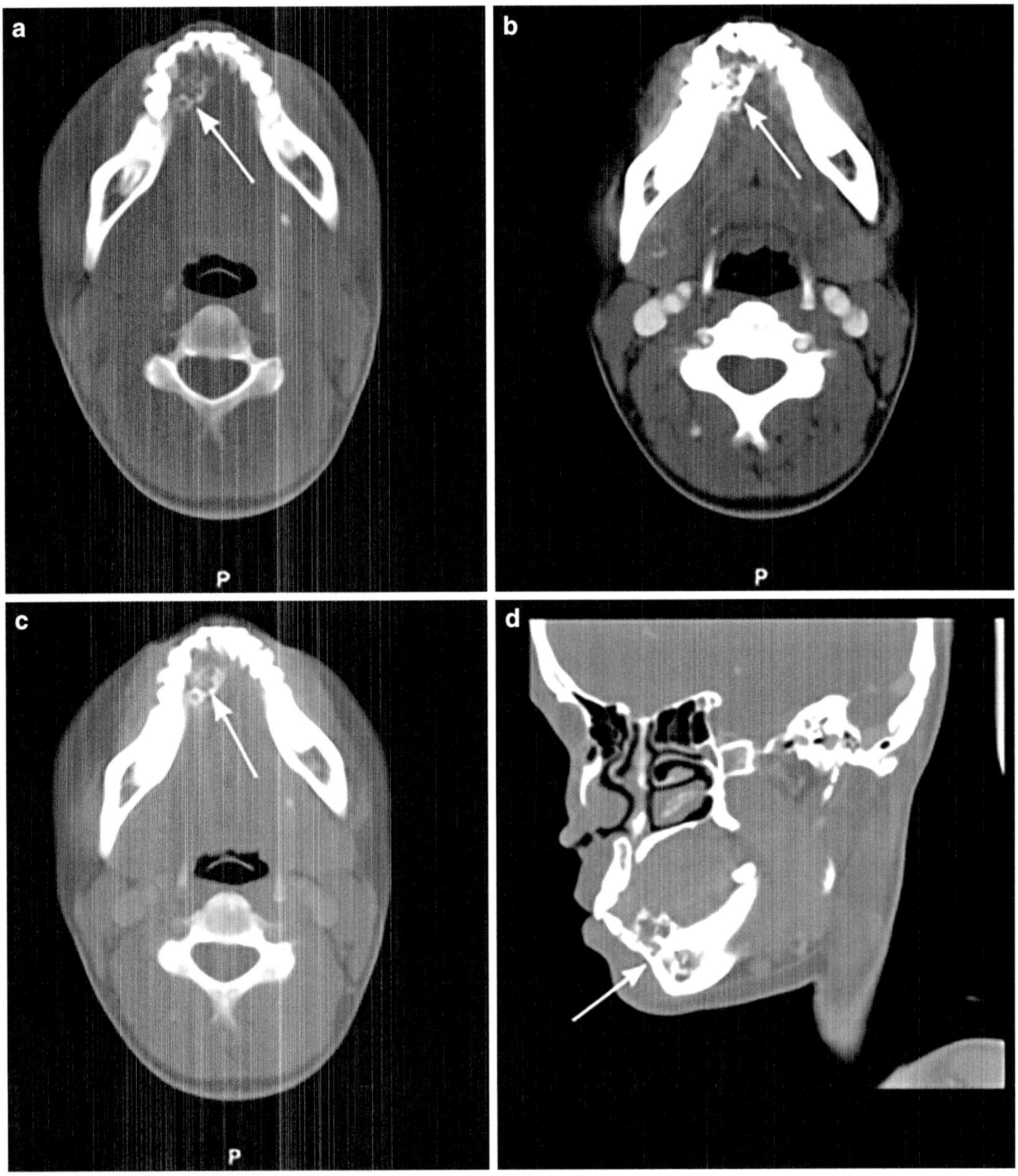

Fig. 45.6 (**a**) CT axial scan: distended bone in the right mandibular anterior region, multilocular structure. (**b**, **c**) CT enhanced axial scan: No significant enhancement of the mass and thinning of the adjacent cortical bone. (**d**) CT enhanced sagittal reconstruction: lingual distension

ble for 2 cm, and the gingival flap was elevated for surgical exposure of the mass at the lingual side of teeth 31–45. The mandible was dissected at teeth 34 and 46, respectively to completely excise the mass and truncated mandible. Intraoperative frozen pathological examination suggested chondroid tissue of the "'mandible," tending to be chondro-osseous tumor or chondrogenic tumor. Hard tissue was difficult to generate panoramic radiographs, so please refer to paraffin pathological examination results. All incisional margins tested were negative (−).The left fibula flap was made, shaped and reconstructed to restore the continuity of the mandible and the occlusal relationship, and vascular anastomosis of the fibula and right facial arte-

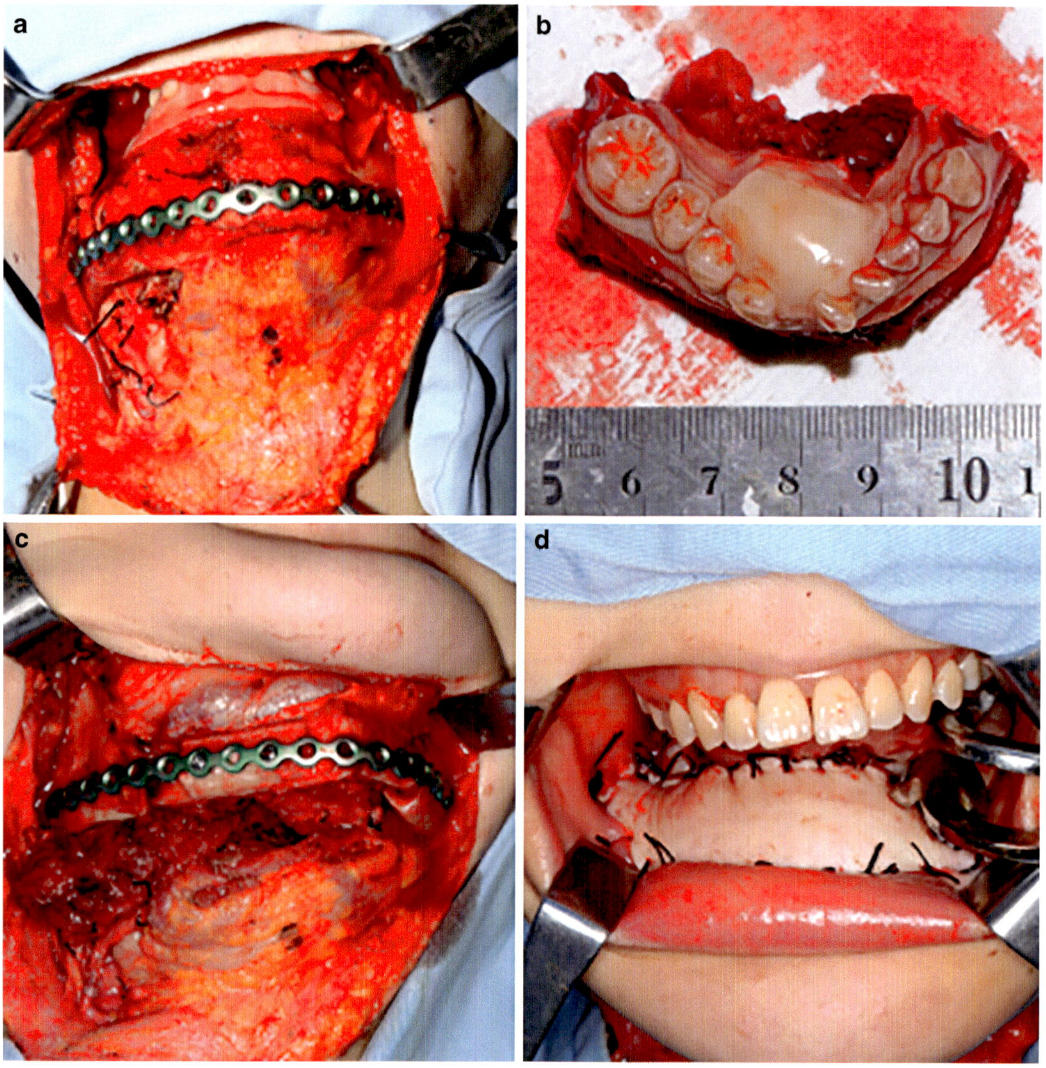

Fig. 45.7 (**a**) Exposure of the mandible and pre-bending to shape the reconstructed titanium plate. (**b**) Isolated mandible with the swelling convex to the lingual side. (**c**) Reconstruction of the fibula to restore mandibular continuity. (**d**) Myoepithelial island to repair intraoral tissue defect

riovenous vessels was performed. The wound was rinsed and thoroughly hemostatic, negative pressure drainage tube was indwelled, and layered suture was performed to close the wound (Fig. 45.7).

[Pathological Examination] Gross pathological examination revealed a part of the mandibular tissue, 6.5 cm × 5.4 cm × 4 cm in size, with nine attached teeth. A mass of 2.5 cm × 2.4 cm was found on the lingual side of the anterior teeth region, which was gray white and hard. The microscopic examination showed chondroid tissue hyperplasia, with lobulated appearance, cell atypia, dikaryocytes, and mitosis occasionally (Fig. 45.8).

[Pathological Diagnosis] Grade I chondrosarcoma of the "mandible," with ICD-O code: 9220/3.

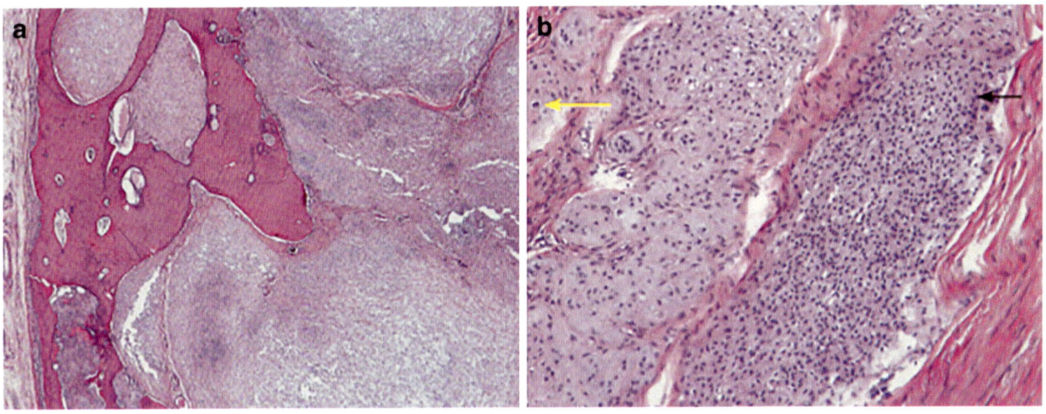

Fig. 45.8 (**a**) The tumor was lobulated and involved interosseous tissue (40x). (**b**) The tumor cells are abundant, and some of the cells are surrounded by cartilage lacunae (yellow arrow). The tumor nucleus was atypical, with bicarbonated cells (black arrow). The pericellular cartilage matrix lessened with mucous degeneration (200x)

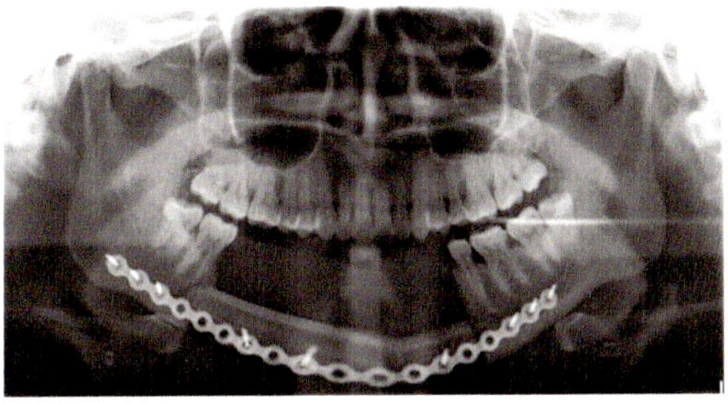

Fig. 45.9 Postoperative changes in the mandible, with bone defects partially, good healing of the bone stump, no significant displacement of the condyles bilaterally, and good restoration of the occlusal relationship of the posterior teeth

[Follow-Up] The patient healed uneventfully. The postoperative 3-month follow-up exhibited no reoccurrence of tumor, with good recovery of the occlusal relationship between the bilateral posterior teeth, and mandibular contour function (Fig. 45.9).

45.4 Key Points of Diagnosis and Treatment

Chondrosarcoma is a rare malignant tumor that occurs in the pelvis, chest wall, scapula, and long bones of the limbs. First reported in 1958, it is rare in the maxillofacial bones, accounting for only 1% to 3% of all chondrosarcomas. Chondrosarcoma is locally aggressive. Chondrosarcoma in the jaw often invades vital craniofacial structures and is difficult to be completely removed by surgical treatment. Therefore, the prognosis of chondrosarcomas in the jaw is worse than that in other parts of the body.

Clinical Manifestations Chondrosarcoma of the jaws can occur at any age, with the average age about 30 years old, showing no significant gender difference. Chondrosarcoma is more common in the mandible than the maxilla, and mostly occur in the posterior mandible and anterior maxilla. The most common clinical symptoms are slowly increasing painless hard mass, possibly accompanied by tooth loosening and loss, lower lip numbness, nasal symptoms, restricted mouth opening, etc. The most common distant metastasis is lung, followed by liver, kidney, and brain. Regional lymph node metastasis is rare.

Pathological Characteristics According to the pathological origin, chondrosarcoma can be divided into primary chondrosarcoma and secondary chondrosarcoma. The former originates from undifferentiated chondroblasts, and the latter from chondroma or chondrogenic exostosis; according to the degree of differentiation of tumor cells, chondrosarcoma can be divided into Grade I, Grade II, and Grade III; according to the location, chondrosarcoma can be divided into central chondrosarcoma and peripheral chondrosarcoma, with peripheral chondrosarcoma rarer than chondrosarcoma of the jaws; histologically, chondrosarcoma can be divided into common type, clear cell type, mesenchymal type, mucoid type, and dedifferentiation type.

Imaging Characteristics For chondrosarcoma of the jaws, the imaging findings are varied and nonspecific, and well circumscribed or poorly circumscribed on transmitted or non-transmitted X-rays. It is difficult to distinguish chondrosarcoma of the jaws from other osteosarcomas (such as osteosarcoma, osteofibrosarcoma, chondrosarcoma). The widening of the periodontal space in the lesion area is considered to be one of the X-ray features. The typical CT findings of chondrosarcoma are bone destruction, chondrogenic calcification, and soft tissue mass. Intrafocal calcification is relative characteristic of chondrogenic tumor.

Pathological Characteristics Microscopic examination shows that chondrosarcoma has a variety of morphologies. The tumor is lobulated and composed of tumor cartilage and cartilage stroma, without osteoid structure. The chondrocytes are mostly clustered at the edge of the lobules, with a sparse center and a partially calcified stroma. The nuclei of the tumor cells are hypertrophic, triangular, round or ovoid, coarse and granular, deeply stained, with obvious nucleoli, and a large number of binucleated and multinucleated giant tumor cells can be seen. Immunohistochemistry of chondrosarcoma of the jaws usually shows strong positivity for S-100 and D2-40 and negative for AE1, AE3, EMA, GFAP, β-cat, and CEA.

Differential Diagnosis Due to the lack of specificity in clinical and imaging manifestations, the diagnosis of the chondrosarcoma of the jaws depends on pathological examination. During diagnosis of the chondrosarcoma of the jaws, the differential diagnosis mainly includes but is not limited to mesenchymal chondrosarcoma, osteosarcoma, chondroblastoma, mandible fibrosarcoma, central maxillary carcinoma, ameloblastoma, and jaw metastasis,.

Treatment Now, there is a lack of clear treatment guideline for chondrosarcoma of the jaws internationally. Since chondrosarcoma is not sensitive to radiotherapy or chemotherapy, the main therapy is radical surgical excision. Because of the aggressive nature, it should be noted to leave adequate safety margins, and where possible, the tumor should be resected at least 2–3 cm outside the tumor border. Maxillary resection should be performed for the chondrosarcoma that occurs in the maxilla. Chondrosarcoma is mainly metastasized to lung, liver, kidney, and brain through direct spread to adjacent bones and advanced hematologic metastasis. Regional lymph node metastasis rarely occurs. Selective cervical dissection should not be performed in case of no evidence of regional lymph node metastasis clinically. Adjuvant radiotherapy is recommended for patients with positive surgical margins and local recurrence.

Prognosis It has been reported that most chondrosarcomas are slow-growing, with a 5-year survival rate of 41–76% and a 10-year survival rate of 35–49%. The median time to postoperative metastasis is greater than 12 years, and long-term follow-up is recommended.

References

1. Prado FO, Nishimoto IN, Perez DE, et al. Head and neck chondrosarcoma: analysis of 16 cases [J]. Br J Oral Maxillofac Surg. 2009;47(7):555–7.
2. Izadi K, Lazow SK, Solomon MP, et al. Chondrosarcoma of the anterior mandible: a case report [J]. N Y State Dent J. 2000;66(7):32–4.
3. Zhang X. Chondrosarcoma of the head and neck [J]. Lin Chung Er Bi Yan Hou Tou Jing Wai Ke Za Zhi. 2015;29(24):2111–3.
4. Ngo QX, Ngo DQ, Tran TD, et al. Chondrosarcoma of the Maxilla [J]. Ear Nose Throat J. 2020:145561320942358.
5. Cuevas-Gonzalez JC, Reyes-Escalera JO, Gonzalez JL, et al. Primary maxillary chondrosarcoma: a case report [J]. World J Clin Cases. 2020;8(1):126–32.
6. Han Z, Guanning S. Status of clinical diagnosis and treatment of chondrosarcoma [J]. Chinese Journal of Surgical Oncology. 2017;9(04):268–70, 75.
7. Majumdar S, Boddepalli R, Uppala D, et al. Mesenchymal chondrosarcoma of mandible [J]. J Oral Maxillofac Pathol. 2016;20(3):545.
8. Almansoori AA, Kim HY, Kim B, et al. Chondrosarcoma of the jaw: a retrospective series [J]. Oral Surg Oral Med Oral Pathol Oral Radiol. 2019;128(2):106–11.
9. Kunpeng Z, Bin S, Hong Z. Treatment of chondrosarcoma in different pathological subtypes of maxillary bone [J]. Medical Medicine. 2019;48(10):1726–31.

46 Mesenchymal Chondrosarcoma

Yue He, Hui Shan Ong, Zhen Tian, Lin Zhu, and Min Ruan

46.1 Introduction

Mesenchymal chondrosarcoma is a rare malignant tumor, accounting for 3–9% of all sarcomas [1–5]. It can occur in the parts of cranial and maxillofacial cartilage, and is prevalent in 20–30-year-olds, without obvious gender tendency. Due to lack of specific clinical and imaging manifestations, the diagnosis requires histopathological examination [6, 7]. Radical extensive excision is an effective method for the treatment of mesenchymal chondrosarcoma. Due to its high rate of late recurrence, long-term postoperative follow-up is recommended.

46.2 Case 88

A 33-year-old woman received chemotherapy for chondrosarcoma of the right infratemporal fossa for 2 weeks.

[History of Present Illness] About 3 months ago, the patient felt discomfort in the right eye and numbness in the infrorbital area. MRI and other examinations revealed malignant space occupying in the right maxilla and infratemporal fossa. Puncture biopsy suggested mesenchymal chondrosarcoma of infratemporal fossa. CT scan in superior hospital suggested malignant tumor of the right mandible (osteosarcoma possible), involving middle cranial fossa and intracranial. After three courses of chemical therapy in the oncology department, the tumor was reduced partially and the patient transferred to our department for surgical treatment.

[Specialty Examination] The face was asymmetrical with a left protuberance in the right maxillofacial region. The skin was normal in integrity, color, and temperature. Examination revealed slight discomfort in the right eye, no obvious visual loss, free eye movement, no double vision, numbness in the right suborbital region, palpation discomfort in the right maxillofacial region, no obvious tenderness. There was no abnormality in mouth opening range and mouth opening pattern. Intraoral examination revealed permanent dentition, normal occlusal relationship, intact right maxillary mucosa, with no obvious rupture and exudation. No significant enlargement of cervical lymph nodes was observed.

[Auxiliary Examination]

1. Maxillofacial enhanced CT scan suggested a soft tissue mass in the infratemporal fossa, which was poorly circumscribed and inhomogeneous in density. Multiple calcifications were seen inside, with a maximum cross-

Y. He · H. S. Ong (✉) · Z. Tian · L. Zhu · M. Ruan
Department of Oral Maxillofacial-Head & Neck Oncology, Shanghai Ninth People's Hospital, Shanghai Jiao Tong University School of Medicine, Shanghai, China

Y. He (ed.), *Inflammatory and Neoplastic Diseases of Craniofacial Bones*,
https://doi.org/10.1007/978-981-97-4155-7_46

section of approximately 4.4 cm × 4.0 cm, C– of 59 Hu, 296 Hu, and C+ of 68 Hu, 417 Hu. The lesions involved pterygomandibular space, pterygopalatine fossa, round foramen, and intracranial temporal, and bone destruction was observed in the right pterygoid lamina. No enlarged cervical lymph nodes were observed (Fig. 46.1).

2. Maxillofacial Enhanced CT scan suggested a soft tissue mass in the infratemporal fossa, which was poorly circumscribed and about 4.3 cm in diameter. The signal was not uniform, with moderate signal on T1WI, slightly high signal on T2WI, low signal on T1WI mixed with T2WI. The enhanced scan showed obvious inhomogeneous enhancement in density. The lesions involved pterygomandibular space, pterygopalatine fossa, round foramen, and intracranial temporal, and bone destruction was observed in the right pterygoid lamina. The ADC value of the mass was about 1.2×10^{-3} mm^2/s, and the TIC was N-type. No enlarged cervical lymph nodes were observed (Fig. 46.2).

[Preliminary Diagnosis] Postchemotherapy for mesenchymal chondrosarcoma of the infratemporal fossa.

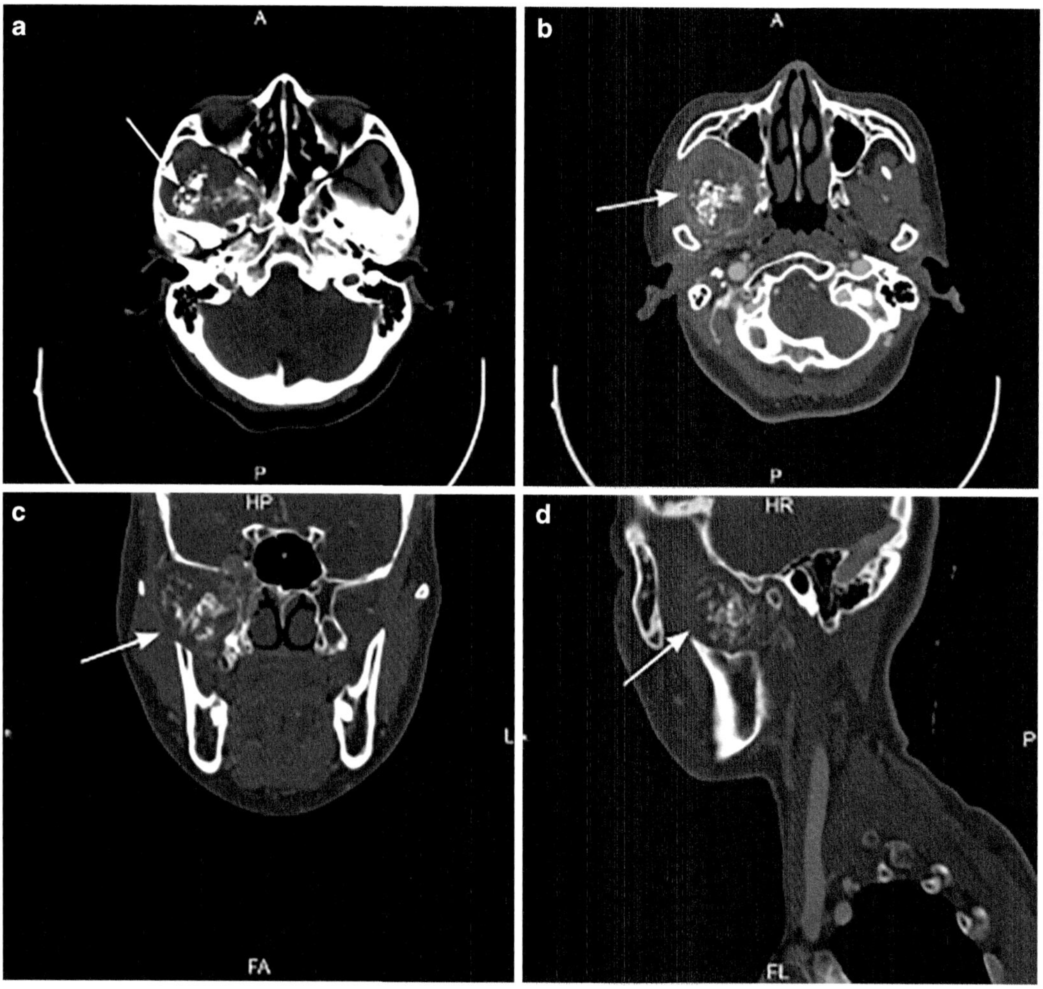

Fig. 46.1 (**a**) CT axial scan: well-circumscribed mass with multiple calcifications. (**b**) CT enhanced axial scan: marked enhancement of the mass. (**c**) CT enhanced coronal reconstruction: upward invasion of the mass into the skull through the cavernous sinus. (**d**) CT enhanced sagittal reconstruction

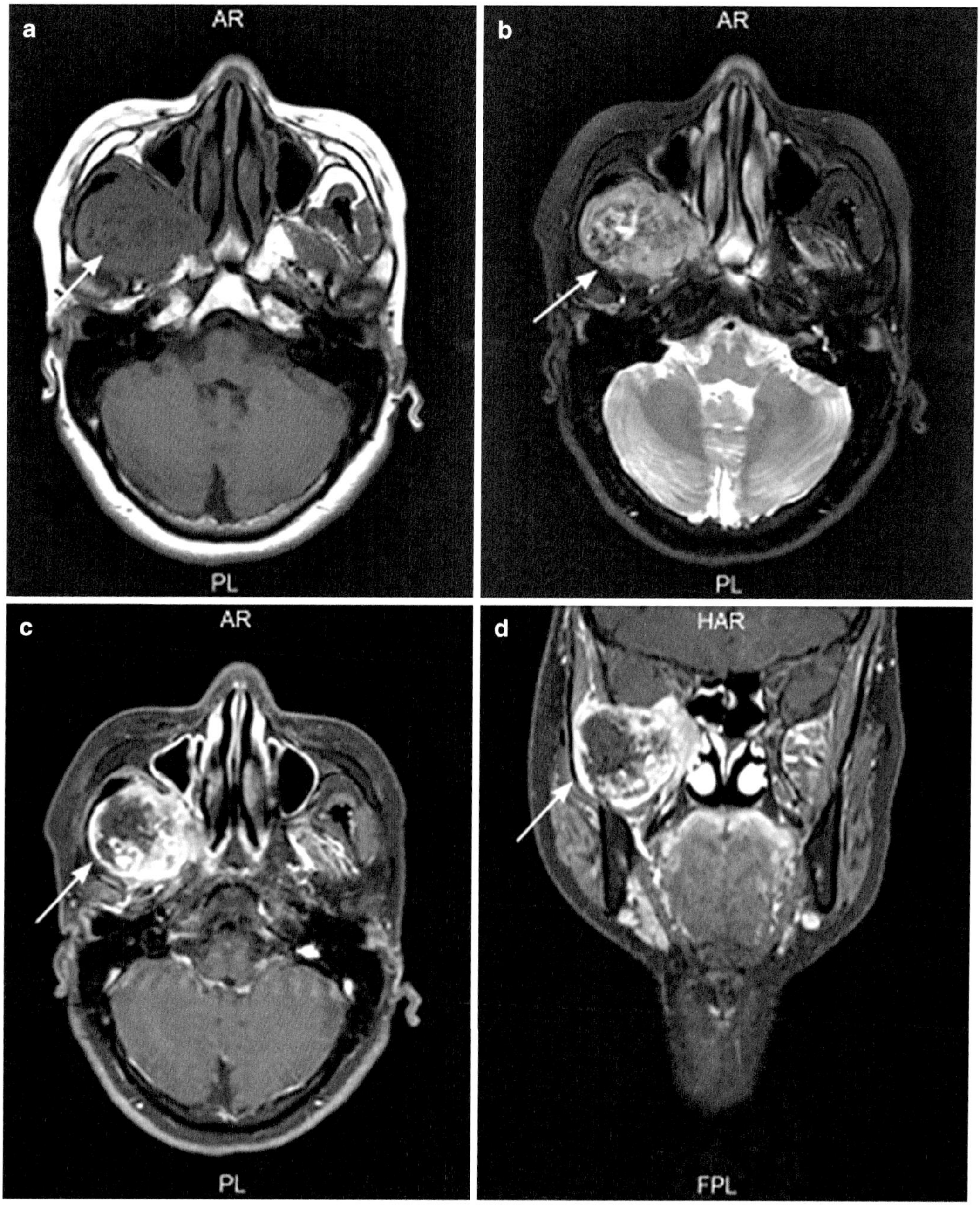

Fig. 46.2 (**a**) T1W axial scan. (**b**) fsT2WI axial scan. (**c**) T1W enhanced axial scan: Tumor enhancement with involvement of cavernous sinus. (**d**) T1WI coronal scan: tumor penetration of skull base and intracranial involvement

[Treatment]

1. Preoperative neoadjuvant chemotherapy (3 courses).
2. "Radical craniomaxillofacial resection with facial nerve anatomy, temporal muscle flap transfer, and condylar reduction and internal fixation" was performed under general anesthesia: a right semi-coronal + anterior and posterior ear incision was made, and the gingival flap was elevated for surgical exposure of the basicranial tumor in the right maxilla. The deep lobe attachment of the epicranial aponeurosis was dissoci-

ated from the temporalis, and the superficial lobe attachment of the temporalis muscle was preserved and prepared for flap transfer. The zygomatic root and external orbital bone were isolated. The tumor was located in the infratemporal fossa, skull base, and medial aspect of the mandibular ramus. The zygomatic arch, coronoid process, and medial wall of the maxillary sinus were removed, and the mandibular condyle was temporarily dissected. The lower, inner, and outer circumscriptions of the tumor were fully dissociate along the periphery of the tumor for 1 cm. At neurosurgery department, the craniotomy from the right temporal area was performed for surgical exposure of the epidural basitemporal. The basitemporal tumor, located in the epidural area, caused a bone destruction in the basitemporal and temporal pole; the basitemporal was resected along the foramen ovale, the pterygoid sinus was exposed, the root of the pterygoid process and the cranial bone of the temporal pole were severed, the tumor boundary was separated outside the tumor capsule until it was dissociated, and the tumor was resected entirely outside the capsule in cooperation with the oral-maxillofacial-head and neck oncology department. The temporal pole near the cavernous sinus dura tumor adhesion site was subject to extensive thorough bipolar electroparaffin pathology. No other abnormal lesions were found in the operative area after tumor resection. After field hemostasis, the temporal skull was repositioned, and the titanium plate and nail were strongly fixed internally. The intraoperative frozen section examination suggested chondroblast dominated malignant tumor of the "right infratemporal fossa," with mesenchymal chondrosarcoma to be excluded, please refer to paraffin pathological examination results. The temporarily disconnected condyle was repositioned, and the titanium plate and nail were strongly fixed internally. The wound was rinsed and thoroughly hemostatic. The right maxillofacial defect was repaired with occlusal muscle and other tissue flap transfer. Negative pressure drainage tube was indwelled, and layered suture was performed to close the wound.

3. Postoperative chemotherapy.

[Pathological Examination] Gross pathological examination revealed bone tissue, 5 cm × 5 cm × 4.5 cm, grayish white, soft, and poorly circumscribed with the surrounding residual bone. Histopathology revealed the tumor was lobulated and invaded into adjacent bone tissue, while a small amount of residual bone tissuex in the tumor. The tumor was composed of dense and sparse areas with a clear boundary. In the sparse area, lamellar hyaline cartilage islands were observed, with good differentiation. In the dense area, the cells were fusiform or oval, with deeply stained nuclei, cell atypia, and mitosis visible. Thin-walled vascular fissure can be seen between tumor cells, showing hemangiopericytoma features (Fig. 46.3).

[Pathological Diagnosis] Mesenchymal chondrosarcoma of the "right infratemporal fossa," ICD-O code: 9240/3.

[Follow-up] The patient healed uneventfully. The postoperative oncology consultation exhibited continuing chemotherapy.

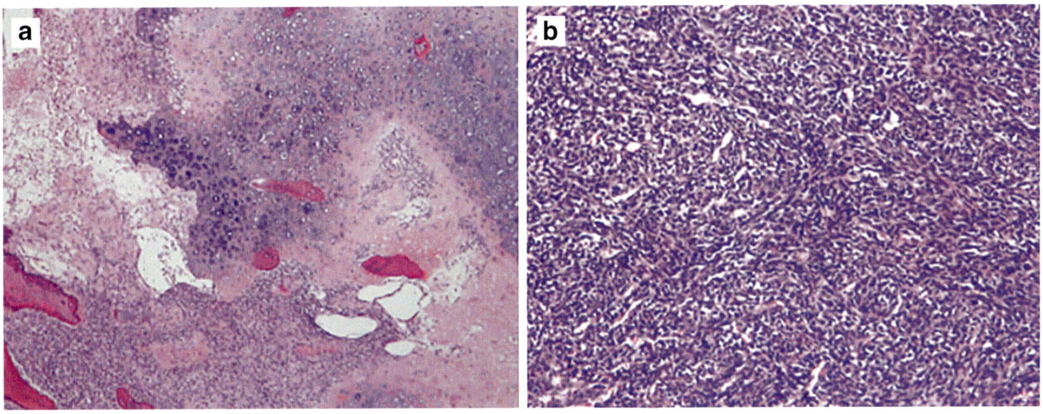

Fig. 46.3 (**a**) The tumor involved bone tissue, partially hypercellular and partially hypocellular, (upper left and lower right), accompanied by a large amount of chondroid tissue formation. The bone tissue buried was residual host bone, not tumor bone (100x). (**b**) Abundant tumor cells, thin-walled fissure blood vessels, similar hemangiocytoma view (200x)

46.3 Key Points of Diagnosis and Treatment

Mesenchymal chondrosarcoma is a rare malignant tumor characterized by bidirectional differentiation, accounting for 3–9% of all sarcomas. With the features of focal chondrogenic differentiation, it can occur in the parts of the cranial and maxillofacial cartilages, such as the maxillofacial bones, skull base, and nasopharynx. The age of onset is 5–74 years old, and 60% of the patients are 20–30 years old, with no obvious gender orientation.

Most patients present with progressive maxillofacial swelling as initial symptom, sometimes with nasal obstruction, nasal bleeding, and loosening and displacement of teeth. The tumor may protrude from the peripheral bone, infiltrate and destroy the surrounding soft tissues such as the buccal fat pad and pterygoid muscle.

The mesenchymal chondrosarcoma lacks characteristic imaging findings. MRI shows the extent of the tumor better than CT, and T2-weighted images show a bicomponent structure of calcified and uncalcified areas in mesenchymal chondrosarcoma. Unevenly enhanced calcified and uncalcified areas can be seen on T1-weighted images after contrast injection.

The diagnosis of mesenchymal chondrosarcoma requires histopathological examination, supplemented with immunohistochemical studies and molecular diagnostic techniques. The typical histological features are small, round, or spindle-shaped mesenchymal cells distributed in the hyaline cartilage. Immunohistochemical findings show positive for CD99, SOX9, and vimentin, and negative for Fli-1 and EMA. The cartilage component is well differentiated and resembles mature hyaline cartilage. Insufficient sampling may lead to misdiagnosis. In the diagnosis of mesenchymal chondrosarcoma, the differential diagnosis includes, but is not limited to, common chondrosarcoma, dedifferentiated chondrosarcoma, clear cell chondrosarcoma, and endosseous small cell malignant tumor.

Radical resection is an effective therapy for mesenchymal chondrosarcoma and should ensure negative margins whenever possible. Adjuvant postoperative radiotherapy and/or chemotherapy is recommended for patients with positive margins for mesenchymal chondrosarcoma. Studies have shown 5- and 10-year survival rates of 82% and 56%, respectively, for patients with mesenchymal chondrosarcoma of the jaws. Mesenchymal chondrosarcoma has a tendency for late local recurrence and metastasis. So long-term postoperative follow-up of at least 10 years is recommended.

References

1. Xu J, Li D, Xie L, et al. Mesenchymal chondrosarcoma of bone and soft tissue: a systematic review of 107 patients in the past 20 years [J]. PLoS One. 2015;10(4):e0122216.
2. Shabani S, Kaushal M, Kaufman B, et al. Intracranial extraskeletal mesenchymal chondrosarcoma: case report and review of the literature of reported cases in adults and children [J]. World Neurosurg. 2019;129:302–10.
3. Mendenhall WM, Reith JD, Scarborough MT, et al. Mesenchymal chondrosarcoma [J]. Int J Part Ther. 2016;3(2):300–4.
4. Majumdar S, Boddepalli R, Uppala D, et al. Mesenchymal chondrosarcoma of mandible [J]. J Oral Maxillofac Pathol. 2016;20(3):545.
5. Uppaluri SA, Yin LH, Goh GH. Maxillary mesenchymal chondrosarcoma presenting with epistaxis in a child [J]. J Radiol Case Rep. 2015;9(8):33–8.
6. Shakked RJ, Geller DS, Gorlick R, et al. Mesenchymal chondrosarcoma: clinicopathologic study of 20 cases [J]. Arch Pathol Lab Med. 2012;136(1):61–75.
7. Tansir G, Rastogi S, Barwad A, et al. Long lasting response with trabectedin monotherapy in relapsed metastatic mesenchymal chondrosarcoma [J]. Clin Sarcoma Res. 2020;10:16.

47 Postirradiation Sarcoma of Jaws

Yue He, Hui Shan Ong, Zhen Tian, Lin Zhu, and Xing Zhou Qu

47.1 Introduction

Postirradiation sarcoma of jaws is a rare mesenchymal malignant tumor that occurs in the mandible and is closely associated with a history of mandibular radiation therapy. The incidence of postirradiation sarcoma of the head and neck ranges from 0.06% to 0.17%, with 47.5% occurring in the mandible and a male-to-female ratio of 1.7:1 [1–7]. Osteosarcoma accounts for the majority of pathological types, followed by fibrosarcoma and chondrosarcoma. Postirradiation sarcoma of the mandible occurs mostly in the mandibular ramus, and the interval with the radiotherapy for primary disease is 8–12 years on average [5–10] The clinical manifestations are mainly local swelling and pain, lower lip numbness, or abnormal sensation. The postirradiation sarcoma of the mandible has a poor prognosis, with a 5-year survival rate of approximately 12.3%. Radical surgical resection is the most important means of prolonging survival.

Y. He · H. S. Ong (✉) · Z. Tian · L. Zhu · X. Z. Qu
Department of Oral Maxillofacial-Head & Neck Oncology, Shanghai Ninth People's Hospital, Shanghai Jiao Tong University School of Medicine, Shanghai, China

47.2 Case 89

A 62-year-old woman suffered from right facial swelling and pain for 4 months.

[History of Present Illness] The patient received radiotherapy for nasopharyngeal carcinoma 9 years ago at other hospital at an unknown dose, and has not seen any recurrence of the tumor since then. Four months ago, she felt pain in the right temporomandibular joint area, and 3 months ago, she had swelling in the right face, with blurred vision in the right eye, restricted mouth opening, and numbness in the right lower lip. The maxillofacial enhanced CT suggested a bone destruction in the right mandible with soft tissue mass, considered as radiogenic intraosseous carcinoma possibly, with radiogenic osteosarcoma to be excluded. MRI was recommended. Multiple small abnormal lymph nodes were observed in the neck bilaterally.

The face was asymmetrical, with swelling on the right face, posteriorly to the posterior edge of the mandibular branch, anteriorly to the anterior edge of the bite muscle, superiorly to the inferior orbit and inferiorly to the inferior edge of the mandible. Radiotherapy caused skin hyperpigmentation, but skin temperature was normal. The swelling was medium to hard, and poorly circumscribed, with local tenderness (+). Numbness occurred in the right lower lip and chin. The right temporomandibular joint was painful, the mouth

Y. He (ed.), *Inflammatory and Neoplastic Diseases of Craniofacial Bones*, https://doi.org/10.1007/978-981-97-4155-7_47

opening was about 0.5 cm, and the mouth opening pattern was downward. Intraoral examination revealed permanent dentition. The right mandibular swelling, hard and poorly circumscribed, was accessible from the right gingival-buccal sulcus but not from cavum oris proprium (Fig. 47.1a, b). No significant enlargement of submandibular and cervical lymph nodes was observed bilaterally.

[Auxiliary Examination]

1. Panoramic radiographs suggested an obvious bone destruction in the right mandible body, angle, ascending ramus, coracoid process, and condyle, with wormy appearance, poor circumscription, teeth 46–48 involvement, and no obvious resorption in tooth root (Fig. 47.1c).
2. Maxillofacial enhanced CT scan suggested an obvious bone destruction in the right mandibular body, angle, ascending ramus, coracoid process, and condyle, with wormy appearance. A soft tissue mass involving adjacent masticatory muscles was seen, approximately 4.8 cm × 5.5 cm in range, with a C− of 50 Hu and C+ of 59 Hu and 88 Hu. Multiple lymph nodes less than 1 cm in diameter were observed in the neck bilaterally, with significant enhancement. The left mandible, bilateral maxilla, pterygoid, and temporal bone marrow cavity were diffusely increased in density with uneven surface (Fig. 47.2).
3. Maxillofacial enhanced MR suggested an obvious bone destruction in the right mandibular body, angle, ascending ramus, coracoid process, and condyle, with wormy appearance. A soft tissue mass of approximately 74 mm × 52 mm × 80 mm involving adjacent masticatory muscles was seen, approximately 4.8 cm × 5.5 cm in range. T1WI showed isosignal, T2WI weighted high and low signal. The lesion was obviously inhomogeneously enhanced after enhancement (Fig. 47.3).

[Preliminary Diagnosis] Malignant tumor of the right mandible.

[Treatment] "Left mandible resection with anterolateral thigh flap transfer and tracheotomy" was performed under general anesthesia:

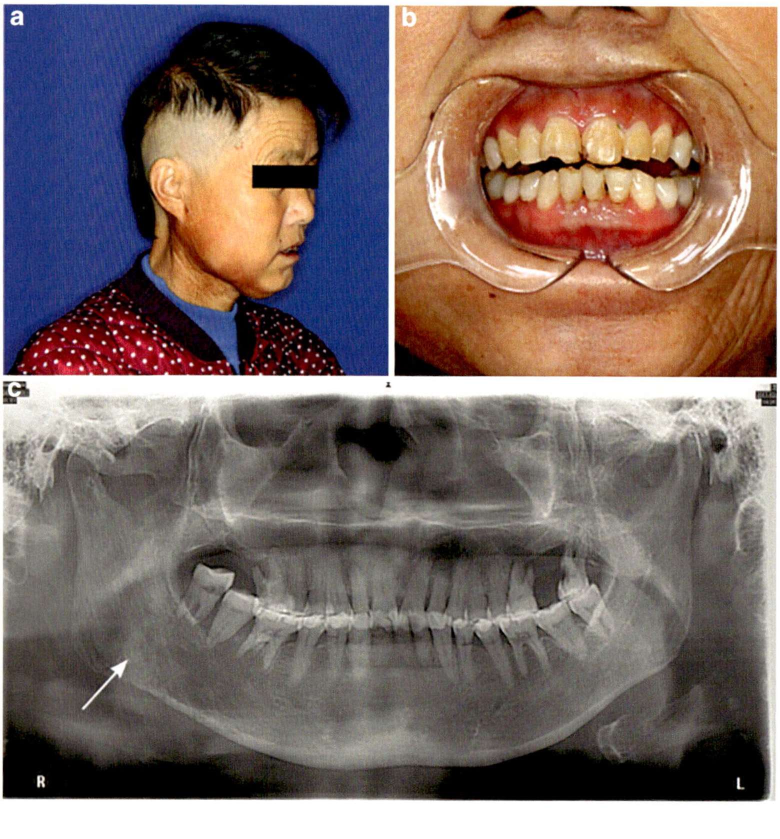

Fig. 47.1 (**a**) Facial asymmetry, swelling of the right face, skin pigmentation. (**b**) Severe restriction of mouth opening. (**c**) Obvious bone destruction in the right mandibular body, angle, ascending ramus, coracoid process, and condyle, showing wormy appearance with poor circumscription, teeth 46–48 involved, and no obvious resorption in tooth roots

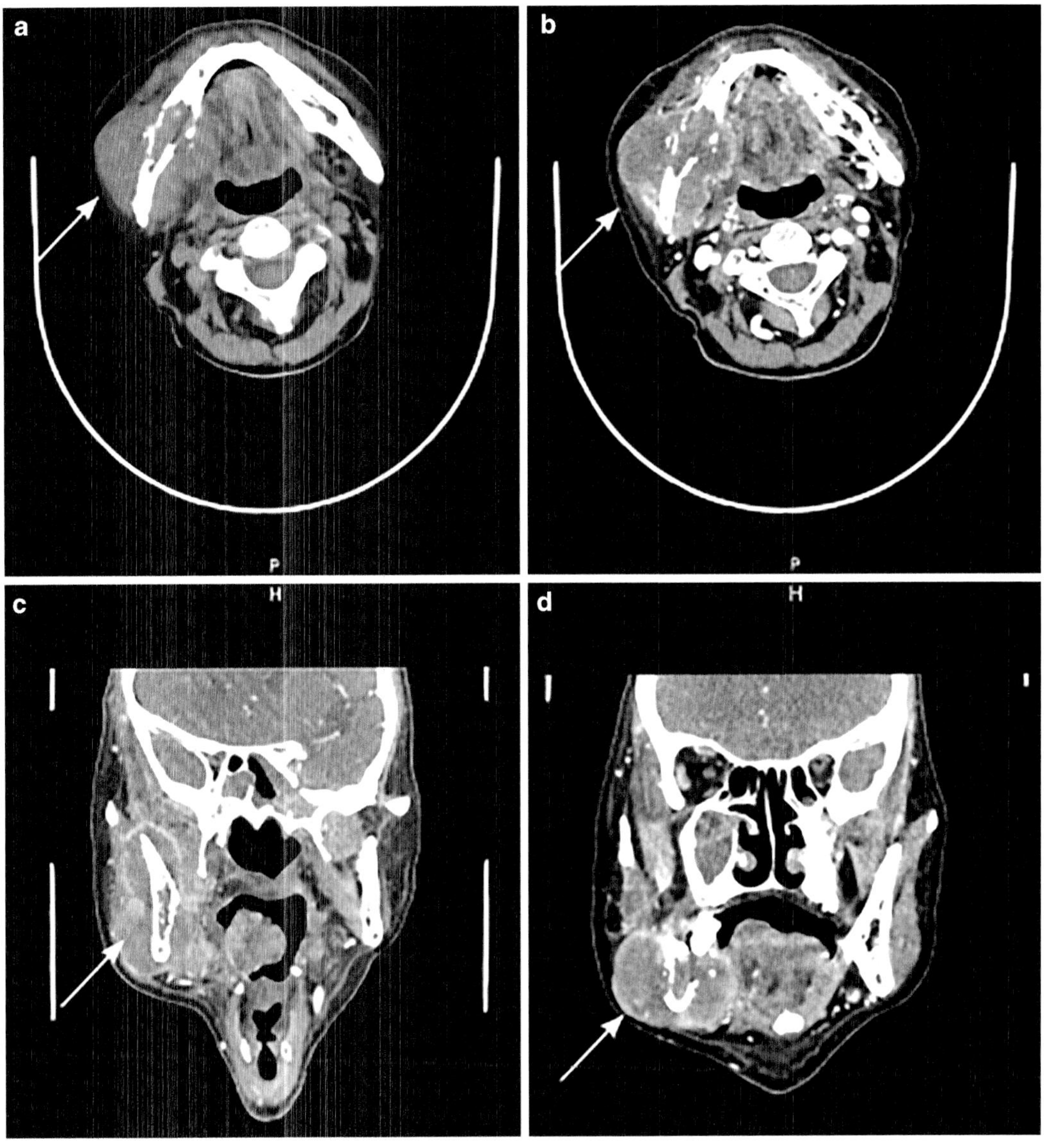

Fig. 47.2 (**a**) CT axial scan: bone destruction in right mandibular body and angle, with wormy appearance, and soft tissue mass around. (**b**) Enhanced CT axial scan: inhomogeneous enhancement of the mass, mainly marginal enhancement. (**c**, **d**) Enhanced CT coronal reconstruction: involvement of the right mandibular ramus, coracoid process, condyle process, and adjacent masticatory muscle

an incision was made along the lower margin of the mandible for 1–2 cm, and the gingival flap was elevated for surgical exposure of the destruction of right mandibular ramus, and the poorly circumscribed mass involving masseter, medial pterygoid, lateral pterygoid, and temporal muscles. The mandible was truncated at tooth 42, and the mandible, including the condyle, and the swelling were removed completely within the range of normal tissue. Intraoperative frozen pathological examination showed "spindle cell lesion" in the right mandible, cell focal atypia, visible mitosis and a few pathological mitosis, tendency to malignity, but to be determined with paraffin section and enzyme-labeled immunoassay. Incisional margins were negative (−).The anterolateral thigh flap was routinely prepared and anasto-

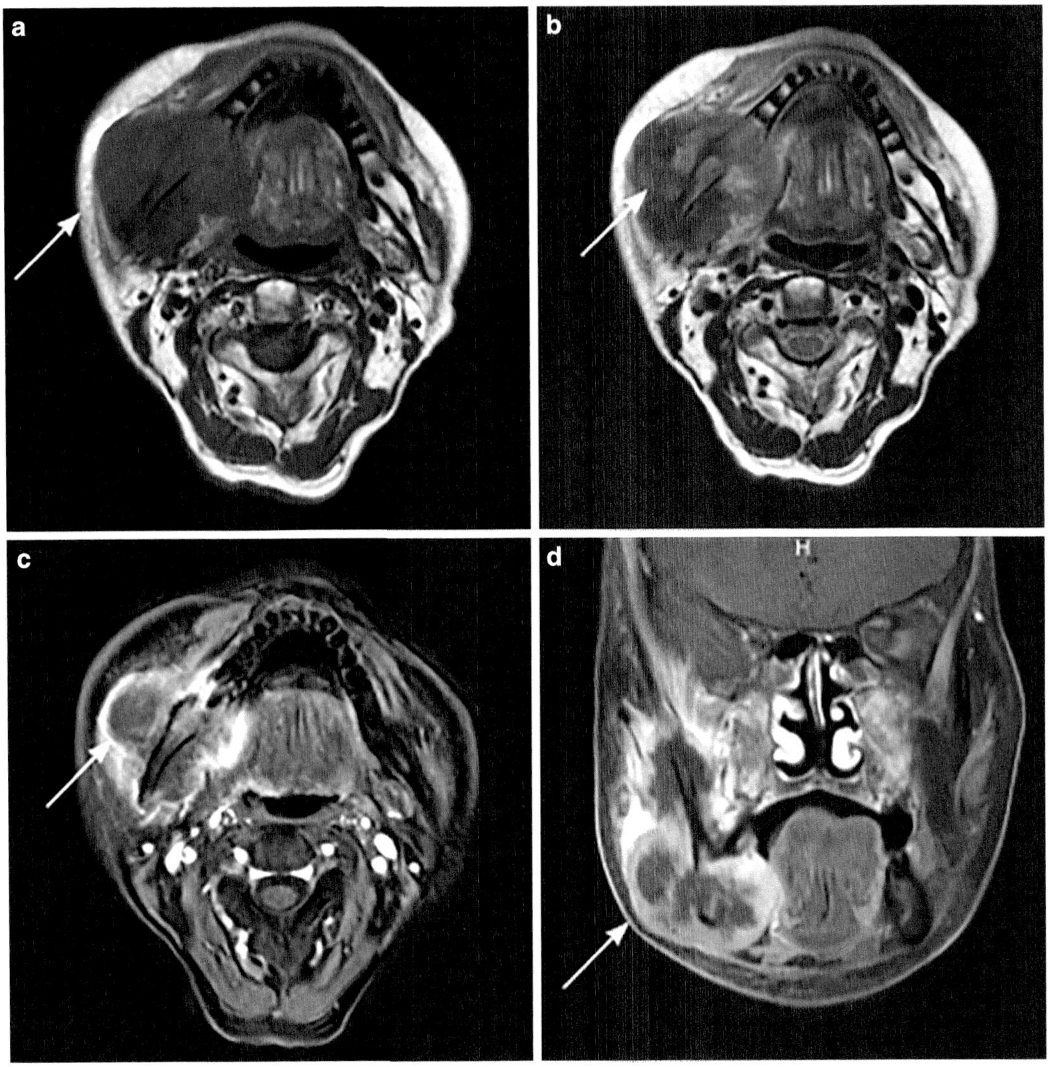

Fig. 47.3 (**a**, **b**) T1WU, T2WI axial scan: Bone destruction of the right mandibular body, angle and ascending ramus, accompanied by soft tissue mass. (**c**, **d**) T1WI enhanced axial and coronal views: the lesion showed inhomogeneous enhancement, with marginal enhancement predominating

mosed to the superior thyroid artery and common facial vein, respectively. The flap was sutured to the body of the tongue and the mucosa of the mouth floor and buccal area. The wound was rinsed and thoroughly hemostatic, negative pressure drainage tube was indwelled, and layered suture was performed to close the wound (Fig. 47.4).

[Pathological Examination] Gross pathological examination revealed the mandibular bone, 12 cm × 6 cm × 8 cm in size, with four teeth attached and a buccolingual protuberance. Microscopically, the tumor cells were spindle-shaped or short spindle-shaped, with obvious cell heterogeneity and bundle-like staggered arrangement, and vacuolated nuclei with obvious nucleoli and mitosis (Fig. 47.5).

[Pathological Diagnosis] Postirradiation sarcoma of the "right mandible."

[Follow-Up] The patient healed uneventfully. The postoperative 6-month follow-up exhibited no recurrence of tumor, with normal opening and

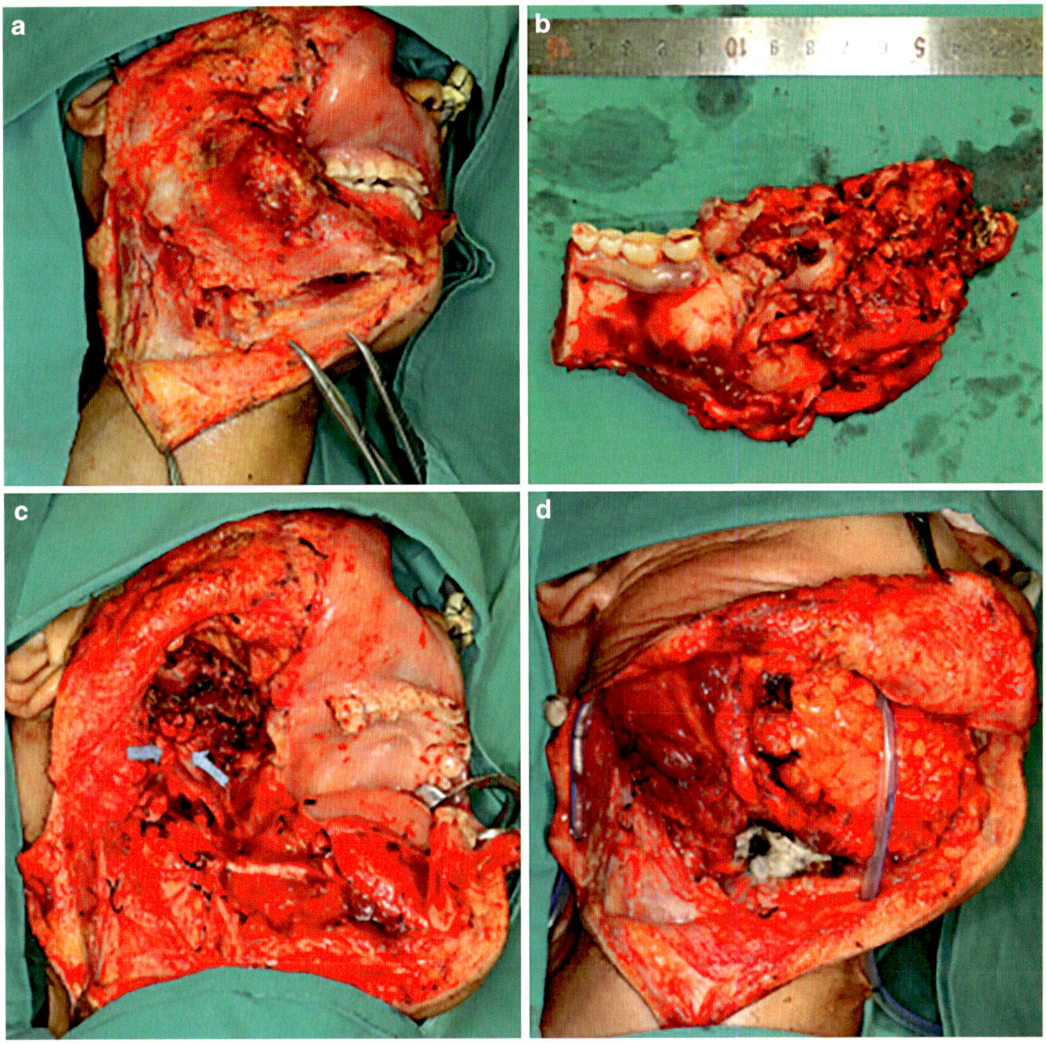

Fig. 47.4 (**a**) Exposure of the mandibular body and ascending ramus, with irregular bony expansion seen. (**b**) Discrete mandible. (**c**) Preservation of the internal carotid artery. (**d**) Anterolateral femoral flap to repair mandibular and intraoral tissue defects

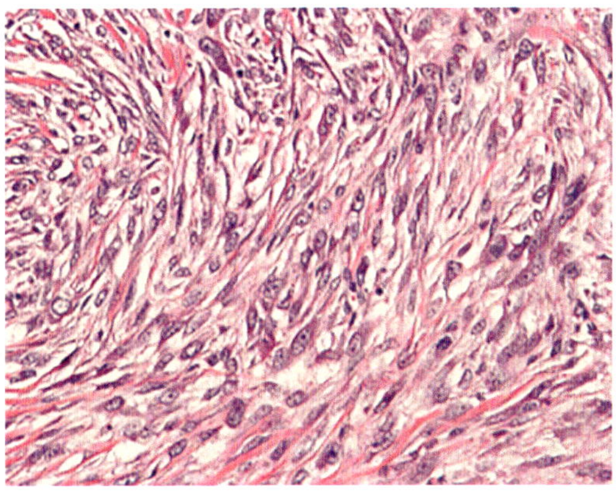

Fig. 47.5 The tumor cells were fusiform with obvious nuclear atypia, clear nucleoli, and delicate chromatin. Filamentous collagen fibers between tumor cells (400x)

closing function, and good recovery of contralateral occlusal relationship, and mandible appearance and function.

47.3 Key Points of Diagnosis and Treatment

Warren and Sommer first reported postirradiation sarcoma in 1936, and less than 500 cases of postirradiation sarcoma of the head and neck have been reported in the literature. In China, due to the high incidence of nasopharyngeal carcinoma in southern China and the long survival period of patients with nasopharyngeal carcinoma, postirradiation sarcoma of the jaw is commonly seen in patients after radiotherapy for nasopharyngeal carcinoma, and may also happen to the patients after radiotherapy for lymphoma, head and neck cancer, and other diseases. About 87% of postirradiation sarcoma cases occur within 15 years after radiotherapy, with approximately 45% occurring 5–10 years after radiotherapy, and the time interval between radiotherapy and the development of postirradiation sarcoma can be up to 30 years or more. Postirradiation sarcoma often occurs in the areas exposed to high levels of radiation, and the risk of postirradiation sarcoma is generally considered to be significantly higher at the level of radiation above 55 Gy. The diagnostic criteria for postirradiation sarcoma include: (1) history of previous radiotherapy; (2) tumor occurrence within the original field of radiotherapy; (3) at least 3 years between the onset of tumor and the end of radiotherapy; and (4) pathological diagnosis of sarcoma.

Clinical Manifestations Postirradiation sarcoma of the mandible is most common in the mandibular ramus, presenting as well-circumscribed mass, generally hard in texture, accompanied by local swelling and pain, or local numbness, numbness of the lower lip, etc. Due to the history of radiotherapy in patients, severe local soft tissue fibrosis makes early detection of tumor difficult. When patients complain of swelling, numbness, and other symptoms in the field of radiotherapy, attention should be paid and careful examination should be given to strengthen the follow-up of patients after radiotherapy, which is conducive to the early detection and diagnosis of the disease.

Imaging Characteristics CT shows a space occupying of soft tissue in postirradiation sarcoma of the mandible, with heterogeneous density and significant enhancement of tumor tissues after enhancement. Most tumors have a poor circumscription and often extensively invade the surrounding tissue space, with obvious bone destruction. CT also shows new bone formation in osteoblastic osteosarcoma. Postirradiation sarcoma of the mandible shows a mixed-signal soft tissue space occupying in T1- and T2-weighted MRI, and most of the tumors show high-signal images in T2-weighted MRI. Compared with general osteosarcoma, postirradiation sarcoma of the mandible has no specific imaging findings.

Diagnosis and Differential Diagnosis The diagnostic criteria for postirradiation sarcomas of the mandible are as described above. Compared with general sarcomas, postirradiation sarcomas of the mandible have no specific clinical or radiographic findings. The clinical diagnosis of postirradiation sarcoma of the mandible should be considered in conjunction with a history of previous radiotherapy when the mandible is clinically found to be space occupying, hard in texture, and accompanied by symptoms of swelling, pain, or numbness.

Treatment and Prognosis Radical resection is the main therapy for postirradiation sarcoma of the mandible. If the tumor invades vital structures such as carotid artery and skull base and cannot be completely resected, radiotherapy or chemotherapy can be used, but the effect of radiotherapy and chemotherapy is poor. It is widely believed at home and abroad that radical surgical excision is the most important treatment method to improve the survival of patients. Surgical resection of tumor should be performed at a sufficient safe distance to cross anatomic landmarks. For example, for a postirradiation sarcoma in the angle of the mandible, the resection should span at least the ipsilateral sigmoid notch and chin hole. Besides, due to the strong invasion and growth characteristics of sarcoma, attention should be paid to the removal of the starting and ending points of the muscles attached to the mandible. For example, in the removal of the occlusal muscle, it is important to follow up the occlusal muscle to the attachment point of zygomatic arch to prevent the tumor cells from contracting below the zygomatic arch with the muscle, resulting in the recurrence of tumor in the infratemporal space. Due to the difficulty in early detection of for postirradiation sarcoma of the mandible, the prognosis of patients is poor. The 3-year overall survival (OS), 3-year disease-free survival (DFS), and 5-year overall survival (OS) are reported to be about 19.1%, 11.1%, and 12.3%, respectively.

References

1. Yang Q, Mo Y, Zhao Q, et al. Radiation-induced sarcomas of the head and neck in post-radiation nasopharyngeal carcinoma [J]. Radiol Med. 2017;122(1):53–60.
2. de Souza LL, Pontes HAR, Santos-Silva AR, et al. Oral radiation-induced sarcomas: systematic review [J]. Head Neck. 2020;42(9):2660–8.
3. Cahan WG, Woodard HQ. Sarcoma arising in irradiated bone : report of 11 cases [J]. Cancer. 1948;1(1):3–29.
4. Koyama T, Kobayashi T, Maruyama S, et al. Radiation-induced undifferentiated high-grade pleomorphic sarcoma (malignant fibrous histiocytoma) of the mandible: report of a case arising in the background of long-standing osteomyelitis with a review of the literature [J]. Pathol Res Pract. 2014;210(12):1123–9.
5. Xi M, Liu MZ, Wang HX, et al. Radiation-induced sarcoma in patients with nasopharyngeal carcinoma: a single-institution study [J]. Cancer. 2010;116(23):5479–86.
6. Chan JY, Wong ST, Lau GI, et al. Postradiation sarcoma after radiotherapy for nasopharyngeal carcinoma [J]. Laryngoscope. 2012;122(12):2695–9.
7. Patel SG, See ACH, Williamson PA, et al. Radiation induced sarcoma of the head and neck [J]. Head Neck. 1999;21(4):346–54.
8. Thiagarajan A, Iyer NG. Radiation-induced sarcomas of the head and neck [J]. World J Clin Oncol. 2014;5(5):973–81.
9. Cai PQ, Wu YP, Li L, et al. CT and MRI of radiation-induced sarcomas of the head and neck following radiotherapy for nasopharyngeal carcinoma [J]. Clin Radiol. 2013;68(7):683–9.
10. Chung J, Lee V, Tsang R, et al. Treatment outcomes of postradiation second head and neck malignancies managed by a multidisciplinary approach [J]. Head Neck. 2015;37(6):815–22.

48 Ewing Sarcoma

Yue He, Hui Shan Ong, Zhen Tian, Lin Zhu, and Ji Ping Ding

48.1 Introduction

Ewing sarcoma is a rare and highly malignant tumor that occurs in adolescents and children. It presents clinically as a painful, local mass and pathologically as a small round cell malignancy with varying degrees of neuroectodermal differentiation. The diagnosis should be made with a combination of clinical manifestations, imaging, and pathologic findings, but specific chromosomal translocations, such as EWS-ETS family gene fusion and FUS-ETS gene fusion, have become important diagnostic indicators [1–4]. Fusion gene is not only vital in diagnosis and differential diagnosis but also provides a reference for targeted therapy and prognostic evaluation. For local Ewing sarcoma, radiotherapy is the traditional treatment. Surgical resection is a suitable therapy for small local Ewing sarcoma, and for larger localized Ewing sarcoma, surgery combined with radiotherapy is an option. No breakthrough has been made in the treatment of recurrent, refractory, metastatic Ewing sarcoma. Current studies have demonstrated that PARP inhibitors and tyrosine kinase inhibitors have targeted killing and inhibiting effects on Ewing sarcoma cells, but their clinical applications remain to be verified in more clinical trials [5, 6].

Y. He · H. S. Ong (✉) · Z. Tian · L. Zhu · J. P. Ding
Department of Oral Maxillofacial-Head & Neck Oncology, Shanghai Ninth People's Hospital, Shanghai Jiao Tong University School of Medicine, Shanghai, China

48.2 Case 90

A 5-year-old boy suffered from a left lower tooth pain for about 1 month, accompanied by mandibular swelling for more than half a month.

[History of Present Illness] The patient's parent complained that the patient had pain in the left lower tooth nearly a month ago, which was not taken seriously at that time, and the local pain was relieved spontaneously, so the patient did not receive treatment. Half a month ago, the swelling in the left mandible was found, and panoramic radiographs suggested "low density shadow in the D–E root of the left mandibular deciduous tooth," and the maxillofacial CT scan suggested "the possibility of odontogenic benign space occupying and ameloblastoma."

[Specialty Examination] The face was asymmetrical, with well-coordinated 1/3 proportion of upper, middle, and lower face. A local swelling was found in the left mandible, with tenderness (−). The temporomandibular joint had no obvious snapping and tenderness. The opening of the mouth was about three transverse fingers, with a downward opening pattern, and the left lower papillary teeth D–E were locally distended near

Y. He (ed.), *Inflammatory and Neoplastic Diseases of Craniofacial Bones*,
https://doi.org/10.1007/978-981-97-4155-7_48

the floor of the mouth, and the tongue was centered. No enlargement of submandibular, submental, or cervical lymph nodes were observed bilaterally.

[Auxiliary Examination]

1. Panoramic radiographs suggested a low density shadow in the left mandible body with poor circumscription and no obvious bone alba line (Fig. 48.1).
2. Maxillofacial CT scan suggested a bony protuberance from left mandible chin to angle. Multilocular cyst solid abnormal density shadow was observed, and the buccal-lingual cortex was significantly thinner, local continuity was interrupted, with uniform density and CT values between 2 and 14 Hu (Fig. 48.2).

[Preliminary Diagnosis] Mass of left mandible.

[Treatment]

1. Biopsy under general anesthesia: Pathological examination revealed a small round cell tumor of the "left mandible," which was considered to be Ewing sarcoma /PNET based on the enzyme label and molecular results.
2. Chemotherapy: Six courses of chemotherapy were performed in other hospital. Review of panoramic radiographs (Fig. 48.3) and MRI (Fig. 48.4) indicated a bone destruction in the left mandible after PNET surgery, with no significant change seen.
3. Surgery: "Mandibular tumor resection with anterolateral thigh flap transfer and tracheotomy" was performed under general anesthesia: an incision was made along the lower margin of the mandible for 1–2 cm, and the gingival flap was elevated for surgical exposure and dissection of the submaxillary triangle. Osteotomy was performed from 81 distal to the left condylar neck, preserving the condyle and removing the mandible and the mass together. Intraoperative frozen pathological examination showed that the gingiva of the posterior region of the left mandible was chronic inflammation of the mucosa and small salivary glands, and no obvious tumor was seen. The bone of jaws had a protuberance which was hard I texture and could not be taken by freezing for panoramic radiographs. Paraffin pathology was pending. All incisional margins were negative (−). A left anterolateral femoral flap, approximately 11 cm × 4 cm in size, was routinely prepared to repair the defect in the mandible and the floor of the mouth, and the vessels were anastomosed with the superior thyroid artery and external jugular vein, respectively. The wound was rinsed, thoroughly hemostatic and sutured in layers, and negative pressure drainage tube was indwelled.
4. Postoperative radiotherapy + chemotherapy.

[Pathological Examination] Gross pathological examination revealed three tissues, 1.5 cm × 1.0 cm × 0.2 cm, grayish white. Microscopically, small round cells with round, regular nuclei were seen, and the chromatin was meticulously uniform or densely stained, with rare mitosis and sparse or unclear cytoplasm. Immunohistochemistry showed that the tumor cells expressed CD99 and Fli-1. Fluorescence in situ hybridization (FISH) showed EWSR1 gene splitting (Fig. 48.5).

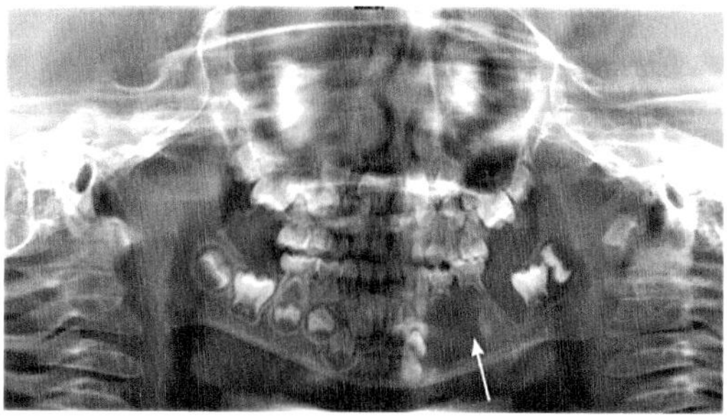

Fig. 48.1 Low-density shadow in the left mandible body with poor circumscription and no obvious bone alba line (preoperative)

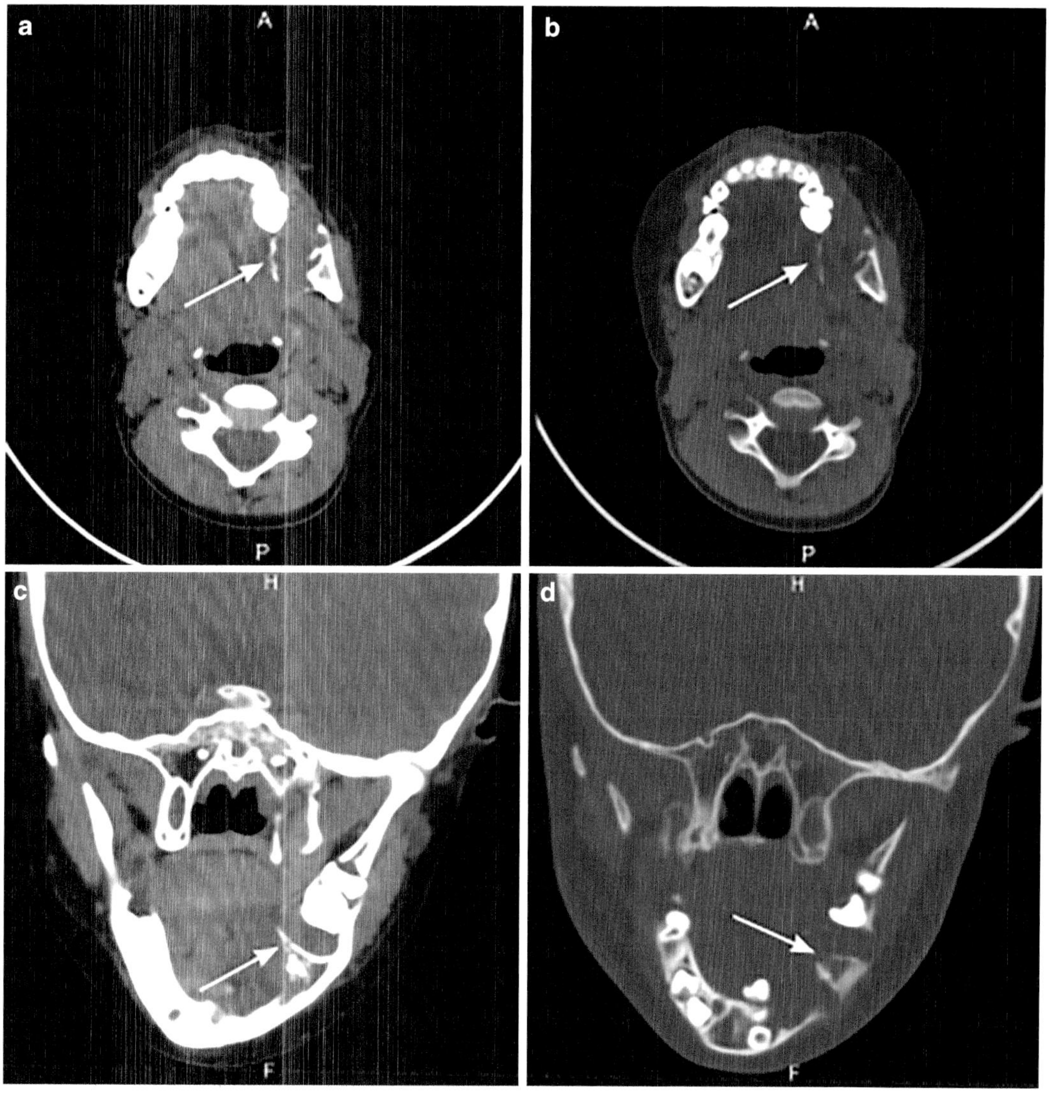

Fig. 48.2 (**a**, **b**) CT axial scan: bony protuberance from chin to angle of the left mandible, solid abnormal density shadow of multilocular cyst, obviously thinning of buccal and lingual bone skin, local continuity interrupted, inhomogeneous density, CT values between 2 and 14 Hu. (**c**, **d**) Coronal reconstruction of soft tissue and bone

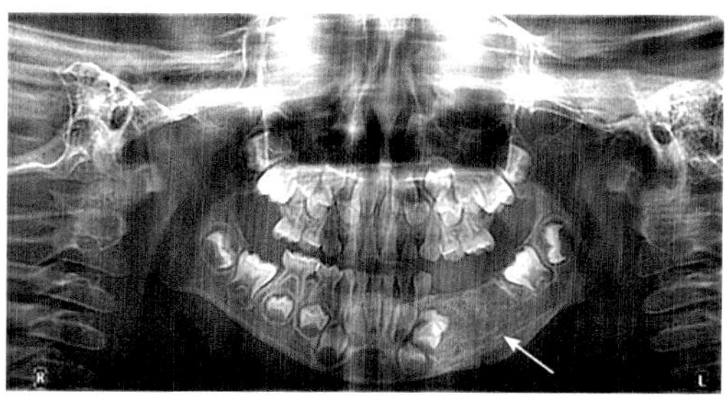

Fig. 48.3 Changes after left mandible biopsy and chemotherapy, with no significant decrease in the lesion scope

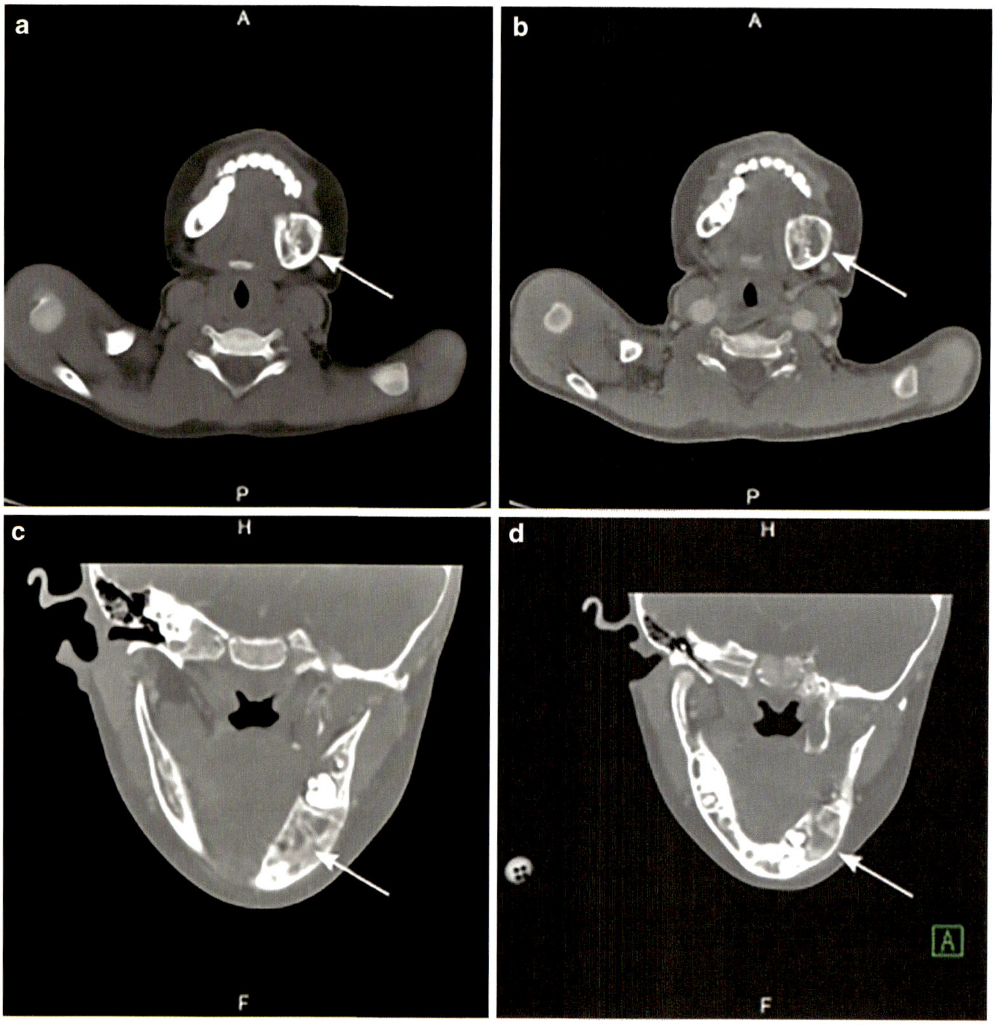

Fig. 48.4 (**a**, **b**) CT plain scan and enhanced axial scan: (after treatment for the left mandible) bony protuberance in the left mandibular chin and body with irregular shape, discontinued buccal bone, slight soft tissue density shadow, inhomogeneous enhancement after enhancement. (**c**, **d**) Coronal reconstruction: no abnormity in the skull base structure

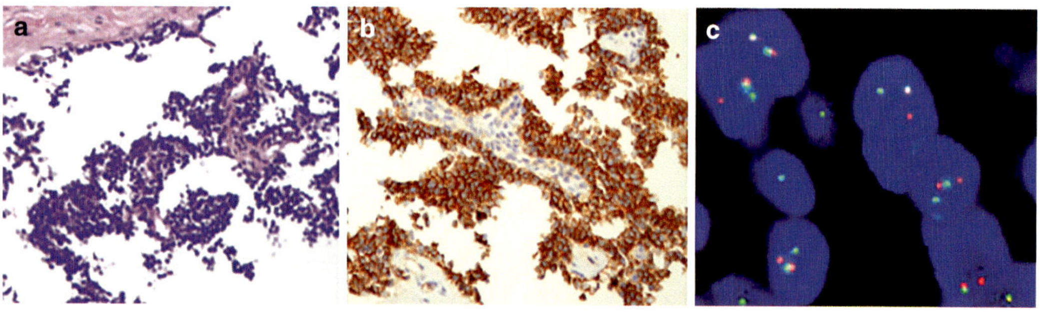

Fig. 48.5 (**a**) Small round cell neoplasms with little or no cytoplasm and rare mitosis (400x). (**b**) Tumor cells showed diffuse strong positive membrane expression of CD99 (400X). (**c**) The detection of EWSR1 fracture probe FISH showed the separation of red and green signals in tumor nucleus, suggesting the fracture and rearrangement of EWSR1 gene

[Pathological Diagnosis] Small round cell tumor in the left mandible, considered as Ewing sarcoma/primary neuroectodermal tumor combined with enzymatic and molecular findings, ICD code: M9260/3.

48.3 Key Points of Diagnosis and Treatment

Ewing sarcoma, first reported by James Ewing in 1921, is the second most common bone tumor in children and adolescents and is a highly malignant tumor that often occurs within and around the bones. Only about 2–7% of patients develop Ewing sarcoma in the oral and maxillofacial region, mostly in the mandible and temporal bone.

Clinical Manifestations Pain is the most common clinical symptom. About 2/3 of patients suffer intermittent pain, which is not severe at first, but rapidly develops to persistent pain. The local pain spreads with the spread of tumor. With the increase of pain, a local mass will appear at the site of the tumor, which is rapidly growing and obviously tender. Ewing sarcoma is often accompanied with systemic symptoms, such as fever, fatigue, loss of appetite, and anemia. In addition, depending on the location of the tumor, it may also affect the surrounding tissues and organs, causing different clinical symptoms. The diagnosis of Ewing sarcoma requires a combination of clinical symptoms and imaging findings. Pathological diagnosis serves as the gold standard and the specific diagnostic basis is not described again.

Molecular Genetic Characteristics Now, the specific chromosomal translocations of Ewing sarcoma have served as important auxiliary diagnostic indicators, such as EWS–ETS family gene fusion, FUS–ETS gene fusion, and some rare fusion subtypes (EWSR1–PATZ1, EWSR1–POU5F1, etc.). EWS and FUS fall in the TET protein family with transcriptional activation domain and RNA binding domain. In case of TET genes fusion, corresponding transcriptional functions are activated, leading to activation of downstream signal transduction pathways. The family members of ETS transcription factor, including FLI1, ERG, ETV1, E1AF, and FEV, are vital in cell proliferation, differentiation, apoptosis, migration, tissue remodeling, and angiogenesis.

Treatment Molecular genetics is also of guiding significance for targeted therapy of Ewing sarcoma. Although the current therapeutic regimen of radiotherapy and chemotherapy combined with surgery has raised the survival of patients to some extent, the prognosis of patients with recurrence and metastasis remains to be improved, with a 5-year survival rate of less than 30%. Targeted therapy is effective with high specificity, and is expected to constitute an important part of combination therapy for Ewing sarcoma in the future. Current studies have shown that PARP inhibitors and tyrosine kinase inhibitors have therapeutic effects on Ewing sarcoma. For example, the olaparid, a PARP1 inhibitor, is capable of targeted killing of Ewing's sarcoma cells with the EWS-FLI1 fusion gene; Ewing sarcoma is less sensitive to olaparid after radiotherapy. The combination of Bcl-2 and BCL-XL inhibitor navitoclax with olaparib can further reduce the tumor volume effectively. IGF-1R inhibitors in the tyrosine kinase family have also been shown to significantly inhibit tumor growth in cellular and animal studies.

In general, for small local Ewing sarcoma, surgical treatment is usually preferred, and for large Ewing sarcoma, surgery combined with radiotherapy is usually preferred. Patients with recurrent, refractory, or metastatic Ewing sarcoma have a poor prognosis and should be treated with standard chemotherapy and/or chemotherapy in combination with treatment of the primary lesion. Targeted therapy is a new therapeutic method that has achieved some results, but its safety and clinical efficacy remain to be verified by more clinical trials.

References

1. Brenner JC, Feng FY, Han S, et al. PARP—1 Inhibition as a targeted strategy to treat Ewing's sarcoma [J]. Cancer Res. 2012;72(7):1608–13.
2. Tanaka M, Yamazaki Y, Kanno Y, et al. Ewing's sarcoma precursors are highly enriched in embryonic osteochondrogenic progenitors [J]. J Clin Invest. 2014;124(7):3061.
3. Li H, Batth IS, Qu X, et al. IGF-IR signaling in epithelial to mesenchymal transition and targeting IGF-IR therapy: overview and new insights [J]. Mol Cancer. 2017;16(1):6.
4. Tanner JM, Bensard C, Wei P, et al. EWS/FLI is a master regulator of metabolic reprogramming in Ewing sarcoma [J]. Mol Cancer Res. 2017;15(11):1517–30.
5. Sujing J, Guannan, et al. Comparison of clinical features and outcomes in patients with extraskeletal vs skeletal Ewing sarcoma: an SEER database analysis of 3178 cases [J]. Cancer Manage Res. 2018;10:6227–36.
6. Jin W. The role of tyrosine kinases as a critical prognostic parameter and its targeted therapies in Ewing sarcoma [J]. Front Cell Dev Biol. 2020;8:613.

49 Primary Intraosseous Squamous Cell Carcinoma

Yue He, Hui Shan Ong, Zhen Tian, Lin Zhu, and Jun Jian Jiang

49.1 Introduction

Primary intraosseous squamous cell carcinoma (PIOSCC), also known as central squamous cell carcinoma of the jaw, is a histopathologic type of primary intraosseous carcinoma. PIOSCC accounts for about 1–2% of oral cancers, and is common in the posterior dental region of the mandible, mostly occurring to middle-aged and elderly male [1–10]. Primary intraosseous carcinoma consists of three histopathologic types: salivary adenocarcinoma, odontogenic carcinoma, and squamous cell carcinoma [11–17]. Primary intraosseous squamous cell carcinoma is the most common type. PIOSCC, first reported in 1913, is a rare malignancy of jaw that may originate from odontogenic epithelial cells. The diagnostic criteria for PIOSCC are as follows: ① exclusion of the invasion of adjacent oral mucosa; ② no tumor at the site of pathological changes; ③exclusion of metastasis of malignant tumors in other parts of the body; and ④ pathological diagnosis as squamous cell carcinoma [13–15, 18–23].

Y. He · H. S. Ong (✉) · Z. Tian · L. Zhu · J. J. Jiang
Department of Oral Maxillofacial-Head & Neck Oncology, Shanghai Ninth People's Hospital, Shanghai Jiao Tong University School of Medicine, Shanghai, China

49.2 Case 91

A 51-year-old gentleman suffered from right facial swelling for 3 months.

[History of Present Illness] The patient developed right facial swelling without obvious inducement 3 months ago, and was diagnosed as "pericoronitis of right mandibular wisdom tooth" at the hospital. After anti-inflammatory treatment, the patient underwent "extraction of right mandibular third molar" more than 2 months ago, but the tooth extraction wound did not heal after surgery, and repeated dressing changes did not lead to a significant improvement. Half a month ago, the patient was diagnosed as "right mandibular osteomyelitis" at a superior hospital. "Curettage of the right mandibular osteomyelitis lesion" was performed under general anesthesia in the hospital. Intraoperative frozen examination showed "squamous cell carcinoma," and mandibulectomy was recommended.

[Specialty Examination] The face was asymmetrical with a right maxillofacial swelling and tenderness. The mouth opening degree was about one transverse finger, with no abnormality in the mouth opening pattern and no tenderness in the bilateral temporal regions. The right lower lip was numb. Wound surface, iodoform tamponade, and vestibular groove protuberance were seen in

Y. He (ed.), *Inflammatory and Neoplastic Diseases of Craniofacial Bones*,
https://doi.org/10.1007/978-981-97-4155-7_49

the right lower posterior tooth zone. The tongue could move freely without numbness and congestion. The secretion of salivary gland duct was normal. Enlarged lymph nodes were palpated under the right jaw.

[Auxiliary Examination]
Maxillofacial enhanced CT scan suggested a lytic bone damage in the right mandible (46 distal), the mandibular ramus sigmoid notch, and the oronoid process; the buccal lingual cortex was discontinuous; periosteal reaction was observed; soft tissue density mass shadow was observed in the space between buccal lingual masticatory muscles, with poor circumscription; the lesion was slightly enhanced after enhancement, with C− of 50 Hu and C+ of 74 Hu; striated dense shadow (possibly tampon) was observed inside. Multiple enhanced lymph nodes were observed in the right cervical I, b, n regions, and masseter anterior edge, some of which were unevenly enhanced (Fig. 49.1).

[Preliminary Diagnosis] Primary intraosseous squamous cell carcinoma of the right mandible.

[Treatment]
1. Preoperative induction chemotherapy (two cycles) N-TP regimen chemotherapy. The specific regimen was: 28 mg of Nimotuzumab on the 1st, 8th, 15th, and 23rd days, 130 mg of docetaxel + 130 mg of cisplatin on the 2nd day, with necessary adjuvant treatment. The treatment proceeded well, with no serious adverse reaction of chemotherapy such as bone marrow suppression. Posttreatment evaluation (PD) was performed.
2. "Right mandible resection with modified radical right neck dissection, left anterolateral thigh flap transfer, and tracheotomy" were performed under general anesthesia: an incision was designed along the lower margin of the mandible for 1–2 cm to make an S-shaped incision from the posterior margin of sternocleidomastoid muscle to the midpoint of the clavicle. The gingival flap was elevated to perform modified radical right neck dissection and en bloc resection of the right mandible. The mass and cervical lymph nodes were completely removed within the normal tissue at 2.0 cm from the outer margin of the mass. Intraoperative frozen pathological examination on incisal margin suggested "squamous cell carcinoma" of the right mandible, and the margins were negative (−). The left anterolateral femoral flap, approximately 22 cm × 7 cm in size, was shaped and folded to repair the defects in the mandible, floor of the mouth, and cheek, and the vessels were anastomosed to the superior thyroid artery and internal jugular vein branches, respectively. The wound was rinsed and thoroughly hemostatic, negative pressure drainage tube was indwelled, and layered suture was performed to close the wound.
3. Postoperative adjuvant radiotherapy.

[Pathological Examination] Gross pathological examination revealed segmental resected mandibular tissue and surrounding soft tissues, approximately 12.5 cm × 8 cm × 6 cm, with three teeth attached. The section of the mandible showed a grayish-white mass, 7 cm × 5 cm × 3 cm, with poor circumscription and peripheral bone destruction. Microscopically, heterogeneous squamous cells were seen in a nest-like invasive growth, involving the surrounding muscle tissue. The tumor cells were abundant in cytoplasm, eosinophilic, and intercellular bridges were visible, with few keratin pearls within the nests (Fig. 49.2).

[Pathological Diagnosis] Central squamous cell carcinoma of "right mandible," a type pf primary intraosseous carcinoma (NOS), ICD-O code: 9270/3.

[Differential Diagnosis Cases]
Carcinoma of Maxillary Sinus

Carcinoma of maxillary sinus is a type of paranasal sinus cancer. Paranasal sinus cancer accounts for about 3% of all head and neck cancers, of which about 80% are carcinoma of maxillary sinus. Squamous cell carcinoma is the most common pathological type of carcinoma of maxillary

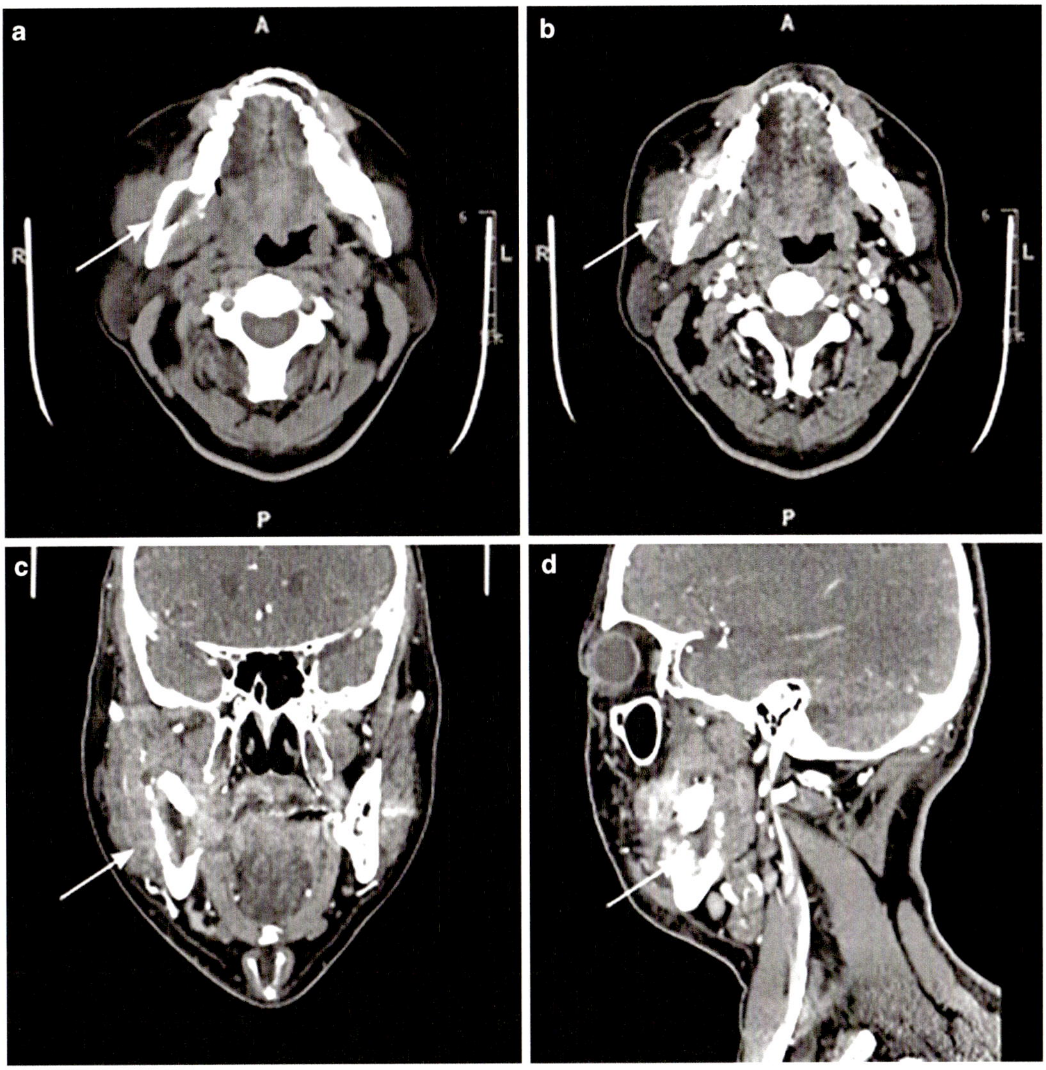

Fig. 49.1 (**a**, **b**) CT axial scan: Lytic bone destruction in the bone body, angle, and ascending ramus of the right mandible, discontinuous buccal lingual cortex, periosteal reaction, soft tissue density mass shadow in the space between buccal lingual masticatory muscles, with poor circumscription. (**b**) Enhanced CT axial scan: mild enhancement of the lesion. (**c**, **d**) Coronal and sagittal reconstruction: condyle involvement, dense striated shadow (possibly tampon)

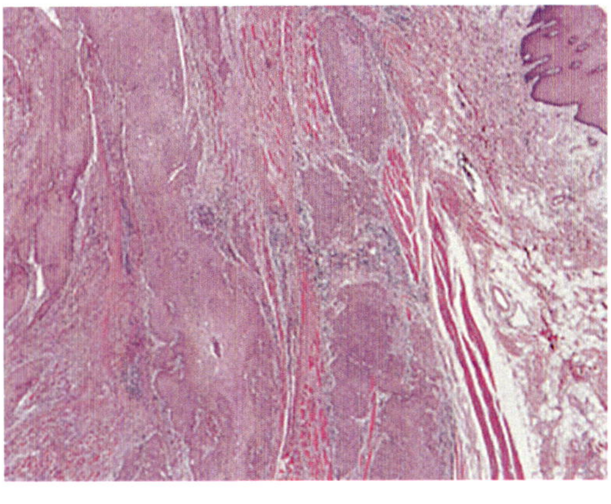

Fig. 49.2 Heterotypic squamous cells were distributed in nests and have invaded the muscle tissue; the upper right mucosal epithelium had no obvious heterotype (40x)

sinus, accounting for about 60–90% of the cases, followed by adenoid cystic carcinoma, adenocarcinoma, and undifferentiated carcinoma.

In China, carcinoma of maxillary sinus usually occurs at the age of 50–60, with more males than females. Carcinoma of maxillary sinus occurs in the mucous membrane of maxillary sinus and is hidden in location, making early detection difficult. With the progression of the tumor, the inner wall, the parietal wall, the posterior wall, the anterior wall, and the basal wall of the maxillary sinus are damaged, invading the corresponding tissue structure, and resulting in symptoms such as nasal congestion, nasal bleeding, eyeball protrusion, restricted mouth opening, numbness in the infraorbital region, and tooth loosening. Therefore, most patients are already in the advanced stage of clinical treatment. Radiotherapy and surgery are the main therapies for carcinoma of maxillary sinus. Radiotherapy combined with radical surgical resection is the main treatment therapeutic regimen at present, leading to the highest survival of patients. Despite great advances in radiotherapy and surgical techniques in recent decades, the overall survival rate for carcinoma of maxillary sinus is still less than 60%, and even lower in patients at advanced stage.

49.3 Case 92

A 42-year-old woman suffered from right upper posterior tooth loosening with right facial numbness for more than 4 months.

[History of Present Illness] The patient had a loose right upper molar with unknown pathogenesis 4 months ago, and the pain persisted without relief, accompanied by numbness on the right face. The oral examination revealed a protuberance of about 3.0 cm in diameter in the right upper palate, and the patient was suggested to visit a superior hospital for treatment. The maxillofacial CT examination in the clinic 1 week ago showed malignant space occupying of the right maxillary sinus. Biopsy of the "right upper palate mass" was performed at other hospital. The pathological diagnosis showed tumor cells, which tended to be poorly differentiated carcinoma.

[Specialty Examination] The face was asymmetrical, with well-coordinated 1/3 proportion of upper, middle, and lower face. The skin of the right infraorbital region, zygomatic face, and cheek was intact, with normal color and texture, mild numbness, no blurred vision or double vision, normal bilateral eye movements, and a sense of nasal obstruction on the right side. There was no abnormality in mouth opening range and mouth opening pattern. The right palatal swelling was about 3.0 cm × 3.0 cm in size, with intact mucosa, no obvious rupture or exudation. Palpation showed localized palatal plate bone destruction, soft tissue mass which was hard in texture. Intraoral examination revealed permanent dentition, tooth 16 movement for 1°, teeth 16 and 17 sensitive to percussion (−), and numbness in the right palatal and gingival mucosa. The tongue moved freely without numbness and other sensory abnormalities at the tip of the tongue. No abnormal enlargement of submandibular and cervical lymph nodes was observed bilaterally.

[Auxiliary Examination]
Maxillofacial enhanced CT scan suggested a soft tissue density mass in the right maxillary sinus, with a lesion size of approximately 3.2 cm × 3.0 cm and a CT value of approximately 35 Hu. The lesion involved the nasal cavity inward and the hard palate downward, with adjacent bone destruction of the right maxillary sinus wall, maxillary alveolar process and hard palate, and involvement of the palatine foramen magnum (Fig. 49.3).

[Preliminary Diagnosis] Carcinoma of right maxillary sinus

[Treatment]
1. Preoperative radiotherapy: 36 Gy/18Fx; synchronous chemotherapy with docetaxel 100 mg intravenous drip, Tegafur Gimeracil Oteracil Potassium Capsule, two tablets twice a day, d1-14/q3w oral chemotherapy;

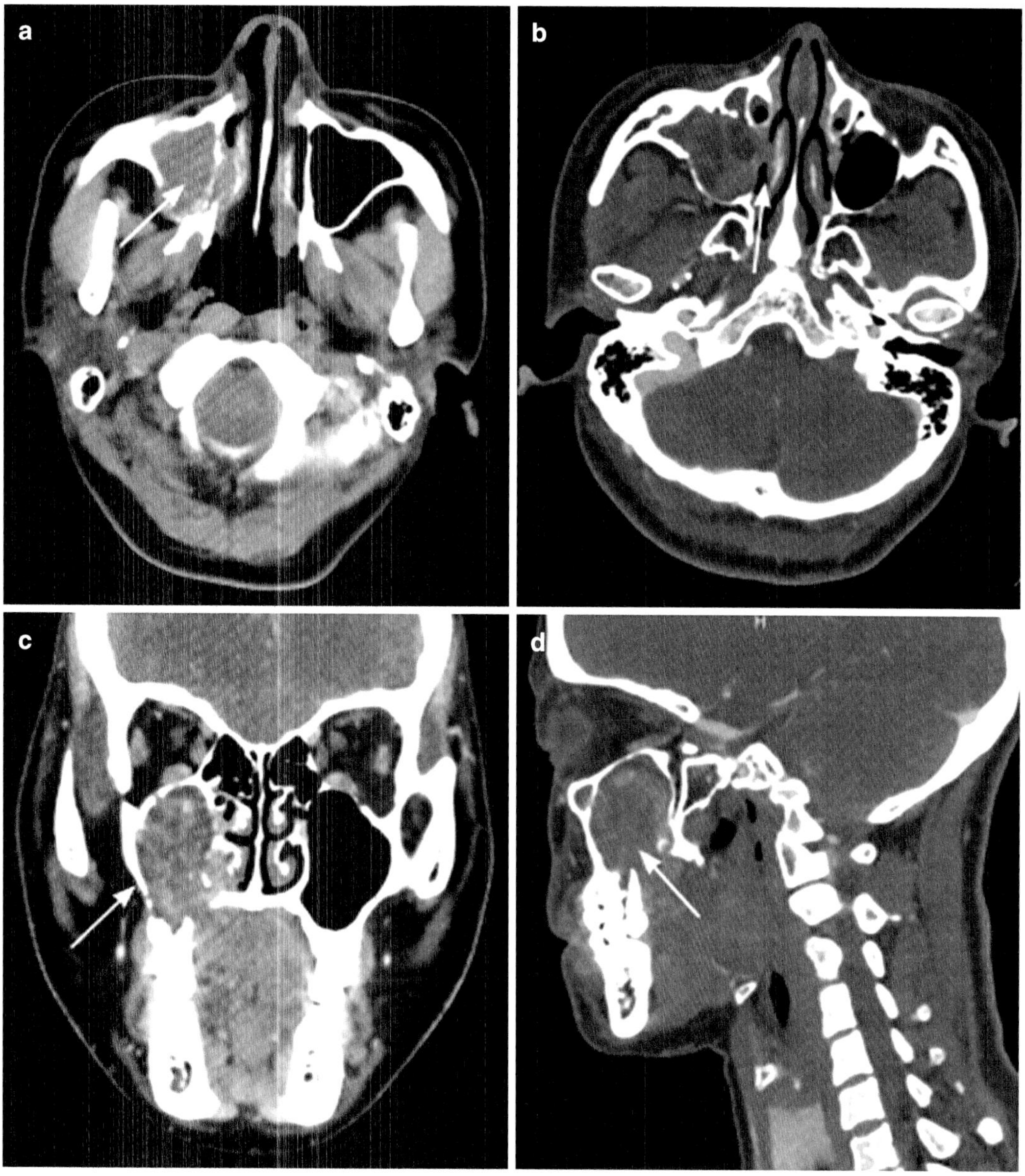

Fig. 49.3 (**a**) CT axial scan: soft tissue density mass in the right maxillary sinus, with a lesion size of approximately 3.2 cm × 3.0 cm and a CT value of approximately 35 Hu. (**b**) Enhanced CT axial scan: significant enhancement of the lesion, with inhomogeneous density. (**c**, **d**) Enhanced CT coronal and sagittal scan: The lesion involved the nasal cavity inward and the hard palate downward, with adjacent bone destruction of the right maxillary sinus wall, maxillary alveolar process, and hard palate, and involvement of the palatine foramen magnum

Nimotuzumab 100 mg/qw intravenous drip for targeted therapy. Imaging examination showed that the tumor was significantly reduced after treatment.

2. Surgery: "Right maxillary subtotal ectomy with right zygoma partial resection, right suprascapular hyoid cervical lymph node dissection, left anterolateral femoral flap transfer and tracheotomy" was performed under general anesthesia: an incision was made along the lower margin of the mandible for 1–2 cm, and the gingival flap was

elevated. Right suprascapular hyoid cervical lymph node dissection was performed to dissect and protect the proximal end of the external maxillary artery and the branches of the internal jugular vein for vascular anastomosis. An extraoral Weber incision was made and the gingival flap was elevated for truncation of connections of the maxilla. The tumor, which involved the pterygoid sinus and the lateral wall of the nasal cavity, was carefully excised from the sinus, and the lateral wall of the nasal cavity was removed along with the turbinate tissue. Intraoperative frozen pathological examination on incisal margin showed spindle cell tumor of the "right maxillary sinus," with cell atypia, loose interstitium, and local bone tissue for malignant tendency. The mesenchymal tumor could not be excluded, with pending paraffin and enzyme labeling. Frozen section examination showed no tumor cells (−). Sharp bone margin was trimmed, rinsed and hemostatic. The left anterolateral femoral flap, approximately 10 cm × 7 cm in size, was routinely prepared and anastomosed with the external maxillary artery and internal jugular vein branches, respectively. The flap was shaped and folded to repair the defects in the right maxillary tissue. Negative pressure drainage tube was indwelled, and layered suture was performed to close the wound. A nasal support catheter was indwelled in the right nasal cavity (Fig. 49.4).

3. Postoperative radiotherapy: 24 Gy/12 Fx.

[Pathological Examination] Gross pathological examination revealed a part of maxilla and surrounding tissues, 7 cm × 6.5 cm × 6 cm, with six attached teeth. A grayish yellow region was found in maxillary sinus, 3.5 cm × 2.5 cm × 2.5 cm, and locally hard. The microscopic examination showed focal keratin and a few squamous epithelial clusters in the background of hyperplastic fibrous tissue with heterogeneous cells and surrounding inflammatory cell infiltration (Fig. 49.5).

[Pathological Diagnosis] Squamous cell carcinoma of the right maxillary sinus (after radiotherapy), ICD code: 8071/3.

[Follow-Up] The patient healed uneventfully after treatment, with normal visual acuity in the right eye. The postoperative six-month follow-up exhibited no abnormality in the operative region.

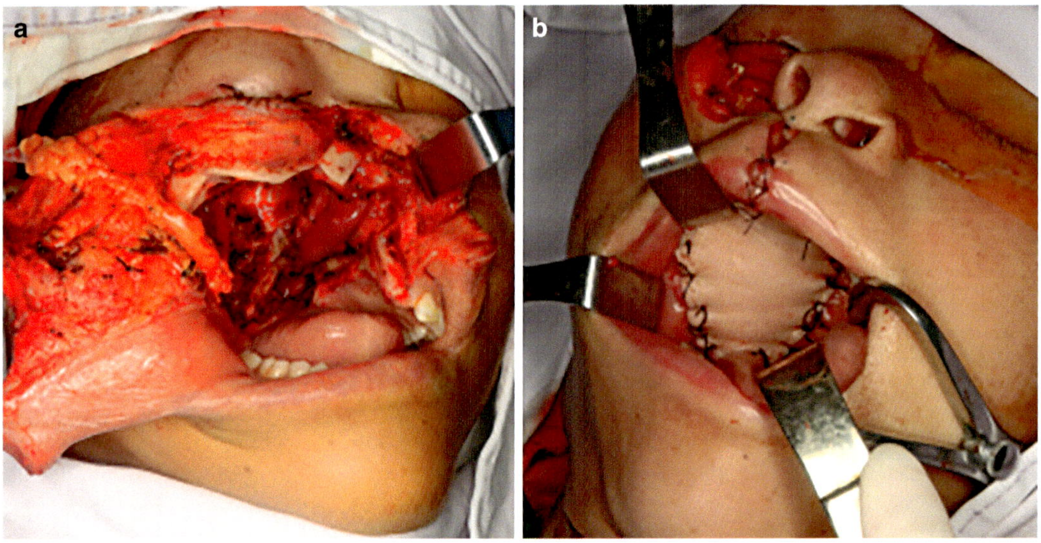

Fig. 49.4 (**a**) Subtotal resection of the right maxilla, preserving the orbital floor and dissecting the sinus cavity mucosa. (**b**) Anterolateral femoral flap to repair the defect in the right maxillary and palatal tissue

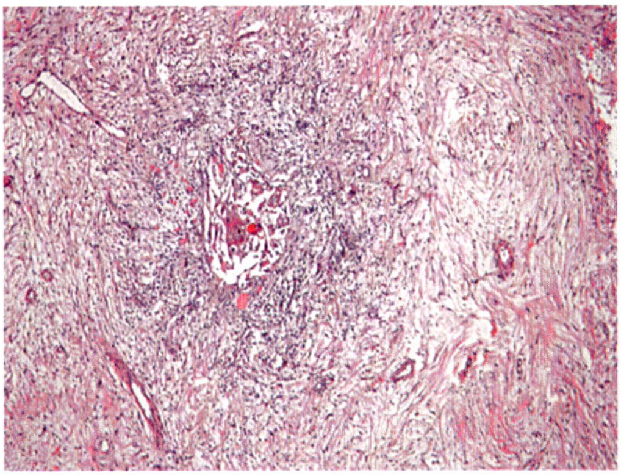

Fig. 49.5 Small focal nests of tumor cells with squamous differentiation and a small amount of filamentous keratinization in the fibrous tissue background with surrounding inflammatory cell infiltration (100x)

49.4 Key Points of Diagnosis and Treatment

Since PIOSCC was first reported in 1913, scholars have published case reports successively, but retrospective statistical analysis of a great number of cases is still lacking. PIOSCC accounts for about 1–2% of oral cancers, and its clinical and pathological features differ from squamous cell carcinoma of oral mucosa. PIOSCC is more common in male, accounting for about 2/3, with middle-aged and elderly males aged 50–70 years old being the majority. The minimum age of PIOSCC cases reported in the literature is 5 years old, but patients under 18 years old are rare. PIOSCC mainly occurs in the mandible, especially in the posterior dental region of the mandible, but rarely in the anterior dental region. The ratio of mandibular to maxillary cases was (3–7): 1.

Clinical Manifestations PIOSCC is difficult to detect in the early stages because it occurs in the jaws. Local pain and sensory nerve abnormalities are usually the initial symptoms, with lower lip numbness being the most common clinical symptom of PIOSCC of the mandible. As the disease progresses, local jawbone swelling and mucosal rupture may happen. When the tumor invades into the teeth, it can cause loose teeth while the surface mucosa keeps intact. Therefore, it is common in clinical patients that the tooth wound does not heal after the extraction of loose teeth or the soft tissue mass grows from the tooth wound. For large tumor, pathological fractures of the mandible can also happen.

Imaging Characteristics PIOSCC is mainly characterized by low-density osteolytic destruction of the lesion area, with irregular and poorly circumscribed low-density shadow in the jaw bone on X-ray and CT. CT shows the destruction of peripheral bone tissue and invasion of surrounding structures, such as the destruction of the inferior alveolar neural tube, which is common in PIOSCC of the mandible. On panoramic radiographs, PIOSCC presents a low-density shadow with a "small mouth and a large base," which is distinct from the low-density shadow with a "small base of the mouth" when the jaw is destroyed by gingival cancer.

Differential Diagnosis Clinically, PIOSCC needs to be distinguished from gingival carcinoma and carcinoma of maxillary sinus. Gingival carcinoma is manifested as soft tissue space occupying of the gingival tissue, and may be exophytic (most common), ulcerative, or invasive. Gingival cancer generally does not cause neurological symptoms such as loose tooth and lower lip numbness; however, X-ray may show a decrease in the roof of the alveolar ridge in the early stage, but show low-density shadow of "large mouth and small floor" at the later stage. Carcinoma of maxillary sinus originates from the mucosa of the maxillary sinus. As carcinoma of maxillary sinus occurs in the mucosa of the maxillary sinus, it is difficult to be detected in the early stage, so most patients are already in the late clinical stage when clinical symptoms appear. If carcinoma of maxillary sinus invades the alveolar process, it is difficult to distinguish it from PIOSCC because of the destruction of jawbone and loosening of teeth. In contrast, PIOSCC center is located in the jawbone and may not involve the maxillary sinus cavity or may be seen to invade the maxillary sinus cavity. MRI usually show T1-weighted low signal or iso-signal images and T2-weighted high signal images for carcinoma of maxillary sinus. Radiotherapy and surgery are the main therapies for carcinoma of maxillary sinus, and the rate of cervical lymph node metastasis is 15–35%. Cervical lymph node dissection is recommended for patients with advanced clinical stage.

Treatment and Prognosis PIOSCC has a 2-year overall survival rate of about 60–70%, and a 5-year overall survival rate of 30–40%. Pathological grading is the main factor affecting the prognosis, and radical surgical resection is the main means to cure PIOSCC. It has been reported that the rate of cervical lymph node metastasis rate in PIOSCC is ranged from 12.8% to 25%, and cervical lymph node metastasis is closely related to the recurrence of tumor, so cervical lymph node dissection is required along with resection of the primary tumor. Postoperative radiation therapy is recommended for pathologically confirmed cervical lymph node metastases. There is a lack of international staging system and treatment guidelines for PIOSCC. Some scholars believe that since the survival rate of PIOSCC patients is comparable to that of stage IV oral cancer, it is proper to refer to the clinical treatment strategy of stage T3N0 oral cancer. In addition, a retrospective study reveals that tumor larger than 4 cm is an independent risk factor for local recurrence and poor prognosis, so more aggressive clinical treatment strategy should be preferred.

References

1. de Morais EF, Carlan LM, de Farias Morais HG, et al. Primary intraosseous squamous cell carcinoma involving the jaw bones: a systematic review and update [J]. Head Neck Pathol; 2020.
2. Woolgar JA, Triantafyllou A, Ferlito A, et al. Intraosseous carcinoma of the jaws: a clinicopathologic review. Part III: primary intraosseous squamous cell carcinoma [J]. Head Neck. 2013;35(6):906–9.
3. Bodner L, Manor E, Shear M, et al. Primary intraosseous squamous cell carcinoma arising in an odontogenic cyst: a clinicopathologic analysis of 116 reported cases [J]. J Oral Pathol Med. 2011;40(10):733–8.
4. El-Naggar AK, Chan JKC, Takata T, et al. The fourth edition of the head and neck World Health Organization blue book: editors' perspectives [J]. Hum Pathol. 2017;66:10–2.
5. Kikuchi K, Ide F, Takizawa S, et al. Initial-stage primary intraosseous squamous cell carcinoma derived from odontogenic keratocyst with unusual keratoameloblastomatous change of the maxilla: a case report and literature discussion [J]. Case Rep Otolaryngol. 2018:7959230.
6. Van der Waal I, Rauhamaa R, Van der Kwast WA, et al. Squamous cell carcinoma arising in the lining of odontogenic cysts: report of 5 cases [J]. Int J Oral Surg. 1985;14(2):146–52.
7. Huang JW, Luo HY, Li Q, et al. Primary intraosseous squamous cell carcinoma of the jaws: clinicopathologic presentation and prognostic factors [J]. Arch Pathol Lab Med. 2009;133(11):1834–40.
8. Naruse T, Yanamoto S, Sakamoto Y, et al. Clinicopathological study of primary intraosseous squamous cell carcinoma of the jaw and a review of the literature [J]. J Oral Maxillofac Surg. 2016;74(12):2420–7.
9. Wenguang X, Hao S, Xiaofeng Q, et al. Prognostic factors of primary intraosseous squamous cell carcinoma (PIOSCC): a retrospective review [J]. PLoS One. 2016;11(4):e0153646.
10. Shen Q, Chen Y, Gokavarapu S, et al. Primary intraosseous squamous cell carcinoma of the mandible: locoregional control and survival is significantly reduced if the tumour is more than 4 cm in size [J]. Br J Oral Maxillofac Surg. 2018;56(1):48–53.
11. Ranasinghe VJ, Stubbs VC, Reny DC, et al. Predictors of nodal metastasis in sinonasal squamous cell carcinoma: a national cancer database analysis [J]. World J Otorhinolaiyngol Head Neck Surg. 2020;6(2):137–41.
12. Takes RP, Ferlito A, Silver CE, et al. The controversy in the management of the N0 neck for squamous cell carcinoma of the maxillary sinus [J]. Eur Arch Otorhinolaryngol. 2014;271(5):899–904.
13. Martinez-Rodriguez N, Barona Dorado C, Cortes-Breton Brinkmann J, et al. Dental considerations in diagnosis of maxillary sinus carcinoma: a patient series of 24 cases [J]. J Am Dent Assoc. 2018;149(11):976–82.
14. Yi KI, Kim SD, Mun SJ, et al. Therapeutic efficacy of regional and systemic chemotherapy in advanced maxillary sinus cancer [J]. Head Neck. 2019;41(8):2732–40.
15. Wang Y, Yang R, Zhao M, et al. Retrospective analysis of 98 cases of maxillary sinus squamous cell carcinoma and therapeutic exploration [J]. World J Surg Oncol. 2020;18(1):90.
16. Crawford KL, Jafari A, Qualliotine JR, et al. Elective neck dissection for T3/T4 cN0 sinonasal squamous cell carcinoma [J]. Head Neck. 2020;42(12):3655–62.
17. Abe T, Saito S, Iino M, et al. Results of definitive radiotherapy with concurrent chemotherapy for maxillary sinus carcinomas with neck lymph node metastasis [J]. J Radiat Res. 2021;62(1):104–9.

18. Kano S, Hayashi R, Homma A, et al. Effect of local extension sites on survival in locally advanced maxillary sinus cancer [J]. Head Neck. 2014;36(11):1567–72.
19. Homma A, Hayashi R, Matsuura K, et al. Lymph node metastasis in t4 maxillary sinus squamous cell carcinoma: incidence and treatment outcome [J]. Ann Surg Oncol. 2014;21(5):1706–10.
20. Ferrari M, Ioppi A, Schreiber A, et al. Malignant tumors of the maxillary sinus: prognostic impact of neurovascular invasion in a series of 138 patients [J]. Oral Oncol. 2020;106:104672.
21. Nishino H, Takanosawa M, Kawada K, et al. Multidisciplinary therapy consisting of minimally invasive resection, irradiation and intra-arterial infusion of 5-fluorouracil for maxillary sinus carcinomas [J]. Head Neck. 2013;35(6):772–8.
22. Wang F, Ren M, Wu J, et al. Definitive radiation therapy versus postoperative radiation therapy for patients with maxillary sinus cancer invading the upper jaw [J]. J Craniofac Surg. 2019;30(4):1234–8.
23. Kawaguchi M, Kato H, Tomita H, et al. Imaging characteristics of malignant sinonasal tumors [J]. J Clin Med. 2017;6(12):116.

50 Primary Intraosseous Mucoepidermoid Carcinoma of Jaws

Yue He, Hui Shan Ong, Zhen Tian, Lin Zhu, and Feng Shuo Zhu

50.1 Introduction

Mucoepidermoid carcinoma (MEC) is the most common malignant tumor originating in salivary glands. Ectopic MECs may occur in any part of the body, but only 2–4% of MECs occur in the jaw bone, which is known as primary intraosseous mucoepidermoid carcinoma (PIMC) [1–5]. PIMC is usually low or medium grade, and its lesion needs to be distinguished from ameloblastoma and odontogenic cysts on imaging findings. Since PIMC may recur long after surgery, long-term follow-up is required for patients with PIMC.

50.2 Case 93

A 49-year-old woman suffered from a protuberance in the mandibular anterior dental region with tooth loosening for 5 months.

[History of Present Illness] Five months ago, the patient felt gingival distension in the mandibular anterior dental area loosening, accompanied by loose tooth, which gradually worsened without any other obvious discomfort. The patient was admitted to the hospital and was considered to have "ameloblastoma," but received no treatment.

[Specialty Examination] The face was symmetrical, with no abnormality in facial skin, mouth opening range, and mouth opening pattern. Intraoral 34–42 lingual and 34–35 buccal bony protuberance was found, with clear circumscription, intact surface mucosa, no tenderness, no obvious rupture or abnormal exudation (Fig. 50.1a). The tongue could move freely. Intraoral examination revealed free movement of the tongue, clear bilateral parotid ductal secretion, and absence of tooth 36. No enlargement of cervical and submandibular lymph nodes was observed bilaterally.

[Auxiliary Examination]

1. Panoramic radiographs suggested an irregular abnormal density shadow in 35–43 tooth roots, with inhomogeneous attenuation in bone density, visible bone spacing, poor circumscription, and no obvious resorption in the affected tooth roots (Fig. 50.1b).
2. Maxillofacial enhanced CT scan suggested a bony protuberance in the chin of the mandible, slightly bulged to the buccal-lingual side, with multiple bony partitions inside; inhomogeneous enhancement, no root resorption, thinning of peri-lesion cortical bone, interruption of local continuity, and poor circumscription with surrounding soft tissue. No enlarged

Y. He · H. S. Ong (✉) · Z. Tian · L. Zhu · F. S. Zhu
Department of Oral Maxillofacial-Head & Neck Oncology, Shanghai Ninth People's Hospital, Shanghai Jiao Tong University School of Medicine, Shanghai, China

Y. He (ed.), *Inflammatory and Neoplastic Diseases of Craniofacial Bones*,
https://doi.org/10.1007/978-981-97-4155-7_50

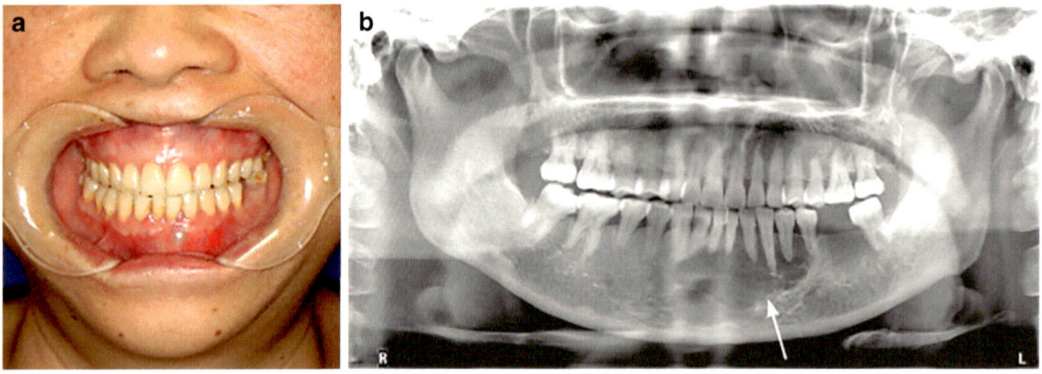

Fig. 50.1 (**a**) Bony protuberance at 34–42 lingual side and 34–35 buccal side, with clear circumscription, intact surface mucosa, no tenderness, no obvious rupture, or abnormal exudation. (**b**) Irregular abnormal density shadow in 35–43 teeth roots, with inhomogeneous attenuation in bone density, visible bone spacing, poor circumscription, and no obvious resorption in the affected tooth roots (preoperative)

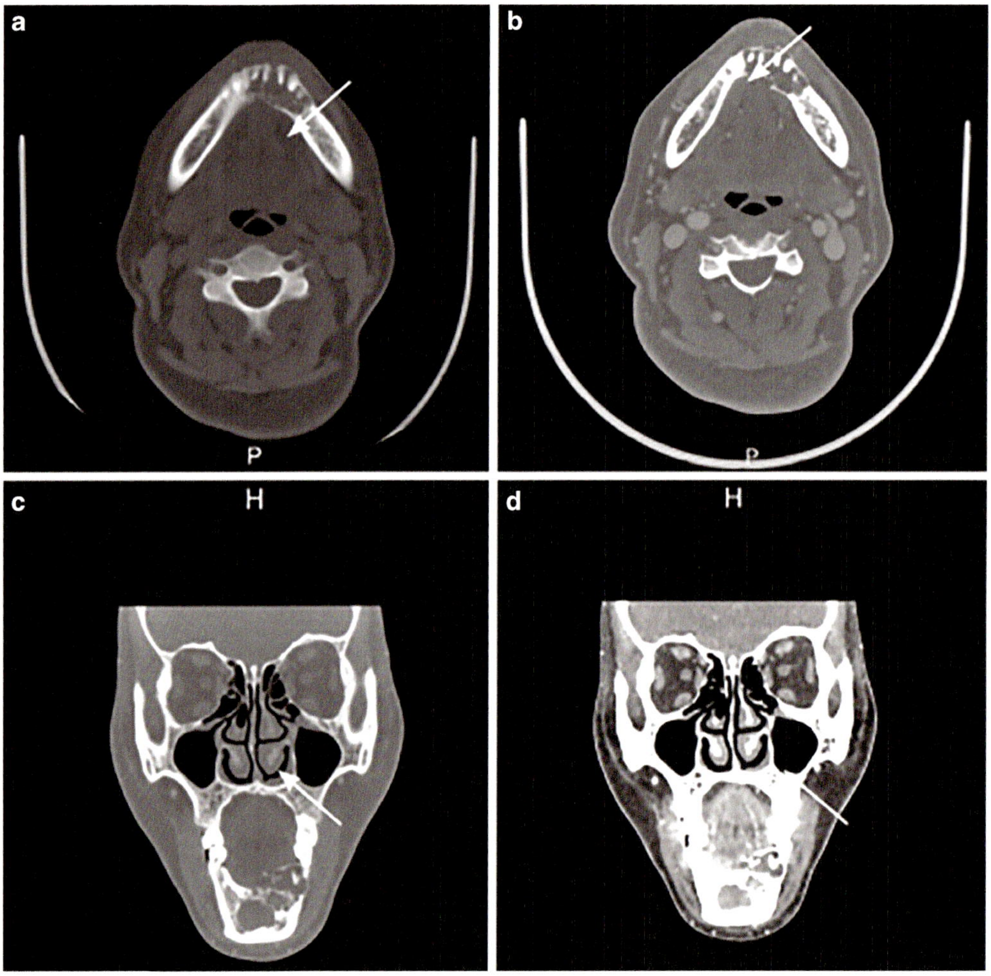

Fig. 50.2 (**a**) CT axial scan: bony protuberance in the chin of the mandible, slightly bulged to the buccal-lingual side, with multiple bony partitions inside. (**b**) Enhanced CT axial scan: inhomogeneous mild enhancement. (**c**, **d**) Coronal reconstruction

cervical lymph nodes were observed bilaterally. Nodules were seen in the left thyroid gland (Fig. 50.2).

3. Maxillofacial enhanced MR suggested a bony protuberance in the chin of the mandible, slightly bulged to the buccal-lingual side, with multiple bony partitions inside; inhomogeneous enhancement, no obvious adjacent root resorption, thinning of peri-lesion cortical bone, interruption of local continuity, and poor circumscription with surrounding soft tissue (Fig. 50.3).

[Preliminary Diagnosis] Mandibular mass.

[Treatment] "Extensive mandible resection with fibular flap transfer and tracheotomy" was performed under general anesthesia: an incision was made along the lower margin of the mandible for 1–2 cm, and the gingival flap was elevated for surgical exposure of the mass located between teeth 34 and 42, with buccolingual expansion. A part of the mass protrudes from the bone cortex and invaded the periosteum. The mandible was truncated at teeth 36 and 44 respectively, and the truncated mandible and the tumor were completely removed within the range of normal tissue. Intraoperative frozen pathological examination suggested the "mandible" lesion was considered to be a mucoepidermoid carcinoma of low grade. The fibular flap was routinely prepared and shaped to restore mandibular continuity and occlusal relationship, and the fibular artery and vein were anastomosed with the external maxillary artery and the common facial vein, respectively. The wound was rinsed and thoroughly hemostatic, negative pressure drainage tube was indwelled, and layered suture was performed to close the wound (Fig. 50.4).

[Pathological Examination] Gross pathological examination revealed a part of the mandibular tissue, 5 cm × 4.4 cm × 2.5 cm in size, with six teeth attached. The section showed cystic space, irregular shape, and bone septa. The microscopic examination showed multiple cystic spaces of varying sizes and neoplastic epithelial clusters, and residual bone tissue inside. Epithelial hyperplasia was observed in the lining of the cyst cavity, with no obvious cell atypia, and a small amount of mucus cells. Some of the tumor cells were rich in cytoplasm, eosinophilic and squamous, and appeared to be epidermoid cells, while some are small with clear cytoplasm (Fig. 50.5).

[Pathological Diagnosis] Polycystic lesion of the mandible, considered as mucoepidermoid carcinoma, low grade. Note: In this case, the MAML2 FISH indicated no splitting of MAML2 gene.

[Follow-Up] The patient healed uneventfully. The postoperative 6-month follow-up exhibited no recurrence of the tumor, with normal function and good recovery of bilateral posterior teeth occlusal relationship.

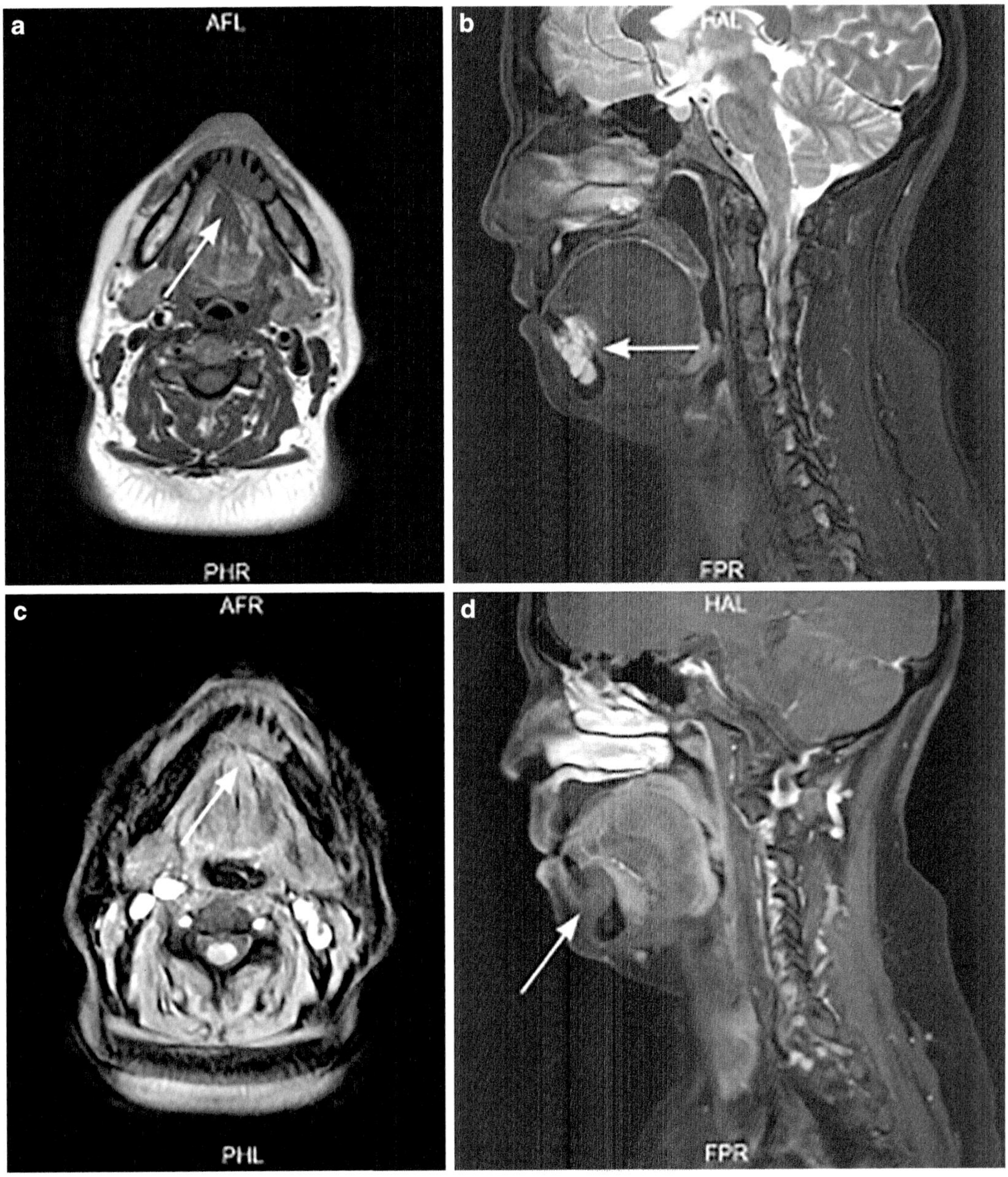

Fig. 50.3 (**a**) T1W1 axial scan: bony protuberance in the chin of the mandible, with multiple bony partitions inside. (**b**) fsT2W sagittal scan: multiple bony partitions inside the lension. (**c**, **d**) T1W enhanced axial and sagittal scan: inhomogeneous enhancement of the mass

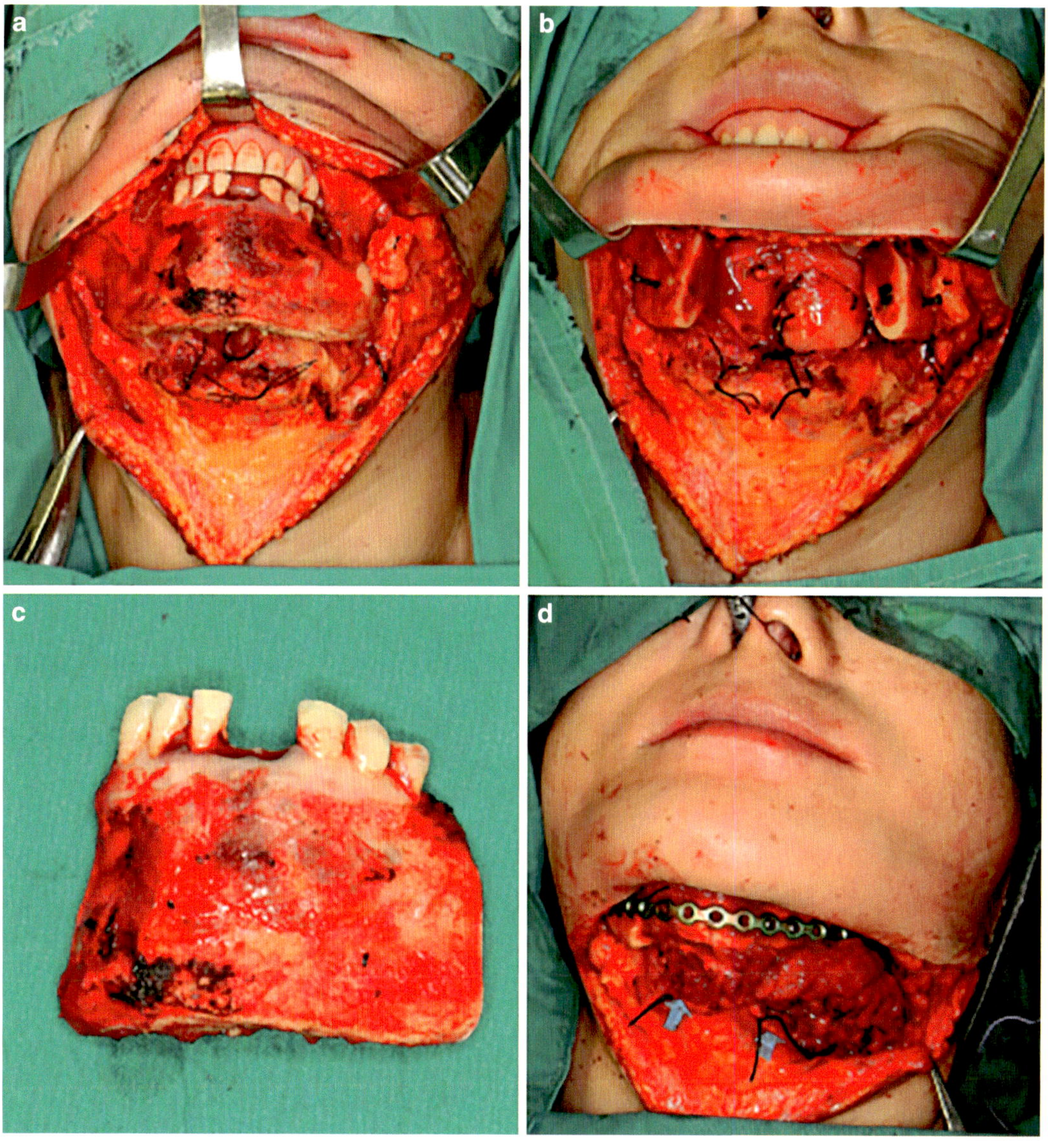

Fig. 50.4 (**a**) Exposed bilateral mandibular body to show chin bone distension. (**b**) Defect in the operative region after amputation of the mandible. (**c**) Isolated mandible and mass. (**d**) Fibula reconstruction to restore mandibular continuity

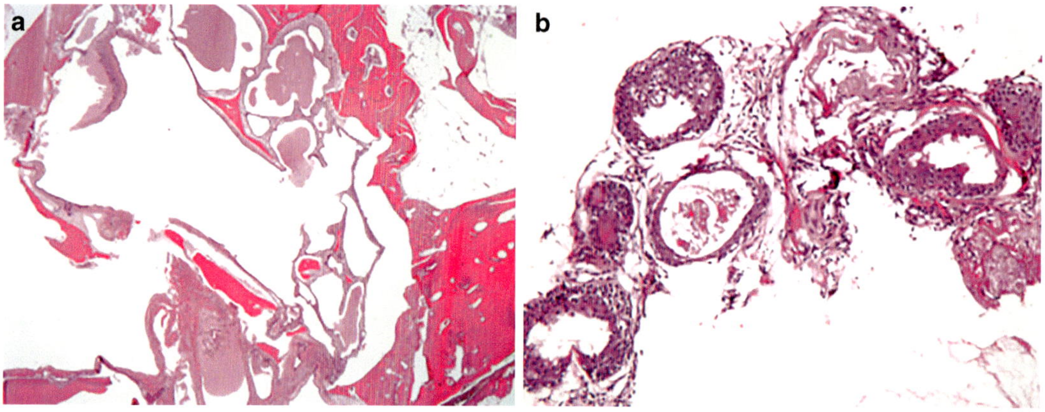

Fig. 50.5 (**a**) Multiple cystic cavities of different sizes in the bone tissues, interspersed between the bone tissues, with certain aggressiveness (200x). (**b**) Some of the tumor cells were rich in cytoplasm, and appeared to be epidermoid cells, while some are small with clear cytoplasm (200x)

50.3 Key Points of Diagnosis and Treatment

Clinical Manifestations The main clinical symptom of PIMC is painless swelling, and PIMC is usually characterized by local tissue infiltration, but metastasis rarely occurs. It is reported that approximately 9% of patients with PIMC develop metastases. Metastases happen mainly in the cervical lymph nodes and rarely in other distant organs.

Imaging Characteristics Imaging findings show that PIMC is characterized by well-circumscribed unilocular or multilocular projection, mainly affecting the molar and mandibular ramus regions. Unilocular lesion resembles odontogenic keratocyst, while multilocular lesion has a honeycomb-like internal structure and should be differentiated from enameloblastomas.

Diagnosis The diagnosis of PIMC should be based on histopathology and imaging findings. For the diagnosis of PIMC, pathology examination should confirm the following points: exclusion of primary MEC in salivary glands and other tissues, no odontogenic tumor, the histological structure of MEC, positive mucin staining, as well as bone destruction on imaging.

Treatment and Prognosis The therapies for PIMC include conservative surgery and radical surgery. Although PIMC is described as a low-grade malignancy in many publications, conservative treatment including curettage and enucleation has a recurrence rate of approximately 40%. Therefore, radical jaw surgery should be the preferred. Cervical lymph node dissection and postoperative adjuvant radiotherapy should depend on the presence or absence of regional lymph node metastases. It is difficult to predict the prognosis of PIMC, as different surgical approaches and biologic specificities produce different outcomes. PIMC is characterized by the possibility of recurrence and metastasis, so long-term follow-up of patients is necessary.

References

1. Li X, Wang F, Wang Y, et al. An unusual case of intraosseous mucoepidermoid carcinoma of the mandible: A case report and literature review [J]. Medicine (Baltimore). 2018;97(51):e13691.
2. Merna C, Kita A, Wester J, et al. Intraosseous mucoepidermoid carcinoma: Outcome review [J]. Laryngoscope. 2018;128(5):1083–92.
3. Abt NB, Lawler ME, Zacharias J, et al. Primary intraosseous mucoepidermoid carcinoma of the mandible: radiographic evolution and clinicopathological features [J]. BMJ Case Rep. 2019;12(4):e224612.
4. Nallamilli SM, Tatapudi R, Reddy RS, et al. Primary intraosseous mucoepidermoid carcinoma of the maxilla [J]. Ghana Med J. 2015;49(2):120–3.
5. Raut D, Khedkar S. Primary intraosseous mucoepidermoid carcinoma of the maxilla: a case report and review of literature [J]. Dentomaxillofac Radiol. 2009;38(3):163–8.

Primary Intraosseous Adenoid Cystic Carcinoma of Jaws

51

Yue He, Hui Shan Ong, Zhen Tian, Lin Zhu, and Chen Ye

51.1 Introduction

Adenoid cystic carcinoma (ACC) is an epithelial malignant tumor of salivary gland origin, about 70–90% in sublinguial gland, 15–32% in parotid gland, and also in submandibular gland and other small salivary glands [1–5]. Primary intraosseous adenoid cystic carcinoma (PIACC) originating in jaw bone is extremely rare and usually occurs in people aged between 40 and 50 years [6, 7]. Due to the lack of relevant clinicopathological data, statistical data on gender difference is absent. PIACC occurs mostly in the mandible body (posterior dental region), presenting as osteolytic destruction [8–11]. When it invades nerve, it may cause numbness in the lower gum, lip and chin, etc., which should be regarded as one of the differential diagnoses of osteolytic tumors in the jaw.

51.2 Case 94

A 43-year-old woman suffered from spontaneous pain in left anterior teeth for 1 year with radicular mass for more than 5 months.

[History of Present Illness] One year ago, the patient developed weakness in the left lower anterior teeth with unknown pathogenesis, and occasionally had spontaneous parochial dull pain. The periapical film examination more than 5 months ago showed low density shadow in the left lower anterior teeth with no special abnormalities in the affected teeth, and referral to the oral surgery department was recommended. Further CT examination showed bone destruction in the left lower anterior teeth with no obvious abnormal mass detected, considered to be "apical cyst." The patient underwent referral to the endodontics department for "root canal therapy," and then to the oral surgery department 1 month ago for reexamination, which suggested no great improvement in the symptom of tooth weakness, involving the right lower anterior teeth, with slight pain and discomfort in the left mandible at night, no facial skin numbness, tongue numbness and motion discomfort, etc. Panoramic radiographs showed a shadow of the root tip in the mandibular anterior teeth region, and the range was slightly increased.

[Specialty Examination] The face was symmetrical, with well-coordinated 1/3 proportion of upper, middle, and lower face. There was no abnormality in mouth opening range and mouth opening pattern. Intraoral examination showed no obvious protuberance or tenderness in the mandibular anterior teeth; no abnormality in tongue movement; 1° movement at teeth 31, 32,

Y. He · H. S. Ong (✉) · Z. Tian · L. Zhu · C. Ye
Department of Oral Maxillofacial-Head & Neck Oncology, Shanghai Ninth People's Hospital, Shanghai Jiao Tong University School of Medicine, Shanghai, China

Y. He (ed.), *Inflammatory and Neoplastic Diseases of Craniofacial Bones*, https://doi.org/10.1007/978-981-97-4155-7_51

41, and 42; percussion (−); dull at teeth 31 and 32 in vitality test; red and swollen gingival papillae, BOP (+), PD 2 ~ 4 mm; loss of teeth 18 and 28; meso-impacted at teeth 38 and 48; 6 maxillofacial amalgum restoration, and intact oral mucosa. No significant enlargement of submental, submandibular, and cervical lymph nodes was observed bilaterally.

[Auxiliary Examination]

1. Periapical film suggested a low-density shadow in the 31, 32, and 41 teeth apical region, with poor circumscription and cloudy shape. No alae bone line was observed, and the shadows disappeared in the periodontal space (Fig. 51.1a).
2. Maxillofacial enhanced CT scan suggested a resorption and destruction of alveolar bone in the 32–41 teeth apical area of the mandible, with C− of 70 Hu. No obvious soft tissue mass was observed around, so further enhancement examination was recommended to exclude the possibility of malignancy (Fig. 51.2).
3. Panoramic radiographs suggested a low-density shadow in the 33–42 teeth apical region, well circumscribed, 31, 32 root canals in place closely, 38, 48 meso-impacted, 28 residual root, and 18 absent (Fig. 51.1b).

[Preliminary Diagnosis] Mandibular mass (malignant to be excluded).

[Treatment] "Expanded resection of mandibular mass" was performed under general anesthesia: an incision was made along the gingiva of 33–43 teeth, and the gingival flap was elevated for surgical exposure of the destruction in the buccal lamina of the mandibular anterior region. The mass was solid, brittle in texture and locally fish-like, without intact capsule, and the mass was completely resected including the buccal periosteum. Intraoperative frozen pathological examination suggested the possibility of adenoid cystic carcinoma. The surrounding bone was trimmed, the remaining bone cavity was cauterized with carbolic acid, and the cavity was filled with iodoform gauze. Postoperative radiotherapy, 60 Gy in total.

[Pathological Examination] Gross pathological examination revealed two fragments of tissue, 1.6 cm × 0.8 cm × 0.5 cm in size, grayish yellow. The microscopic examination showed that the tumor was composed of glandular epithelial cells and mutated myoepithelial cells, arranged in ethmoidal and tubular shapes, invading the surrounding bone tissue. Duct-like structures were observed in the tumor nest, with glandular epithelium lining around the catheter lumen.

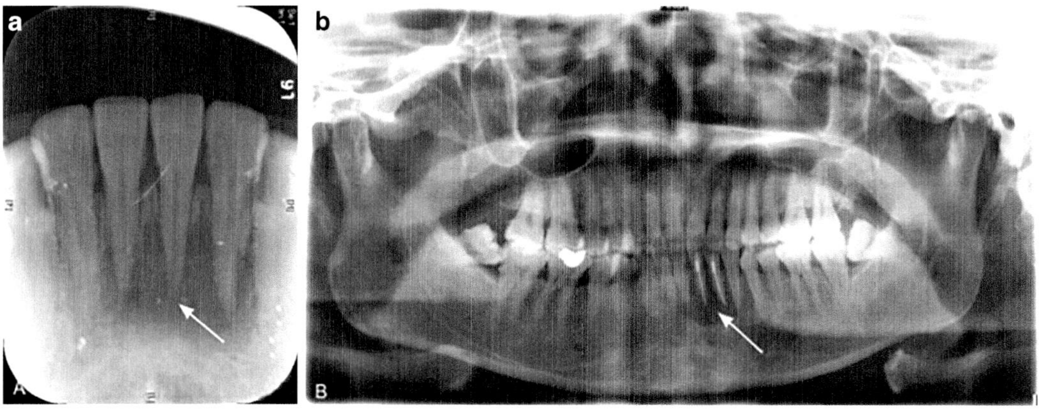

Fig. 51.1 (**a**) Low-density shadow in the 31, 32, and 41 teeth apical region, with poor circumscription and cloudy shape. No alae bone line was observed, and the shadows disappeared in the periodontal space. (**b**) low-density shadow in the 33-42 teeth apical region, well circumscribed, 31, 32 root canals in place closely, 38, 48 teeth meso-impacted, 28 residual root, and 18 tooth absent

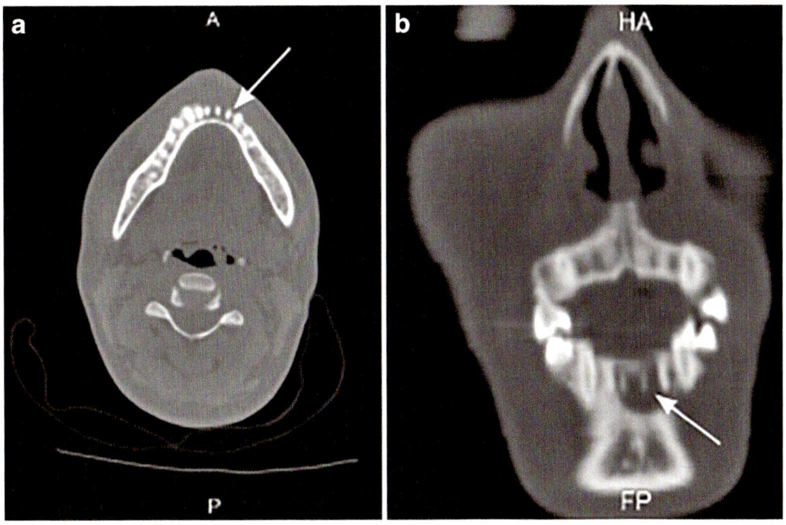

Fig. 51.2 (**a**) CT axial scan: resorption and destruction of alveolar bone in the 32–41 teeth apical area of the mandible, with C− of 70 Hu. No obvious soft tissue mass was observed around. (**b**) Coronal reconstruction

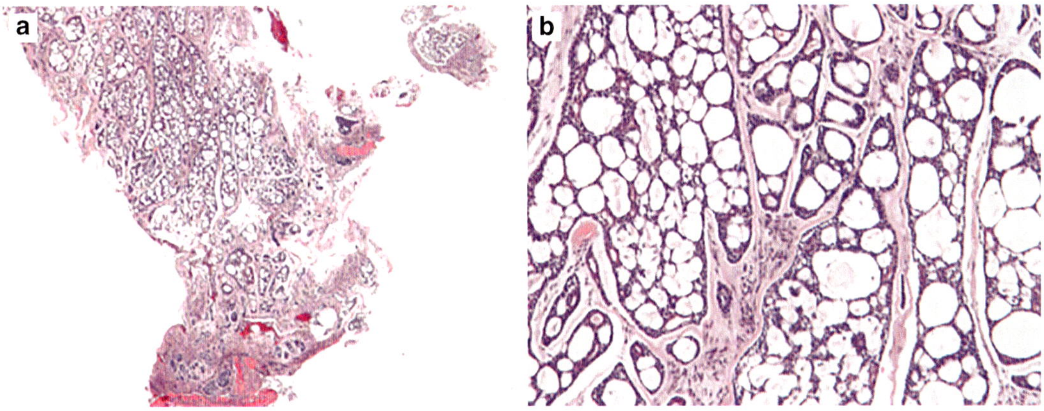

Fig. 51.3 (**a**) The tumor cells were arranged in ethmoid and tubular patterns with aggressive growth and remaining bone tissue visible (40x). (**b**) The classic clathrate structure was pseudoglandular lumen of variable size enclosed by variant myoepithelial cells. A number of true ductal structures (indicated by arrows), usually with small lumen and eosinophilic surrounding glandular epithelial cytoplasm (200x), were also observed

Eosinophilic basophilic basaloid cells surrounded the cytoplasm, with small cells and few mitosis (Fig. 51.3).

[Pathological Diagnosis] Adenoid cystic carcinoma of the mandible, mainly ethmoid type, low grade.

[Follow-Up] The patient healed uneventfully after surgery, and developed an oral fistula in the operative region of the lower anterior teeth after radiotherapy without discharge of pyorrhea. The 5-year follow-up exhibited no cancer relapse. However, an oral fistula was found during the follow up, curettage biopsy reported as radioactive osteonecrosis of the mandible. The postoperative pathological examination indicated adenoid cystic carcinoma. The "extended mandibulectomy with fibula flap transplantation reconstruction" was performed, and the patient healed uneventfully after surgery (Fig. 51.4).

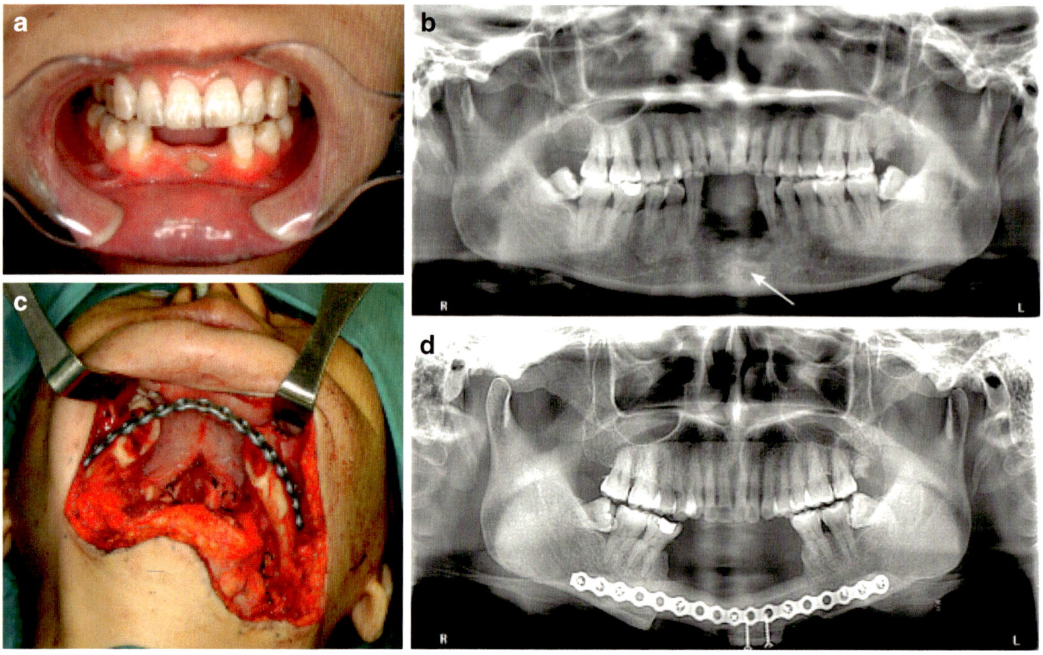

Fig. 51.4 (**a**) Oral fistula in the operative region of the lower anterior teeth after radiotherapy without discharge of pyorrhea. (**b**) At the 5th year after treatment, panoramic radiographs suggested destruction of bone erosion in the operative region of the mandible, with poor circumscription. (**c**) The mandibular bone was resected and fibula was reconstructed to restore the continuity of the mandible. (**d**) Postoperative changes of the mandible showed good healing of the fibula

51.3 Key Points of Diagnosis and Treatment

The possible pathogenesis of PIACC is as follows: ① the epithelial cells of salivary glands proliferate ectopically and are encapsulated in the bone marrow cavity to form granulation tissue; ② Odontogenic epithelial cells were induced to transform into mucous cells under specific microenvironment. The main clinical manifestation of PIACC is painless and progressive distension of the jaw. When it invades the nerve, it may cause numbness in the lower gum, lip, and chin. PIACC should be differentiated from jaw cyst, ameloblastoma/carcinoma, primary squamous cell carcinoma of jaw and osteosarcoma on imaging findings. Pathologically, PIACC can be divided into three types, namely, ethmoid type (main type), tubular type, and solid type. ACC occurring in salivary glands has no obvious histological and cytological difference. The diagnostic criteria of PIACC include the following: ① osteolytic lesion on imaging findings, ② complete cortical bone in the mandible, ③ no primary tumors found in the salivary glands, and ④pathologically confirmed as ACC.

The main therapy for PIACC is also surgical treatment, with postoperative adjuvant radiotherapy. Extended resection of the mandible and surrounding soft tissues to obtain negative margins is the key to ensure good prognosis. However, due to the neurophilic and vascular biology of ACC, it is difficult to achieve negative margins intraoperatively, which makes postoperative adjuvant radiotherapy particularly important. Patients with ACC have the 5-year and 10-year survival rates of 77% and 57% respectively after radical surgery in combination with adjuvant radiotherapy. It is now believed that PIACC is less likely to have cervical lymph node metastases, while distant metastases are 40–60%, with pulmonary metastases in most cases but extensive bone metastases in a few cases. For patients with distant metastases, chemotherapy or concurrent radiotherapy is the best treatment option. Despite distant metastases, patients can survive with tumor for a long time.

In general, PIACC is a rare intraosseous malignant tumor that is often difficult to distinguish from maxillary cysts, benign tumors, or other malignant tumors because of the absence of clinical and imaging features. Intraoperative frozen pathological examination is vital in supplementing and improving the therapeutic regimen. Radical surgery with adjuvant radiotherapy is currently the most common therapeutic regimen. Close follow-up is required after treatment, and early intervention is needed to improve the survival rate in case of local recurrence, cervical lymph node metastasis, and lung metastasis.

References

1. Li Y, Li LJ, Huang J, et al. Central malignant salivary gland tumors of the jaw: retrospective clinical analysis of 22 cases [J]. J Oral Maxillofac Surg. 2008;66(11):2247–53.
2. Chen YK, Chen CH, Lin CC, et al. Central adenoid cystic carcinoma of the mandible manifesting as an endodontic lesion [J]. Int Endod J. 2004;37(10):711–6.
3. Brookstone MS, Huvos AG. Central salivary gland tumors of the maxilla and mandible: a clinicopathologic study of 11 cases with an analysis of the literature [J]. J Oral Maxillofac Surg. 1992;50(3):229–36.
4. Martinez-Madrigal F, Pineda-Daboin K, Casiraghi O, et al. Salivary gland tumors of the mandible [J]. Ann Diagn Pathol. 2000;4(6):347–53.
5. Capodiferro S, Scully C, Macaita MG, et al. Bilateral intraosseous adenoid cystic carcinoma of the mandible: report of a case with lung metastases at first clinical presentation [J]. Oral Dis. 2005;11(2):109–12.
6. Alexander RW, Dupuis RH, Holton H. Central mucoepidermoid tumor (carcinoma) of the mandible [J]. J Oral Surg. 1974;32(7):541–7.
7. Black KM, Fitzpatrick PJ, Palmer JA. Adenoid cystic carcinoma of the salivary glands [J]. Can J Surg. 1980;23(1):32–5.
8. Savithri V, Suresh R, Janardhanan M, et al. Primary intraosseous adenoid cystic carcinoma with widespread skeletal metastases showing features of high-grade transformation [J]. Head Neck Pathol. 2020;
9. Deng RX, Xu X, Zhang CP, et al. Primary intraosseous adenoid cystic carcinoma of the jaw: clinical and histopathologic analysis [J]. J Oral Maxillofac Surg. 2014;72(4):835.
10. Hu HY, Liu YY, Wang H, et al. Primary intraosseous adenoid cystic carcinoma of the mandible: a comprehensive review with analysis of 2 additional cases [J]. J Oral Maxillofac Surg. 2017;75(8):1685–701.
11. You L, Chunjie L, Fanglong W, et al. Primary adenoid cystic carcinoma of mandible: a case report [J]. Chin J Stomatol. 2015;33(5):548–50.

Metastatic Malignant Tumor in Jaws

52

Yue He, Hui Shan Ong, Zhen Tian, Lin Zhu, and Zhong Long Liu

52.1 Introduction

Oral metastases are rare, accounting for approximately 1% of all oral malignancies, and occur more frequently in the jaws than in the soft tissues. Metastases to the jaws occur mainly in the posterior ascending rami and condyles of the mandible, which were rich in red bone marrow. Maxillary metastases are rare, accounting for 20% of all metastatic tumors in jaws. The ratio of male to female patient is almost equal, with a ratio of 1–1.1 [1–5]. The average age of patients is 45 years. The primary lesions occur usually in the breast, genitalia, thyroid, and kidney for female patients, but mainly in the lung, prostate, kidney, bone, large intestine, and adrenal gland for male patients. Diffusion through the valveless vertebral venous system is the main route of oral metastasis. Histologically, the primary focus is usually cancer, especially adenocarcinoma. Adenocarcinoma usually arises from metastasis of primary lesions in the breast in women or in the lungs, digestive tract, or prostate in men. Oral metastases are a complication of malignancy, which usually happen in the advanced stages of cancer.

52.2 Case 95

A 56-year-old woman suffered from pain and discomfort in the left maxillofacial region with increasingly restricted mouth opening for 3 months.

[History of Present Illness] The patient developed left maxillofacial pain with unknown pathogenesis 3 months ago, involving the left upper and lower jaw regions. The pain was intermittent, accompanied by increasingly restricted mouth opening, affecting daily diet. CT examination one month ago revealed osteolytic destruction in the left mandibular ramus involving the sphenoid bone. There was no headache, dizziness, syncope history, lip numbness, tooth loosening or loss, nasal bleeding or abnormal secretions, or double vision. Maxillofacial enhanced CT showed multiple maxillary destruction, considered as malignant tumor. ECT results suggested a partial defect of the left iliac crest. Puncture examination showed a tendency to adenoid cystic carcinoma.

[Specialty Examination] The face was asymmetrical, with bony protuberance in the mandibular ramus under the left zygomatic arch. The skin was normal in color, with no rupture or congestion. Palpation did not show ping-pong sensation or wave sensation, but with mild tenderness. The mouth opening was about 2.5 cm, and the occlusal relationship was generally normal, with-

Y. He · H. S. Ong (✉) · Z. Tian · L. Zhu · Z. L. Liu
Department of Oral Maxillofacial-Head & Neck Oncology, Shanghai Ninth People's Hospital, Shanghai Jiao Tong University School of Medicine, Shanghai, China

Y. He (ed.), *Inflammatory and Neoplastic Diseases of Craniofacial Bones*,
https://doi.org/10.1007/978-981-97-4155-7_52

out movement or loss of teeth (Fig. 52.1b). The lip had no sensory disorders, and the tongue could move normally, with no numbness and other sensory abnormalities. The mucosa of the left pterygnathic ligament was normal in color, without redness and swelling, and no obvious protuberance was found on palpation. The temporomandibular joint movement was normal, with no void in the articular fossa. No significant enlargement of submandibular and cervical lymph nodes was observed bilaterally.

[Auxiliary Examination]

1. Panoramic radiographs suggested multiple bone destructions in the left mandibular angle, ascending rami, and condyle, with density attenuation and poor circumscription (Fig. 52.1b).
2. Maxillofacial enhanced CT scan suggested a bone destruction in the left mandibular ramus and condyle, with abnormal soft tissue density shadow observed locally. After enhancement, the lesion was significantly enhanced with inhomogeneous density, with C− of 37.2 Hu, C+ of 103.9 Hu and 48.5 Hu. In the left mandibular angle and ascending ramus, multiple round low-density shadows with less than 1 cm in diameter were also observed. Multiple bone destructions were seen in the left great wing of sphenoid bone and temporal bone, as well as abnormal soft tissue density shadows (Fig. 52.2).

[Preliminary Diagnosis] ① Multiple myeloma; ②ACC metastases to be excluded.

[Treatment] "Excision biopsy of left mandible tumor" was performed under general anesthesia: a left pretragal S-shaped incision was made, and the gingival flap was elevated to dissect facial nerve buccal branches carefully and expose the mandible and the mass. The mass tissue was cut and sent to the intraoperative frozen examination and paraffin pathology. The frozen pathological results showed that the adenocarcinoma was prone to metastasis. The wound was rinsed and thoroughly hemostatic. Layered suture was performed to close the wound. Further examination such as PET/CT was recommended to identify the source of the tumor.

[Pathological Examination] Gross pathological examination revealed a part of soft tissue, 1.2 cm × 0.9 cm × 0.5 cm, dark red. The microscopic examination showed that tumor cells were observed with clear cytoplasm, atypia, and rare mitosis. Immunohistochemical staining showed positive expressions of CD10 and vimentin in tumor cells (Fig. 52.3).

[Pathological Diagnosis] Considered as "mandibular mass" metastatic renal clear cell carcinoma, combined with the medical history and enzyme label results.

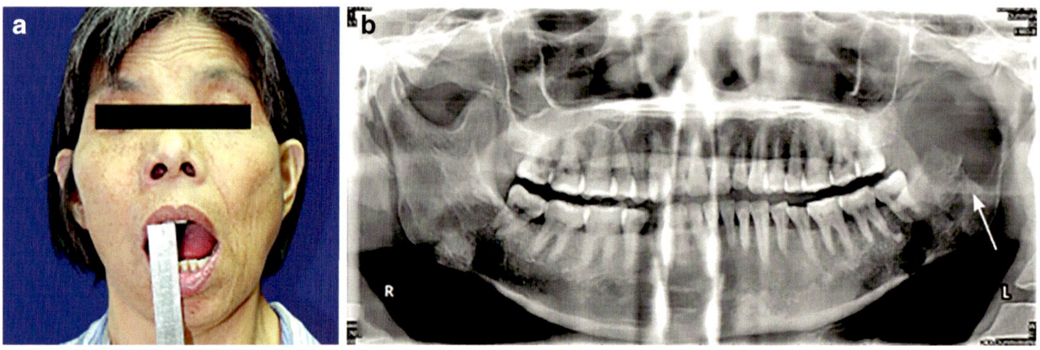

Fig. 52.1 (**a**) Restricted mouth opening with a mouth opening degree of about 2.5 cm. (**b**) Multiple bone destructions in the left mandibular angle, ascending rami, and condyle, with density attenuation and poor circumscription (preoperative)

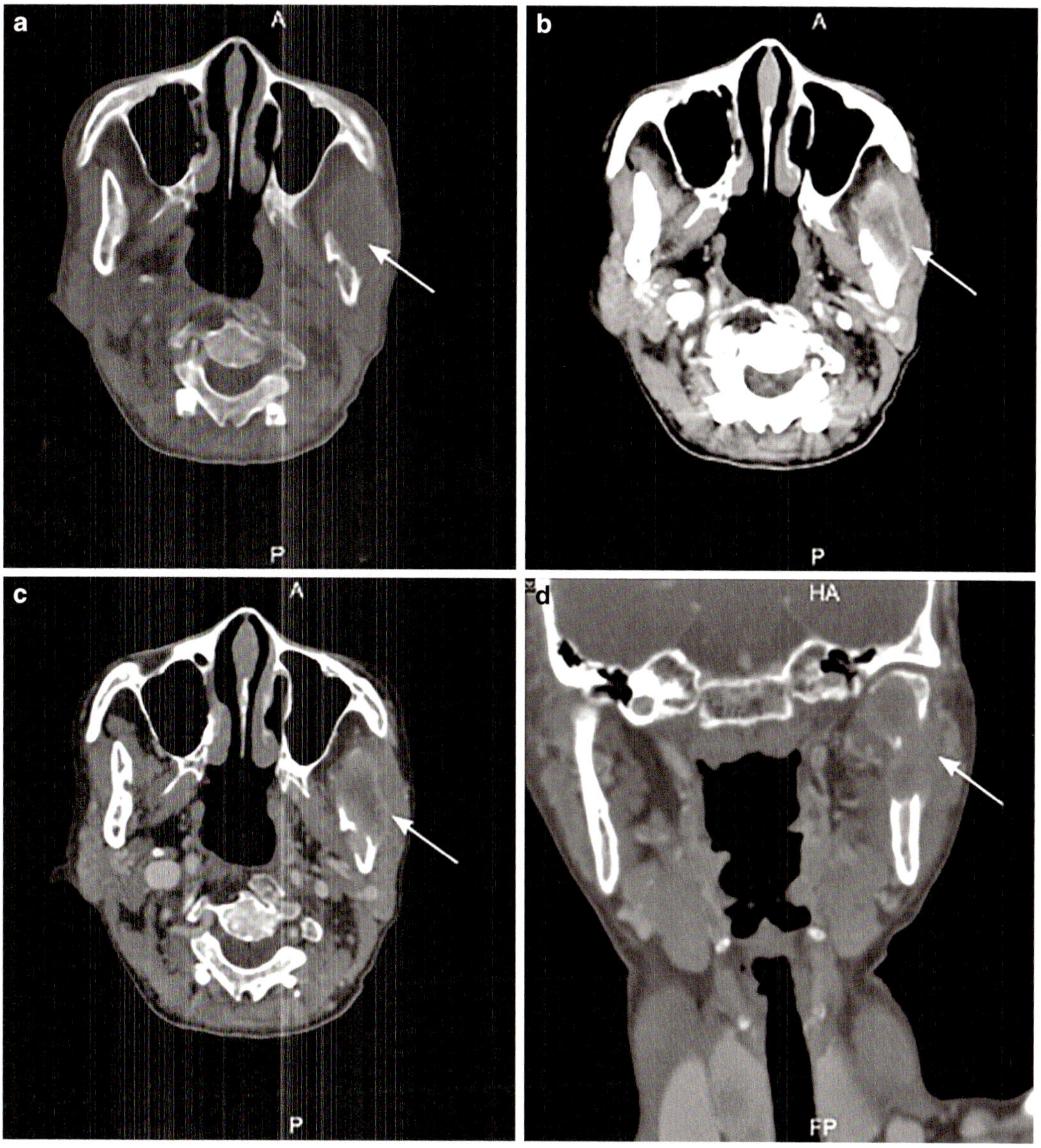

Fig. 52.2 (**a**) CT axial scan: bone destruction in left mandibular ramus. (**b**, **c**) Enhanced CT axial scan: Abnormal soft tissue mass with significant enhancement and inhomogeneous density after enhancement. (**d**) Enhanced CT coronal reconstruction: No obvious abnormality in the left temporomandibular joint space

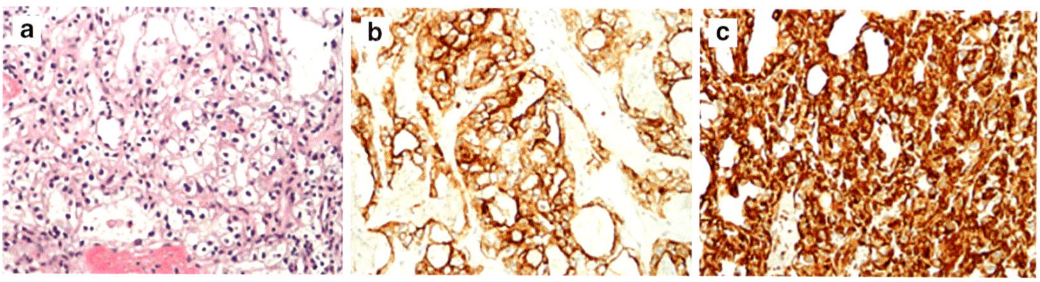

Fig. 52.3 (**a**) Large tumor cells with clear cytoplasm and rare mitosis (400x). (**b**, **c**) Diffuse strong positive expression of CD10 (**b**) and vimentin (**c**) in tumor cells (400x)

52.3 Key Points of Diagnosis and Treatment

Metastatic carcinoma in jaws has the main symptoms of pain, numbness, and swelling of the lower lip and chin, and tooth loosening. According to X-ray findings, metastatic carcinoma in jaws can be divided into three categories: osteolytic, osteoblastic, and mixed. Low-density irregular lytic destruction is the most common manifestation of metastatic carcinoma in jaws, with few osteogenic lesions. Most metastatic lesions on imaging examination present as transmission region with poor circumscription. The mean time from diagnosis of primary tumor to jaw metastasis is 40 months. Metastatic carcinoma in jaws has a poor prognosis, and the mean survival time of 6–7 months after diagnosis. Metastatic lesions should be treated with radiotherapy, chemotherapy, and surgery. Palliative care can help relieve suffering, reduce the size of the tumor, and preserve oral function.

References

1. Irani S. Metastasis to the Jawbones: a review of 453 cases [J]. J Int Soc Prev Community Dent. 2017;7(2):71–81.
2. Zachariades N. Neoplasms metastatic to the mouth, jaws and surrounding tissues [J]. J Craniomaxillofac Surg. 1989;17(6):283–90.
3. Irani S. Metastasis to the oral soft tissues: a review of 412 cases [J]. J Int Soc Prev Community Dent. 2016;6(5):393–401.
4. Friedrich RE, Abadi M. Distant metastases and malignant cellular neoplasms encountered in the oral and maxillofacial region: analysis of 92 patients treated at a single institution [J]. Anticancer Res. 2010;30(5):1843–8.
5. Singh H, Kumar P, Nirwan A, et al. Possible pathogenetic mechanisms and overview of metastatic tumours to the oral cavity [J]. Internet J Oncol. 2010;8:1–6.

53 Solitary Plasmacytoma of Bone

Yue He, Hui Shan Ong, Zhen Tian, Lin Zhu, and Xiao Guang Li

Plasmacytoma is a malignant tumor formed by monoclonal proliferation of mature B cells secreting clonal immunoglobulin with light chain inhibition at the end of differentiation. Plasmacytoma includes multiple myeloma (MM) and solitary plasmacytoma (SP) [1–5]. Unlike MM, SP has limited lesions and often has no abnormal bone marrow changes. Depending on location, SP is further classified into solitary plasmacytoma of bone (SPB) and extramedullary plasmacytoma (EMP). SPB in the mandible is rare, involving the mandible more than the maxilla. As the most active hematopoietic region, the mandibular ramus, angle, and molar region are the most common sites of occurrence [3–5].

53.1 Case 96

A 61-year-old woman suffered from a growing swelling of the right mandible for 6 months.

[History of Present Illness] Six months ago, the patient developed a swelling of the right mandible with unknown pathogenesis, which gradually worsened, without bleeding, numbness, or occasional pain. Follow-up medical history showed the patient had a history of osteoporosis, treated with alenalphosphate sodium, alfacalcalcitol, and calcium acetate.

[Specialty Examination] The face was asymmetrical, with an obvious swelling on the right face. The mass occurred in the mandibular ramus and body, and was about 3 cm × 3 cm in size, hard, immobile, with smooth surface, clear circumscription, and no obvious adhesion to the surrounding tissues (Fig. 53.1a). The opening range was normal but the opening pattern was rightward. Intraoral examination revealed NAD (no abonormality detected), no swelling, no congestion, no obvious tenderness or tenderness. No significant enlargement of cervical lymph nodes was observed.

[Auxiliary Examination]

1. Panoramic radiographs suggested a density attenuation of the right mandibular ramus and condyle, and a bone destruction with poor circumscription; defect in mandibular dentition, and moderate and severe resorption of upper mandibular alveolar bone (Fig. 53.1b).
2. Maxillofacial enhanced CT scan suggested a bone destruction in the right mandibular ramus and condyle, and a mass shadow of soft tissue, about 3.4 cm × 3.3 cm. After enhancement, the lesion was significantly enhanced with inho-

Y. He · H. S. Ong (✉) · Z. Tian · L. Zhu · X. G. Li
Department of Oral Maxillofacial-Head & Neck Oncology, Shanghai Ninth People's Hospital, Shanghai Jiao Tong University School of Medicine, Shanghai, China

Y. He (ed.), *Inflammatory and Neoplastic Diseases of Craniofacial Bones*, https://doi.org/10.1007/978-981-97-4155-7_53

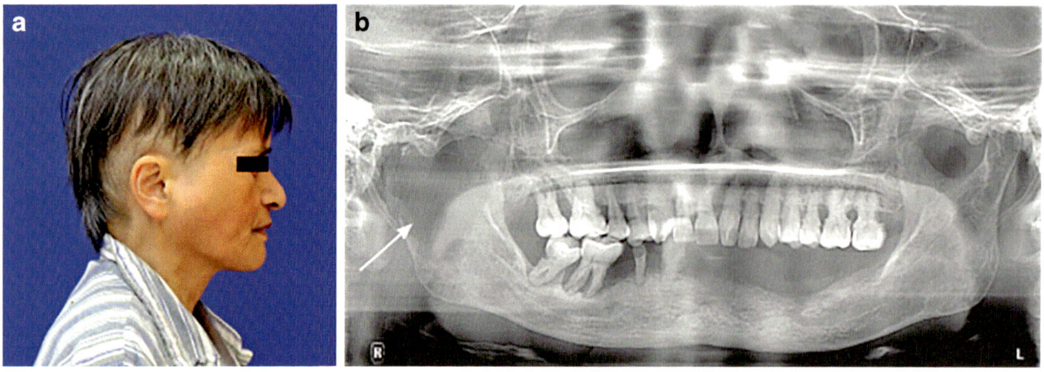

Fig. 53.1 (**a**) Asymmetrical face, with a large swelling in the right mandibular ramus region, about 3.0 cm in diameter. (**b**) Density attenuation of the right mandibular ramus and condyle, and bone destruction, with poor circumscription; mandibular dentition defect with moderate and severe resorption of alveolar bone of upper mandible (preoperative)

mogeneous density, and C− of 63 Hu and C+ of 125 Hu. There was resorption in the local alveolar bone of maxilla and mandible, and multiple osteoporosis in the cranial maxillofacial bone and cervical vertebra. Soft tissue density shadow was observed in bilateral maxillary sinus, part of ethmoid sinus and frontal sinus. No significant enlargement of cervical lymph nodes was observed bilaterally (Fig. 53.2).

[Preliminary Diagnosis] Mass of right mandible.

[Treatment] "Right segmental mandibulectomy" was performed under general anesthesia: a right mandibular incision was made, and the gingival flap was elevated for truncation of the mandible at the right mandibular angle. The diseased mandible, including the condyle, and the tumor were completely removed. Intraoperative frozen pathological examination showed small round cell hyperplasia of the "right mandible" accompanied by plasmacytoid differentiation, with lymphohematopoietic system tumor to be excluded. Ligation was performed for inferior alveolar nerve vascular bundle. The wound was rinsed and thoroughly hemostatic, negative pressure drainage tube was indwelled, and layered suture was performed to close the wound.

[Pathological Examination] Gross pathological examination revealed a fragment of tumor tissue and two fragments of hard bone tissue. The mass was tender with smooth surface, and the section was gray and yellow. Hard tissue suffered a partial defect. Microscopically, the tumor cells were distributed in sheets and arranged closely, with consistent cell morphology, round cell shape, rich and eosinophilic cytoplasm, eccentric nuclei, and rare mitosis. Besides, the tumor cells had less interstitial components and more thin-walled blood vessels. Immunohistochemical staining showed that tumor cells expressed plasma cell markers CD38 and CD138 (Fig. 53.3).

[Pathological Diagnosis] Plasma cell tumor of the "right mandible," combined with immunohistochemical results, ICD-O code: 9731/3.

[Follow-Up] The patient healed uneventfully. The postoperative 6-month follow-up exhibited no tumor recurrence, with slight mandibular deviation, and mandibular dentition loss (Fig. 53.4).

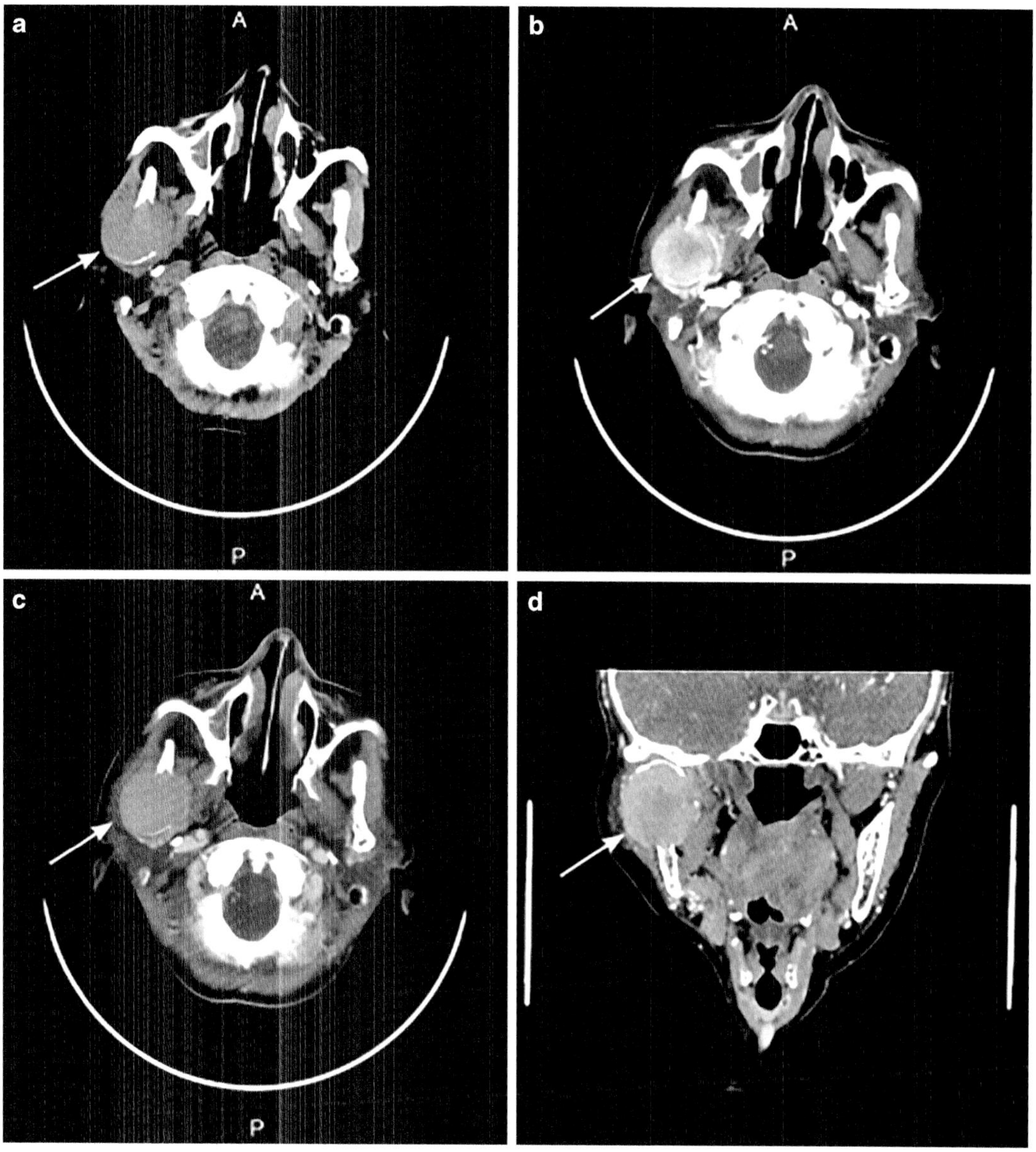

Fig. 53.2 (**a**) CT axial scan: Bone destruction in the right mandibular ramus and condyle, and mass shadow of soft tissue. (**b**, **c**) Enhanced CT axial scan: The lesions were significantly enhanced with inhomogeneous density. (**d**) CT enhanced coronal reconstruction

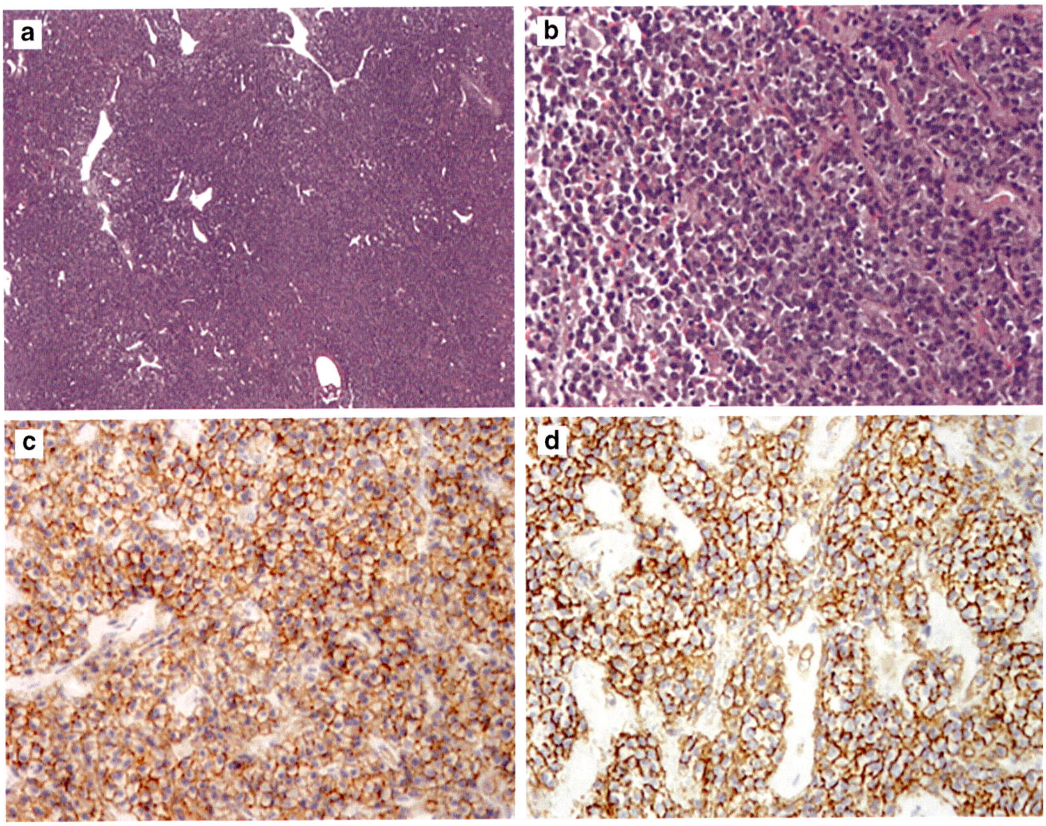

Fig. 53.3 (**a**) The tumor cells grew diffusedly in sheets with slit-like parenchyma blood (40x). (**b**) The tumor cells were homogeneous with eosinophilic cytoplasm, and eccentric nuclei (400x). (**c**, **d**) The tumor cells showed positive CD38 (**c**), CD138 (**d**) membranes (400x)

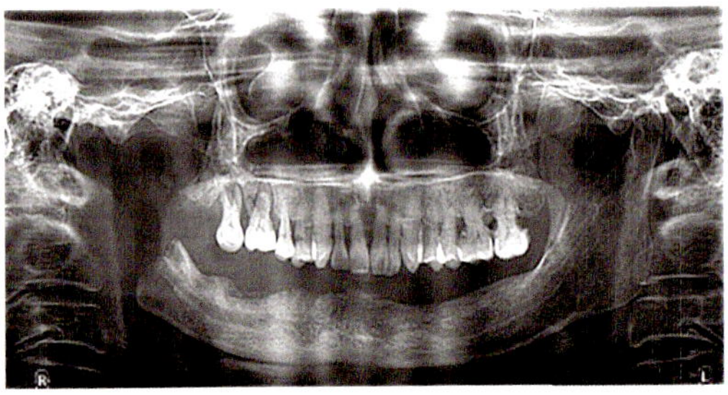

Fig. 53.4 Postoperative changes in the right mandible, with absence of ascending rami and mandibular dentition

53.2 Key Points of Diagnosis and Treatment

SPB usually presents as solitary osteolytic lesion without involvement of the bone marrow or with plasmacytosis. SPB mostly occurs in the long bones and vertebrae, but rare in the jaws, only 4%. SPB mainly affects the marrow-rich regions (mandibular body, angle, and ramus). The most common clinical symptoms of SPB in jaws are pain in jaws and teeth, limitation of jaw movement, loosening of teeth, pathological fractures, swelling, and bleeding. On X-ray, SPB appears as a well-circumscribed, unilocular or multilocular, round, translucent region with no periosteal reaction.

Differential Diagnosis

1. Cystic lesions of jaws: including ameloblastoma, odontogenic keratocyst, odontogenic jaw cyst, and aneurysmal bone cyst. These lesions tend to be maxillary swelling, with mild pain symptom. Bone white line around lesion and multiple lesion teeth or ambush

teeth existed, with no osteoporosis symptoms. Laboratory examination showed no abnormality in blood and urine.

2. Central hemangioma of jaws or arteriovenous malformation: the arteriovenous malformation of jaws is a poorly circumscribed osteoporotic region which was honeycomb or soap bubble-like translucent. The bone trabeculae have hyperplastic reactions. Thickened mandibular canal may happen in the mandibular cases if hemangioma occurs in the mandible. This method cannot be used to differentiate between these two diseases because a large amount of blood can also be extracted during SPB puncture. Imaging and DSA angiography can be used to easily identify them.
3. Metastatic cancer of jaws: rare, manifested as destructive bone resorption, but with no typical SPB lesions; mostly with clear primary focus.

SP may develop to MM, which is more likely to happen in patients with SPB than in patients with EMP. It is reported that 35–85% of SPBs will develop to MM within a few months to a few years. At present, the risk factors of SPB to MM remains unclear. Therefore, the plasma globulin and urine Bence-Jones protein levels in patients with SPB should be monitored regularly after treatment.

References

1. Agostini T, Sacco R, Bertolai R, et al. Solitary plasmacytoma of the jaw [J]. J Craniofac Surg. 2011;22(6):e2–e10.
2. Lombardo EM, Maito FLDM, Heitz C. Solitary plasmacytoma of the jaws: therapeutical considerations and prognosis based on a case reports systematic survey [J]. Braz J Otorhinolaryngol. 2018;84(6):790–8.
3. Chittemsetti S, Guttikonda VR, Sravya T, et al. Solitary plasmacytoma of mandible: a rare entity [J]. J Oral Maxillofac Pathol. 2019;23(1):136–9.
4. Tsang RW, Gospodarowicz MK, Pintilie M, et al. Solitary plasmacytoma treated with radiotherapy: impact of tumor size on outcome [J]. Int J Radiat Oncol Biol Phys. 2001;50(1):113–20.
5. Dimopoulos MA, Moulopoulos LA, Maniatis A, et al. Solitary plasmacytoma of bone and asymptomatic multiple myeloma [J]. Blood. 2000;96(6):2037–44.

Part XIII

Miscellaneous

54 Retiform Hemangioendothelioma

Yue He, Hui Shan Ong, Zhen Tian, Lin Zhu, and Zhong Long Liu

54.1 Introduction

Retiform hemangioendothelioma (RH) is a rare vascular tumor first reported by Calonje et al in 1994. RH is classified as locally aggressive or borderline vascular tumor by the International Society for the Study of Vascular Anomalies (ISSVA) in 2018 [1–5]. The mean age of the patients is 37.8 years, with the age range from 6 to 78 years. RH is more common in female, with a male to female ratio of 1:2 [4–6].

54.2 Case 97

A 56-year-old woman suffered from a painless mass in the right mandible for 3 weeks.

[History of Present Illness] The patient happened to find a painless mass in the right mandible 3 weeks ago, without other discomfort symptoms. Maxillofacial enhanced CT showed a right mandibular mass, possibly osteosarcoma. Puncture biopsy was performed at outer hospital, indicating that few lymphocytes were found, but with no tumor cells. Follow-up medical history suggested that the patient experienced numbness in the right lower lip and chin 1 year ago.

[Specialty Examination] The face was asymmetrical, with a swelling mass in the right mandibular angle and ramus. The mass was 2.5 cm × 2.5 cm in size, hard, immobile, poorly circumscribed with no tenderness, and no sense of infiltration. There was numbness in the right chin and lower lip. Bilateral temporomandibular joint was free from tenderness and snapping. There was no abnormality in mouth opening range and mouth opening pattern. Intraoral examination revealed general oral hygiene. Mandibular prosthesis was performed with fixed porcelain crown from teeth 36 to 46, and the mucosa of the gum of the right jaw was intact without obvious rupture, redness, swelling, and exudation (Fig. 54.1a, b). The tongue movement was normal. No significant enlargement of submandibular and cervical lymph nodes was observed bilaterally.

[Auxiliary Examination]

1. Panoramic radiographs suggested elliptic low-density shadow in the right mandibular angle and ramus; bone destruction, with poor circumscription locally; porcelain crown restoration in the mandible, and loss of maxillary dentition (Fig. 54.1c).
2. Maxillofacial enhanced CT scan suggested an elliptic mass in the right mandibular angle and ramus, about 2.8 cm × 2.5 cm × 3.3 cm in size,

Y. He (✉) · H. S. Ong · Z. Tian · L. Zhu · Z. L. Liu
Department of Oral Maxillofacial-Head & Neck Oncology, Shanghai Ninth People's Hospital, Shanghai Jiao Tong University School of Medicine, Shanghai, China

Y. He (ed.), *Inflammatory and Neoplastic Diseases of Craniofacial Bones*,
https://doi.org/10.1007/978-981-97-4155-7_54

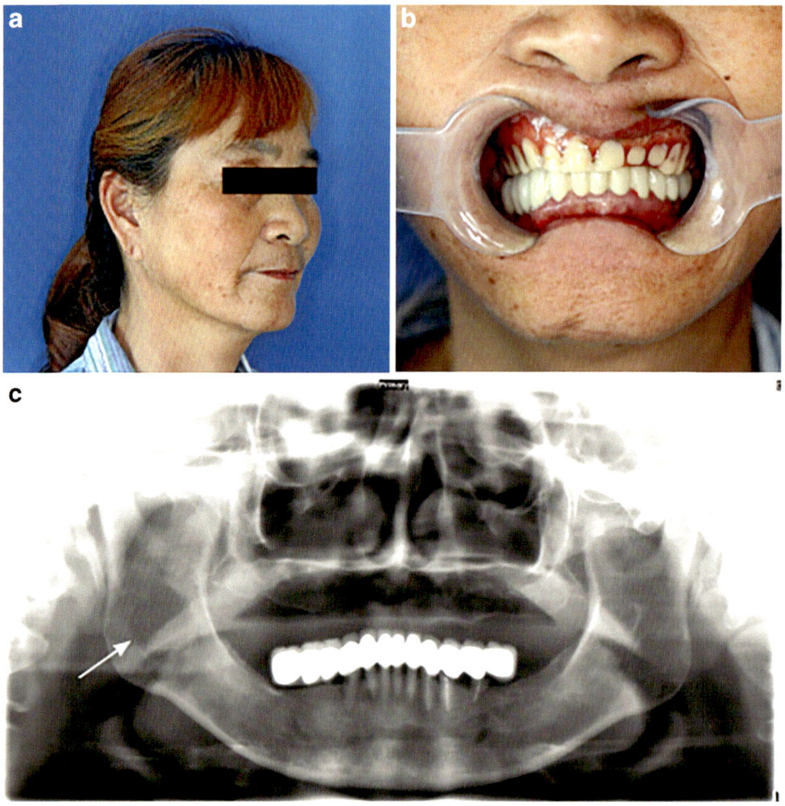

Fig. 54.1 (**a**) Distension in the left mandibular angle and masseter region. (**b**) Mandibular porcelain union crown restoratory, with intact gingival mucosa, and no obvious rupture and new organisms. (**c**) Elliptic low-density shadow in the right mandibular angle and ramus; bone destruction, with poor circumscription locally; porcelain crown restoration in the mandible, and loss of maxillary dentition

with clear circumscription. The plain CT value was about 43 Hu, and C+ was 75–191 Hu, showing a significant enhancement after enhancement. Obvious bone resorption destruction in the right mandible and radial periosteal reaction at the margin were observed, involving right mandibular nerve (with more oral metal artifacts at some levels, which was not satisfactory). No enlargement of cervical lymph nodes were observed (Fig. 54.2).

[Preliminary Diagnosis] Mass of right mandible (nature to be determined).

[Treatment] "Extensive resection of right mandibular mass" was performed under general anesthesia: an incision was made along the lower margin of the mandible for 1–2 cm, and the gingival flap was elevated for surgical exposure of the mass in the right mandibular angle and ramus. The mass was considered to be aneurysmal bone cyst. The right external carotid artery was ligated. Frozen pathological examination suggested proliferative fibers and vascular tissues in the "right mandible," which appeared as cystoid arrangement and contained deposition of hemosiderin. No positive evidence of malignancy was found (−), with pending paraffin examination. The right inferior alveolar artery was ligated and the mass was removed completely. The bone surface was smoothed. The wound was rinsed and thoroughly hemostatic, negative pressure drainage tube was indwelled, and layered suture was performed to close the wound.

[Pathological Examination] Gross pathological examination revealed clot issue, 2.7 cm × 2.2 cm × 1.3 cm, dark red, with grayish-yellow cystoid tissue inside. The microscopic examination showed that the tumor was poorly circumscribed, thin blood vessels interwoven into a network, the lumen was lined with monolayer endothelial cells, with sparse cytoplasm and nucleus located apically in a characteristic hobnail pattern. Lymphocyte infiltration was seen in the vascular lumen and stroma. Local thick-walled vessels dilated, presenting venous malformations (Fig. 54.3).

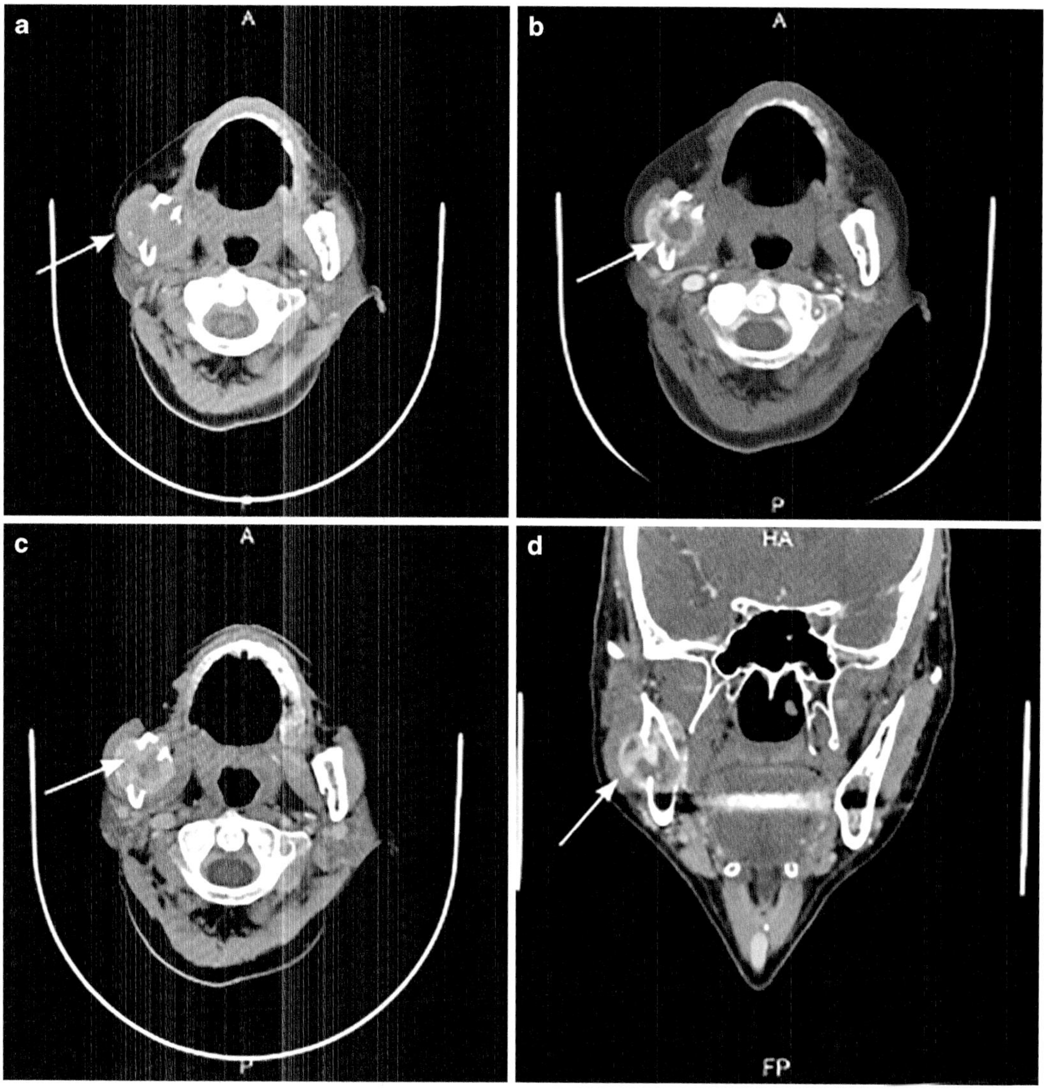

Fig. 54.2 (**a**) Plain CT axial scan: Elliptic mass in the right mandibular angle and ramus, with clear circumscription. Obvious bone resorption destruction in the right mandible and radial periosteal reaction at the margin. (**b**, **c**) Enhanced CT axial scan: marked enhancement of the lesion. (**d**) Enhanced CT coronal reconstruction

[Pathological Diagnosis] Vascular tumour of the "right mandible," intermediate type, prone to retiform hemangioendothelioma, ICD code: M9712/3.

[Follow-Up] The patient healed uneventfully. The postoperative 2-year follow-up exhibited no tumor recurrence and no special abnormalities in the operative region (Fig. 54.4).

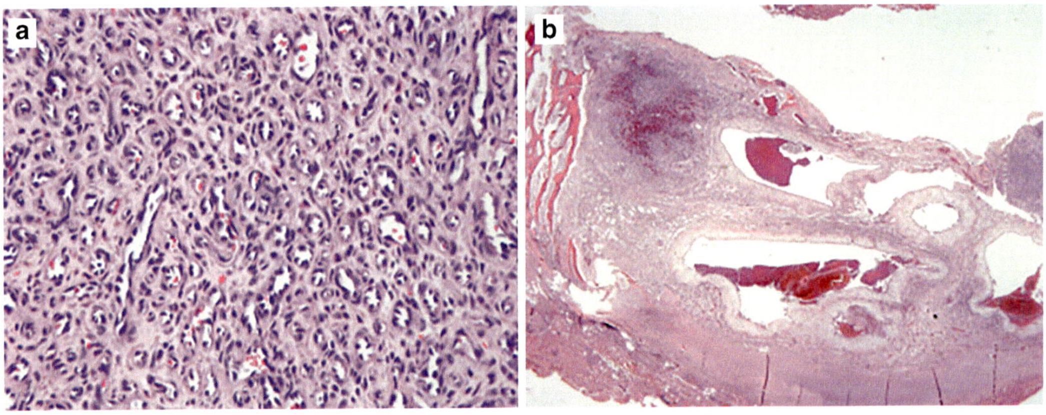

Fig. 54.3 (**a**) The vascular lumen was lined with monolayer hobnail endothelial cells (400x). (**b**) Local vascular hyperplasia, malformed distention, thick vascular wall, venous malformation (20x)

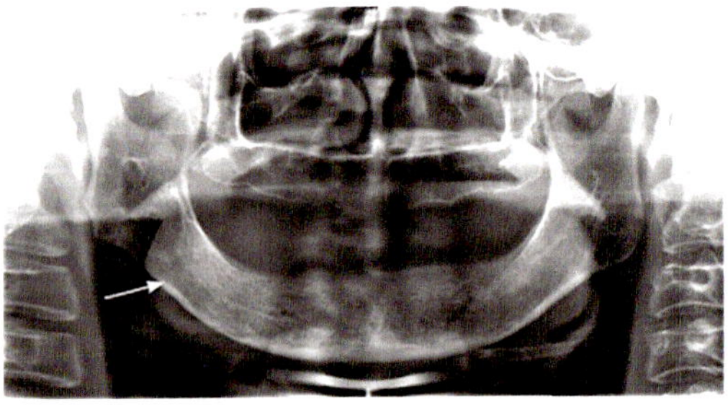

Fig. 54.4 Postoperative changes of the right mandibular angle and ramus, with dental erosion, upper mandibular dentition loss, and no obvious coarse margin

54.3 Key Points of Diagnosis and Treatment

Diagnosis Only about 50 cases of RH have been reported. The patient in this case is the first case of RH in the mandible. Most RHs originate from blood vessels in superficial parts of the body, including skin or subcutaneous tissue. It is difficult to make a definite diagnosis of RH clinically and needs to be differentiated from osteosarcoma of the mandible, aneurysmal bone cysts, and intra-maxillary arteriovenous malformations. Histopathological examination is the only reliable method to diagnose RH. RH pathological characteristics fall in between benign and malignant hemangiomas, and present as a large number of slender and dendritic thin-walled vascular channels intertwined in a network, similar to normal testicular tissue. Lymphocytic infiltration is common, while cellular anisotropy and nuclear schizophrenia are rare. Immunohistochemistry was positive for CD31, CD34, and VIII factor-associated antigen in the endothelial cells and negative for SMA in the vascular wall.

Treatment Now, there is a lack of standard therapy for RH. The existing treatment options include radiotherapy, chemotherapy, radiotherapy combined with chemotherapy, and surgery. For the first patient with RH in the jaws, surgical curettage was performed, and the postoperative 2-year follow-up exhibited no signs of recurrence. However, it is reported that RH is a recrudescent tumor, and the suitability of curettage for patients with RH remains to be studied.

References

1. Calonje E, Fletcher CD, Wilson-Jones E, et al. Retiform hemangioendothelioma: a distinctive form of low-grade angiosarcoma delineated in a series of 15 cases [J]. Am J Surg Pathol. 1994;18:115–25.
2. Jiang J, Li X, Zhu F, et al. Retiform hemangioendothelioma of the mandible: a case report [J]. Oral Oncol. 2020;17:105120.

3. Nobeyama Y, Ishiuji Y, Nakagawa H. Retiform hemangioendothelioma treated with conservative therapy: report of a case and review of the literature [J]. Int J Dermatol. 2016;55(2):238–43.
4. Hirsh AZ, Yan W, Wei L, et al. Unresectable retiform hemangioendothelioma treated with external beam radiation therapy and chemotherapy: a case report and review of the literature [J]. Sarcoma. 2010:756246.
5. Kim IK, Cho HY, Jung BS, et al. Retiform hemangioendothelioma in the infratemporal fossa and buccal area: a case report and literature review [J]. J Korean Assoc Oral Maxillofac Surg. 2016;42(5):307–14.
6. Requena L, Kutzner H. Hemangioendothelioma [J]. Semin Diagn Pathol. 2013;30(1):29–44.

Langerhans Cell Histiocytosis

55

Yue He, Hui Shan Ong, Zhen Tian, Lin Zhu, and Jing Jing Sun

55.1 Introduction

Langerhans cell histiocytosis (LCH) is a disease characterized by an abnormal clonal proliferation and infiltration of dendritic cells [1–3]. The report on the study of Hand-Schuller-Christian Syndrome, Letterer-Siwe disease, and eosinophilic granuloma was published by Schuller and Christian in 1915–1920. Despite great difference in clinical manifestations, the three diseases show the same microcellular origin under microscope and ultrastructure. LCH may occur at any age, with the peak age of 1–4 years old. The incidence of LCH in children is (2–9)/1,000,000. LCH is more common in male than female, with a male to female ratio of about (1.2–1.4):1. The pathogenesis of LCH remains unknown, and its clinical manifestations are heterogeneous [4–6]. Moreover, it can invade multiple organs and systems of the whole body, even threatening life in severe cases.

Y. He (✉) · H. S. Ong · Z. Tian · L. Zhu · J. J. Sun
Department of Oral Maxillofacial-Head & Neck Oncology, Shanghai Ninth People's Hospital, Shanghai Jiao Tong University School of Medicine, Shanghai, China

55.2 Case 98

A 12-year-old boy suffered from a left mandibular swelling with pain for more than 1 month.

[History of Present Illness] The patient developed swelling and pain in the left mandible with unknown predisposing factors more than 1 month ago, with no symptoms such as restricted opening of the mouth or numbness of the lower lip. Anti-inflammatory symptomatic treatment did not lead to an obvious relief. Maxillofacial Plain CT scan showed a bone destruction from the body to the left mandibular angle with possible pathological fracture.

[Specialty Examination] The face was asymmetrical, and the left mandible was swollen, which was intact and normal in color and temperature, with obvious tenderness. The bony protuberance was accessible to the left mandibular angle, about 2.5 cm × 2.5 cm in size, poorly circumscribed, with local cortical bone defect. There was no abnormality in mouth opening range and mouth opening pattern. Intraoral examination revealed permanent dentition, eruption of teeth 36 and 37, probing (−), percussion (−), loosening (−). A buccal vestibular groove bulge was observed, with intact

Y. He (ed.), *Inflammatory and Neoplastic Diseases of Craniofacial Bones*,
https://doi.org/10.1007/978-981-97-4155-7_55

mucosa and no obvious redness, swelling, and exudation. One enlarged lymph node was seen in the left submaxillary region, about 1.5 cm × 1.0 cm in size, with clear circumscription, good motion, smooth surface, and no tenderness.

[Auxiliary Examination]

1. Panoramic radiographs suggested a bone destruction in the left mandibular body, angle and ramus, irregular and poorly circumscribed, involving 36, 37 tooth roots and 38 dental germ (Fig. 55.1).
2. Maxillofacial enhanced MRI suggested a bone destruction of the left mandibular body to the ascending rami, irregular mass shadow, isosignal on T1WI, mixed high signal on T2WI, about 3.2 cm × 2.6 cm × 3.2 cm in size, poorly circumscribed, uneven enhancement after enhancement. ADC was about (0.8–1.8) × 10^{-3} mm^2/s, TIC curve was flat. The swelling involved the left masseter muscle, with patchy high signal intensity and uneven enhancement on T2WI. No skull base bone destruction was observed. Several lymph node shadows less than 1 cm in diameter were observed in the submandibular, upper and middle neck, and postpharyngeal region bilaterally (Fig. 55.2).
3. Maxillofacial enhanced CT scan suggested a bone protuberance in the left mandible body and ramus. An irregular mass shadow was observed, which was poorly circumscribed, and 1.7 cm × 2.6 cm × 3.5 cm in size. Mild enhancement, with C− 48 Hu and C+ 62 Hu. Local discontinuity of the marginal cortical bone was observed, with obvious periosteum reaction. The lesion is poorly circumscribed with the surrounding masticatory muscle. There was no obvious abnormality in skull base structure. No significantly enlarged lymph nodes were found in the neck (Fig. 55.3).

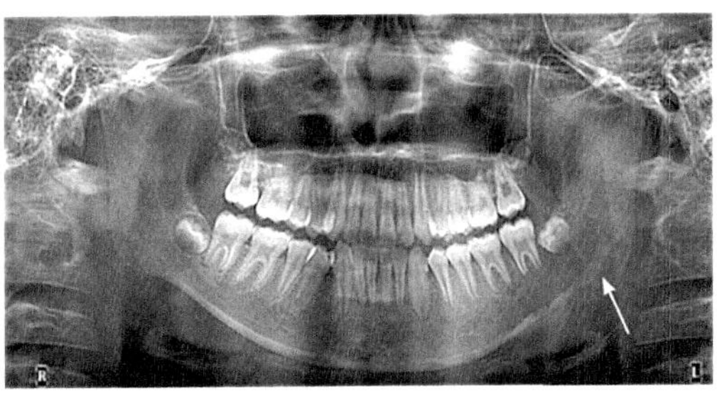

Fig. 55.1 Bone destruction in the left mandibular body, angle and ramus, irregular and poorly circumscribed, involving 36, 37 tooth roots and 38 dental germ

[Preliminary Diagnosis] Mass of left mandible (nature to be determined).

[Treatment]

1. "Left mandibular mass excision biopsy with extraction of tooth 37" was performed under general anesthesia: a gingival margin incision was made and the gingival flap was elevated for extraction of tooth 37. The tumor was found to be solid. Intraoperative frozen pathological examination suggested diffuse monocytic cells and a small number of cytomegalosis infiltration in the left mandible, with Langerhans cell histiocytosis or giant cell lesion to be excluded, and paraffin and enzyme labeling in the pending. The operative region was hemostatic, and layered suture was performed to close the wound.
2. Paraffin and enzyme labeling results indicated Langerhans cell histiocytosis. After MDT consultation, intensity modulated radiation therapy was performed in the radiotherapy department: left mandibular mass region DT 30 Gy/10 Fx; subclinical region DT 20 Gy/10 Fx.

[Pathological Examination] Gross pathological examination revealed a fragment of tissue, 0.8 cm × 0.4 cm × 0.3 cm in size, grayish yellow. Microscopic examination showed that the lesions were composed of Langerhans cells, histiocytes, eosinophils, and other inflammatory cells. Langerhans cells were arranged sparsely, with eosinophilic cytoplasm and characteristic nuclear grooves. Eosinophils, lymphocytes, and multinucleated giant cells appeared. Langerhans cells showed positive expression of S100 and CD1a (Fig. 55.4).

[Pathological Diagnosis] Langerhans cell histiocytosis of the "left mandible," ICD code: D76.003.

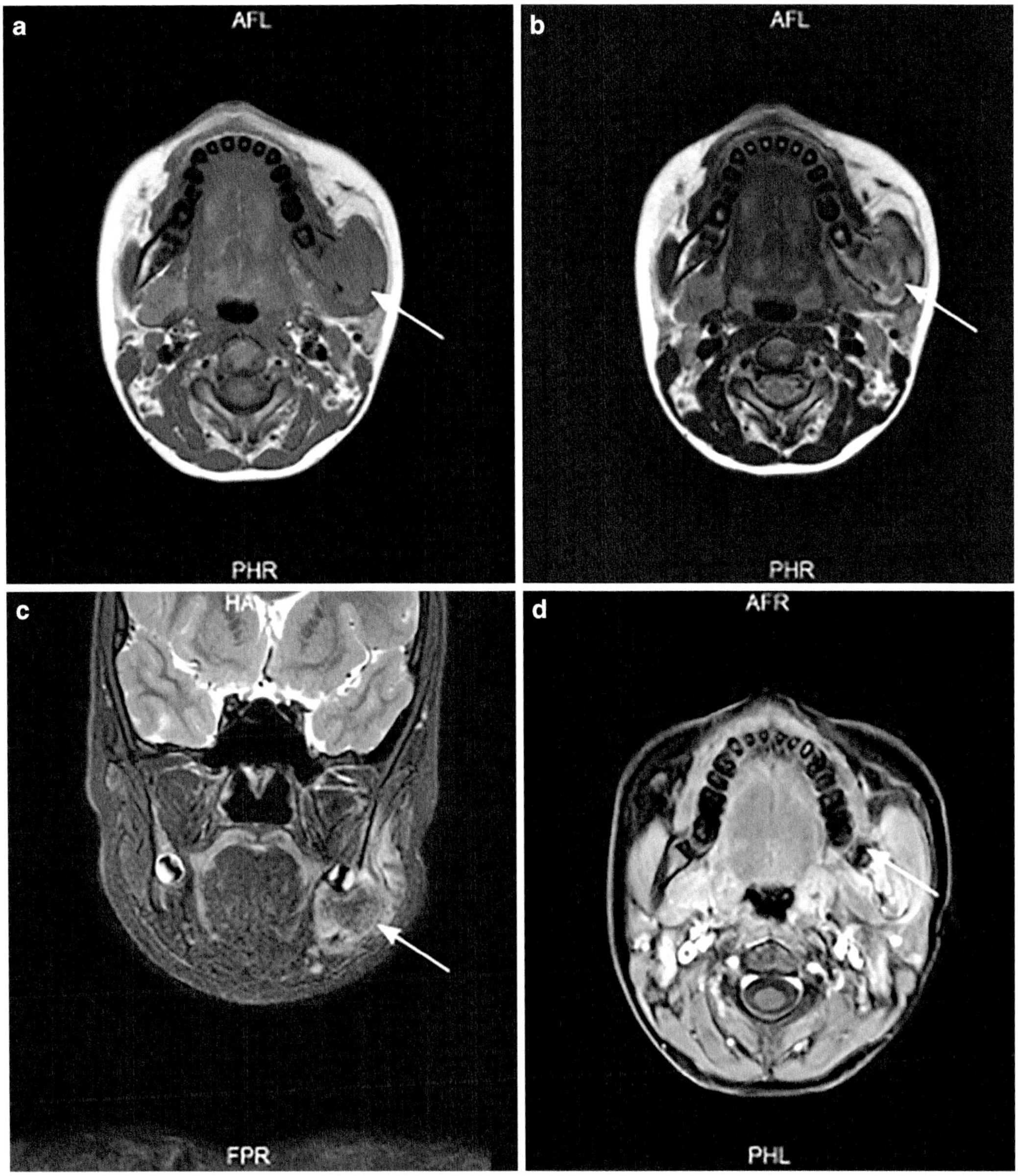

Fig. 55.2 (**a**) MRI T1WI axial scan: Bone destruction in the left mandibular ramus, poorly circumscribed, with abnormal soft tissue signal. (**b**) Axial scan on T2WI: mixed signal of the lesion. (**c**) Coronal scan on T2WI: left masseter muscle involved swelling with high signal. (**d**) Enhanced axial scan on T1WI: heterogeneous enhancement of the lesion

[Follow-Up] The patient's soft tissue mass was significantly reduced after radiotherapy, and the further consultation 3 months later exhibited face symmetry, with a decrease in the range of low density shadow in the left mandible, and no abnormality in mouth opening range and mouth opening pattern (Fig. 55.5).

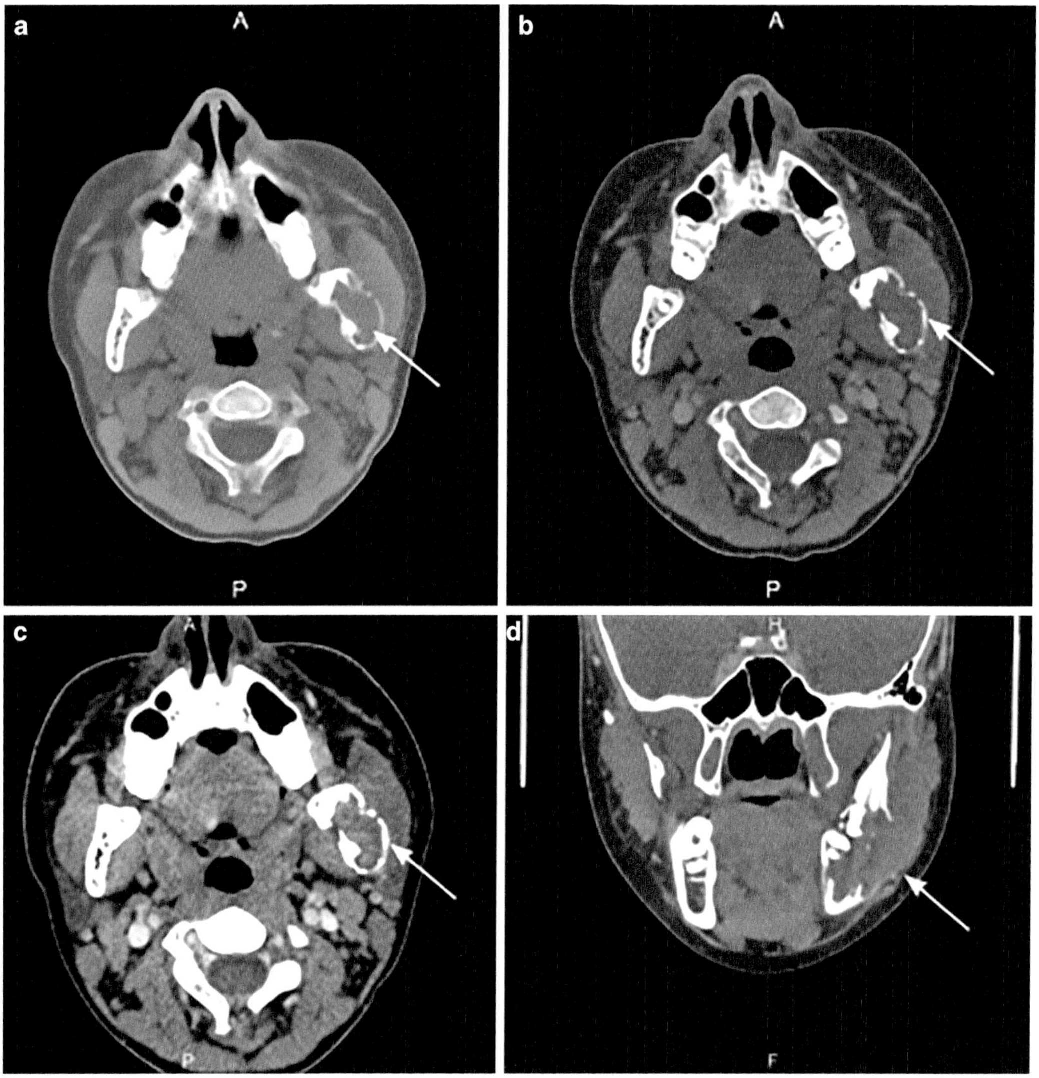

Fig. 55.3 (**a**) Plain CT axial scan: Expansive destruction of bone from the left mandibular body to the ascending ramus with soft tissue mass. (**b**, **c**) Enhanced CT axial scan: mild enhancement of the mass. (**d**) Enhanced CT coronal reconstruction: Poorly circumscribed between lesion and surrounding masticatory muscle

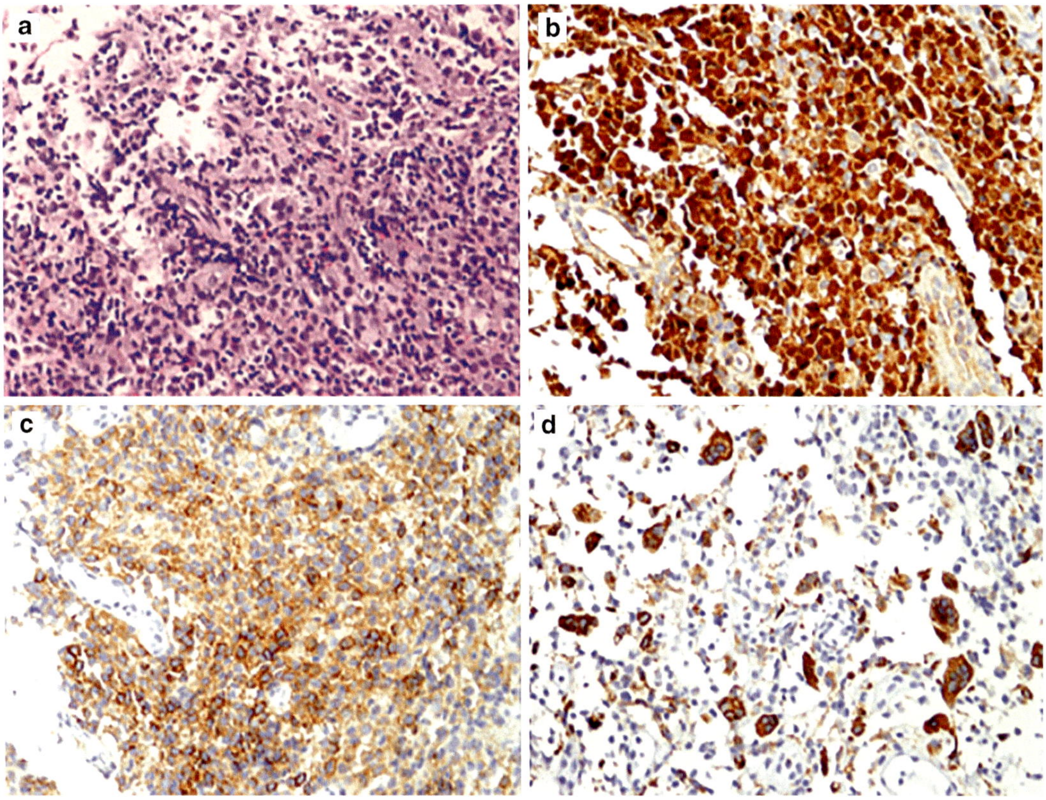

Fig. 55.4 (**a**) The lesions were composed of Langerhans cells, eosinophils, lymphocytes, etc. (400x). (**b**, **c**) Positive expression S100 (**b**) and CD1a (**c**) in tumor cells (40000x). (**d**) Positive expression of PGM1 in histiocytes and multinucleated giant cells (400x)

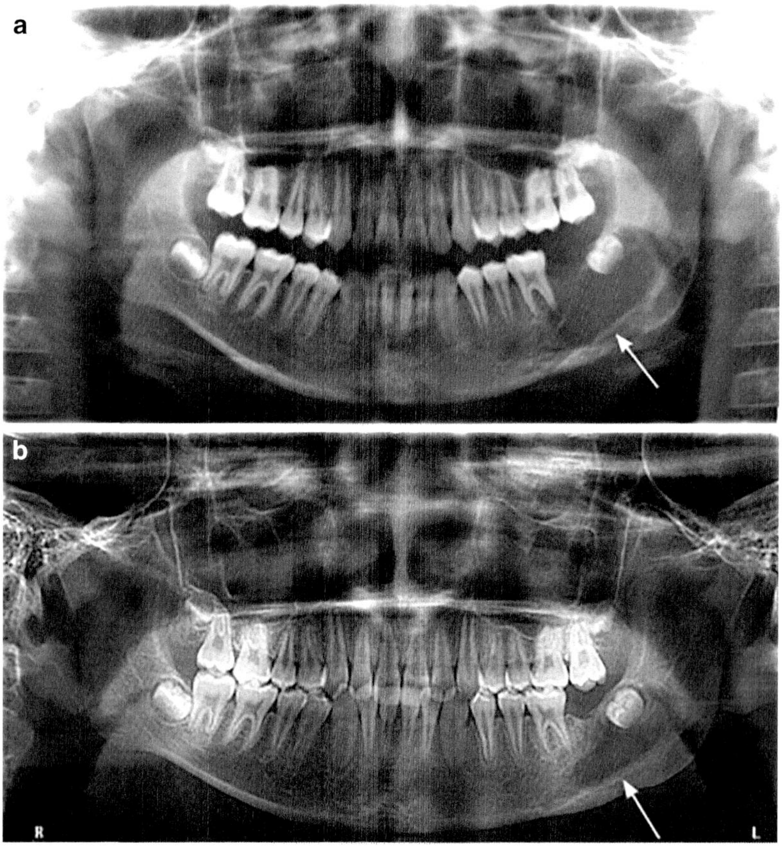

Fig. 55.5 (**a**) Review of panoramic radiograph after radiotherapy. (**b**) The range of low-density shadow of the left mandible decreased significantly 3 months after the end of radiotherapy

55.3 Key Points of Diagnosis and Treatment

Diagnosis Among the three manifestations of LCH, the most common one is eosinophilic granuloma, accounting for about 50–60%, which mainly manifests as intraosseous lesion with good prognosis. In bone tissue, LCH may be solitary (70–75%) or multiple (25–30%), and mainly affects males, older children, and young adults, aged 10–30 years. LCH that occurs in the oral cavity usually causes gingivitis, tooth loosening, and nonhealing of the wound after tooth extraction. On X-ray, bone resorption is the manifestation of jaw bone, regardless of solitary or multiple lesions. After resorption, teeth are floating with clear circumscription. LCH that occurs in long bones may cause pathologic fractures. In addition to the jaws and long bones, LCH often involves the skull, ribs, spine, pelvis, and scapula, and the masses are often nodular in shape. The X-ray film shows a circular bone defect with clear circumscription, often accompanied by pain and swelling and the invasion of the corresponding parts. The definitive diagnosis of LCH requires the observation of ultrastructure of Birbeck's particles or positive CD1α or Langerhans on immunohistochemistry.

Treatment For solitary LCH of the jaws, lesion excision may be performed, and the patients who are not suitable for surgery can be treated with radiotherapy. For patients with multifocal LCH, systemic therapy is required. Now, there is a lack of standard therapy, but the combination of vincristine and prednisolone is a recommended option. In recent years, cases of targeted therapy for LCH have been reported. Imatinib is a tyrosine kinase inhibitor that targets receptors expressed in LCH and is reported to be effective in patients with refractory LCH. Vemurafenib (a BRAF inhibitor) has shown efficacy in LCH patients with BRFAF-V6(8)E mutation, but serious adverse events have been reported, including the development of squamous cell carcinoma. What's more, early recurrence appears in most patients after discontinuation of therapy. Targeted therapy for LCH remains to be further studied.

References

1. El Demellawy D, Young JL, de Nanassy J, et al. Langerhans cell histiocytosis: a comprehensive review [J]. Pathology. 2015;47(4):294–301.
2. Zinn DJ, Chakraborty R, Allen CE. Langerhans cell histiocytosis: emerging insights and clinical implications [J]. Oncology (Williston Park). 2016;30(2):122–32, 39.
3. Horibe K, Saito AM, Takimoto T, et al. Incidence and survival rates of hematological malignancies in Japanese children and adolescents (2006–2010): based on registry data from the Japanese society of pediatric hematology [J]. Int J Hematol. 2013;98(1):74–88.
4. Cardoso E, Mercier T, Wagner AD, et al. Quantification of the next-generation oral anti-tumor drugs dabrafenib, trametinib, vemurafenib, cobimetinib, pazopanib, regorafenib and two metabolites in human plasma by liquid chromatography-tandem mass spectrometry [J]. J Chromatogr B Analyt Technol Biomed Life Sci. 2018;15(1083):124–36.
5. Heritier S, Helias-Rodzewicz Z, Lapillonne H, et al. Circulating cell-free BRAFV600E as a biomarker in children with Langerhans cell histiocytosis [J]. Br J Haematol. 2017;178(3):457–67.
6. Kolenova A, Schwentner R, Jug G, et al. Targeted inhibition of the MAPK pathway: emerging salvage option for progressive life-threatening multisystem LCH [J]. Blood Adv. 2017;1(6):352–6.

Osteopetrosis

56

Yue He, Hui Shan Ong, Zhen Tian, Lin Zhu, and Zhou Zhu

56.1 Introduction

Osteosclerosis, also known as marble bone disease or Albers-Schonberg disease, is a genetic bone disease characterized by increased bone density and impaired resorption of osteoclasts. It can be divided into autosomal dominant osteosclerosis (ADO), autosomal recessive osteosclerosis (ARO), and rare X-linked osteosclerosis (XLO) according to clinical manifestations and causative genes [1–6]. The average incidence is 5/100000 for ADO, 1/250000 for ARO, and even lower for XLO. Osteosclerosis has extensive heterogeneity in clinical features: some patients may present with fatal clinical manifestations such as anemia, pancytopenia, septicopyemia, and secondary hepatosplenomegaly; some patients may also be asymptomatic or have mild symptoms, which can only be detected by skeletal imaging [3–6]. Imaging diagnosis is mainly used, and further typing can also be achieved in combination with genetic testing. Treatment requires a multidisciplinary approach for symptomatic treatment of some serious complications. The main treatment options are vitamin D medication, steroids, and bone marrow transplantation, etc.

Y. He (✉) · H. S. Ong · Z. Tian · L. Zhu · Z. Zhu
Department of Oral Maxillofacial-Head & Neck Oncology, Shanghai Ninth People's Hospital, Shanghai Jiao Tong University School of Medicine, Shanghai, China

56.2 Case 99

A 12-year-old girl suffered from a swelling in the left mandible for 6 months.

[History of Present Illness] Half a year ago, the patient underwent orthodontic treatment for irregular dentition in a hospital. Intraoral examination suggested a swelling in the left mandible, with no discomfort symptoms such as numbness of the lower lip. CT examination revealed widespread abnormal density in the left mandible. Panoramic radiographs showed an increase in the density of the left mandible.

[Specialty Examination] The face was slightly asymmetrical, with a mild swelling in the left mandible. There was no abnormality in mouth opening range and mouth opening pattern. Intraoral examination revealed mixed dentition. The 31–36 buccal vestibular groove was slightly swollen, which was poorly circumscribed, hard, and no tenderness. The lower lip had no obvious numbness. (Fig. 56.1a, b). No abnormal enlargement of submandibular and cervical lymph nodes was observed bilaterally.

Y. He (ed.), *Inflammatory and Neoplastic Diseases of Craniofacial Bones*,
https://doi.org/10.1007/978-981-97-4155-7_56

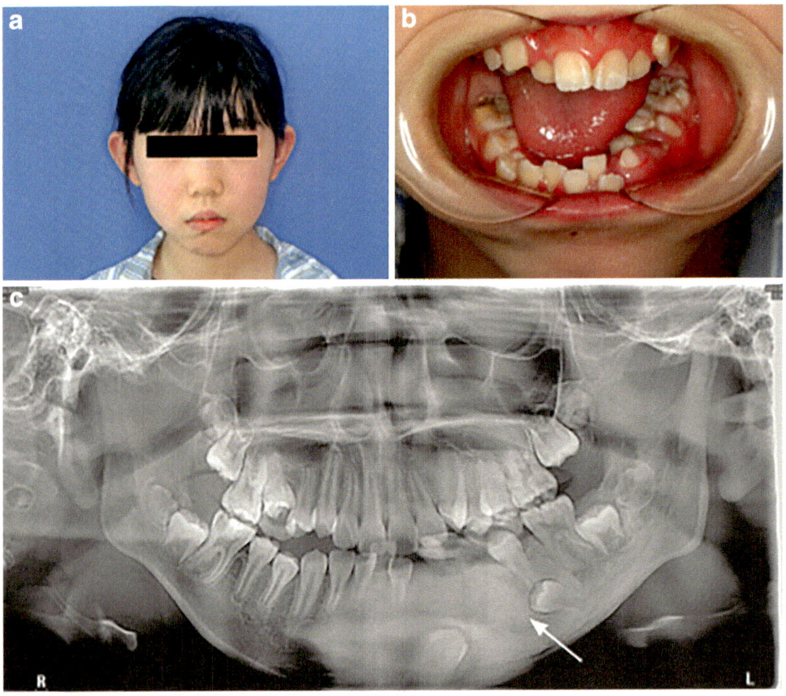

Fig. 56.1 (**a**) Facial asymmetry, slight distention of the left mandible. (**b**) Mixed dentition, left mandibular vestibular sulcus slightly distended. (**c**) Abnormal higher density of the left mandible, not well-circumscribed

[Auxiliary Examination]

1. Panoramic radiographs suggested an abnormal increase in bone density of the left mandible, with poor circumscription (Fig. 56.1c).
2. Maxillofacial enhanced CT scan suggested an expansive change of bone in the left mandible and an inhomogeneous increase in the density from the left mandibular body to the condyle, with ground-glass appearance partially. No obvious abnormal thickening or enhancement was observed in the adjacent soft tissues. An enlargement of left retropharyngeal and cervical lymph nodes was observed (possible reactive hyperplasia) (Fig. 56.2).

[Preliminary Diagnosis] Osteosclerosis of left mandible.

[Treatment] "Segmentectomy of the left mandible with fibular flap transfer" was performed under general anesthesia: an incision was made along the lower margin of the mandible for 1–2 cm, and the gingival flap was elevated. As per the preoperative osteotomy guide (Virtual Surgical Planning), the left mandible was osteotomise at 43 and left sigmoid notch, the mandibular angle can be preserved. The left peroneal muscle flap with vascular pedicle was prepared. The peroneal bone about 12 cm long was cut according to the preoperatively designed peroneal osteotomy plate. The fibular flap was taken and reconstructed to restore mandibular continuity and occlusal relationship. Peroneal, facial, and lateral cervical arteriovenous anastomosis was performed. The wound was rinsed and thoroughly hemostatic, negative pressure drainage tube was indwelled, and the wound was closed with layered sutures (Fig. 56.3).

[Pathological Examination] Gross pathological examination revealed a part of the mandibular tissue, 8 cm × 6 cm × 3 cm, with local bone slightly swollen and hard. Microscopic examination showed the lamellar bone was hyperplastic and compact, the bone marrow cavity got smaller, with a lack of fibroadipose bone marrow between the bone tissues (Fig. 56.4).

[Pathological Diagnosis] Left mandibular osteopetrosis.

[Follow-Up] The patient healed uneventfully. The postoperative 6-month follow-up exhibited satisfactory reconstruction of the mandible and good recovery of contralateral occlusal relationship.

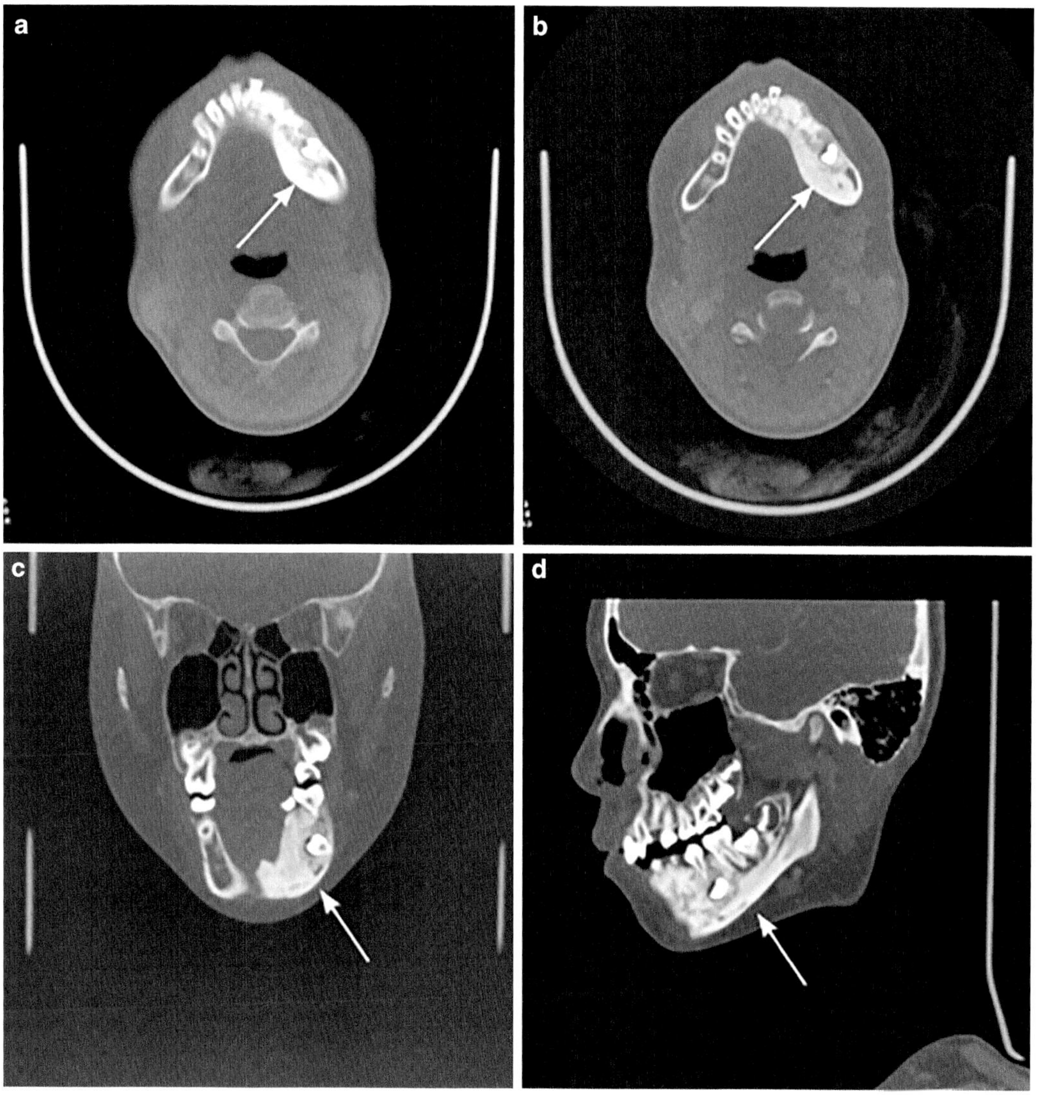

Fig. 56.2 (**a**) CT axial scan: bony expansion of the left mandible, heterogeneous increase in the density of the left mandible from the body to the condyle, with ground-glass attenuation seen in part. (**b**) Enhanced CT axial scan: no abnormal thickening of adjacent soft tissue, and no abnormal hypodensity. (**c**, **d**) Coronal and sagittal reconstruction images

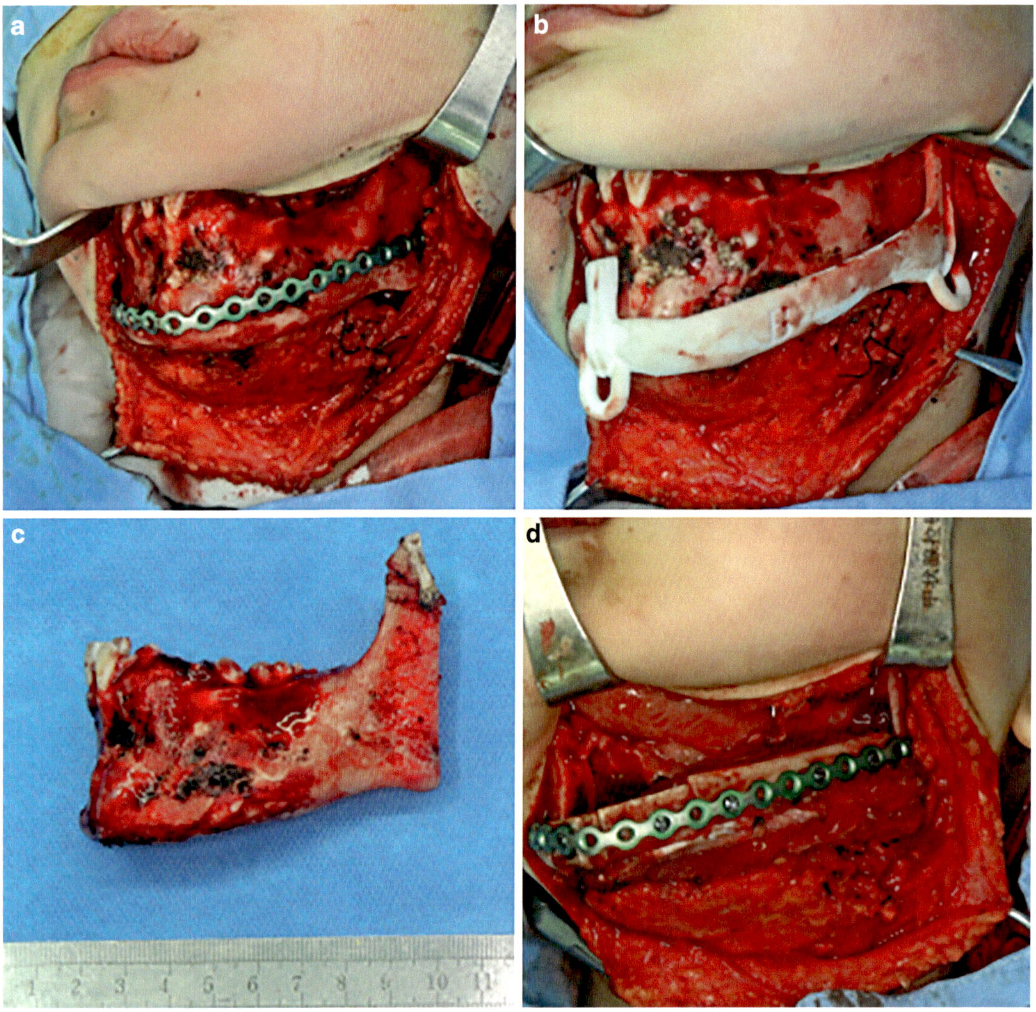

Fig. 56.3 (**a**) Pre-bending reconstruction of titanium plate. (**b**) Design the osteotomy line according to the digital model. (**c**) Pathological mandible in vitro. (**d**) Fibular reconstruction to restore mandibular continuity

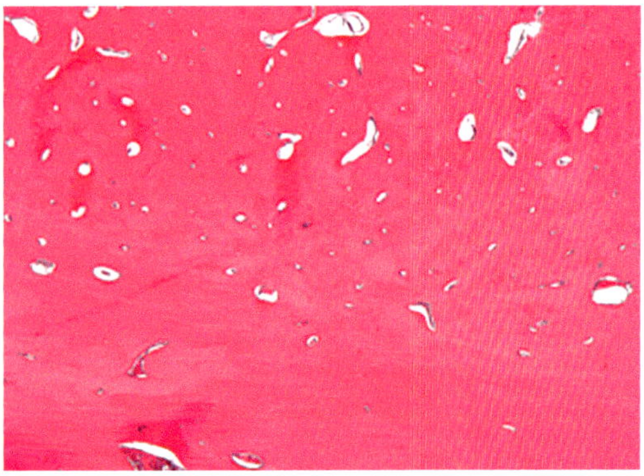

Fig. 56.4 Compact bone tissue, small bone marrow cavity, lack of normal bone marrow tissue (4x)

56.3 Key Points of Diagnosis and Treatment

Osteopetrosis is a hereditary bone disease caused by osteoclast resorption dysfunction. Normal human bone tissue maintains a dynamic balance between osteoclasts and osteoblasts through bone resorption/osteogenesis. Imbalance between osteoclasts and osteoblasts, such as deficiency of cytokines M-CSF and RANKL, will lead to abnormal bone disease. Currently, the causative genes for osteosclerosis have been found to be *a3-V-ATPase, CLCN7, OSTM1, PLEKHM1, CAII, RANKL, RANK*, etc. Pathogenic mechanisms vary from causative genes.

Clinical Manifestations Osteopetrosis is clinically manifested as highly heterogeneous, with some patients presenting fatal clinical signs, such as anemia, hematopenia, sepsis, and secondary hepatosplenomegaly. Some patients may also have mild or no symptoms. In the oral and maxillofacial region, patients with osteopetrosis usually have specific clinical manifestations, such as dental retardation, crowded dentition, hypocalcemia, maxillofacial deformity, peculiar facial features, and osteomyelitis of the jaws.

Diagnosis and Differential Diagnosis Osteopetrosis diagnosis is mainly based on imaging data, which can be combined with gene detection to distinguish it from other osteosclerotic diseases with different complications. Osteopetrosis should be differentiated from cementoma, ossifying fibroma, fibrodysplasia, and other jaw diseases.

Treatment Osteopetrosis is a systemic bone metabolism disease, and therefore it should be treated with the patient's systemic condition taken into account. According to the expert consensus published by UCLA in 2017, the following treatments are recommended. (1) Ca and vitamin D are used as first-line medicines to treat hypocalcemia with secondary hyperparathyroidism. (2) Red blood cell transfusion is adopted after consultation with the hematology department when symptomatic anemia and low hemoglobin are present to the point of transfusion indication. (3) IFNγ-1b may be used as an experimental treatment for osteopetrosis. Current studies show that osteoclasts bone resorption rely on superoxide and osteoclasts in patients with osteopetrosis exhibit a defect in the formation of oxygen free radicals, and the use of IFNγ-1b in the treatment of chronic sarcoidosis has shown an increase in superoxide and a clinical improvement in patients. Therefore, researchers conducted a clinical trial of IFNγ in patients with pediatric osteopetrosis and results showed an increase in leukocyte superoxide dismutase activity and a decrease in trabecular bone size after 18 months of treatment. However, due to limited clinical experience with such therapy, further clinical trials are needed to elucidate the role of IFNγ-1b in patients with non-pediatric osteopetrosis. (4) Cortisol hormones may be used as second-line therapy in patients who are not candidates for bone marrow transplantation. (5) Bone marrow transplantation: Being younger than 1 year of age and loss of bone marrow function are the primary indications for consideration of bone marrow transplantation. Gene detection for relevant mutations may suggest a clinical prognosis for bone marrow transplantation, but in general, bone marrow transplantation is not a common treatment modality. Multidisciplinary consultation is needed to evaluate patients prior to bone marrow transplantation. (6) Osteomyelitis of the jaws may be secondary to osteopetrosis in the maxillofacial region, often occurring in the mandible, usually caused by post-extraction infection. Antibiotic treatment and surgical debridement are often used in this group of patients. Surgery is not the standard therapy for osteosclerosis, but for patients with maxillofacial deformity that seriously affects the appearance and function of the jaws, surgical resection with simultaneous peroneal muscle flap restoration is a good therapeutic strategy.

References

1. Key LL, Ries WL, Rodriguiz RM, et al. Recombinant human interferon gamma therapy for osteopetrosis [J]. J Pediatr. 1992;121(1):119.
2. Frattini A, Vezzoni P, Villa A. The genetics of dominant osteopetrosis [J]. Drug Discov Today Dis Mech. 2005;2(4):503–9.
3. Balemans W, Wesenbeeck LV, Hul WVJCTI. A clinical and molecular overview of the human osteopetroses [J]. Calcif Tissue Int. 2005;77(5):263–74.
4. Davachi B, Nemati S, Johari M. Dental radiographic findings of malignant osteopetrosis: report of four cases [J]. Iran J Radiol. 2009;41(3)
5. Sobacchi C, Schulz A, Coxon FP, et al. Osteopetrosis: genetics, treatment and new insights into osteoclast function [J]. Nat Rev Endocrinol. 2013;9(9):522–36.
6. Wu CC, Econs MJ, Dimeglio LA, et al. Diagnosis and management of osteopetrosis: consensus guidelines from the osteopetrosis working group [J]. J Clin Endocrinol Metab. 2017;102(9):3111–23.

57 Hemophilic Pseudotumor

Yue He, Hui Shan Ong, Zhen Tian, Lin Zhu, and Jing Jing Sun

57.1 Introduction

Hemophilia is a hereditary disease caused by a deficiency of coagulation factors VIII or IX. Hemophilic pseudotumor is a rare but serious complication of hemophilia, which often occurs in femur, pelvis, iliac bone, and other parts of the body, but rare in skull and jawbone [1–7]. Its main clinical manifestations are repeated bleeding in extra-articular bone or soft tissue, resulting in intra-articular blood accumulation, and the continuous enlargement of the capsule cavity to compress and destroy the adjacent tissues; patients usually have no obvious symptoms in the early stage, but after the involvement of the adjacent tissues, specific symptoms appear. The clinical diagnosis is based on the history of traumatic bleeding and X-ray, ultrasonography, CT, and MRI examinations. Treatment includes factor replacement therapy, radiotherapy, and surgery (including local suction/drainage, surgical resection, and amputation).

Y. He (✉) · H. S. Ong · Z. Tian · L. Zhu · J. J. Sun
Department of Oral Maxillofacial-Head & Neck Oncology, Shanghai Ninth People's Hospital, Shanghai Jiao Tong University School of Medicine, Shanghai, China

57.2 Case 100

A 5-year-old boy suffered from left facial swelling for 1 month.

[History of Present Illness] One month ago, the patient presented with left facial enlargement with no pathogenic factor, which gradually aggravated, no obvious symptoms of pain and discomfort, no restriction of mouth opening, difficulty in eating, and other abnormalities. CT examination revealed bone destruction on the left mandible, possibly ameloblastoma. The patient was advised to transfer to a higher level hospital for treatment.

[Past Medical History] History of hemophilia A, controlled with factor VIII when bruising occurs.

[Specialty Examination] Bilateral asymmetry of the maxillofacial region was observed, with obvious swelling and distention of the left face and submandibular region, intact surface skin, color, and skin temperature. Palpation suggested the bone of the mandible was swollen and hard in texture. There was no abnormality in mouth opening range and mouth opening pattern. Intraoral examination revealed mixed dentition, 36 odontosis, 75 lingual displacement, and obvious buccal and lingual expansion of the left mandible, involving the

Y. He (ed.), *Inflammatory and Neoplastic Diseases of Craniofacial Bones*, https://doi.org/10.1007/978-981-97-4155-7_57

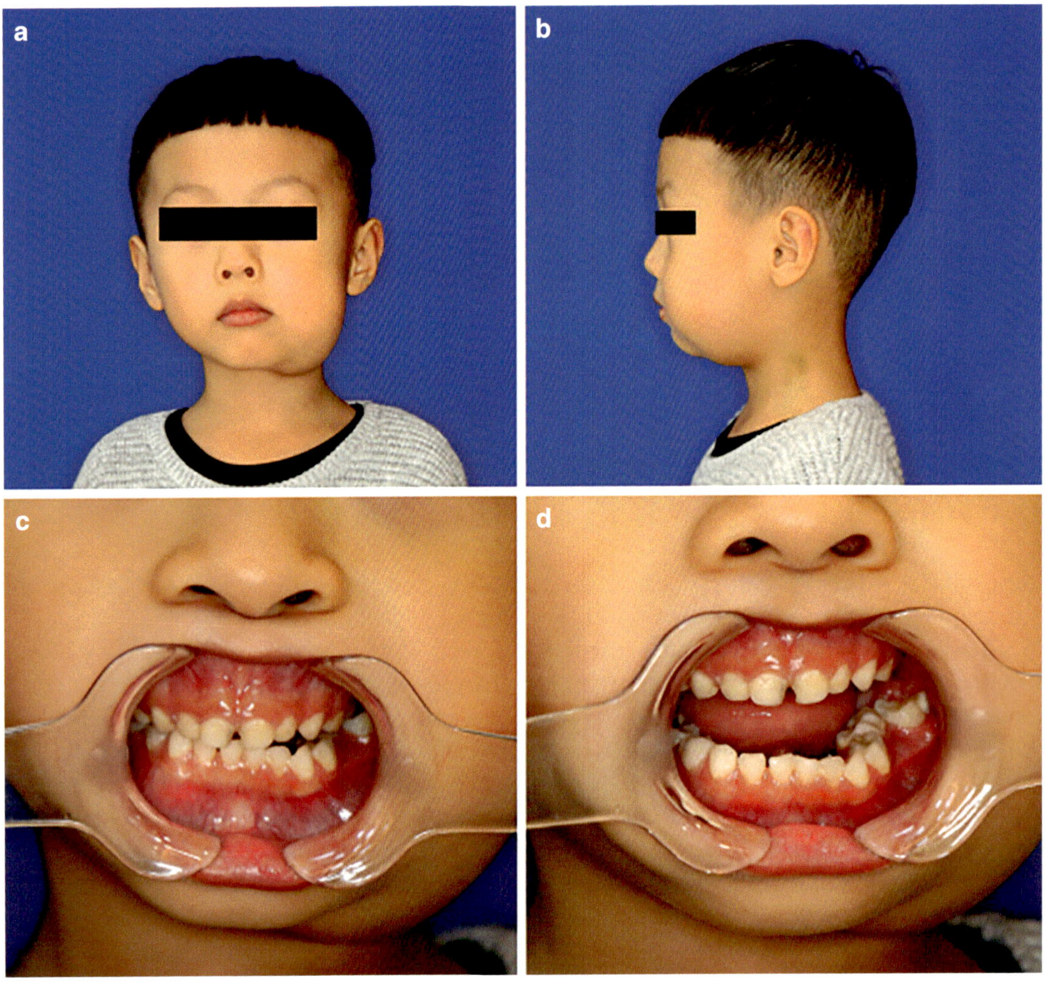

Fig. 57.1 (**a**, **b**) Visible swelling of the left face and jaw. (**c**, **d**) Mixed dentition, heterogeneous occlusion, left mandibular distension, 75 lingual displacement and inclination

left mandibular molar region and the postmolar region. The swelling was hard, with no ping-pong sensation. The mucosa did not show any ulceration, erythema, or congestion (Fig. 57.1). No submaxillary and cervical lymph node enlargement was observed.

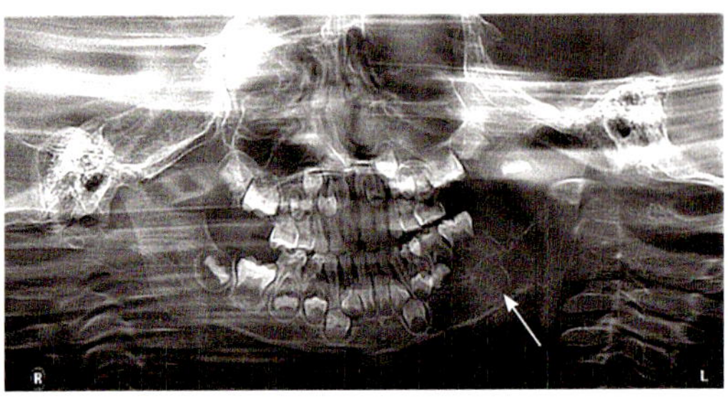

Fig. 57.2 Distensible change in the left mandible, thin bone cortex, bone density attenuation

[Auxiliary Examination]

1. Panoramic radiographs suggested distensible change in the left mandible, thin bone cortex and bone density attenuation (Fig. 57.2).

2. Maxillofacial enhanced CT scan suggested bony distention of left mandibular body angle and ascending bone, density attenuation and soft tissue-like changes, expanding buccally and lingually, with multiple bony segments; C− 50 Hu, partially enhanced, C+ 41 Hu and 154 Hu, heterogeneously enhanced; thinning of peripheral cortex of the lesion, local discontinuity, and well circumscribed from the surrounding soft tissues. No significant bilateral cervical lymph node enlargement was observed (Fig. 57.3).

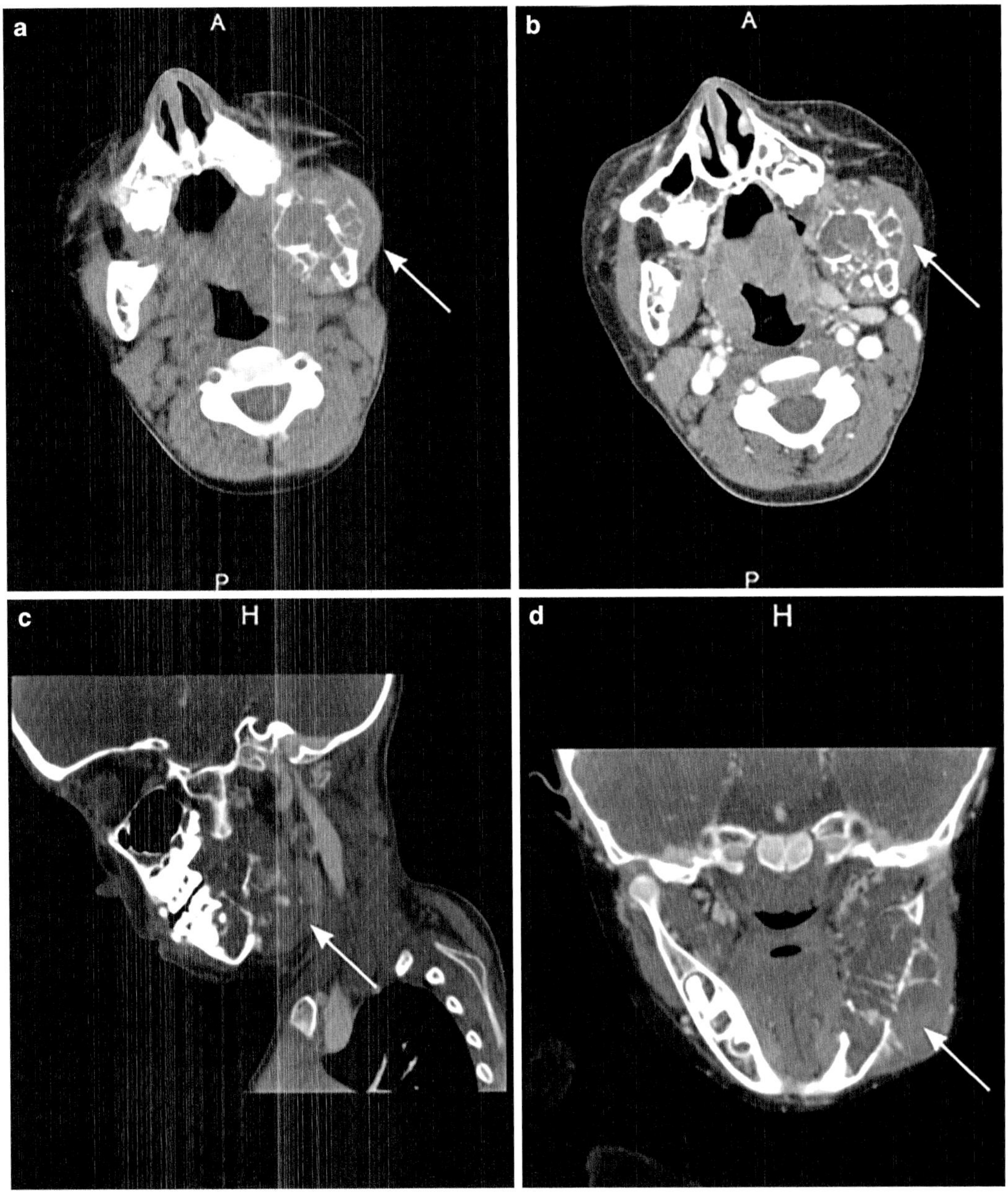

Fig. 57.3 (**a**) CT axial scan: Bony distention of left mandibular body angle and ascending bone with soft tissue mass, buccolingual expansion, with multiple septa inside. (**b**) Enhanced CT axial scan: lesion with heterogeneous density, obvious cystic change, thinning of peripheral cortex of the lesion, local discontinuity, and well circumscribed from the surrounding soft tissues. (**c**, **d**) Oblique sagittal and coronal reconstruction

3. Maxillofacial enhanced MR scan suggested bony distention of left mandibular body angle and ascending bone with soft tissue mass, buccolingual expansion, with multiple septa inside; T1WI isosignal, T2WI high signal, unevenly enhanced after enhancement; obvious cystic change, thinning of peripheral cortex of the lesion, local discontinuity, and well circumscribed from the surrounding soft tissues (Fig. 57.4).

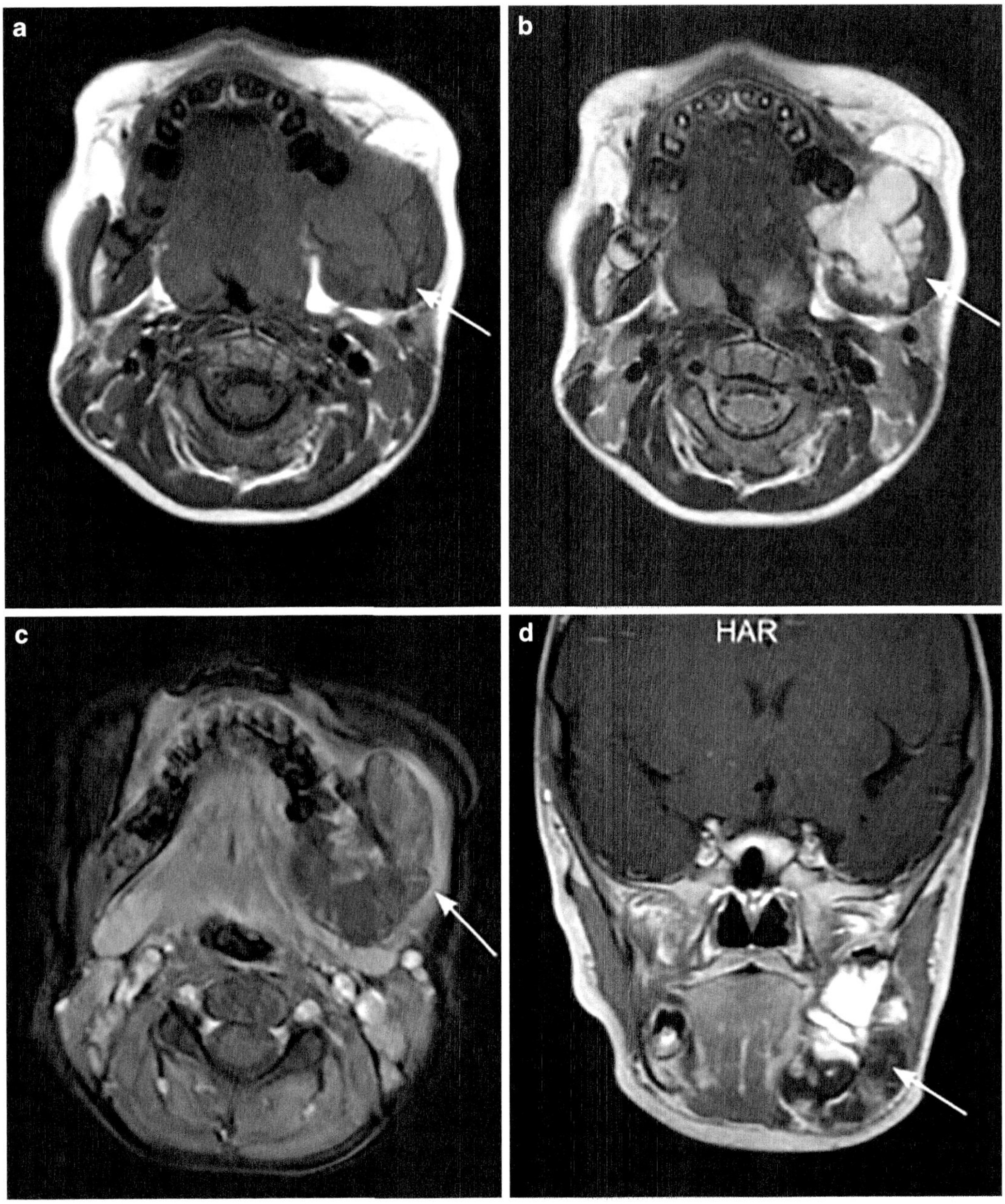

Fig. 57.4 (**a**, **b**) T1WI and T2WI axial scan: bony distention of left mandibular body angle and ascending bone with soft tissue mass, buccolingual expansion, with multiple septa inside. (**c**, **d**) Enhanced T1WI axial and coronal scan: lesion heterogeneously enhanced, obvious cystic change

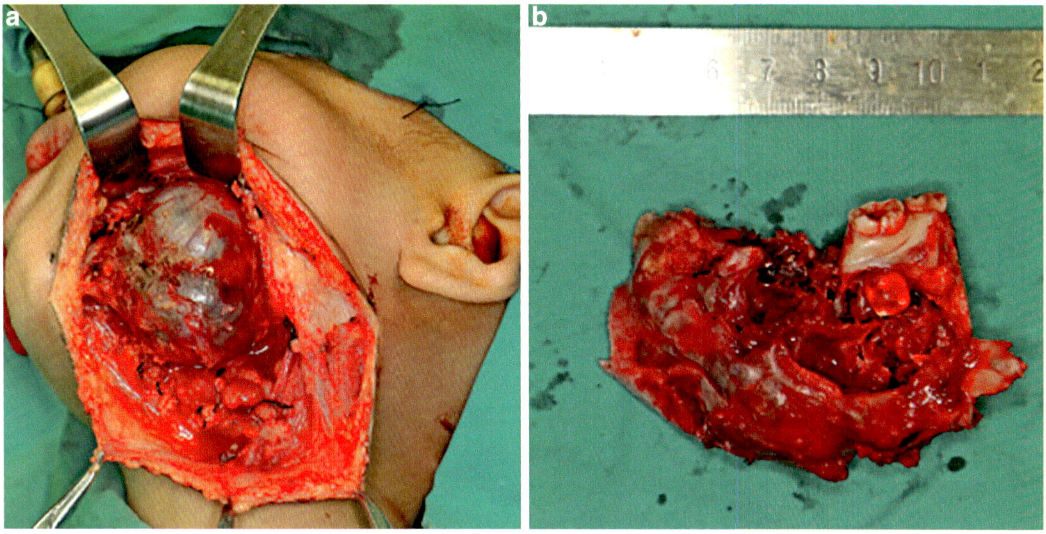

Fig. 57.5 (**a**) Expose the mandibular body and ascending branch, with obvious bone swelling seen and dark red. (**b**) Mandibular bone destruction, polycystic, containing bloody inclusions

[Preliminary Diagnosis] Mass of the left mandible.

[Treatment] "Left mandibulectomy" was performed under general anesthesia: after intraoral extraction 36, significant bleeding happened and part of the tissue was submitted for intraoperative frozen pathology, showing hemophilic pseudotumor to be excluded. An incision was designed along the inferior border of the mandible for 2 cm, and the gingival flap was elevated to reveal a bulging mandibular body with a dark red color and severe buccolingual bone destruction. The osteotomy was performed from the posterior aspect of the chin foramen of the left mandible to the neck of the condylar process, and the mandibular bone and mass were completely removed and sent for pathologic examination. The wound was rinsed and thoroughly hemostatic, negative pressure drainage tube was indwelled, and layered suture was performed to close the wound (Fig. 57.5).

[Pathological Examination] Gross pathological examination revealed a part of mandibular tissue with local expansion and bone destruction, multicystic profile containing bloody inclusions. Microscopic examination exhibited a cystic cavity in the center of the lesion, showing hematomatous change, with surrounding fibrous histiomatous hyperplasia, accompanied by reactive new bone formation (Fig. 57.6).

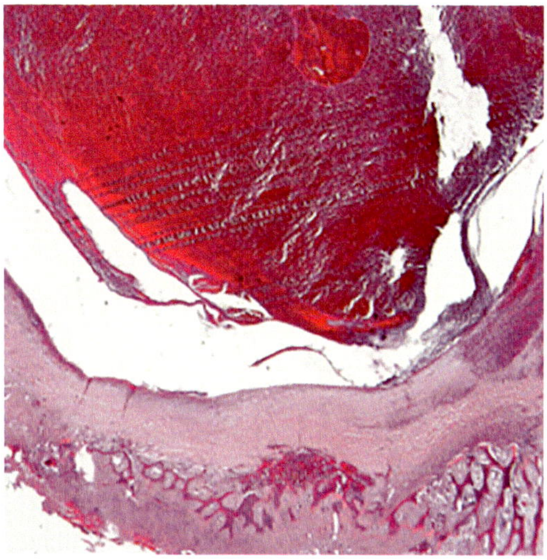

Fig. 57.6 Polycystic lacunae of varying sizes in the jaw bone, with unlined epithelium, blood as cyst content, and reactive new bone formation in the cyst wall (20x)

[Pathological Diagnosis] Hemophilic pseudotumor of the "left mandible."

[Follow-Up] The patient healed uneventfully. The postoperative 6-month follow-up exhibited that the wound healed well and the mandible was slightly skewed.

57.3 Key Points of Diagnosis and Treatment

Hemophilia is an X-chromosome-linked recessive disease that is a coagulation dysfunction caused by the deficiency of coagulation factor VIII or IX. Patients with hemophilia tend to bleed from bones and joints. Repeated bleeding may lead to the formation of cystic cavities in the bones and joints and their progressive enlargement, thus compressing the muscles and even involving the bone, which manifests as a tumor-like lesion of the bone, i.e., hemophilic pseudotumor, firstly reported by Starker in 1918. From an epidemiologic perspective, Buchowski et al. believed that the incidence rate of hemophilic pseudotumor ranged from 1% to 2%. However, a single-center retrospective study of hemophilia cases from 1983 to 2004 in China showed that there were 14 cases of hemophilic pseudotumor among 1248 hemophiliacs, with incidence rate approximately 1.12%. Hemophilic pseudotumor mostly occurs in the femur, pelvis, and ilium, and but is rare in skull and jawbone.

Clinical Manifestations Hemophilic pseudotumor is predispositional to men between 20 and 70 years of age, and patients may remain asymptomatic or stable for a long period of time, with symptoms appearing only when the tumor increases in size and invades adjacent tissues, but the pseudotumor itself manifests no specific clinical manifestations. There is one pseudotumor case in the pelvis, compressing the sciatic nerve and manifesting severe sciatica.

Diagnosis and Differential Diagnosis Clinical diagnosis requires a combination of hemophilia-related tests and history, and imaging examinations such as CT to evaluate trabecular bone, periosteal reaction of the bone cortex, and the proximity of the pseudotumor to localized blood vessels and nerves. Hemophilic pseudotumor should be differentiated from jaw cyst, giant-cell tumor of bone, and Ewing sarcoma.

Treatment There is a lack of standardized diagnostic and therapeutic measures for hemophilic pseudotumor because of its rarity. WFH (World Federation of Hemophilia) guidelines state that the treatment of hemophilic pseudotumor depends on the location, size, growth rate, and impact on the surrounding tissues. Treatment options include factor replacement therapy, radiotherapy, and surgery (local suction/drainage, surgical resection, amputation). Conservative therapy, i.e., limb immobilization with factor replacement therapy, is effective in pediatric cases occurring at the distal limb, but recurrence rate is high. In addition to conservative treatment, radiotherapy can also be effective. For example, Subasi reported a case of a 14-year-old boy with hemophilic pseudotumor in the left digit and pinkie finger, who was treated with 2 weeks of radiotherapy alone, and had relief of symptoms after 4 months.

Most scholars believe that conservative treatment in adult patients is ineffective, failing to stop the progression of the disease, and that surgical resection should be the first choice of treatment. The main indications for surgery are large pseudotumor in soft tissue, ineffective conservative treatment with skin necrosis or nerve or vascular compression, and the possibility of pathological fracture. Patients should be well prepared for the perioperative period, such as supplementing with adequate factor replacement therapy before surgery to prevent intraoperative and postoperative bleeding and other surgical complications. No consensus has been reached so far on whether complete resection of the pseudotumor is necessary. Some scholars declared that if the not completely removed hematoma may cause bleeding again and result in recurrence or other complications. In 2020, one case of secondary venous malformation following surgical removal of hemophiliac pseudotumor of the maxilla was reported. However, for deep-seated pseudotumors, some scholars hold that complete excision may cause massive haemorrhage. The exact extent of resection should depend on the actual situation of the patient, combined with conservative treatment and radiotherapy. The dominant view is that surgical resection with guaranteed factor levels can achieve a more ideal therapeutic effect, but nonsurgical treatment can also be used as a combination therapy for patients who do not meet the indications for surgery. Not all of the 12 reported cases of hemophilic pseudotumor of the jaws were treated surgically; some patients were treated with embolization only, and a follow-up CT scan 5 months later showed new bone formation.

References

1. Buchowski JM, Cascio BM, Streiff MB, et al. Resection and reconstruction of a massive femoral hemophilic pseudotumor [J]. Clin Orthop Rolat Res. 2005;430:237–42.
2. Cox DP, Solar A, Huang J, et al. Pseudotumor of the mandible as first presentation of hemophilia in a 2-year- old male: a case report and review of jaw pseudotumors of hemophilia [J]. Head Neck Pathol. 2011;5(3):226–32.
3. Srinivasan K, Gadodia A, Bhalla AS, et al. Magnetic resonance imaging of mandibular hemophilic pseudotumor associated with factor IX deficiency: report of case with review of literature [J]. J Oral Maxillofac Surg. 2011;69(6):1683–90.
4. Xue F, Sun C, Sui T, et al. Hemophilic pseudotumor in Chinese patients: a retrospective single-centered analysis of 14 cases [J]. Clin Appl Thromb Hemost. 2011;17(3):279–82.
5. Yoshitake Y, Nakayama H, Takamune Y, et al. Haemophilic pseudotumour of the mandible in a 5-year-old patient [J]. Int J Oral Maxillofac Surg. 2011;40(1):120–3.
6. Otsuka H, Ozeki M, Kanda K, et al. Complete bone regeneration in hemophilic pseudotumor of the mandible [J]. Pediatr Int. 2016;58(5):406–8.
7. Cai X, Yu JJ, Tian H, et al. Intraosseous venous malformation of the maxilla after enucleation of a hemophilic pseudotumor: a case report [J]. World J Clin Cases. 2020;8(19):4644–51.

GPSR Compliance

The European Union's (EU) General Product Safety Regulation (GPSR) is a set of rules that requires consumer products to be safe and our obligations to ensure this.

If you have any concerns about our products, you can contact us on ProductSafety@springernature.com

In case Publisher is established outside the EU, the EU authorized representative is:

Springer Nature Customer Service Center GmbH
Europaplatz 3
69115 Heidelberg, Germany

Batch number: 10756353

Printed by Printforce, the Netherlands